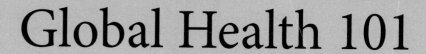

Global Health 101

THIRD EDITION

Richard Skolnik
Lecturer in Public Health
Department of Health Policy and Management
Yale School of Public Health
New Haven, CT

Lecturer in the Practice of Management
Yale School of Management
New Haven, CT

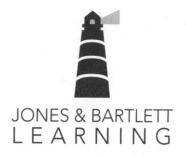

JONES & BARTLETT
LEARNING

World Headquarters
Jones & Bartlett Learning
5 Wall Street
Burlington, MA 01803
978-443-5000
info@jblearning.com
www.jblearning.com

Jones & Bartlett Learning books and products are available through most bookstores and online booksellers. To contact Jones & Bartlett Learning directly, call 800-832-0034, fax 978-443-8000, or visit our website, www.jblearning.com.

04538-3

Production Credits
VP, Executive Publisher: David D. Cella
Publisher: Michael Brown
Associate Editor: Lindsey Mawhiney
Associate Editor: Nicholas Alakel
Production Manager: Tracey McCrea
Senior Marketing Manager: Sophie Fleck Teague
Manufacturing and Inventory Control Supervisor: Amy Bacus
Composition: Cenveo® Publisher Services
Cover Design: Kristin E. Parker
Rights & Media Manager: Joanna Lundeen
Rights & Media Research Coordinator: Mary Flatley
Media Development Editor: Shannon Sheehan
Cover Image: © Randy Plett/Stone/Getty Images
Printing and Binding: RR Donnelley
Cover Printing: RR Donnelley

Library of Congress Cataloging-in-Publication Data
Skolnik, Richard L., author.
 Global health 101 / Richard Skolnik.—Third edition.
    p. ; cm.
 Global health one hundred one
 Global health one hundred and one
 Includes bibliographical references and index.
 ISBN 978-1-284-05054-7 (pbk.)
 I. Title. II. Title: Global health one hundred one. III. Title: Global health one hundred and one.
 [DNLM: 1. Global Health. 2. Health Services Accessibility. 3. Public Health. WA 530.1]
 RA441
 362.1—dc23
                          2015014288
6048

Printed in the United States of America
19 18 17 16 15   10 9 8 7 6 5 4 3

Contents

Part III   The Burden of Disease

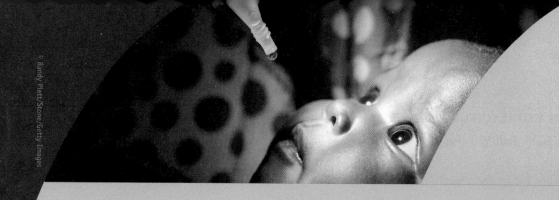

Essential Public Health Series

*Log on to **www.essentialpublichealth.com** for the most current information on the series.*

<u>CURRENT AND FORTHCOMING TITLES IN THE *ESSENTIAL PUBLIC HEALTH* SERIES:</u>

Public Health 101: Healthy People–Healthy Populations, Enhanced Second Edition Includes Navigate Advantage Access—Richard K. Riegelman, MD, MPH, PhD & Brenda Kirkwood, MPH, DrPH

Epidemiology 101—Robert H. Friis, PhD

Global Health 101, Third Edition Includes Navigate Advantage Access—Richard Skolnik, MPA

Essentials of Public Health, Third Edition Includes Navigate Advantage Access—Bernard J. Turnock, MD, MPH

Essentials of Health Policy and Law, Third Edition—Joel B. Teitelbaum, JD, LLM & Sara E. Wilensky, JD, MPP

Essentials of Environmental Health, Second Edition—Robert H. Friis, PhD

Essentials of Biostatistics in Public Health, Second Edition—Lisa M. Sullivan, PhD

Essentials of Health Behavior: Social and Behavioral Theory in Public Health, Second Edition—Mark Edberg, PhD

Essentials of Health, Culture, and Diversity: Understanding People, Reducing Disparities—Mark Edberg, PhD

Essentials of Planning and Evaluation for Public Health Programs Includes Navigate Advantage Access—Karen Marie Perrin, MPH, PhD

Essentials of Health Information Systems and Technology Includes Navigate Advantage Access—Jean A. Balgrosky, MPH, RHIA

Essentials of Public Health Communication—Claudia Parvanta, PhD; Patrick Remington, MD, MPH; Ross Brownson, PhD; & David E. Nelson, MD, MPH

Essentials of Public Health Ethics—Ruth Gaare Bernheim, JD, MPH; James F. Childress, PhD; Richard J. Bonnie, JD; & Alan L. Melnick, MD, MPH, CPH

Essentials of Management and Leadership in Public Health—Robert Burke, PhD & Leonard Friedman, PhD, MPH

Essentials of Public Health Preparedness—Rebecca Katz, PhD, MPH

Essentials of Global Community Health—Jaime Gofin, MD, MPH & Rosa Gofin, MD, MPH

ACCOMPANYING CASE BOOKS AND READINGS

Essential Case Studies in Public Health: Putting Public Health into Practice—Katherine Hunting, PhD, MPH & Brenda L. Gleason, MA, MPH

Essential Readings in Health Behavior: Theory and Practice—Mark Edberg, PhD

ABOUT THE EDITOR

Richard K. Riegelman, MD, MPH, PhD, is Professor of Epidemiology-Biostatistics, Medicine, and Health Policy, and Founding Dean of The George Washington University Milken Institute School of Public Health in Washington, DC. He has taken a lead role in developing the Educated Citizen and Public Health initiative which has brought together arts and sciences and public health education associations to implement the Institute of Medicine of the National Academies' recommendation that "…all undergraduates should have access to education in public health." Dr. Riegelman also led the development of The George Washington's undergraduate major and minor and currently teaches "Public Health 101" and "Epidemiology 101" to undergraduates.

The Importance of Global Health

Why should we care about the health of other people, especially that of people in other countries? Actually, for a number of critical reasons, the health of people everywhere must be an important concern for all of us.

First, diseases do not respect boundaries. Human immunodeficiency virus (HIV) has spread worldwide. A person with tuberculosis can infect 15 people a year, wherever they are. The West Nile Virus came from Egypt but occurs today in many countries. In addition, there is an important risk of a worldwide epidemic of influenza. Clearly, the health of each of us increasingly depends on the health of others.

Second, there is an ethical dimension to the health and well-being of other people. Many children in poor countries get sick and die needlessly of nutrition-related causes or from diseases that are preventable and curable. Many adults in poor countries die because they lack access to medicines that are customarily available to people in rich countries. Is this just? Are we prepared to accept such deaths without taking steps to prevent them?

Third, health is closely linked with economic and social development in an increasingly interdependent world. Children who suffer from undernutrition may not reach their full mental potential and may not enroll in or stay in school. Sick children from low- and middle-income countries are less likely than healthy children to become productive adults who can contribute to the economic standing of their family, community, or country. Adults who suffer from AIDS, tuberculosis, malaria, and other diseases lose income while they are sick and out of work, which contributes in many ways to keeping their families in an endless cycle of poverty.

Finally, the health and well-being of people everywhere have important implications for global security and freedom. High rates of HIV/AIDS have contributed to destabilizing some countries, as more teachers and health workers died than were trained, and as insufficient numbers of rural workers grew and harvested crops. Outbreaks of other diseases, such as cholera, the plague, SARS (Severe Acute Respiratory Syndrome), and Ebola, for example, threaten people's ability to engage freely in economic pursuits and can have devastating economic and social consequences. An outbreak of cholera in 1991 cost Peru about $1 billion, the plague in 1994 cost India about $2 billion, and SARS in Asia in 2003 cost the economies of Asia a staggering $18 billion in lost economic activity.

Indeed, these factors have increased interest in global health both within universities and among university students. The aim of this book, therefore, is to examine the most critical global health topics in a clear and engaging manner. The book will provide the reader with an overview of the importance of global health in the context of development, examine the most important global health issues and their economic and social consequences, and discuss some of the steps that are being taken to address these concerns. It will also provide numerous "success stories," as examples of effectively dealing with important global health problems.

This book is intended to provide an introduction to global health for all students. This includes students who have never studied public health before and who will not take additional public health courses in the future. However, it also includes those students, whether they have studied public health before or not, who may wish to pursue additional studies in public health later.

This book is largely based on an undergraduate global health course that I taught at The George Washington University in Washington, DC and now teach at Yale. The text seeks to "speak" to the reader in a manner one would find in an exciting and motivating classroom. In addition to covering key concepts in global health and frameworks for the analysis of global health issues, this book also contains numerous examples of on-the-ground experiences in addressing key global health problems.

Very few introductory materials on global health are available to students or their professors. Hopefully, this book will help to close that gap by providing a foundation for enhanced studies in public health, global health, and economic and social development.

THE ORGANIZATION OF THE BOOK

This book is organized in several parts that closely follow the topics mentioned previously. Part I introduces the reader to the basic principles of global health, key measures of health, and the concepts of the health and the development link. Chapter 1 introduces readers to some key principles, themes, and goals of global health. Chapter 2 examines the determinants of health, how health is measured, and how health conditions change over time and as countries develop economically. Chapter 3 looks at the links between health and development, touching upon the connections between health and education, equity, and poverty.

Part II reviews cross-cutting themes in global health. Chapter 4 examines human rights and ethical issues in global health. Chapter 5 covers health systems. This chapter reviews the purpose and goals of health systems and how different countries have organized their health systems. The chapter also reviews the key challenges that health systems face, the costs and consequences of those challenges, and how some countries have addressed health system challenges. Culture plays an extremely important part in health, and Chapter 6 examines the links between culture and health. This chapter reviews the importance of culture to health, how health is perceived in different groups, the manner in which different culture groups seek health care and engage in health practices, and how one can promote change in health behavior.

Part III reviews the most important causes of illness, disability, and death, particularly in low- and middle-income countries. The chapters in this part of the book examine environmental issues, nutrition, women's health, child health, and adolescent health. The book then looks at communicable diseases, noncommunicable diseases, and unintentional injuries.

Part IV examines how cooperative action can address global health issues. Chapter 15 reviews the impact on health of conflicts, natural disasters, and other health emergencies. Chapter 16 examines how different actors in the global health field work both individually and cooperatively to address key global health problems. Chapter 17 reviews how science and technology have helped to improve public health and how further advances in science and technology could help to address some of the most important global health challenges that remain.

Part V focuses on careers in the global health field. Chapter 18 examines the types of careers in global health; the skills, knowledge, and experience needed to pursue these careers; and how you can get those skills, knowledge, and experience. The book ends with Chapter 19, which includes profiles of 21 actors in the global health field whose personal stories are meant to inspire you, as well as provide guidance about pursuing a career in global health if that is your interest.

Each of the chapters, other than those on working in global health and on profiles of global health actors, follows a similar outline. The chapters begin with vignettes that relate to the topic to be covered and which are intended to make the topic "real" for the reader. Some of these vignettes are not true in the literal sense. However, each of them are based on real events that occur regularly in the countries discussed in this book. Most chapters then explain key concepts, terms, and definitions. The chapters that deal with cross-cutting issues in the second and fourth parts of the book then examine the importance of the topic to enhancing global health, some key challenges in further improving global health, and what can be done to address those challenges.

The chapters that focus on health conditions look at the burden of disease related to these conditions; who is most affected by these issues; major risk factors for these burdens; and, the costs and consequences of these issues for individuals, communities, and the world. These chapters then examine what has been learned about how to deal with these health burdens in the most cost-effective ways, the future challenges in each of these areas, and some specific cases of successful efforts at addressing such challenges.

Most chapters contain "policy and program briefs" that are meant to briefly introduce you to and illustrate important global health topics, actors, and organizations.

Most chapters also contain several case studies. Some of these deal with well-known cases that have already proven to be models for global health efforts. Others, however, are based on experiences that show good promise, both for success and for providing lessons, but which have not yet proven themselves.

Each chapter concludes with a summary of the main messages in the chapter and a set of study questions that can assist the reader in reviewing the materials included in the chapter. Each chapter also contains endnotes with citations for the data that are used in the book. The book does not contain any additional lists of reference materials. Those wishing to explore topics in greater depth will find ample suggestions for additional reading in the endnotes.

The reader should note that the chapters are not in order of importance. Nutrition, for example, is fundamental to all health concerns. However, it only makes sense to cover nutrition in this book after establishing the context for studying global health and after covering some cross-cutting global health issues. In addition, you will note that there is no chapter called "globalization and health." Rather, you will find that the relationships between globalization and health are integrated into all of the chapters. Some students may also wish to read Chapter 16 on global health policy, actors, and actions before they cover many of the other chapters. This may help them understand at an earlier stage how different actors have organized themselves to address key global health issues.

THE PERSPECTIVE OF THE BOOK

The book will take a global perspective to all that it covers. Although the book includes many country case studies, topics will be examined from the perspective of the world as a whole. The book also pays particular attention to the links between poverty and health and the relationship between health, equity, and health disparities. Special attention will also be given to gender and ethnicity and their relation to health. Another theme that runs through the book is the connection between health and development.

The book follows the point of view that health is a human right. The book is written with the presumption that governments have an obligation to try to ensure that all of their people have access to an affordable package of healthcare services and that all people should be protected from the costs of ill health. The book is also based on the premise, however, that the development of a health system by any country, as discussed further in Chapter 5, is inextricably linked to the value system and the political structure of that country.

The book covers key global health topics, including those that affect high-income countries. However, the book pays particular attention to low- and middle-income countries and to poor people within them. The rationale for this is that improving health status indicators within and across countries can only be accomplished if the health of the poor and other disadvantaged groups is improved. In addition, the idea of social justice is at the core of public health.

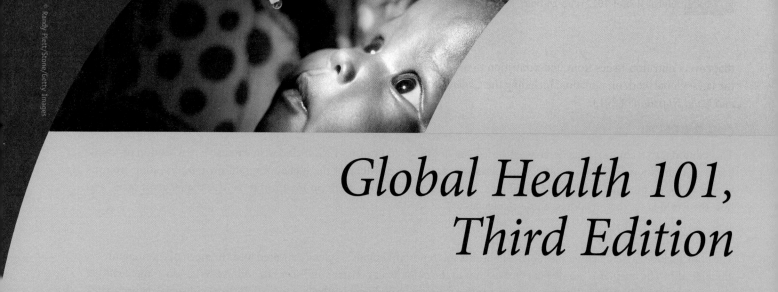

Global Health 101,
Third Edition

What's New in the *Third Edition?*

OVERVIEW

The third edition of *Global Health 101* contains an extensive amount of new and revised information, while maintaining its clarity, simplicity, and ease of use by faculty and students.

The aim of the revision is to bring the book in line with the latest burden of disease data, offer unique content on key topics that are often insufficiently covered in introductory materials, such as immunization and adolescent health, and to make the book increasingly attractive to students and teachers alike with the addition of more case studies and profiles of global health actors.

The major substantive changes to the book are given below.

THE BURDEN OF DISEASE AND OTHER HEALTH DATA

One of the foundations for the book is data on the burden of disease. The third edition has updated all data on the burden of disease and related risk factors, largely using information from the *Global Burden of Disease Study 2010*, which was published in 2013.

Considerable progress continues to be made in many countries in improving health. This edition uses health statistics from 2012 or later, whenever possible, for all key data. This data is taken largely from WHO, UNICEF, the World Bank, and UNAIDS.

The reader will find that almost all tables and figures in the book that relate to the burden of disease and risk factors have been completely updated.

HEALTH SYSTEMS

This edition of the book includes revised, updated, and expanded comments about health systems in a number of settings.

HEALTH DISPARITIES

Equity and inequality are essential public health concerns. This edition explores equity and inequality issues for a variety of groups more deeply than the earlier editions.

NUTRITION

The place of nutrition in health has changed dramatically, with considerable growth in the share of populations that are over-weight and obese, even in low- and middle-income countries. This edition features a completely redone chapter on nutrition that covers nutrition issues from undernutrition to overweight and obesity in a single chapter. In doing so, it takes account of the latest global work on nutrition, including the *Global Nutrition Report* of November 2014 and the *Lancet Series on Maternal and Child Nutrition* of 2013.

CHILD HEALTH

This edition also features a considerably expanded chapter on child health, which includes an extensive new section on childhood immunization. The comments on immunization feature the history of the global program on immunization from its inception to the present. This section highlights the status of the world's work on immunization, the challenges it faces, and how the world is seeking to address those challenges.

ADOLESCENT HEALTH

The book includes a new chapter on adolescent health, an important but insufficiently covered topic in much of the literature on global health. The chapter is parallel in construction to the child health chapter and seeks to address: What do adolescents get sick, disabled, and die from? Which adolescents suffer from these problems? What are the risk factors and social determinants for these problems? What are their consequences? What have we learned can be done to address these issues?

PHARMACUETICALS

Pharmaceuticals are an especially important issue for all health systems. This edition includes a new section on pharmaceuticals.

NONCOMMUNICABLE DISEASES

The share of the burden of disease that is noncommunicable has continued to grow. This edition features considerable additional information on noncommunicable diseases broadly, and on cancer, mental health, and essential surgery, in particular.

SCIENCE AND TECHNOLOGY

Science and technology continue to be used in increasingly diverse ways to meet Global Health needs. This edition features a range of new policy and program briefs on science and technology. These include, for example, new briefs on the use of mobile technologies for Global Health, telemedicine in India, and on new drugs and diagnostics for TB.

WORKING IN GLOBAL HEALTH

This edition continues to include two chapters on careers in Global Health. The chapter on working in global health has been updated. Eight new profiles of Global Health actors have been added to the chapter on Profiles of Global Health Actors.

CASE STUDIES AND POLICY AND PROGRAM BRIEFS

Case studies and policy and program briefs bring topics to life for students and faculty. This edition includes more than 25 additional "Policy and Program Briefs" of about 750 to 1,000 words each, which cover the range of key topics in the book. Some of the new briefs in this edition, for example, cover:

- Product development partnerships, such as AERAS for the development of TB vaccines;
- Vaccines, such as for polio and measles;
- Emerging infectious diseases, such as the Ebola virus and Cryptococcus in AIDS patients in Africa;
- Noncommunicable diseases, such as diabetes in the Pacific;
- Essential Surgery, as described in a recent *Lancet* Commission report;
- Mental Health, including comments on the gap between needs and action globally and on the growing numbers of people with dementia.

BLOG ON TEACHING GLOBAL HEALTH

The author will once again be preparing a monthly blog on teaching global health. The blog contains information about resources for teaching global health. It also includes lessons that the author is learning from his teaching of Global Health at three levels, as well as lessons that others have shared with him about their teaching experiences.

Prologue: *Global Health 101, Third Edition*

In the prologue to the previous editions, I wrote: "The issues of global health have finally arrived in the consciousness of the developed world through a unique union of efforts by former presidents, software pioneers, and rock stars. It is now time that students have a textbook . . . that systematically leads them through the issues of global health from basic principles, to the burden of disease, to examples of successful efforts to improve lives and livelihoods." *Global Health 101* has fulfilled these expectations and more. It has become the classic textbook of global health and is now being used in a wide range of countries.

What can you as students and faculty expect from the third edition of *Global Health 101*? The third edition builds upon the strengths of the previous editions and provides substantial new and updated material.

Expanded chapters keep the textbook up to date and state of the art. The share of the burden of disease that is noncommunicable has continued to grow. The third edition features considerable additional information on noncommunicable diseases broadly and on cancer, mental health, and essential surgery. Pharmaceuticals are an especially important issue for all health systems. This edition includes a new section on pharmaceuticals. The place of nutrition in health has changed dramatically, with considerable growth in the share of populations that are obese, even in low- and middle-income countries. This edition features a substantially revised nutrition chapter, which deals with obesity as well as undernutrition. This edition also features a new major section on immunization and a new chapter on adolescent health.

Equity is essential to all public health concerns. This edition explores equity issues for a variety of groups more deeply than the earlier editions. Science and technology continue to be used in increasingly diverse ways to meet global health needs. This edition features new sections on the use of mobile technologies for global health.

As students you'll enjoy and learn from the engaging videos, expand your knowledge using the web links, and test your understandings using the interactive questions and answers. The expanded chapters on careers in global health bring to life the opportunities provided by this growing and dynamic field.

For faculty, there are an abundance of additional resources to help broaden and deepen students' understanding of global health.

Whether you are taking a global health course as part of general education, a major or minor in public health or global health, as part of your health professions education, or as part of your interest in international affairs, you will find the third edition an exhilarating experience that opens your mind and your heart to the world of global health.

Richard Riegelman, MD, MPH, PhD
Essential Public Health Series Editor

Foreword

The world has made enormous progress against some of the leading causes of premature death and disability. The number of children under 5 years of age who die each year has fallen substantially, but there are still more than 6 million child deaths each year. Despite substantial gains against diseases such as measles, almost 150,000 children still die of measles each year, as well. Progress has also been made against disability-causing infections such as polio, for which there are now fewer than 500 new cases a year, and it is hoped that eradication is in sight. The number of women dying a maternal death has also declined to below 300,000 per year and the number of new HIV infections in the world each year is also falling. Life expectancy at birth for the world as a whole is at its highest point ever and, as many have commented, never before have so many people lived so long. However, these gains still remain out of reach of the world's poor living in both industrialized and developing countries, and health inequalities must be addressed.

There is thus a substantial unfinished agenda in global health:

- Although the deaths of children under 5 have declined substantially, for example, who can accept that more than 6 million children a year still die before their fifth birthday? Although the number of maternal deaths has declined, as well, who can accept that almost 300,000 women die each year during or just after childbirth? Why has it taken the world 60 years after the development of polio vaccines to make this progress? And why are there are still 2.1 million new HIV infections and 9 million new people who fall ill with tuberculosis each year?

- In addition to this, the world faces continuing threats from emerging and reemerging infectious diseases, such as the Ebola virus, which has caused a major epidemic in West Africa. The world has also failed to make sufficient progress in addressing the threats of resistance to medicines that treat bacterial, viral, and parasitic infections; in developing new medicines to replace those becoming less effective; and in developing vaccines that can prevent these infections. Moreover, we are also seeing the effects of climate change and increasing globalization on health, with the spread, for example, of the dengue and Chikungunya viruses.

- At the same time, an increasing share of the world's population is at risk of noncommunicable diseases, including those who live in low- and middle-income countries. More and more people are living longer, but many of them are also living longer with disabilities. Will we be able to keep tobacco consumption from continuing to increase in today's low-income countries as most higher income countries have done? Can all countries, including those that are low income, create an environment that will enable their people to avoid as much as possible the other "lifestyle" diseases that are spreading worldwide?

Many students flock to the study of global health to celebrate and learn from the progress made to date and to commit to addressing the important gaps that remain. Other students understand that a knowledge of global health is critical in today's interconnected and globalized world. For both reasons, the demand for studies in global health has continued to grow worldwide and the need for coherent resources to help these students gain a solid foundation in the study of global health is critical.

In light of the progress in global health, the large unfinished agenda, the remarkable demand for learning about global health, and the ever-changing global health landscape, I am pleased to see this third edition of Richard Skolnik's book on global health.

Richard has laid out the fundamental concepts of global health studies in a clear and coherent manner that is data and evidence based and well illustrated. Most important, the book stresses issues of equity, social justice, a deep concern for the poor and marginalized, and the importance of value for money from investments in health. Grounding the book in the latest data on the burden of disease is invaluable and including in the book an increasing number of case studies and policy and program briefs helps to bring the contents of the book alive for students who are learning about global health for the first time, as well as those who already are familiar with or are practitioners of global health.

Richard brings to the writing of the book his personal experience of more than 30 years of work in global health; and another 13 years of teaching global health to undergraduates, graduate students in public health, and students in business and other professional schools.

The first two editions of Richard's book have been widely used, both in the United States and internationally. I am confident that this substantially updated and enlarged third edition will likewise be widely used by students who wish to gain basic understanding of key global health issues and by those who wish to obtain a strong foundation for further studies in global health.

David L. Heymann, M.D.
March 2015

Dr. Heymann is a professor of infectious disease epidemiology at the London School of Hygiene and Tropical Medicine and head and senior fellow of the Centre on Global Health Security, Chatham House (London). Dr. Heymann spent 15 years working with the U.S. Centers for Disease Control and Prevention (CDC) in disease control programs based in Africa and Asia and 10 years working on secondment from the CDC to the World Health Organization. He began this work with 2 years on smallpox eradication in India. He then worked in sub-Saharan Africa, beginning in 1976 in Yambuku, Democratic Republic of the Congo, where he was a member of the team that investigated the first Ebola outbreak. Dr. Heymman stayed on in Africa for 13 years to investigate future outbreaks of Ebola and other African infectious diseases. Following that, Dr. Heymann began a 22-year career at the World Health Organization, 10 of those on secondment from the CDC, beginning as a medical epidemiologist in the newly developed AIDS program. He then set up and directed the program on emerging infections and finally became assistant director-general in charge of infectious diseases.

Dr. Heymann is an elected member of the United States Institute of Medicine and the United Kingdom Academy of Medical Sciences. He has also received a variety of awards for his work in public health and infectious diseases, including the American Public Health Association Award for Excellence. In addition, Dr. Heymann has been named Commander of the Order of the British Empire (CBE) for excellence in public health.

Acknowledgments

This third edition of *Global Health 101* would not have been possible without the exceptional help provided to me in the development of the first and second editions. Thus, I repeat here the acknowledgements for those editions, before acknowledging those who helped with this edition.

THE FIRST EDITION

Many people graciously assisted me with the preparation of the first edition of this book, which could never have been completed without their help.

Four colleagues prepared initial chapter drafts and were the coauthors of the chapters indicated: Victor Barbiero for Communicable Diseases, Michael Doney for Unintentional Injuries, Heidi Larson for Child Health, and John Tharakan for Ethics and Human Rights. Vic also provided the Quotable Quotes at the beginning of the book.

A large number of individuals contributed case studies to the first edition. Florence Baingana prepared the case study on mental health in Uganda in Chapter 12. Sadia Chowdhury provided the case study on oral rehydration in Bangladesh in Chapter 5. Ambar Kulshreshtra prepared the case study of Kerala in Chapter 2. Nancy J. Haselow and Musa Obadiah, assisted by Julia Ross, prepared the case study on vitamin A and Ivermectin in Chapter 5. Peter J. Hotez, Ami Shah Brown, and Kari Stoever provided the case study on the Human Hookworm Vaccine Initiative in Chapter 16 of the first edition. Orin Levine prepared the case study on pneumococcal vaccine that is also in Chapter 16 of the first edition. Andrea Thoumi, a student at Tufts University, provided drafts of the case studies on fistula, the earthquake in Pakistan, refugees in Goma, motorcycle helmets in Taiwan, and speed bumps in Ghana. Andrea also prepared drafts of cases on cataract blindness in India and vitamin A in Nepal, based on *Case Studies in Global Health: Millions Saved.*

A large number of friends and colleagues also reviewed and commented on different book chapters, always adding great value as they did so. These people included Ian Anderson, Alan Berg, Florence Baingana, Stephanie Calves, Roger-Mark de Souza, Wafaie Fawzi, Charlotte Feldman-Jacobs, Adrienne Germain, Reuben Granich, Robert Hecht, Judith Justice, James Levinson, Kseniya Lvovsky, Venkatesh Mannar, William McGreevey, Anthony Measham, Tom Merrick, Elaine Murphy, Rachel Nugent, Kris Olson, Ramanan Laxminarayanan, Rudy van Puymbroeck, Richard Southby, Ron Waldman, and Abdo Yazbeck.

Several of my former students at The George Washington University, including Yvonne Orji, Sapna Patel, David Schneider, and Melanie Vant, provided background information for the first edition and reviewed various book chapters. Pamela Sud, then a student at Stanford University, also reviewed a number of chapters.

Andrea Thoumi not only helped me to prepare cases, as noted previously, but also provided background materials, helped with citations, and reviewed a number of chapters.

Jessica Gottlieb, Molly Kinder, and Ruth Levine, then of the Center for Global Development, were especially helpful to the preparation of this book. I am very grateful to them and to the center for agreeing to make *Case Studies in Global Health:*

Millions Saved the companion reader to my book. In addition, my book includes abbreviated versions of 16 of the 20 cases in *Millions Saved*, 14 of which the center graciously prepared for me. Jessica, Molly, and Ruth also reviewed many of the chapters of my book and Jessica Pickett, who then worked with the center, also commented on a chapter.

Jessica Roeder, my former colleague at the Harvard School of Public Health, was kind enough to take on a second job at night to help me prepare tables and figures.

I am also especially grateful to my daughter, Rachel, who worked with me almost full time for many months and assisted in preparing background information, tables, figures, and citations and reviewing and editing each chapter of the first edition.

Barry Bloom, then dean of the Harvard School of Public Health, was kind enough to prepare the preface for the first edition, for which I remain very appreciative.

I remain grateful, as well, to Sir George Alleyne, Dean Jamison, and Adrienne Germaine who very kindly wrote advance praise for the first edition. I am honored, of course, that three such distinguished people would do so.

The staff of Jones & Bartlett Learning, especially Katey Birtcher, Mike Brown, Sophie Fleck, and Rachel Rossi, were also immensely helpful to the preparation of the first edition.

THE SECOND EDITION

The second edition would also have been impossible without the extensive assistance of many people.

Roger Glass, the director of the Fogarty International Center of the United States National Institutes of Health, has honored me by preparing the foreword for this edition.

Elizabeth H. Bradley, professor of public health and faculty director, Global Health Leadership Institute at Yale University, and Prabhat Jha, Canada Research Chair in Health and Development and Director, Centre for Global Health Research at the Li Ka Shing Knowledge Institute, St. Michael's Hospital and Dalla Lana School of Public Health, University of Toronto, prepared advance praise for the book.

Joe Millum, of the National Institutes of Health, graciously coauthored the chapter on ethics and global health. Joe did marvelous work revising, expanding, and illuminating the text of the first edition to make the chapter more coherent, more enlightening, and more vibrant.

This edition of the book includes 30 new Policy and Program Briefs, many of which were written with the assistance of friends and professional colleagues who provided drafts of the briefs or other major inputs to the brief writing process. These people included Kate Acosta and Luzon Pahl of TOSTAN; Soji Adeyi of the Affordable Medicines Facility—malaria; Faruque Ahmed of BRAC; Lisa Beyer from the International AIDS Vaccine Initiative (IAVI); Aya Caldwell and Kris Olson of Massachusetts General Hospital; Susan Higman of the Global Health Council, Peg Willingham of Aeras; Dan Kammen, of the University of California, Berkeley and the World Bank, who prepared the draft of the brief on cookstoves; Linda Kupfer of the Fogarty International Center of the National Institutes of Health; Anjana Padmanabhan of The Global Network on Neglected Tropical Diseases; Jennifer Staple-Clark of Unite for Sight; Eteena Tadjiogueu from the Human Hookworm Vaccine Initiative; and Karen Van der Westhuizen and Patrizia Carlevaro of the Eli Lilly Corporation. Josephine Francisco and her mentor, Tom Davis, allowed me to prepare a brief about breastfeeding in Burundi that was based on Josie's master of public health research project. Josie also kindly reviewed the draft of the brief we prepared from her work.

Many former colleagues at the World Bank, World Health Organization, and Population Reference Bureau, as well as other friends, helped me assemble data and other resources for the book. These included John Briscoe, Dave Gwatkin, Rob Hecht, Dean Jamison, Pete Kolsky, Joel Lamstein, Kseniya Lvovsky, Colin Mathers, Kris Olson, Eduardo Perez, David Peters, and Abdo Yazbeck.

A number of colleagues and friends were also kind enough to review sections of the book or whole book chapters, including Leslie Elder of the World Bank, Robert Hecht of the Results for Development Institute, Peter Hotez of The George Washington University, Susan Higman of the Global Health Council, and Rachel Nugent of the Center for Global Development.

I am also exceptionally grateful to the friends and colleagues for whom I have so much respect and who allowed me to prepare a profile of them for the chapter we have added to the second edition called "Profiles of Global Health Actors." These wonderful people gave much of their time and energy to help us develop a profile about them. Their names appear in Chapter 18.

It would have been impossible, over any time frame, to have prepared this edition without the many former students I was sensible enough to employ for this effort. Laura Chambers, Becky Crowder, Lindsay Gordon, and Emma Morse served as principal research assistants for the second edition. Lindsay and Laura gathered research materials and data, prepared graphs and tables, and drafted countless policy and program briefs, with which Emma also helped. Lindsay and Laura also developed the initial drafts of most of the profiles in Chapter 18. Becky and Emma reviewed each chapter of the book at each stage of writing and production. Becky, Emma, Laura, and Lindsay were instrumental to the preparation of the book and a delight to work with at all times.

The same enjoyment and many valuable inputs came from working with another group of former students who put in a substantial number of hours on data collection; the review of draft chapters, copyedited chapters, and page proofs; and the preparation of materials for the website. These major contributors to the book included Shannon Doyle, Elizabeth Gomes, Tae Min Kim, and Sara Walker.

A number of former students also assisted me with data collection for the book and the website, including Ahsan Butt, Tanvi Devi, Jenny Durina, David Hidalgo, and Mara Leff. Lisa Hendrickson commented on the brief on Calcutta Kids. Demitsa Rakitsa prepared the initial draft of the brief on HIV financing in Cambodia and South Africa. Candace Martin helped gather data, prepared references and materials for both the book and the website, and also helped to prepare the brief on sanitation in Indonesia.

My thanks also go to former students who allowed me to put on the book's website the policy briefs they wrote for my classes. Their names appear on their briefs on the website, unless they preferred to make their contributions anonymously.

Richard Riegelman, my former dean at the George Washington University, friend, and editor of the series of which my book is a part, provided irreplaceable help throughout the preparation of the first and second editions.

The staff of Jones & Bartlett Learning was a delight to work with and immensely helpful, including Mike Brown, Sophie Fleck, Maro Gartside, Catie Heverling, Nicole LaLonde, Carolyn Rogers, and Teresa Reilly.

THE THIRD EDITION

A number of colleagues, friends, former colleagues, and former students have been especially helpful to the development of this edition, including some who assisted with the earlier editions.

Richard Riegelman has been a wonderful editor of the series to which this book belongs. He has provided an enormous amount of assistance in the development of all three editions, across a range of areas. He also prepared the prologue for this edition.

David Heymann, the former assistant director-general of the World Health Organization, honored me by writing the foreword to this book, as well as allowing me to profile him in Chapter 19.

Joe Millum, a bioethicist at the National Institutes of Health, in his personal capacity, was the co-author of the chapter on ethics for the second edition. Joe also reviewed and helped me revise the ethics chapter for this edition.

Aviva Musicus, a former student, co-authored the nutrition chapter. She drafted the sections on overweight and obesity and worked closely with me to refine the chapter and to make it a coherent one.

Amy Davis, another former student, prepared the major new section on immunization.

Ian Anderson helped in the preparation of the Policy and Program Brief on diabetes in the Pacific, which was based on his own excellent work.

Lew Barker updated the Policy and Program Brief on AERAS.

Robert Davis reviewed in detail the new immunization section.

Tom Davis assisted in the preparation of the Policy and Program Brief on CARE groups.

Gregg Gonsalves reviewed the entire book, with a particular focus on human rights and social justice. Gregg's comments were extremely helpful to the preparation of the third edition.

Reuben Granich reviewed and provided valuable comments on the treatment of HIV/AIDS in the book.

Robert Hecht assisted in the development and review of a number of Policy and Program Briefs on the financing of global health activities.

Sue Horton provided me access to forthcoming publications on the economics of nutrition, so that I might benefit from them in preparing the nutrition chapter of this book.

Peter Hotez and his colleagues assisted me in the preparation of Policy and Program Briefs on the Global Network on Neglected Tropical Diseases and on the Human Hookworm Vaccine Initiative.

Steve Hyman reviewed a Policy and Program Brief on mental health based on some of his own excellent research and writing.

Prabhat Jha, and his colleagues at the University of Toronto assisted me in the preparation of a Policy and Program Brief on their Million Deaths Study on India.

As she did so ably on the first and second editions, my daughter, Rachel Skolnik Light, provided substantial editorial help on this edition.

Greg Martin reviewed the career chapters of the book and offered keen insights into how they could be improved.

Rachel Nugent provided an enormous amount of help with the book, by pointing me to resources, introducing me to people who could help me with the book, and reviewing a number of parts of the book, including the new sections on overweight and obesity.

Diana Weil reviewed and provided valuable comments on the sections in the book that refer to tuberculosis.

In addition, as on the first and second edition, I employed a substantial number of other former students to assist in a variety of efforts related to the book. These students, from Yale College and the Yale School of Public Health, are identified next, as is a student I employed from the George Mason University.

Hilary Rogers worked with me in conceiving the third edition, reviewing the entire second edition as a basis for the third, collecting data, preparing figures and tables, drafting some of the Policy and Program Briefs and Profiles, drafting some revisions to the book, and editing much that I wrote. Hilary, along with Stephanie Siow, also made major inputs to the new chapter on adolescent health.

Lindsey Hiebert took over Hilary Rogers' work when Hilary moved on to postgraduation employment. Lindsey worked tirelessly on the book in remarkable ways, no matter what other demands faced her. Among other things, Lindsey was exceptionally helpful in finding resources, reviewing the second edition for needed changes, drafting many Policy and Program Briefs, drafting an excellent new section on cancer, and putting together—literally—scores of tables and figures. Lindsey also reviewed all of my writing and many copyedited chapters and helped us to assemble the book into what I hope is a coherent one.

Michealla Baker, Stephanie Heung, and Rachel Wilkinson also played a major role in the preparation of the book. They drafted Policy and Program Briefs and tables and figures and reviewed numerous copyedited chapters of the book. Michealla also worked extensively on the web based materials for the book, including finalizing the video list. Rachel also made special inputs to the chapter on adolescent health and to the web-based bibliography.

Lauren Tronick and Laura Anderson also assisted me in the development of the book's web materials. Among other things, they reviewed and annotated countless videos. They also helped put together the extensive bibliography on global health resources. Laura also drafted several Policy and Program Briefs, including initiating the one on essential surgery.

Kevin Boehm, Emily Briskin, and Vivek Vishwanath also drafted Policy and Program Briefs for the book.

Justin Mendoza drafted a major new addition to the book on pharmaceuticals.

Katherine McDaniel, carefully read the entire second edition and kindly provided me with notes on errors, omissions, and phrases that needed editing before inclusion in the third edition.

Shannon Taylor, a graduate student at The George Mason University, drafted a Policy and Program Brief on oral health, incorporating materials on which Laura Anderson had also assisted.

I am also very grateful to the many people who gave so freely of their time so that I could include a profile or an updated profile of them in this edition.

The staff of Jones & Bartlett Learning was exceptionally helpful and continued to be a delight to work with and included Mike Brown, Sophie Fleck Teague, Chloe Favilene, Lindsey Mawhiney, Nicholas Alakel, and Tracey McCrea.

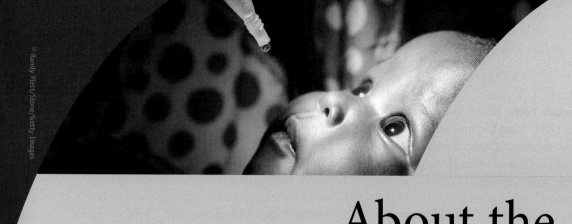

About the Author

Richard Skolnik has worked for more than 40 years in education, health, and development and is one of the world's most experienced teachers of global health. Richard is now a lecturer in the Department of Health Policy and Management at the Yale School of Public Health. He is also a lecturer in the practice of management at the Yale School of Management.

At Yale, Richard teaches an introductory global health course for undergraduates. He also teaches an undergraduate seminar, Case Studies in Global Health, that uses case studies to teach about combatting communicable diseases, reforming health systems, and making those systems better serve the poor. In addition, Richard teaches a course on global health to the MBA for Healthcare Executives Course at the Yale School of Management and a graduate-level introduction to global health at the Yale School of Public Health.

From 2001 to 2004 and from 2009 until 2011, Richard was a part-time lecturer in the Department of Global Health at the George Washington University (GWU), where he taught four courses per year of an introductory global health course for undergraduates. At GWU, Richard also supervised final research projects for master of public health students.

In 2007 and 2008, Richard was the vice president for international programs at the Population Reference Bureau (PRB). In 2005 and 2006, he served as the executive director of the Harvard School of Public Health PEPFAR program for AIDS treatment in Botswana, Nigeria, and Tanzania.

Until 2014, while teaching at GWU and Yale, Richard also worked as a consultant, largely with the Results for Development Institute and mostly working on the financing of HIV in Cambodia, India, and Nigeria.

Richard worked at the World Bank from 1976 to 2001, last serving as the director for health and education for the South Asia region. His work at the World Bank focused on health systems development, family planning and reproductive health, child health, the control of communicable diseases, and nutrition in low-income countries. He was also deeply engaged with tuberculosis (TB), HIV, leprosy, and cataract blindness control projects in India.

Richard has also participated extensively in policy making and program development at the international level. Richard coordinated the World Bank's international work on TB for 5 years, was deeply involved in the establishment of STOP TB, represented the World Bank with the Global Polio Eradication Initiative, served on a number of World Health Organization working groups on TB, and served three rounds on the Technical Review Panel of the Global Fund. Richard led two evaluations of the International AIDS Vaccine Initiative and also led an evaluation of the Global Alliance to Eliminate Leprosy.

In addition, Richard has served on advisory groups and faculty for the Harvard Humanitarian Initiative, the development of a women's health program at Harvard University, and the Global Health Leadership Institute at Yale University. He was also a member of an expert panel that reviewed the Framework Program of the Fogarty Center of the United States National Institutes of Health. He also served 3 years on the advisory board for the College of Health and Human Services at George Mason University. He now serves on the editorial advisory committee for *Disease Priorities in Developing Countries, third edition.*

Richard was an Undergraduate Public Health Teacher of the Year at The George Washington University and was asked in 2009 to deliver a lecture in the GWU "Last Lecture" series. Richard has given numerous guest lectures in a variety of forums and, in May 2011, was the commencement speaker for the George Mason University College of Health and Human Services.

Richard attended high school in Dayton, Ohio. He received a bachelor of arts degree from Yale University and a master's of public affairs from the Woodrow Wilson School of Princeton University. At Yale, he participated in the Experimental Five-Year BA Program, under which he spent 1 year teaching high school biology in Laoag City, Philippines, living with the same family with whom he had lived as an exchange student in 1966. Upon graduation from Yale, Richard was selected for a fellowship by the Yale–China Association and spent 2 years teaching at The Chinese University of Hong Kong. In the summer between his 2 years at the Woodrow Wilson School, Richard was a research fellow at the Institute of Southeast Asian Studies in Singapore, where he authored a monograph on education and training in Singapore.

Richard has worked on health issues in Africa, Latin America and the Caribbean, the Middle East and North Africa, South Asia, and Southeast Asia. He has also studied and learned to varying degrees Cantonese, French, Ilocano, Mandarin, Spanish, and Tagalog.

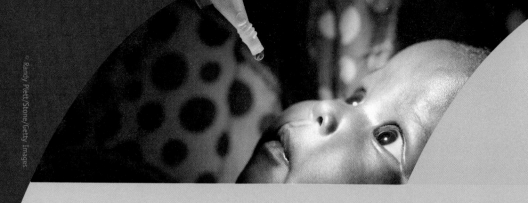

Quotable Global Health Quotes

Health is a state of complete physical, mental and social well-being and not merely the absence of disease or infirmity. The enjoyment of the highest attainable standard of health is one of the fundamental rights of every human being without distinction of race, religion, political belief, economic or social condition.

World Health Organization*

Public health . . . represents an organised response to the protection and promotion of human health and encompasses a concern with the environment, disease control, the provision of health care, health education and health promotion.

Research Unit in Health and Behavioural Change, University of Edinburgh**

Public health is the science and art of promoting health. It does so based on the understanding that health is a process engaging social, mental, spiritual and physical well-being. Public health acts on the knowledge that health is a fundamental resource to the individual, to the community and to society as a whole and must be supported by soundly investing in living conditions that create, maintain and protect health.

Ilona Kickbusch

Prevention is better than cure.

Desiderius Erasmus

Every patient carries her or his own doctor inside.

Albert Schweitzer

The doctor of the future will give no medicine, but will interest his patients in the care of the human frame, in diet and in the cause and prevention of disease.

Thomas A. Edison

Of all forms of inequality, injustice in health care is the most shocking and inhumane.

Martin Luther King, Jr.

It is health that is real wealth and not pieces of gold and silver.

Mohandas K. (Mahatma) Gandhi

. . . class differences in health represent a double injustice: life is short where its quality is poor.

Richard G. Wilkinson

Where once it was the physician who waged bellum contra morbum, the war against disease, now it's the whole society.

Susan Sontag

Health consists of having the same diseases as one's neighbors.

Quentin Crisp

Be careful about reading health books. You may die of a misprint.

Mark Twain

---

*World Health Organization. (2015). *Constitution of WHO: principles*. Retrieved from http://www.who.int/about/mission/en/.

**Research Unit in Health and Behavioural Change, University of Edinburgh. (1995). *Changing the Public Health*. Chichester: John Wiley & Sons.

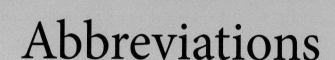

Abbreviations

TERM	DEFINITION
ADB	Asian Development Bank
AfDB	African Development Bank
AIDS	acquired immune deficiency syndrome
APOC	African Programme for Onchocerciasis Control
ARI	acute respiratory infection
ART	antiretroviral therapy
AusAID	Australian Agency for International Development
BCG	Bacillus Calmette-Guérin (the tuberculosis vaccine)
BMI	body mass index
BOD	burden of disease
CDC	The U.S. Centers for Disease Control and Prevention
CFR	case fatality ratio
CHE	complex humanitarian emergency
CMR	crude mortality rate
CVD	cardiovascular disease
DALY	disability-adjusted life year
DANIDA	Danish International Development Agency
DFID	Department for International Development of the United Kingdom
DHS	Demographic and Health Survey
DTP	diphtheria, tetanus, and pertussis
EPI	Expanded Program on Immunization
EU	European Union
FAO	Food and Agriculture Organization of the United Nations
FSU	Former Soviet Union

Gavi	The Vaccine Alliance
GBD	*Global Burden of Disease Study 2010*
GDP	gross domestic product
GNP	gross national product
GOBI	growth monitoring, oral rehydration, breastfeeding, and immunization
HALE	health-adjusted life expectancy
Hib	*Haemophilus influenzae* type b
HIV	human immunodeficiency virus
HPV	human papillomavirus
IAVI	International AIDS Vaccine Initiative
IBRD	International Bank for Reconstruction and Development (World Bank)
IDA	International Development Association (the "soft" lending window of the World Bank)
IDB	Inter-American Development Bank
IDD	iodine deficiency disorder
IDP	internally displaced person
IEC	information, education, and communication
IFFIm	International Financing Facility for Immunisation
IHD	ischemic heart disease
IMCI	integrated management of childhood illness
IMF	International Monetary Fund
IMR	infant mortality rate
IND	investigational new drug
IPT	intermittent preventive treatment
IPV	injectable polio vaccine
IQ	intelligence quotient
IRB	institutional review board
ITI	International Trachoma Initiative
ITN	insecticide-treated bednet
IUD	intrauterine device
LMICs	low- and middle-income countries
MCH	maternal and child health
MDG	Millennium Development Goal
MDR	multidrug resistant
MDT	multidrug therapy
MI	The Micronutrient Initiative
MMR	maternal mortality rate
MSF	Doctors Without Borders (Médicins Sans Frontières in French)
NCD	noncommunicable disease
NGO	nongovernmental organization

NID	National Immunization Day
NNMR	neonatal mortality rate
NTD	neglected tropical disease
OCP	Onchocerciasis Control Program
OPV	oral polio vaccine
ORS	oral rehydration solution
ORT	oral rehydration therapy
PAHO	Pan American Health Organization
PDP	product development partnership
PEPFAR	President's Emergency Plan for AIDS Relief
PHC	primary health care
PMTCT	prevention of mother-to-child transmission
PPP	public–private partnership
RBM	Roll Back Malaria
RTI	road traffic injury
SDG	sustainable development goal
SIDA	Swedish International Development Cooperation Agency
SSB	sugar-sweetened beverage
STI	sexually transmitted infection
SWAp	sector-wide approach
TB	tuberculosis
TBA	traditional birth attendant
TFR	total fertility rate
TRIPS	Agreement on Trade-Related Aspects of Intellectual Property Rights
TT	tetanus toxoid
UN	United Nations
UNAIDS	Joint United Nations Programme on HIV/AIDS
UNDP	United Nations Development Programme
UNFPA	United Nations Family Planning Association
UNICEF	United Nations Children's Fund
USAID	U.S. Agency for International Development
WFP	World Food Program
WHA	World Health Assembly of the World Health Organization
WHO	World Health Organization
WHO/TDR	WHO Special Programme for Research and Training in Tropical Diseases
WTO	World Trade Organization
YLD	years lived with disability
YLL	years of life lost

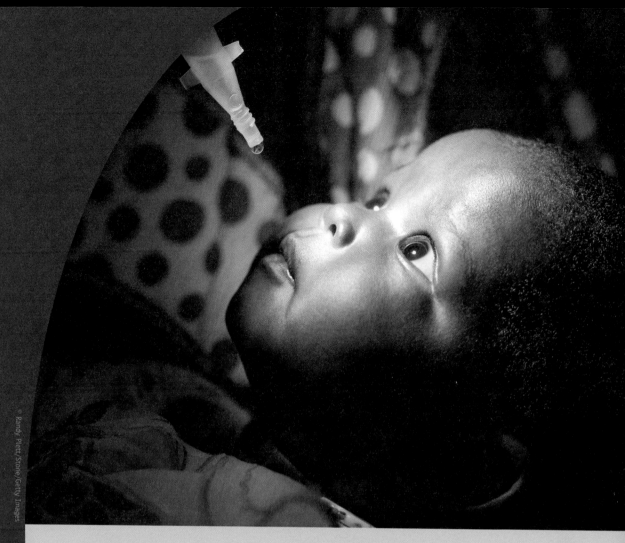

PART I

Principles, Measurements, and the Health–Development Link

CHAPTER 1

The Principles and Goals of Global Health

LEARNING OBJECTIVES

By the end of this chapter the reader will be able to:

- Define the terms *health*, *public health*, and *global health*
- Discuss some examples of public health efforts
- Discuss some examples of global health activities
- Describe some of the guiding principles of public health work
- Describe the Millennium Development Goals and their relation to global health
- Briefly discuss the global effort to eradicate smallpox

VIGNETTES

By 2005, polio was on the verge of being eradicated. That year, however, rumors circulated in northern Nigeria that the polio vaccine was causing sterility. In response to these rumors, some community leaders discouraged people from immunizing their children. Within months, polio cases began to appear in the area. Shortly thereafter, polio cases spread from northern Nigeria to Sudan, Yemen, and Indonesia. The global campaign to eradicate polio had been dealt a major blow, stemming partly from rumors in one country about the alleged side effects of the vaccine.[1]

Getachew is a 20-year-old Ethiopian with HIV. His disease is advanced, but he receives no treatment for it. He has tuberculosis (TB) and much of his mouth is coated with a white, pasty yeast called thrush. He has lost more than 20 percent of his body weight. He stopped going to work some time ago, has no money, and is totally dependent on his family for care and day-to-day needs. Getachew is one of about 760,000 people in Ethiopia with HIV.[2] In fact, in 2013 about 35 million

people were living with HIV worldwide.[3] There are countries in Africa, such as Botswana, Lesotho, and Swaziland, in which about one quarter of the adults are HIV-positive.[3]

Laurie lived in Portsmouth, Virginia, in the United States. She was 50 years old and had always been healthy. Last weekend, she woke up with a headache, a high fever, and a very stiff neck. Laurie was so sick that she went to the emergency room of the local hospital. The physicians diagnosed Laurie as having meningitis, an inflammation of the membrane around the brain and spinal cord,[4] that was caused by the West Nile virus. This virus originated in Egypt in the 1930s and is transmitted by a mosquito. Today, the virus can be found in much of the world.[5]

Jim Smith is a high school student in London, England. Early in the school year, he had a fever and cough that would not go away. He did not feel like eating. He slept badly and woke up every morning in a sweat. Jim had TB. Although many people think that TB has been eliminated from high-income countries, it has not. Rather, the spread of HIV has triggered an increase in TB worldwide. In addition, immigration is helping to spread the disease from lower-income to higher-income countries. In fact, there are urban areas of the United Kingdom in which the rates of TB are higher than the rates in some low- and middle-income countries.[6]

Nirupama is a 50-year-old woman who lives in Chennai, India. "Niru," as her friends call her, has diabetes. She is dependent on a regular supply of insulin, which she picks up monthly at a government clinic. Although she is only 50, she already has suffered some of the circulatory complications of diabetes. There is a common perception that diabetes is a disease that affects only people in high-income countries. This, however, is not the case. Rather, the prevalence of diabetes is growing rapidly in low- and middle-income countries. India now has the largest number of people with diabetes.[7] The highest percentage of an adult population with the disease can be found in the Pacific Island of Nauru, in which 31 percent of adults have diabetes.[7]

WHY STUDY GLOBAL HEALTH

Over the last 50 years, the world has made significant progress in improving human health. From 1950 to 2012, for example, the death rate of children under 5 years fell from 148 deaths per 1,000 children to fewer than 48 deaths per 1,000 children.[8,9] From 1950 to 2010, life expectancy for the world grew from 48 years to 68 years.[9,10] Smallpox has been eradicated, polio has been eliminated in all but a few countries, and great progress has been made in reducing the burden of vaccine-preventable diseases in children and the burden of parasitic infections, such as Guinea worm. One reason to study global health is to gain a better understanding of the progress made so far in addressing global health problems.

Another reason to study global health, however, is to better understand the most important global health challenges that remain and what must be done to address them rapidly, effectively, and efficiently. Despite the important progress in improving human health:

- 289,000 women are estimated to have died of maternal causes in 2013.[11]
- 6.3 million children under 5 years of age died in 2013.[12]
- 1.5 million people died of TB in 2013.[13]
- 1.5 million people died of HIV-related causes in 2013.[14]
- 584,000 people died of malaria in 2013.[15]

In addition, the world is shrinking and the health of people everywhere must be of concern to all of us. This is particularly important because many diseases are not limited by national boundaries. Tuberculosis, HIV, and polio, for example, can spread from one country to the next. Prior to 1960, dengue fever used to be concentrated largely in Southeast Asia and the coast of South America. However, cases are now seen in five continents, as shown in **Figure 1-1**.[16,17]

FIGURE 1-1 The Spread of Dengue Fever/Dengue Hemorrhagic Fever

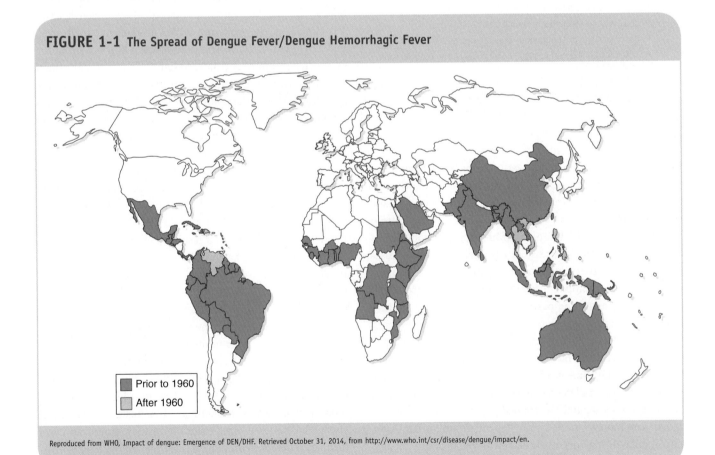

Prior to 1960
After 1960

Reproduced from WHO, Impact of dengue: Emergence of DEN/DHF. Retrieved October 31, 2014, from http://www.who.int/csr/disease/dengue/impact/en.

The "avian flu" first appeared in East Asia, but it, too, is spreading to other regions. Ten years ago, no one in Laurie's neighborhood ever thought of getting West Nile virus. Recently, the chikungunya virus has also been spreading globally.

Besides the central global health challenges noted previously, there are also exceptional disparities in the health of some groups compared to the health of others. Life expectancy in Japan and France, for example, is about 83 years, but it is only 45 years in Sierra Leone.[18] In addition, there are a number of life-saving technologies, such as the hepatitis B vaccine, that have been used in high-income countries for many years that are not yet used as widely in low-income countries. In fact, the previous points raise important ethical and humanitarian questions about the extent to which people everywhere should be concerned about disparities in access to health services and in health status.

The important link between health and development is another reason to pay particular attention to global health. Poor health of mothers is linked to poor health of babies and the failure of children to reach their full mental and physical potential. In addition, ill health of children can delay their entry into school and can affect their attendance, their academic performance, and, therefore, their future economic prospects. Countries with major health problems, such as high rates of malaria or HIV, have difficulty attracting the investments needed to develop their economies. Moreover, having large numbers of undernourished, unhealthy, and ill-educated people in any country is destabilizing and poses a health, economic, and security threat to all countries.

The nature of many global health concerns and the need for different actors to work together to address them are more reasons why we should be concerned with global health. Although locally relevant solutions are needed to address most health problems, some health issues can be solved only with a global approach. In addition, some problems, such as ensuring access to drugs to treat HIV/AIDS, may require more financial resources than any individual country can provide. Still other global health issues require technical cooperation across countries because few countries have the technical capacity to deal with them. Global cooperation might be needed, for example, to establish standards for drug safety, to set protocols for the treatment of certain health problems, such as malaria, or to develop an HIV vaccine that could serve the needs of low-income countries.

The concepts and concerns of global health are also becoming increasingly prominent worldwide. The spread of HIV, the SARS scare, the fear of the avian flu, and a new outbreak of Ebola virus in West Africa have all brought attention to global health. The advocacy efforts, for example, of Doctors Without Borders and the rock star Bono, the establishment of the Millennium Development Goals, and the philanthropy of the Bill & Melinda Gates Foundation have also dramatically raised attention to global health. The topic has become so important that there is a push in many universities throughout the world to ensure that all students have a basic understanding of key global health issues.

HEALTH, PUBLIC HEALTH, AND GLOBAL HEALTH

Health

Before starting our review of global health in greater detail, it will be helpful to establish a set of definitions for *health*, *public health*, and *global health*. Most of us think of "health" from our individual perspective as "not being sick." The World Health Organization, however, set out a broader definition of health in 1948 that is still widely used:

> Health is a state of complete physical, mental and social well-being and not merely the absence of disease or infirmity.[19]

This is the definition of "health" used in this text.

Public Health

Although the World Health Organization (WHO) concept of "health" refers first to individuals, this book is mostly about "public health" and the health of populations. C.E.A. Winslow, considered to be the founder of modern public health in the United States, formulated a definition of public health in 1923 that is still commonly used today. In his definition, public health is:

> the science and the art of preventing disease, prolonging life, and promoting physical health and mental health and efficiency through organized community efforts toward a sanitary environment; the control of community infections; the education of the individual in principles of personal hygiene; the organization of medical and nursing service for the early diagnosis and treatment of disease; and the development of the social machinery to ensure to every individual in the community a standard of living adequate for the maintenance of health.[20]

According to Winslow's definition, some examples of public health activities would include the development of a campaign to promote child immunization in a particular country, an effort to get people in a city to use seat belts when they drive, and actions to get people in a specific setting to eat healthier foods and to stop smoking. In addition, most levels of government also carry out certain public health functions. These include the management of public health clinics, the operation of public health laboratories, and the maintenance of disease surveillance systems. Other examples are shown in **Table 1-1**.

There are a number of guiding principles to the practice of public health that have been articulated, for example, by the American Public Health Association in its public health code of ethics.[21] These principles focus on prevention of disease, respect for the rights of individuals, and a commitment to developing public health efforts in conjunction with communities. They also highlight the need to pay particular attention to disenfranchised people and communities and the importance of evidence-based public health interventions. In addition, they note the importance of taking account of a wide range of disciplines and appreciation for the values, beliefs, and cultures of diverse groups. Finally, they put considerable emphasis on engaging in public health practice in a way that "enhances the physical and social environment" and that builds on collaborations across public health actors.[21]

Many people confuse "public health" and "medicine," although they have quite different approaches. **Table 1-2** outlines these differences.[22] To a large extent, the biggest difference between the medical approach and the public health approach is the focus in public health on the health of populations rather than on the health of individuals. Exaggerating somewhat for effect, we could say, for example, that a physician cares for an individual patient whom he or she immunizes against a particular disease, whereas a public health specialist is likely to focus on how one ensures that the whole community gets vaccinated. A physician will counsel an individual patient on the need to exercise and avoid obesity; a public health specialist will work with a program meant to help a community stay sufficiently active to avoid obesity. In addition, there are branches of public health, such as epidemiology, that focus on studying patterns and causes of disease in specific populations and the application of this information to controlling health problems.[23] Finally, we should note the exceptional attention that public health approaches pay to prevention of health problems.

TABLE 1-1 Selected Examples of Public Health Activities

- The promotion of handwashing
- The promotion of bicycle and motorcycle helmets
- The promotion of knowledge about HIV/AIDS
- Large-scale screening for diabetes and hypertension
- Large-scale screening of the eyesight of schoolchildren
- Mass dosing of children against worms
- The operation of a supplementary feeding program for poorly nourished young children

---

TABLE 1-2 Approaches of Public Health and Medicine

Differentiating Factors	Public Health	Medicine
Focus	Population	Individual
Ethical basis	Public service	Personal service
Emphasis	Disease prevention and health promotion for communities	Disease diagnosis, treatment, and care for individuals
Interventions	Broad spectrum that may target the environment, human behavior, lifestyle, and medical care	Emphasis on medical care

Modified with permission from Harvard School of Public Health. About HSPH: Distinctions Between Public Health and Medicine. Retrieved September 8, 2013, from http://www.hsph.harvard.edu/about/public-health-medicine/.

Global Health

What exactly is *global health*? The U.S. Institute of Medicine defined global health as "health problems, issues, and concerns that transcend national boundaries and may best be addressed by cooperative actions."[24]

Another group defined what we would now call global health as "the application of the principles of public health to health problems and challenges that transcend national boundaries and to the complex array of global and local forces that affect them."[25]

The discussion of the definition of global health has continued. Two groups of distinguished public health scholars and practitioners offered additional commentaries on this matter. One group suggested that we should define global health as:

> an area for study, research, and practice that places a priority on improving health and achieving equity in health for all people worldwide. Global health emphasizes transnational health issues, determinants, and solutions, involves many disciplines within and beyond the health sciences, and promotes interdisciplinary collaboration; and is a synthesis of population based prevention with individual-level clinical care.[26]

In response to this suggestion, however, another panel suggested that one should not distinguish between global health and public health more broadly. They also suggested that the key principles of both are the same: a focus on the public good, belief in a global perspective, a scientific and interdisciplinary approach, the need for multilevel approaches to interventions, and the need for comprehensive frameworks for health policies and financing.[27]

The study and practice of global health today reflects many of the comments made here. *Global health* implies a global perspective on public health problems. It suggests issues that people face in common, such as the impact of a growing and aging worldwide population on health or the potential risks of climate change to health. The topic also relates in important ways to problems that require cooperative action. An important part of global health also covers the growing problem everywhere of noncommunicable diseases, as well as the "unfinished agenda" of the health needs of the poor in poor countries. In practical terms, as a new student to global health, it may be best not to worry much about the definition of *global health*, but rather to see the topic as an important part of public health, which itself has many areas of critical importance.

TABLE 1-3 Selected Examples of Global Health Issues

- Emerging and reemerging infectious diseases
- Antimicrobial resistance
- Eradication of polio
- TB
- Malaria
- HIV
- The increasing cases of diabetes and heart disease globally

---

Some examples of important global health concerns include the factors that contribute to women dying of pregnancy-related causes in so many countries; the exceptional amount of malnutrition among young children, especially in South Asia and Africa; and the burden of different communicable and noncommunicable diseases worldwide and what can be done to control those diseases. The impact of the environment on health globally and the effects of natural disasters and conflicts are also important to global health. Other significant global health issues include how countries can organize and manage their health systems to address the healthiest population possible given the resources available to them, the search for new technologies to address important global health problems, and how different actors can work together to solve health problems that are too significant for any country or actor to solve on their own. Another global health matter of importance is the relationship between globalization and the health of different communities. Some additional global health issues of importance are shown in **Table 1-3**.

CRITICAL GLOBAL HEALTH CONCEPTS

In order to understand and to help address key global health issues like those noted previously, there are a number of concepts concerning global health with which one must be familiar. Some of the most important include:

- The determinants of health
- The measurement of health status
- The importance of culture to health
- The global burden of disease
- The key risk factors for different health conditions
- The demographic and epidemiologic transitions
- The organization and functions of health systems

It is also essential to understand the links among health, education, development, poverty, and equity.

Building on the previous concepts, those interested in global health also need to have an understanding of how key health issues affect different parts of the world and the world as a whole. These include:

- Environmental health
- Nutrition
- Reproductive health
- Child health
- Communicable diseases
- Noncommunicable diseases
- Injuries

Finally, it is important to understand global health issues that are generally addressed through cooperation. Some of these concern conflicts, natural disasters, and humanitarian emergencies. Others relate to the mechanisms by which different actors in global health activities work together to solve global health problems. Harnessing the power of science and technology for global health needs also requires cooperation.

THE ORGANIZATION OF DATA IN THE BOOK

This is a book about global health that has a particular focus on the "health–development link." Thus, data are organized wherever possible by the six World Bank regions:

- Africa
- East Asia and Pacific
- Europe and Central Asia
- Latin America and the Caribbean
- Middle East and North Africa
- South Asia

The Middle East and North Africa region covers essentially the Middle East and the Arabic speaking countries of North Africa. For the sake of clarity and consistent with World Bank data, the Africa region will be referred to as sub-Saharan Africa.

For the most part, the World Bank regions cover only low- and middle-income countries. The World Bank regions are shown in **Figure 1-2**.

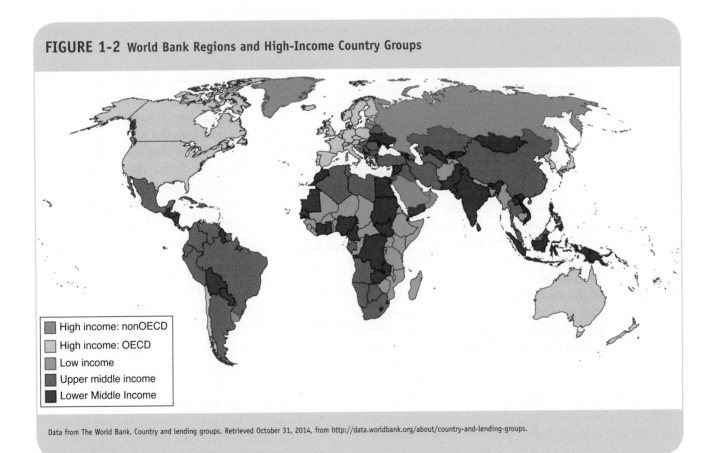

FIGURE 1-2 World Bank Regions and High-Income Country Groups

- High income: nonOECD
- High income: OECD
- Low income
- Upper middle income
- Lower Middle Income

Data from The World Bank. Country and lending groups. Retrieved October 31, 2014, from http://data.worldbank.org/about/country-and-lending-groups.

Some critical data, however, are collected only by region of the World Health Organization (WHO). WHO regions cover all countries. Those regions are:

- Africa
- The Americas
- South-East Asia
- Europe
- Eastern Mediterranean
- Western Pacific

Figure 1-3 shows the WHO regions.

To complement information by World Bank or WHO region, the book also includes information for the high-income countries that are members of the Organization for Cooperation and Development (OECD). The list of countries that belong to the OECD is shown in **Table 1-4**.

The book also speaks of countries in terms of their income and the income group to which they belong. These terms largely follow the definitions used by the World Bank, which divides countries into four income groups, based on their gross national income per person, as shown in **Table 1-5**.[28]

- $1,035 or less—low-income
- $1,036 to $4,085—lower-middle-income
- $4,086 to $12,615—upper-middle-income
- $12,616 or above—high-income

This book contains substantially updated information on the burden of disease and associated risk factors. This information is drawn largely from a study published in 2013 by the Institute of Health Metrics and Evaluations (IHME), *The Global Burden of Disease: Generating Evidence, Guiding Policy*,[29] the extensive website for that study, and a related *Lancet* series on the Global Burden of Disease 2010.[30] The IHME study, *The Global Burden of Disease: Generating Evidence, Guiding Policy*, used 2010 as the base year for its data. It also included a revision of data that was calculated earlier for 1990, to allow for more valid comparisons between 1990

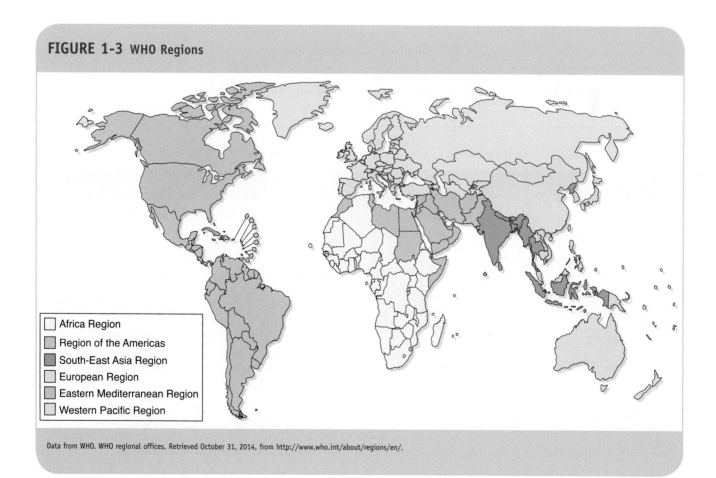

FIGURE 1-3 WHO Regions

- Africa Region
- Region of the Americas
- South-East Asia Region
- European Region
- Eastern Mediterranean Region
- Western Pacific Region

Data from WHO. WHO regional offices. Retrieved October 31, 2014, from http://www.who.int/about/regions/en/.

TABLE 1-4 List of OECD Countries

Country	Country	Country
Australia	Hungary	Norway
Austria	Iceland	Poland
Belgium	Ireland	Portugal
Canada	Israel	Slovak Republic
Chile	Italy	Slovenia
Czech Republic	Japan	Spain
Denmark	Korea	Sweden
Estonia	Luxembourg	Switzerland
Finland	Mexico	Turkey
France	Netherlands	United Kingdom
Germany	New Zealand	United states
Greece		

Data from OECD, List of OECD Member Countries—Ratification of the Convention on the OECD, http://www.oecd.org/about/membersandpartners/list-oecd
-member-countries.htm. Accessed on November 3, 2014.

TABLE 1-5 World Bank Country Income Groups, 2013, Selected Representative Countries

Low-Income	Lower-Middle-Income	Upper-Middle-Income	High-Income
Bangladesh	Bolivia	Botswana	Belgium
Cambodia	Cameroon	Costa Rica	Canada
Ethiopia	Egypt	Panama	Denmark
Haiti	India	South Africa	Italy
Mozambique	Morocco	Turkey	Netherlands
Zimbabwe	Philippines	Venezuela	Portugal
	Swaziland		Singapore
	Vietnam		Switzerland

Data from the World Bank, Country, and Lending Groups. Retrieved August 5, 2014, from http://data.worldbank.org/about/country-and-lending-groups.

and 2010 about trends in the burden of disease. This text will refer to the study and its parts as *The Global Burden of Disease Study 2010*.

The burden of disease data from the IHME study is complemented as needed by data on particular diseases that is published by other organizations such as UNICEF, WHO, and the World Bank. The data are also complemented when necessary by data from earlier burden of disease studies and from data published in *Disease Control Priorities in Developing Countries, Second Edition* and *Third Edition*.[31]

THE MILLENNIUM DEVELOPMENT GOALS

This book makes continuous references to the Millennium Development Goals (MDGs). The MDGs were formulated in 2000 at the United Nations Millennium Summit and were articulated in the Millennium Declaration.[32] There are 8 MDGs and 15 core targets that relate to them. The countries that signed the declaration pledged to meet the MDGs by 2015. The MDGs are important for understanding global health issues because they are an explicit statement of the goals that many countries have set for an important part of their development efforts. The MDGs and their related targets are noted in **Table 1-6**.

All eight of the MDGs relate to health. The goals of reducing child mortality, improving maternal health, and combating HIV/AIDS, malaria, and other diseases directly concern health. However, each of the other goals also relates to health. Hunger and poverty, referred to in goal 1, are intimately linked with health status, both as causes of ill health and as consequences of ill health. The goal of universal primary education can be met only if children are well enough nourished and healthy enough to enroll in school, attend school, and have capacity to learn while they are there. The gender disparities referred to in goal 3 are central to the health issues that affect women globally, many of which relate to their lack of empowerment. Goal 7 is meant to address the need for safe water and sanitation, the lack of which is a major cause of ill health and death. Different actors in global health can work together to help countries improve health status, as indicated in goal 8 on partnerships for development.

The United Nations (UN) has set up a process to develop a new set of global development goals that will build on the MDGs and will be called Sustainable Development Goals. This work is being led by representatives from 70 countries, who share 30 seats on an "Open Working Group," which the UN has established to guide the process.[33,34] It will be important for students of global health to follow the progress in the articulation of the new goals and their relation to health and the determinants of health.

THE CASE STUDIES

Many of the case studies in this book were provided by the Center for Global Development and are elaborated upon further in a companion piece to this book entitled *Case Studies in Global Health: Millions Saved*.[35] That book provides detailed case studies of 20 successful interventions in global health. The cases were carefully selected on the basis of five selection criteria: scale, importance, impact, duration, and cost-effectiveness. When considered together, the cases suggest a number of important lessons that are reflected throughout this book:

- Success in addressing important health problems *is* possible, even in the poorest countries.
- Governments in poor countries *can* manage major public health successes and often can fund them, as well.
- Technology does enable progress in health; however, many successes stem from basic changes in people's behavior, such as filtering water, giving infants oral rehydration for diarrhea, and smoking cessation.
- Cooperation among global health actors can make a major difference to the achievement of health aims.
- It is possible to find evidence of what works and does not work in global health efforts.
- Success comes in all shapes—different types of programs in different types of settings have been and can be successful.

SMALLPOX ERADICATION—THE MOST FAMOUS SUCCESS STORY

It is fitting to end the main part of this introductory chapter with a summary of the most famous public health success story of all, the case of smallpox eradication. This effort was not only a great triumph of public health but also a great accomplishment for mankind. In addition, the history of smallpox eradication is well known to everyone who works in public health, and it provides many lessons that can be applied to other public health efforts.

Background

In 1966, smallpox ravaged over 50 countries, affecting 10 million to 15 million people, of whom almost 2 million died each year.[36] At the time, smallpox killed as many as 30 percent of

TABLE 1-6 The Millennium Development Goals and Their Related Targets

Goal	Targets
Goal 1: Eradicate Extreme Hunger and Poverty	Target 1. Halve, between 1990 and 2015, the proportion of people whose income is less than $1 a day Target 2. Halve, between 1990 and 2015, the proportion of people who suffer from hunger
Goal 2: Achieve Universal Primary Education	Target 3. Ensure that, by 2015, children everywhere, boys and girls alike, will be able to complete a full course of primary schooling
Goal 3: Promote Gender Equality and Empower Women	Target 4. Eliminate gender disparity in primary and secondary education, preferably by 2005, and in all levels of education no later than 2015
Goal 4: Reduce Child Mortality	Target 5. Reduce by two-thirds, between 1990 and 2015, the under-5 mortality rate
Goal 5: Improve Maternal Health	Target 6. Reduce by three-quarters, between 1990 and 2015, the maternal mortality ratio
Goal 6: Combat HIV/ AIDS, Malaria, and Other Diseases	Target 7. Have halted by 2015 and begun to reverse the spread of HIV/AIDS Target 8. Have halted by 2015 and begun to reverse the incidence of malaria and other major diseases
Goal 7: Ensure Environmental Sustainability	Target 9. Integrate the principles of sustainable development into country policies and programs and reverse the loss of environmental resources Target 10. Halve, by 2015, the proportion of people without sustainable access to safe drinking water and basic sanitation Target 11. Have achieved by 2020 a significant improvement in the lives of at least 100 million slum dwellers
Goal 8: Develop a Global Partnership for Development	Target 12. Develop further an open, rule-based, predictable, nondiscriminatory trading and financial system Target 13. Address the special needs of the least developed countries Target 14. Address the special needs of landlocked developing countries and small island developing states Target 15. Deal comprehensively with the debt problems of developing countries through national and international measures in order to make debt sustainable in the long term

Data from Millennium Project: Goals, Targets, and Indicators. Retrieved April 9, 2011, from http://www.unmillenniumproject.org/goals/gti.htm.

those infected. Those who survived could suffer from deep-pitted scars and blindness as a result of their illness.[37]

The Intervention

Although a vaccine against smallpox was created by Edward Jenner in 1798, eradication of smallpox became a practical goal only in the 1950s when the vaccine could be mass produced and stored without refrigeration. A later breakthrough came in the form of the bifurcated needle, a marvel of simple technology that dramatically reduced costs by allowing needles to be reused endlessly after sterilization and by requiring a far smaller amount of vaccine per patient then had previously been the case. The needle also made vaccination easy, thereby reducing the time and effort required to train villagers in its use.

In 1959, WHO adopted a proposal to eradicate smallpox through compulsory vaccination, but the program languished until 1965, when the United States stepped in with technical and financial support. A Smallpox Eradication Unit was established at WHO, headed by Dr. D.A. Henderson of the Centers for Disease Control and Prevention (CDC) in the United States. As part of the smallpox eradication program, all WHO member countries were required to manage program funds effectively, report smallpox cases, encourage research on smallpox, and maintain flexibility in the implementation of the smallpox program to suit local conditions.

The Smallpox Eradication Unit proved to be a small but committed team, supplying vaccines and specimen kits to those countries that still had smallpox. Although wars and civil unrest caused disruptions in the program's progress, momentum was always regained with new methods and extra resources that focused on containing outbreaks by speedily seeking out new cases with motorized teams, isolating new cases, and vaccinating everyone in the vicinity of the new cases.

This military-style approach proved effective even in the most difficult circumstances. It also took practical account of the facts that (1) it would have been extraordinarily difficult to immunize the whole world against smallpox, and (2) the transmission of the smallpox virus could be stopped by focusing vaccination efforts around new cases.

The Impact

In 1977, the last endemic case of smallpox in the world was recorded in Somalia. In 1980, after additional surveillance and searching, WHO declared smallpox the first disease in history to have been eradicated. Smallpox had previously been eliminated in Latin America in 1971 and in Asia in 1975.[38]

Costs and Benefits

The annual cost of the eradication campaign between 1967 and 1979 was $23 million. For the whole campaign, international donors provided $98 million, and $200 million came from the endemic countries.[32] The United States saves the total of all its contributions every 26 days because it no longer needs to spend money on vaccination or treatment, making smallpox eradication one of the best values in health interventions ever achieved.[35] Estimates for economic loss due to smallpox being endemic in a low- or middle-income country are available only for India. Based on these, it has been estimated that low- and middle-income countries as a whole suffered economic losses related to smallpox of about $1 billion each year at the start of the intensified campaign.[39]

Lessons Learned

The success of the smallpox eradication program can be attributed to the political commitment and leadership exemplified in the partnership between WHO and the U.S. Centers for Disease Control and Prevention. Success in individual countries hinged on having someone who was responsible, preferably solely, for the eradication effort. In addition, small WHO teams made frequent field trips to review progress, and a small number of committed people working in the program were able to motivate large numbers of staff. Moreover, in the days before the Internet and email, the program managers held a monthly meeting in which they exchanged information about the progress of the campaign and the lessons learned from working on it in different countries.

No two national campaigns were alike, which makes flexibility essential in program design. The plan for eradicating smallpox used existing healthcare systems, and it also enabled many countries to improve their health services. This benefited immunization programs more generally and also offset the cost of the initial smallpox campaign.

Monitoring standards were established across the program to constantly evaluate progress against agreed benchmarks. Community participation provided strategic lessons for later community-based projects. The value of publicity was highlighted when news about the program's progress triggered large donations in 1974 to complete eradication in five remaining countries. An important discovery made during the campaign was that immunization programs could vaccinate people with more than one vaccination at a time. This helped to pave the way for routine immunization.

The eradication of smallpox continues to inspire efforts against other diseases, but it must be remembered that the particular features of smallpox made it a prime candidate for eradication. The disease was passed directly between people, without an intervening carrier, so there were no reservoirs; the distinctive rash of smallpox made diagnosis easy; survivors gained lifetime immunity; and the severity of symptoms, once the disease became infectious, made patients take to their beds and infect few others. Good vaccination coverage could therefore disrupt transmission entirely. Unfortunately, almost 30 years after eradication, funds are still allocated to precautionary measures against the disease because of the continuing threat of smallpox being used as an agent of bioterrorism.

CENTRAL MESSAGES OF THE BOOK

Because this is the introductory chapter of the book, it does not end with a summary, as the other chapters do. Rather, it is more valuable to end this chapter by highlighting some of the central messages of the book as a whole. They are listed here, without citations or recitation of the evidence behind them. That evidence is provided and cited in the chapters that follow. It is very important to keep these messages in mind throughout the book.

- There are strong links among health, human development, labor productivity, and economic development.
- Health status is determined by a variety of factors, including age, culture, income, education, knowledge of healthy behaviors, social status, sex, genetic makeup, and access to health services. The economic and social conditions under which people live and government policies also have an important influence on people's health.
- Given the wide range in the determinants of health, it is fundamental in setting health policy to think and act broadly—in some respects more like a minister of finance must think and act, rather than how a minister of health would do so.
- There has been enormous progress in improving health status over the last 50 years in many countries. This is reflected in the substantial increases these countries have witnessed in that period, for example, in life expectancy.
- Some of this progress has come about as a result of overall economic development and improvements in income. However, much of it is due to improvements in public hygiene, better water supply and sanitation, and better education. Increased nutritional status has also had a large impact on improvements in health status. Technical progress in some areas, such as the development of vaccines against childhood diseases and the development of antibiotics, has also improved human health.
- The progress in health status, however, has been very uneven. Hundreds of millions of people, especially poor people in low- and middle-income countries, continue to get sick, be disabled by, or die from preventable causes of disease. In many countries, nutritional status and health status of lower-income people have improved only slowly. In addition, HIV caused an earlier decline in health and nutritional status and life expectancy in a number of countries in sub-Saharan Africa.
- There are enormous disparities in health status and access to health services both within and across countries. Wealthier people in most countries have better health status and better access to health services than poorer people. In general, urban dwellers and ethnic majorities enjoy better health status than rural people and disadvantaged ethnic minorities. In addition, women face a number of unique challenges to their health, as do lesbian, gay, bisexual, and transgender people (LGBT), prisoners, and other marginalized people.
- Countries do not need to be high-income to enjoy good health status. By contrast, there are a number of examples, such as China, Costa Rica, Cuba, Kerala state in India, and Sri Lanka, that make clear that low-income countries or low-income areas within countries can help their people to achieve good health, even in the absence of extensive financial resources to invest in health. However, this requires strong political will and a focus on public hygiene, education, and low-cost but high-yielding investments in nutrition and health.
- In this light, when considering health policy, one must always seek value for money and ask: "If I only had $100 to spend, how should I spend it to achieve the maximum health gains for the key groups, at least cost?"
- The burden of disease is evolving in light of economic and social changes, the aging of populations, and scientific and technical progress, among other things. The burden of disease is predominantly communicable only in sub-Saharan Africa. In all of other regions, the burden of disease is predominantly noncommunicable. In the absence of new communicable disease threats of major importance, the burden of disease is expected to shift universally toward noncommunicable disease.
- Some global health issues can be solved only through the cooperation of various actors in global health. This could include, for example, the eradication of polio.

- An important part of health status is determined by an individual's and families' own knowledge of health and hygiene. People and communities have tremendous abilities to enhance their own health status.
- Nonetheless, political circumstances, the quality of governance, and the level of government commitment to equity all have an important bearing on the health of a people.
- The world continues to shrink at a very rapid pace. For health, security, and humanitarian reasons, each of us should be concerned about the health of everyone else.

- Taking account of these points, we could say, in many respects that low-income countries should focus on "burying old people, instead of young people, making the transition as fast as possible, and doing so at least cost."
- Taking account of these points, we could also say, in many respects, that the health goals for all countries are to enable their people, at least cost, to enjoy a healthy life, for as long as possible.

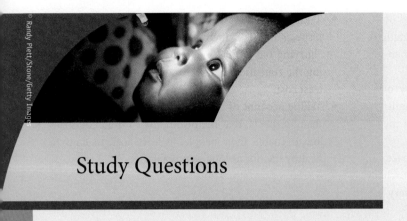

Study Questions

1. What has been among the most important progress in health worldwide over the last 50 years?

2. What are some of the global health challenges that remain to be addressed?

3. How might one define *health*, *public health*, and *global health*?

4. What are some examples of public health activities?

5. What are some examples of global health issues?

6. What are the key differences between the approach of medicine and the approach of public health?

7. What are some of the most important challenges to health globally?

8. Why should everyone be concerned about critical global health issues?

9. What are the Millennium Development Goals, and how do they relate to health?

10. What were some of the keys to the eradication of smallpox? What lessons does the smallpox eradication program suggest for other global health programs?

REFERENCES

1. World Health Organization. (2004, August 24). *New polio cases confirmed in Guinea, Mali and the Sudan.* Retrieved June 10, 2006, from http://www.who.int/mediacentre/news/releases/2004/pr57/en.

2. UNAIDS. (2014). *Ethiopia.* Retrieved August 4, 2014, from http://www.unaids.org/en/regionscountries/countries/ethiopia/.

3. UNAIDS. (2014). *Global report: UNAIDS report on the global AIDS epidemic 2013.* Geneva: UNAIDS.

4. Centers for Disease Control and Prevention. *Meningococcal disease.* Retrieved May 27, 2006, from http://www.cdc.gov/meningococcal/.

5. World Health Organization. (2011). *West Nile virus.* Retrieved August 7, 2014, from http://www.who.int/mediacentre/factsheets/fs354/en/.

6. Health Protection Agency of the United Kingdom. (2006). *Focus on tuberculosis.* Retrieved from http://webarchive.nationalarchives.gov.uk/20130502175630/http://www.hpa.org.uk/webc/HPAwebFile/HPAweb_C/1204100456946

7. International Diabetes Association. (2009). *Latest diabetes figures paint grim global picture.* Retrieved August 4, 2014, from http://www.idf.org/latest-diabetes-figures-paint-grim-global-picture.

8. World Health Organization. (2010). *World health statistics.* Geneva: WHO. Retrieved September 3, 2010 from http://www.who.int/whosis/whostat/EN_WHS10_Full.pdf.

9. World Bank. (2014). *Health.* Retrieved August 4, 2014, from http://data.worldbank.org/topic/health?display=default.

10. United Nations. (2012). *Towards global equity in longevity.* Population facts 2012/2. Retrieved August 7, 2014, from http://www.un.org/esa/population/publications/popfacts/popfacts__2012-2.pdf.

11. World Health Organization. (2014). *Maternal mortality.* Retrieved August 4, 2014, from http://www.who.int/mediacentre/factsheets/fs348/en/.

12. World Health Organization. (2014). *Children: Reducing mortality.* Retrieved February 9, 2015, from http://www.who.int/mediacentre/factsheets/fs178/en/.

13. World Health Organization. (2014). *Tuberculosis.* Retrieved February 9, 2015, from http://www.who.int/mediacentre/factsheets/fs104/en/.

14. UNAIDS. (2014). *Fact Sheet Global Statistics.* Retrieved February 10, 2015, from http://www.unaids.org/en/resources/campaigns/2014/2014gapreport/factsheet.

15. World Health Organization. (2014). *Malaria.* Retrieved February 10, 2015, from http://www.who.int/mediacentre/factsheets/fs094/en/.

16. World Health Organization. *International travel and health: Dengue distribution map.* Retrieved September 5, 2013, from http://gamapserver.who.int/mapLibrary/Files/Maps/Global_DengueTransmission_ITHRiskMap.png.

17. World Health Organization. (2014). *Impact of dengue.* Retrieved August 7, 2014, from http://www.who.int/csr/disease/dengue/impact/en/.

18. World Bank. (2014). *Life expectancy at birth, total (years).* Retrieved August 4, 2014, from http://data.worldbank.org/indicator/SP.DYN.LE00.IN.

19. World Health Organization. (1946). Preamble to the Constitution of the World Health Organization 1946, as adopted by the International Health Conference, New York, 19 June–22 July 1946.

20. Merson, M. H., Black, R. E., & Mills, A. (2001). *International public health: Diseases, programs, systems, and policies* (p. xvii). Gaithersburg, MD: Aspen Publishers.

21. American Public Health Association. *Principles of the ethical practice of public health.* Retrieved November 17, 2014, from http://www.apha.org/~/media/files/pdf/about/ethics_brochure.ashx.

22. Harvard School of Public Health. *Distinctions between medicine and public health.* Retrieved February 8, 2006, from http://www.hsph.harvard.edu/about/public-health-medicine/.

23. Last, J. M. (2001). *A dictionary of epidemiology* (4th ed.). New York: Oxford University Press.

24. Institute of Medicine. (1998). *America's vital interest in global health: Protecting our people, enhancing our economy, and advancing our international interests.* Washington, DC: National Academy Press.

25. Merson, M. H., Black, R. E., & Mills, A. (2001). *International public health: Diseases, programs, systems, and policies* (p. xix). Gaithersburg, MD: Aspen Publishers.

26. Koplan, J. P., Bond, T. C., Merson, M. H., et al. (2009). Towards a common definition of global health. *Lancet, 373*(9679), 1993–1995.

27. Fried, L. P., Bentley, M. E., Buekens, P., et al. (2010). Global health is public health. *Lancet, 375*(9714), 535–537.

28. World Bank. *Country and lending groups.* Retrieved August 5, 2014, from http://data.worldbank.org/about/country-and-lending-groups.

29. Institute of Health Metrics and Evaluation. (2013). *The global burden of disease: Generating evidence, guiding policy.* Seattle, WA: Author.

30. Lancet. (2012, December 15). *The Global Burden of Disease Study 2010.* Retrieved May 31, 2015, from http://www.thelancet.com/journals/lancet/issue/vol380no9859/PIIS0140-6736%2812%29X6053-7

31. Jamison, D. E. A. (Ed.). (2006). *Disease control priorities in developing countries* (2nd ed.). New York, Oxford University Press and the World Bank and Jamison, D. T., R. Nugent, H. Gelband, S. Horton, P. Jha, and R. Laxminarayan, eds. 2015–2016. Disease Control Priorities. Third edition. 9 volumes. World Bank: Washington, DC.

32. United Nations. *55/2. United Nations Millennium Declaration.* Retrieved May 16, 2006, from http://www.un.org/millennium/declaration/ares552e.htm.

33. United Nations. (2014). *Sustainable knowledge platform sustainable development goals.* Retrieved August 5, 2014, from http://sustainabledevelopment.un.org/focussdgs.html.

34. United Nations. (2014). *Beyond 2015 Open Working Group on SDGs.* Retrieved August 5, 2014, from http://www.beyond2015.org/open-working-group-sdgs.

35. Levine, R., & the What Works Working Group. (2007). *Case studies in global health: Millions saved.* Sudbury, MA: Jones and Bartlett.

36. Center for Global Development. *Case 1: Eradicating smallpox.* Retrieved January 31, 2015, from http://www.cgdev.org/page/case-1-eradicating-smallpox.

37. Roberts, M. (2005, July 3). *How doctors killed off smallpox.* Retrieved June 11, 2006, from http://news.bbc.co.uk/1/hi/health/4072392.stm.

38. Fenner, F. (1988). *Smallpox and its eradication.* Geneva: World Health Organization.

39. Brilliant, L. B. (1985). *The management of smallpox eradication in India.* Ann Arbor: University of Michigan Press.

CHAPTER **2**

Health Determinants, Measurements, and Trends

LEARNING OBJECTIVES

By the end of this chapter the reader will be able to:

- Describe the determinants of health
- Define the most important health indicators and key terms related to measuring health status and the burden of disease
- Discuss the concepts of health-adjusted life expectancy (HALE), disability-adjusted life years (DALYs), and the burden of disease
- Describe the leading causes of death and the burden of disease in low-, middle-, and high-income countries
- Describe the leading risk factors for key causes of death and the burden of disease in low-, middle-, and high-income countries
- Describe the demographic and epidemiologic transitions

VIGNETTES

Shawki is a 60-year-old Jordanian man who lives in Jordan's capital of Amman. Unfortunately, Shawki's health has deteriorated in the last year. His blood pressure and cholesterol are too high. He has developed diabetes. He is sometimes short of breath. What are the causes of his ill and declining health? Do these problems stem from any genetic issues? Could they come from a lack of understanding about a healthy lifestyle and diet? Could it be that Shawki lacks the income he needs to eat properly and to ensure that he gets health checkups when he needs them?

Life expectancy in Botswana prior to the spread of HIV/AIDS was about 65 years.[1] In 2013, life expectancy in Botswana was 47 years.[2] Life expectancy in Russia in 1985 was about 64 years for males and 74 years for females. It

then fell by 2001 to about 59 years for males and 72 years for females,[3] before rising again by 2013 to 64 for males and 76 for females.[2] What does life expectancy measure? What are the factors contributing to its decline in both of these countries? What has happened to trends in life expectancy in other countries? Which countries have the longest and shortest life expectancies, and why?

In Cambodia in 2012, families had, on average, 3 children, and their life expectancy was about 62 years.[4] Thirty years ago, the demographic and epidemiologic profile of Thailand looked a lot like Cambodia looks today. In 2012, however, Thai families had on average about 1.6 children and those children on average will live 74 years.[4] What causes these shifts in fertility and mortality? Do they occur consistently as countries develop economically? How long will it take before Cambodia has the same fertility and disease burden that Thailand has today?

In Peru, poor people tend to live in the mountains and be indigenous, less educated, and have worse health status than other people. In Eastern Europe, the same issues occur among their ethnic groups that are of lower socioeconomic status, such as the Roma people. In the United States, there are also enormous health disparities, as seen in the health status of African Americans and Native Americans, compared to white Americans. If one wants to understand and address differences in health status among different groups, then how do we measure health status? Do we measure it by age? By gender? By socioeconomic status? By level of education? By ethnicity? By location?

THE IMPORTANCE OF MEASURING HEALTH STATUS

If we want to understand the most important global health issues and what can be done to address them, then we must understand what factors have the most influence on health status, how health status is measured, and what key trends in health status have occurred historically. We must, in fact, be able to answer the questions that are posed in the narratives at the beginning of the chapter.

This chapter, therefore, covers four distinct, but closely related topics. The first section concerns what are called "the determinants of health." That section examines the most important factors that relate to people's health status. The second section reviews some of the most important indicators of health status and how they are used. The third section discusses the burden of disease worldwide and how it varies across countries. The last section looks at how fertility and mortality change as countries become more developed and what this means for the types of health problems countries face.

THE DETERMINANTS OF HEALTH

Why are some people healthy and some people not healthy? When asked this question, many of us will respond that good health depends on access to health services. Yet, as you will learn, whether or not people are healthy depends on a large number of factors, many of which are interconnected, and most of which go considerably beyond access to health services.

There has been considerable writing about the determinants of health, and one way of depicting these determinants is shown in **Figure 2-1**. This next section largely follows the approach to the determinants of health that is discussed in *What Determines Health* by the Public Health Agency of Canada.[5]

The first group of factors that helps to determine health relates to the personal and inborn features of individuals. These include genetic makeup, sex, and age. Our genetic makeup has much to do with what diseases we get and how healthy we live. One can inherit, for example, a genetic marker for a particular disease, such as Huntington's disease, which is a neurological disorder. One can also inherit the genetic component of a disease that has multiple causes, such as breast cancer. Sex also has an important relationship with health. Males and females are physically different, for example, and may get different diseases. Females face the risks involved in childbearing. They also get cervical and uterine cancers that males do not contract. Females also have higher rates of certain health conditions, such as thyroid and breast

cancers. For similar reasons, age is also an important determinant of health. Young children in low- and middle-income countries often die of diarrheal disease, whereas older people are much more likely to die of heart disease, to cite one of many examples of the relationship between health and age.

Socioeconomic status, which refers to a person's economic, social, and work status, is an important health determinant. People with higher educational attainment have higher socioeconomic status and more control over their lives than people of lower status. As one's socioeconomic status improves, so does his/her health.[6]

The extent to which people get social support from family, friends, and community also has an important link with health.[7] The stronger the social networks and the stronger the support that people get from those networks, the healthier people will be. Of course, culture is also an extremely important determinant of health.[5] Culture helps to determine how one feels about health and illness, how one uses health services, and the health practices in which one engages. In addition, the gender roles that are ascribed to women in many societies also have an important impact on health. In such environments, women may be less well treated than men and this, in turn, may mean that women have less income, less education, and fewer opportunities to engage in employment. All of these militate against their good health.

The environment, both indoor and outdoor, is a powerful determinant of health. Related to this is the safety of the environment in which people work. Although many people know about the importance of outdoor air pollution to health, few people are aware of the importance of indoor air pollution to health. In many low- and middle-income countries, women cook indoors with poor ventilation, thereby creating an indoor environment that is full of smoke and that encourages respiratory illness and asthma. The lack of safe drinking water and sanitation is a major contributor to ill health in poor countries. In addition, many people in those same countries work in environments that are unhealthy. Because they lack skills, socioeconomic status, and opportunities, they may work without sufficient protection from hazardous chemicals, in polluted air, or in circumstances that expose them to occupational accidents.

Education is a powerful determinant of health for several reasons. First, it brings with it knowledge of good health practices. Second, it provides opportunities for gaining skills, getting better employment, raising one's income, and enhancing one's social status, all of which are also related to health. Studies have shown, for example, that the single best predictor of the birthweight of a baby is the level of educational attainment of the mother.[8] Most of us already know

FIGURE 2-1 Key Determinants of Health

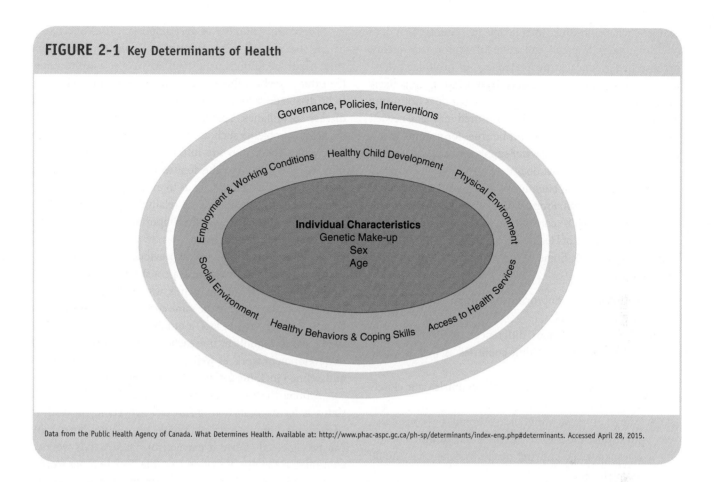

Data from the Public Health Agency of Canada. What Determines Health. Available at: http://www.phac-aspc.gc.ca/ph-sp/determinants/index-eng.php#determinants. Accessed April 28, 2015.

that throughout the world, there is an extremely strong and positive correlation between the level of education and all key health indicators. People who are better educated eat better, smoke less, are less obese, have fewer children, and take better care of their children's health than do people with less education. It is not a surprise, therefore, that they and their children live longer and healthier lives than do less well educated people and their children.

Of course, people's own health practices and behaviors are also critical determinants of their health. Being able to identify when you or a family member is ill and needs health care can be critical to good health. As noted previously, however, one's health also depends on how one eats, or if one smokes, drinks too much alcohol, or drives safely. We also know that being active physically and getting exercise regularly is better for one's health than is being sedentary.

Another important determinant of future health is the way in which families nourish and care for infants and young children. Being born premature or of low birthweight can have important negative consequences on health. There is a strong correlation between the nutritional status of infants

and young children and the extent to which they meet their biological potential, enroll in school, or stay in school. In addition, poor nutritional status in infancy and early childhood may be linked with a number of noncommunicable diseases later in life, including diabetes and heart disease.[9]

Of course, one's health does depend on access to appropriate healthcare services. Even if one is born healthy, raised healthy, and engages in good health behaviors, there will still be times when one has to call on a health system for help. The more likely you are to access services of appropriate quality, the more likely you are to stay healthy. To address the risk of dying from a complication of pregnancy, for example, one must have access to health services that can carry out an emergency cesarean section if necessary. Even if the mother has had the suggested level of prenatal care and has prepared well in all other respects for the pregnancy, in the end, certain complications can only be addressed in a healthcare setting.

The approach that governments take to different policies and programs in the health sector and in other sectors also has an important bearing on people's health. People living in a country that promotes high educational attainment, for example, will be healthier than people in a country that does not promote widespread education of appropriate quality, because better-educated people engage in healthier behaviors. A country that has universal health insurance is likely to have healthier people than a country that does not insure its entire population because the uninsured may lack needed health services. The same would be true, for example, for a country that promoted safe water supply for its entire population, compared to one that does not.

In fact, increasing attention is being paid to the social determinants of health. From 2005 to 2008 the World Health Organization (WHO) constituted a Commission on the Social Determinants of Health. WHO published the commission's report in 2008. Some of the important themes related to the report are:[10]

- Health status is improving in some places in the world but not in others.
- There are enormous differences in the health status of individuals within countries as well as across countries.
- The health differences within countries are closely linked with social disadvantage.
- Many of these differences should be considered avoidable, and they relate to the way in which people live and work and the health systems that should serve them.
- In the end, people's life circumstances, and therefore their health, are profoundly related to political, social, and economic forces.
- Countries need to ensure that these forces are oriented toward improving the life circumstances of the poor, thereby enabling them to enjoy a healthier life, as well. The global community should also work toward this end.

KEY HEALTH INDICATORS

It is critical that we use data and evidence to understand and address key global health issues. Some types of health data concern the health status of people and communities, such as measures of life expectancy and infant and child mortality, as discussed further hereafter. Some concern health services, such as the number of nurses and doctors per capita in a country or the indicators of coverage for certain health services, such as immunization. Other data concern the financing of health, such as the amount of public expenditure on health or the share of national income represented by health expenditure.

There are a number of very important uses of data on health status.[11] We need data, for example, to know from what health conditions people suffer. We also need to know the extent to which these conditions cause people to be sick, to be disabled, or to die. We need to gather data to carry out disease surveillance. This helps us to understand if particular health problems such as influenza, polio, or malaria are occurring, where they are infecting people, who is getting infected, and what might be done to address these conditions. Other forms of data also help us to understand the burden of different health conditions, the relative importance of them to different societies, and the importance that should be attached to dealing with them.

If we are to use data in the previously mentioned ways, then it is important that we use a consistent set of indicators to measure health status. In this way, we can make comparisons across people in the same country or across different countries. There are, in fact, a number of indicators that are used most commonly by those who work in global health and in development work, as well, as noted later. These are listed and defined in **Table 2-1** and are discussed briefly next.

Among the most commonly used indicators of health status is *life expectancy at birth*. Life expectancy at birth is "the average number of additional years a newborn baby can be expected to live if current mortality trends were to continue for the rest of that person's life."[12,p58] In other words, it measures how long a person born today can expect to live, if there were no change in their lifetime in the present rate of death for people of different ages. The higher the life expectancy at birth, the better the health status of a country. In the United States, life expectancy at birth in 2013 was about 79 years; in a middle-income country, such as Jordan, life expectancy was 74 years; in a very poor country, such as Sierra Leone, life expectancy was 46 years.[13] **Figure 2-2** shows life expectancy at birth by World Bank region and for high-income countries.[13]

Another important and widely used indicator is the *infant mortality rate*. The infant mortality rate is "the number of deaths of infants under age 1 per 1,000 live births in a given year."[12,p28] This rate is expressed in deaths per 1,000 live births. In other words, it measures how many children younger than 1 year of age will die for every 1,000 who were born alive that year. Each country seeks as low a rate of infant mortality as possible, but we will see that the rate varies largely with the income status of a country. Afghanistan, for example, had an infant mortality rate in 2013 of 70 infant deaths for every 1,000 live births, whereas in Sweden only about 2 infants die for every 1,000 live births.[14] (See **Figure 2-3**.)

TABLE 2-1 Key Health Status Indicators

Infant mortality rate—The number of deaths of infants under age 1 per 1,000 live births in a given year

Life expectancy at birth—The average number of years a newborn baby could expect to live if current mortality trends were to continue for the rest of the newborn's life

Maternal mortality ratio—The number of women who die as a result of pregnancy and childbirth complications per 100,000 live births in a given year

Neonatal mortality rate—The number of deaths to infants under 28 days of age in a given year per 1,000 live births in that year

Under-5 mortality rate (child mortality rate)—The probability that a newborn baby will die before reaching age 5, expressed as a number per 1,000 live births

Data from Haupt, A., & Kane, T. T. (2004). *Population handbook.* Washington, DC: Population Reference Bureau; World Bank. *Beyond economic growth: Glossary.* Retrieved April 15, 2007, from http://www.worldbank.org/depweb/english/beyond/global/glossary.html.

FIGURE 2-2 Life Expectancy at Birth, by World Bank Region and for High-Income Countries, 2013

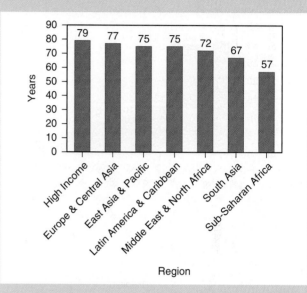

Data from the World Bank. Life expectancy at birth, total (years). Retrieved March 7, 2015, from http://data.worldbank.org/indicator/SP.DYN.LE00.IN/countries/1W-ZG-ZJ-ZQ?display=graph

FIGURE 2-3 Infant Mortality Rates, by World Bank Region and for High-Income Countries, 2013

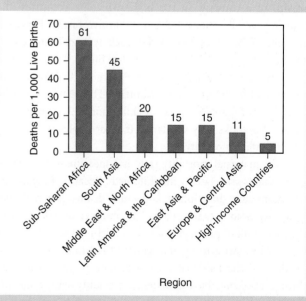

Data from the World Bank. World Development Indicators: Mortality. http://data.worldbank.org/indicator/SH.DYN.MORT/countries/1W-Z4-ZQ-Z7?display=graph. Accessed February 22, 2015.

Although the infant mortality rate is a powerful indicator of health status of a country, most children younger than 1 year of age who die actually die in the first month of life. Thus, the *neonatal mortality rate* is also an important health status indicator. This rate measures "the number of deaths to infants younger than 28 days of age in a given year, per 1,000 live births in that year."[12,p60] Like the infant mortality rate, this rate will generally vary directly with the level of income of different countries. Poorer countries will usually have a much higher neonatal mortality rate than the richer countries. Sierra Leone, among the poorest countries in the world, has a neonatal mortality rate of 44 per 1,000 live births. In Norway, one of the highest income countries in the world, the rate is 2.[14] The neonatal mortality rate by World Bank region and for high-income countries is portrayed in **Figure 2-4**.

The under-5 child mortality rate is also called the *child mortality rate*. This is "the probability that a newborn will die before reaching age five, expressed as a number per 1,000 live births."[15] Like the infant mortality rate, this rate is expressed

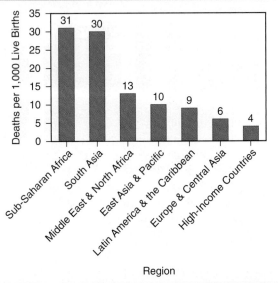

FIGURE 2-4 Neonatal Mortality Rates, by World Bank Region and for High-Income Countries, 2013

Data from the World Bank. World Development Indicators: Mortality. http://data.worldbank.org/indicator/SH.DYN.MORT/countries/1W-Z4-ZQ-Z7?display=graph. Accessed February 22, 2015.

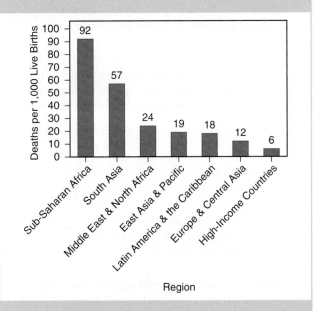

FIGURE 2-5 Under-5 Mortality Rates, by World Bank Region and for High-Income Countries, 2013

Data from World Bank. 2013. World Development Indicators: Mortality. Available at: http://wdi.worldbank.org/table/2.21. Accessed March 20, 2014.

per 1,000 live births. This rate also varies largely with the wealth of a country. In the highest-income countries, the rate is generally about 3–5 per 1,000 live births. However, in some of the poorest countries, such as Angola and Chad, the rate can be over 150 per 1,000 live births.[15] The under-5 child mortality rate is depicted in **Figure 2-5** by World Bank region and for high-income countries. The relative standing of different regions in under-5 child mortality, as shown in Figure 2-5, looks very similar to that for neonatal mortality and for infant mortality.

The maternal mortality ratio is a measure of the risk of death that is associated with childbirth. Because these deaths are more rare than infant and child deaths, the maternal mortality ratio is measured as "the number of women who die as a result of pregnancy and childbirth complications per 100,000 live births in a given year."[12,p28] The rarity of maternal deaths and the fact that they largely occur in low-income settings also contribute to maternal mortality being quite difficult to measure. Very few women die in childbirth in rich countries; for example, the maternal mortality ratio in Sweden is 4 per 100,000 live births. On the other hand, in very poor countries, in which women have low status and there

are few facilities for dealing with obstetric emergencies, the ratios can be over 500 per 100,000 live births, as they are, for example, in Mali, Niger, and Nigeria. In the worst-off country for maternal health, Sierra Leone, the maternal mortality ratio is estimated to be 1,100 per 100,000 live births.[16] As you can see in **Figure 2-6**, the maternal mortality ratio is also very strongly associated with a country's income.

A few other concepts and definitions are important to understand as we think about measuring health status. The first is *morbidity*. Essentially, this means sickness or any departure, subjective or objective, from a psychological or physiological state of well-being. Second is *mortality*, which refers to death. A *death rate* is the number of deaths per 1,000 population in a given year.[12,p25] The third is *disability*. Although some conditions cause people to get sick or die, they might also cause people to suffer the "temporary or long-term reduction in a person's capacity to function."[17,p51]

There will also be considerable discussion in most readings on global health of the *prevalence* of health conditions. This refers to the number of people suffering from a certain health condition over a specific time period. It measures the chances of having a disease. For global health work, one usually

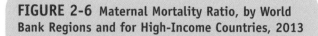

FIGURE 2-6 Maternal Mortality Ratio, by World Bank Regions and for High-Income Countries, 2013

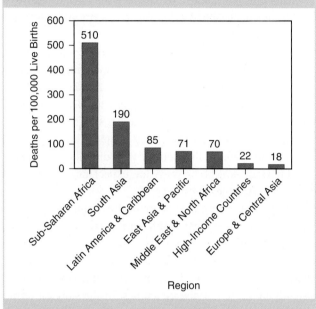

Data from World Bank. Data: Maternal mortality ratio. Data from the World Bank. http://data.worldbank.org/indicator/SH.STA.MMRT/countries/1W-8S-Z4-ZJ-XD-Z7-ZG?display=graph. Accessed March 10, 2015.

refers to "point prevalence" of a condition, which is "the proportion of the population that is diseased at a single point in time."[12,p31] The point prevalence of HIV/AIDS among adults in South Africa, for example, is estimated to be 19.1. This means that today 19.1 percent of all adults between the ages of 15 and 49 in South Africa are estimated to be HIV-positive.[18]

The *incidence rate* is also a very commonly used term. This measures how many people get a disease, for a specified number of people at risk, for given period of time.[12] The denominator for the rate usually depends on how commonly the disease occurs in a year and is often per 1,000 or 100,000 people. In India, for example, the incidence rate for tuberculosis (TB) in 2013 was 171, per 100,000.[19] This means that for every 100,000 people in India, 171 got sick from TB in 2013.

Many people confuse incidence rate and prevalence rate. It may be convenient to think of prevalence as the pool of people with a disease at a particular time and incidence as the flow of new cases of people with that disease each year into that pool. You should note, of course, that the size of the pool will vary as new cases flow into the pool and old cases flow out, as they die or are cured.

Finally, one needs to be familiar with how diseases get classified. When you read about health, there will be discussions of communicable diseases, noncommunicable diseases, and injuries. Communicable diseases are also called infectious diseases. These are illnesses that are caused by a particular infectious agent and that spread directly or indirectly from people to people, animals to people, or people to animals.[17] Examples of communicable diseases include influenza, measles, and HIV. Noncommunicable diseases are illnesses that are not spread by any infectious agent, such as hypertension, coronary heart disease, and diabetes. Injuries include, among other things, road traffic injuries, falls, drownings, poisonings, and violence.[20]

VITAL REGISTRATION

The quality of data on population and health depends in many ways on the extent to which countries maintain a system of vital registration that can accurately record births, deaths, and the causes of death. Unfortunately, this is not the case in many low- and lower-middle-income countries.[21] They generally have only rudimentary systems for vital registration, which cannot fulfill either their statistical or their legal purposes. In addition, access to vital registration systems is highly inequitable, with higher income groups enjoying much better access than less well-off people (**Figure 2-7**).

There are also cultural barriers to timely vital registration because people in many countries wait until a child is a certain age before registering the birth. Coupled with the lack of access to vital registration, this means the existence of some children is never officially known, because they die before their births are registered. There are also enormous difficulties with accurate indications of causes of death in countries that have weak health systems and a limited number of well-trained physicians. This is especially so for causes of death of adults.

The former director-general of WHO, Lee Jong-Wook, noted in a speech to his colleagues: "To make people count, we first need to be able to count people."[22,p1569] To overcome the lack of effective vital registration systems in many low- and middle-income countries, a number of tools, such as surveys and projection models, have been developed. Some, like the Demographic and Health Surveys, have become an important source of information about health, population, nutrition, and HIV in low-income countries.

In the longer term, however, the world would be better served by helping countries further develop their own vital registration systems. This would allow countries and their development partners to more accurately gauge the nature of key demographic and health issues and the progress made toward resolving them. Moving in this direction will require assessments of vital registration systems. It will also require

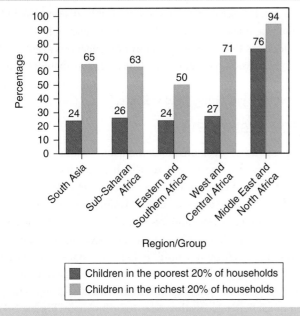

FIGURE 2-7 Percentage of Children Under 5 Whose Births Have Been Registered, by Income Quintile, for Selected UNICEF Regions, 2005–2012

■ Children in the poorest 20% of households
■ Children in the richest 20% of households

Data from UNICEF. 2013. Every Child's Birth Right: Inequities and trends in birth registration. Retrieved April 27, 2015, from http://www.unicef.org/media/files/Embargoed_11_Dec _Birth_Registration_report_low_res.pdf.

programs to improve the organization and functioning of vital registration departments. This will have to include, among other things, strengthening their methods to improve the quality of vital statistics, including for the causes of death, and enhancing their approach to publishing data.[21]

MEASURING THE BURDEN OF DISEASE

The WHO definition of health is "a state of complete physical, mental and social well-being and not merely the absence of disease or infirmity."[23] Those who work on global health have attempted for a number of years to construct a single indicator that could be used to compare how far different countries are from the state of good health. Ideally, such an index would take account of morbidity, mortality, and disability; allow one to calculate the index by age, by gender, and by region; and allow one to make comparisons of health status across regions within a country and across countries.[24] This kind of index would measure what is generally referred to as "the burden of disease."

One such indicator is *health-adjusted life expectancy*, or HALE. It is a health expectancy measure. HALE is the number of years a person of a given age can expect to live in good health, taking account of mortality and disability.[25,p9] This can also be seen as "the equivalent number of years in full health that a newborn can expect to live, based on current rates of ill health and mortality."[26] To calculate the HALE, "the years of ill health are weighted according to severity and subtracted from the overall life expectancy."[27]

WHO has calculated HALEs for most countries, using a standard methodology. **Table 2-2** shows life expectancy at birth in 2010 for a number of low-, middle-, and high-income countries and how it compares with HALEs for those countries in the same year. As you can see from Table 2-2, the greater the number of years that people in any population are likely to spend in ill health or with disability, the greater the difference will be between life expectancy at birth and health-adjusted life expectancy.

The composite indicator of health status that is most commonly used in global health work is called the *disability-adjusted life year*, or DALY. This indicator was first used in conjunction with the *1993 World Development Report* of the World Bank and is a health gap measure. It is now used consistently in burden of disease studies. In the simplest terms, a DALY is:

> The sum of years lost due to premature death (YLLs) and years lived with disability (YLDs). DALYs are also defined as years of healthy life lost.[26,p9]

The DALY is a summary measure of losses due to premature death and years lived with disability in a given population. The calculation of years lost to premature death takes account of the highest life expectancy globally at every age. If a 20-year-old male died in a car accident in Malawi in 2010, for example, he would have 66 years of life lost. This is calculated based on the highest life expectancy for anyone 20 years old, which is 86 years for 20-year-old females in Japan.[26]

The value of years lived with disability is calculated by weighting these years by a disability index. For the *Global Burden of Disease Study 2010*, 14,000 people were surveyed directly and 16,000 people were involved via the Internet in establishing disability weights. If someone lived 30 years with a disability that was given a weight of 0.5, for example (but died at the highest life expectancy possible), then they would have 30 times 0.5, or 15 years of life lived with disability.[27]

If the two people described previously lived in the same society, then the total DALYs for that society would be the total of the years of life lost due to premature death of the first person and the years lived with disability of the second. In this case, the total DALYs lost due to premature death and years lived with disability would be 66 plus 15, or 81.

TABLE 2-2 Life Expectancy at Birth and Health-Adjusted Life Expectancy, Selected Countries, 2010

Country	Life Expectancy/ Health-Adjusted Life Expectancy Males	Life Expectancy/ Health-Adjusted Life Expectancy Females
Afghanistan	58.2/48.5	57.3/46.2
Bangladesh	67.2/57.1	71.0/59.8
Bolivia	69.7/60.1	71.7/61.5
Brazil	70.5/61.1	77.7/66.6
Cambodia	64.6/55.9	70.1/60.0
Cameroon	57.1/49.0	61.1/51.4
China	72.9/65.5	79.0/70.4
Costa Rica	77.1/67.3	81.9/70.5
Cuba	76.1/63.5	79.8/66.9
Denmark	76.8/66.3	81.0/69.5
Ethiopia	59.5/51.4	62.3/53.5
Ghana	63.2/54.5	66.7/56.1
India	63.2/54.9	67.5/57.7
Indonesia	67.7/59.3	71.8/62.5
Jordan	75.7/64.8	75.1/63.2
Malaysia	71.3/62.6	76.5/66.4
Nepal	67.7/57.6	70.6/59.9
Niger	56.9/48.5	58.7/49.4
Nigeria	58.8/50.0	60.4/50.8
Peru	75.2/64.8	77.6/66.6
Philippines	66.6/57.4	73.8/63.2
Sri Lanka	71.6/62.3	79.8/68.6
Turkey	71.2/61.8	77.7/66.0
United States of America	75.9/66.2	80.5/69.5
Vietnam	71.6/62.6	79.6/69.1

Data from Salomon, J. A., Wang, H., Freeman, M. K., et al. (2013). Healthy life expectancy for 187 countries, 1990-2010: A systematic analysis for the Global Burden Disease Study 2010. *Lancet*, *380*(9859), 2144–2162.

In reality, of course, many health conditions produce both disability and premature death. Let us suppose that a man with diabetes has to have a leg amputated at age 45, that the disability index is 0.5 for this condition, and that the man dies at age 47. In this case, he loses 0.5 times 2 years lived with disability, which would be equal to 1 year of life lived with disability. If the longest known life expectancy for a 47 year old were, say, 87, then he would also have 40 years lost due to premature death. This person would have contributed 1 year of life lived with disability, plus 30 years of life lost due to premature death, or 31 total DALYs.

A society that has more premature death, illness, and disability has more DALYs than a society that is healthier and has less illness, disability, and premature death. One of the goals of health policy is to avert these DALYs in the most cost-efficient manner possible. If, for example, a society has many hundreds of thousands of DALYs due to malaria that is not diagnosed and treated in a timely and proper manner, what steps can be taken to avert those DALYs at the lowest cost?

An important point to remember when considering DALYs, compared to measuring deaths, is that DALYs take account of periods in which people are living with disability. By doing this, DALYs and other composite indicators try to give a better estimate than measuring deaths alone of the true health of a population. This is easy to understand. Most mental health problems, for example, are not associated with deaths. However, they cause an enormous amount of disability. Several parasitic infections, such as schistosomiasis, also cause very few deaths, but enormous amounts of illness and disability. If we measured the health of a population with an important burden of schistosomiasis and mental illness only by measuring deaths, we would miss a major component of morbidity and disability and would seriously overestimate the health of that population. The next section on the global burden of disease elaborates on the concept of DALYs and how DALYs compare to deaths for a number of health conditions.

A number of critiques of DALYs have been written.[28] Nonetheless, this text repeatedly refers to DALYs because this measure is so extensively used in global health work. In addition, a considerable amount of important analysis has been carried out that is based on the use of DALYs for measuring overall health status and assessing the most cost-effective approaches to dealing with various health problems.

BURDEN OF DISEASE DATA

As you start a review of global health, it is important to get a clear picture of the leading causes of illness, disability, and death in the world. It is also very important to understand how they vary by age, sex, ethnicity, and socioeconomic status, both within and across countries. Additionally, it is essential to understand how these causes have varied over time and how they might change in the future. These topics are examined next.

A collaboration of seven institutions has taken the lead over the last several years in collecting, analyzing, and disseminating data on the burden of disease globally. The partners in this effort have been Harvard University; Imperial College, London; the Institute for Health Metrics and Evaluation (IHME), the University of Washington; the Johns Hopkins University; the University of Queensland; the University of Tokyo; and the World Health Organization. In late 2012, the *Lancet* published in seven papers the key findings from the *Global Burden of Disease Study 2010* (GBD 2010).[29] In 2013, the IHME published a companion report to the *Lancet* papers: *The Global Burden of Disease: Generating Evidence, Guiding Policy*.[26]

Much of the data in this chapter is based on the findings of the *Global Burden of Disease Study 2010* and the related IHME study.[26,29] It also heavily uses data from interactive data visualizations that IHME has posted on its website. Some of the data used here refer to deaths and some to DALYs. References to the "burden of disease" refer to DALYs. Those readers who wish to explore the burden of disease further are encouraged to review the range of IHME visualizations on this topic. This text will refer to the *Lancet* series and the related IHME paper as the *Global Burden of Disease Study 2010*.

It is important to note that the *Global Burden of Disease Study 2010* categorized its data in a number of ways. This included by country income group, for which it showed at the highest-level data for developing countries, developed countries, and high-income countries. The data from this study that it labeled developing countries is consistently referred to here as data for low- and middle-income countries. The data that it referred to as for high-income countries is referred to by the same name here. This approach has been taken to make the nomenclature of data categories as consistent as possible across this chapter and the book as a whole.

Earlier burden of disease studies broke causes of death and DALYs into three categories:

Group I—communicable, maternal, and perinatal conditions (meaning in the first week after birth) and nutritional disorders

Group II—noncommunicable diseases

Group III—injuries, including, among other things, road traffic accidents, falls, self-inflicted injuries, and violence

The *Global Burden of Disease Study 2010* did not use the groupings as extensively as they had been used earlier.

Nonetheless, such groupings can be valuable to those who are new to the study of the burden of disease. Thus, they are used occasionally here.

Overview of Patterns and Trends in the Burden of Disease

Understanding the patterns and trends in the burden of disease is central to understanding and dealing with key issues in global health. As one examines some of the key data on the burden of disease, therefore, it is critical to understand a number of points:

- People in much of the world are living longer than before
- People in much of the world are dying at lower rates than earlier
- As people live longer, there is an increase in the years people live with disability
- The burden of disease is predominantly noncommunicable in all World Bank regions, except sub-Saharan Africa
- Over the last few decades, the burden of disease has shifted increasingly toward noncommunicable diseases in all World Bank regions
- This shift has been fueled, among other things, by a reduction in communicable diseases and the aging of populations.

The Leading Causes of Deaths and DALYs

Table 2-3 shows the 10 leading causes of death and the 10 leading causes of DALYs for low- and middle-income countries and for high-income countries in 2010. Both deaths and DALYs are ranked in order of importance.

About 58 percent of the deaths in low- and middle-income countries for both sexes and all age groups are from noncommunicable causes, 31 percent from communicable causes, and 11 percent from injuries.[30] Stroke and ischemic heart disease are the leading causes of death in low- and middle-income countries. They are followed by chronic obstructive pulmonary disease (COPD), lower respiratory infections, and diarrheal diseases. HIV/AIDS, malaria, road traffic injury, tuberculosis and diabetes make up the remainder of the 10 leading causes.[31] The importance of noncommunicable diseases is clear, even in low- and middle-income countries. At the same, however, there remains an important unfinished agenda of communicable diseases in these countries. For example, lower respiratory infections, as well as diarrhea, malaria, and HIV/AIDS are still important killers of young children in these countries. Noncommunicable

diseases are also the leading causes of deaths in high-income countries for both sexes and all age groups. However, in other respects, the picture of deaths that emerges in high-income countries is quite different from that in low- and middle-income countries. In high-income countries almost 87 percent of the deaths are from noncommunicable causes, about 7 percent are from communicable diseases, and about 6 percent are due to injuries.[30]

In high-income countries, the first three leading causes of death are stroke, ischemic heart disease, and lung cancer. The fourth, and the only communicable cause among the leading causes of death, is lower respiratory infections, which are associated in high-income countries mostly with death from pneumonia of older people. This is followed by COPD, Alzheimer's disease, colorectal cancer, diabetes, other cardiovascular and circulatory diseases, and chronic kidney disease.[31]

If we look at DALYs, rather than deaths, for both sexes and all age groups for low- and middle-income countries, noncommunicable diseases make up 49 percent of total DALYs, communicable diseases 40 percent, and injuries 11 percent. In this case, communicable diseases are substantially more important and noncommunicable diseases less important in percentage terms than they are for deaths.[30]

The leading individual causes of DALYs for both sexes and all age groups in low- and middle-income countries are lower respiratory infections, diarrheal diseases, and ischemic heart disease. This is followed by malaria, stroke, HIV/AIDS, preterm birth complications, road injury, COPD, and low back pain.[31] This ranking is significant for several reasons. First, it contains four communicable diseases. Second, it reflects the high burden of conditions related to birth in low-resource settings. Third, despite the number of communicable diseases in this ranking, noncommunicable diseases are also significant. Fourth, it is substantially different from the 10 leading causes of DALYs in high-income settings.

For both sexes and all age groups in high-income countries, noncommunicable diseases make up 85 percent of the DALYs, communicable diseases 5 percent, and injuries 10 percent. This is significantly different from the share of deaths by these cause groups only for injuries, whose share of DALYs is greater than the share of deaths.[30] The ranking of the causes of DALYs is especially significant because of the extent to which it reflects the aging of those populations. Musculoskeletal issues and falls, for example, make up 4 of the top 10 causes of DALYs in these settings.[30] The fact that major depressive disorder is the fourth leading cause of DALYs is also especially important and highlights the importance of mental health issues to overall ill health and disability.[31]

TABLE 2-3 Leading Causes of Deaths and DALYs for Low- and Middle-Income and High-Income Countries, 2010

Leading Causes of Deaths			
Low- and Middle-Income Countries		*High-Income Countries*	
Rank	Cause	Rank	Cause
1	Stroke	1	Ischemic heart disease
2	Ischemic heart disease	2	Stroke
3	Chronic obstructive pulmonary disease (COPD)	3	Trachea, bronchus, and lung cancers
4	Lower respiratory infections	4	Lower respiratory infections
5	Diarrheal diseases	5	COPD
6	HIV/AIDS	6	Alzheimer's disease
7	Malaria	7	Colorectal cancer
8	Road injury	8	Diabetes
9	Tuberculosis	9	Other cardiovascular and circulatory diseases
10	Diabetes	10	Chronic kidney disease
Leading Causes of DALYs			
Low- and Middle-Income Countries		*High-Income Countries*	
Rank	Cause	Rank	Cause
1	Lower respiratory infections	1	Ischemic heart disease
2	Diarrheal diseases	2	Low back pain
3	Ischemic heart disease	3	Stroke
4	Malaria	4	Major depressive disorder
5	Stroke	5	Trachea, bronchus, and lung cancers
6	HIV/AIDS	6	COPD
7	Preterm birth complications	7	Other musculoskeletal disorders
8	Road injury	8	Diabetes
9	COPD	9	Neck pain
10	Low back pain	10	Falls

Data from Institute for Health Metrics and Evaluation (IHME). (2013). *GBD heat map*. Seattle, WA: IHME, University of Washington. Retrieved April 28, 2015, from http://vizhub.healthdata.org/irank/heat.php.

Trends in the Cause of Deaths and DALYs, 1990–2010

Table 2-4 indicates changes that have occurred between 1990 and 2010 in the leading causes of deaths and DALYs globally. The table indicates the important extent to which the burden of deaths globally, when considering all age groups and both sexes, has shifted increasingly toward noncommunicable diseases. Road injuries have also become more important. The trend has been similar when looking at this from the point of view of DALYs, with some significant shifts from communicable diseases and other Group I causes to noncommunicable diseases and injuries.

Causes of Death and DALYs by Region

As you would expect, the causes of death and burden of disease vary by region, as shown in **Table 2-5**. In general, the higher the level of income of the countries in a region, the more likely it is that the leading causes of death and DALYs will be noncommunicable. The lower the level of income, the more likely it is that communicable diseases will be important. What is most essential to note is the extent to which the burden of disease in the sub-Saharan Africa region remains dominated by communicable diseases and the continuing importance of communicable diseases in the South Asia region. Of course, these are in the face of a growing burden, even in these regions, of noncommunicable diseases.[31]

Causes of Death by Age

Table 2-6 shows the leading causes of death for children aged 0 to 5 years for low- and middle-income countries and for high-income countries. The leading causes of death of under-5 children in low- and middle-income countries are generally related to conditions of newborns, infections to which newborns are particularly susceptible, or communicable diseases. The leading causes of death of under-5 children in high-income countries are dominated by conditions related to newborns. However, they also include road injury, drowning, and interpersonal violence.[31]

Table 2-7 shows the leading causes of death for children aged 5 to 14. It is striking how the leading causes of death of children 5 to 14 in low- and middle-income countries are preventable or treatable communicable diseases, such as malaria, HIV/AIDS, and diarrheal diseases. Nutritional issues are also prominent. By contrast, in high-income countries, children who die in this age group overwhelmingly die of injuries, cancer, or leukemia.[31]

Table 2-8 examines the leading causes of death and DALYs for both sexes for the age group 15 to 49. In low- and middle-income countries, the leading causes of death are HIV/AIDS, road injury, and tuberculosis. Lower respiratory infections, malaria and maternal causes are also in the top 10 leading causes of death. The importance of stroke, ischemic heart disease, and self-harm must also be noted. When one considers DALYs for both sexes for this age group, HIV/AIDS, TB, and maternal disorders remain important. However, road injury, low back pain, depressive disorders, and interpersonal violence are also important causes of DALYs.[31]

The picture of deaths and DALYS for both sexes in this age group in high-income countries varies substantially from that in low- and middle-income countries. Only one of the top 10 causes of deaths is communicable: HIV/AIDS. The others are all noncommunicable or injuries. In fact, self-harm is the leading cause of death in this age group in high-income countries. When we look at DALYs for both sexes in this age group, the importance of musculoskeletal disorders, neuropsychiatric disorders, and substance abuse disorders is clear and contrasts sharply with the pattern in low- and middle-income countries.[31]

Causes of Death and DALYs by Sex

It is also important to examine deaths and DALYs by sex, as shown in **Table 2-9**, for low- and middle-income countries and for high-income countries for all age groups. It is striking to note that five of the ten leading causes of deaths of females in low- and middle-income countries are communicable and that another leading cause is maternal complications. By contrast, the leading causes of deaths of females in high-income countries are all noncommunicable, except lower respiratory infections, which is overwhelmingly among older people in these countries. The leading causes of DALYs among females in low- and middle-income countries is similar to that for deaths, but also includes preterm birth complications, related to the deaths of so many young people in these countries, major depressive disorders, and low back pain. The leadings causes of DALYs among females in high-income countries is again similar to the causes of death, but also includes low back pain and neck pain and major depressive disorder and anxiety disorders.[31]

The leading causes of death among males in low- and middle-income countries is similar to that for females, but road injury is a leading killer of males but not females. The leading causes of death among males in high-income countries is similar to those for females in those countries, but includes self-harm. The leading cause of DALYs for males in low- and middle-income countries is similar to that for deaths but includes preterm birth complications, again related to young deaths, and low back pain. The leading

TABLE 2-4 Changes in the Leading Causes of Deaths and DALYs Globally, 1990 and 2010

Leading Causes of Deaths in 1990		Leading Causes of Deaths in 2010	
Rank	Cause	Rank	Cause
1	Ischemic heart disease	1	Ischemic heart disease
2	Stroke	2	Stroke
3	Lower respiratory infections	3	COPD
4	COPD	4	Lower respiratory infections
5	Diarrheal diseases	5	Lung cancer
6	Tuberculosis	6	HIV/AIDS
7	Preterm birth complications	7	Diarrheal diseases
8	Lung cancer	8	Road injury
9	Malaria	9	Diabetes
10	Road injury	10	Tuberculosis
Leading Causes of DALYs in 1990		Leading Causes of DALYs in 2010	
Rank	Cause	Rank	Cause
1	Lower respiratory infections	1	Ischemic heart disease
2	Diarrheal diseases	2	Lower respiratory infections
3	Preterm birth complications	3	Stroke
4	Ischemic heart disease	4	Diarrheal diseases
5	Stroke	5	HIV/AIDS
6	COPD	6	Malaria
7	Malaria	7	Low back pain
8	Tuberculosis	8	Preterm birth complications
9	Protein-energy malnutrition	9	COPD
10	Neonatal encephalopathy	10	Road injury

Data from Institute for Health Metrics and Evaluation (IHME). (2013). *GBD heat map*. Seattle, WA: IHME, University of Washington. Retrieved April 28, 2015, from http://vizhub.healthdata.org/irank/heat.php.

TABLE 2-5 Leading Causes of DALYs by World Bank Regions and for High-Income Countries, 2010

East Asia and Pacific	
Rank	Cause
1	Stroke
2	Ischemic heart disease
3	Road injury
4	COPD
5	Low back pain
6	Major depressive disorder
7	Trachea, bronchus, and lung cancers
8	Lower respiratory infections
9	Diabetes
10	Liver cancer

Latin America and Caribbean	
Rank	Cause
1	Ischemic heart disease
2	Exposure to forces of nature
3	Interpersonal violence
4	Road injury
5	Major depressive disorder
6	Low back pain
7	Stroke
8	Lower respiratory infections
9	Diabetes
10	Preterm birth complications

Europe and Central Asia	
Rank	Cause
1	Ischemic heart disease
2	Stroke
3	Low back pain
4	Major depressive disorder
5	Lower respiratory infections
6	Road injury
7	HIV/AIDS
8	COPD
9	Self-harm
10	Trachea, bronchus, and lung cancers

Middle East and North Africa	
Rank	Cause
1	Ischemic heart disease
2	Lower respiratory infections
3	Stroke
4	Low back pain
5	Major depressive disorder
6	Preterm birth complications
7	Congenital anomalies
8	Road injury
9	Diabetes
10	Diarrheal diseases

(continues)

TABLE 2-5 Leading Causes of DALYs by World Bank Regions and for High-Income Countries, 2010 (*continued*)

South Asia	
Rank	*Cause*
1	Lower respiratory infections
2	Preterm birth complications
3	Diarrheal diseases
4	Ischemic heart disease
5	COPD

South Asia	
Rank	*Cause*
6	Neonatal encephalopathy
7	Tuberculosis
8	Sepsis and other infectious disorders of the newborn
9	Iron-deficiency anemia
10	Road injury

Sub-Saharan Africa	
Rank	*Cause*
1	Malaria
2	HIV/AIDS
3	Lower respiratory infections
4	Diarrheal diseases
5	Protein-energy malnutrition

Sub-Saharan Africa	
Rank	*Cause*
6	Preterm birth complications
7	Sepsis and other infectious disorders of the newborn
8	Meningitis
9	Neonatal encephalopathy
10	Road injury

High-Income Countries	
Rank	*Cause*
1	Ischemic heart disease
2	Low back pain
3	Stroke
4	Major depressive disorder
5	Trachea, bronchus, and lung cancers

High-Income Countries	
Rank	*Cause*
6	COPD
7	Other musculoskeletal disorders
8	Diabetes
9	Neck pain
10	Falls

Data from Institute for Health Metrics and Evaluation (IHME). (2013). *GBD heat map.* Seattle, WA: IHME, University of Washington. Retrieved April 28, 2015, from http://vizhub.healthdata.org/irank/heat.php.

TABLE 2-6 Leading Causes of Death in Children Under 5, Low- and Middle-Income Countries and High-Income Countries, 2010

Low- and Middle-Income Countries	High-Income Countries
1. Lower respiratory infections	1. Preterm Birth Complications
2. Preterm birth complications	2. Congenital anomalies
3. Malaria	3. Neonatal encephalopathy
4. Diarrheal diseases	4. SIDS
5. Sepsis and other infectious disorders of the newborn	5. Sepsis and other infectious disorders of the newborn
6. Neonatal encephalopathy	6. Lower respiratory infections
7. Congenital anomalies	7. Road injury
8. Protein-energy malnutrition	8. Drowning
9. Meningitis	9. Interpersonal violence
10. HIV/AIDS	10. Meningitis

Data from Institute for Health Metrics and Evaluation (IHME). (2013). *GBD heat map*. Seattle, WA: IHME, University of Washington. Retrieved April 28, 2015, from http://vizhub.healthdata.org/irank/heat.php.

TABLE 2-7 Leading Causes of Death in Children Ages 5–14, Low- and Middle-Income Countries and High-Income Countries, 2010

Low- and Middle-Income Countries		High-Income Countries	
Rank	Cause	Rank	Cause
1	Diarrheal diseases	1	Road injury
2	HIV/AIDS	2	Leukemia
3	Road injury	3	Brain and nervous system cancers
4	Malaria	4	Congenital anomalies
5	Lower respiratory infections	5	Drowning
6	Drowning	6	Self-harm
7	Typhoid and paratyphoid fevers	7	Interpersonal violence
8	Meningitis	8	Lower respiratory infections
9	Congenital anomalies	9	Fire
10	Protein-energy malnutrition	10	Other transport injuries

Data from Institute for Health Metrics and Evaluation (IHME). (2013). *GBD heat map*. Seattle, WA: IHME, University of Washington. Retrieved April 28, 2015, from http://vizhub.healthdata.org/irank/heat.php.

TABLE 2-8 Leading Causes of Deaths and DALYs Ages 15–49, Low- and Middle-Income Countries and High-Income Countries, 2010

Leading Causes of Deaths			
Low- and Middle-Income Countries		*High-Income Countries*	
Rank	Cause	Rank	Cause
1	HIV/AIDS	1	Self-harm
2	Road injury	2	Road injury
3	Tuberculosis	3	Ischemic heart disease
4	Self-harm	4	Cirrhosis
5	Ischemic heart disease	5	Interpersonal violence
6	Interpersonal violence	6	Drug use disorders
7	Stroke	7	Trachea, bronchus, and lung cancers
8	Lower respiratory infections	8	Stroke
9	Maternal disorders	9	Breast cancer
10	Malaria	10	HIV/AIDS
Leading Causes of DALYs			
Low- and Middle-Income Countries		*High-Income Countries*	
Rank	Cause	Rank	Cause
1	HIV/AIDs	1	Low back pain
2	Road injury	2	Major depressive disorder
3	Low back pain	3	Drug use disorders
4	Major depressive disorder	4	Road injury
5	Tuberculosis	5	Neck pain
6	Self-harm	6	Self-harm
7	Ischemic heart disease	7	Other musculoskeletal disorders
8	Interpersonal violence	8	Anxiety disorders
9	COPD	9	Migraine
10	Maternal disorders	10	Ischemic heart disease

Data from Institute for Health Metrics and Evaluation (IHME). (2013). *GBD heat map*. Seattle, WA: IHME, University of Washington. Retrieved April 28, 2015, from http://vizhub.healthdata.org/irank/heat.php.

TABLE 2-9 Leading Causes of Deaths and DALYs by Sex, Low- and Middle-Income Countries and High-Income Countries, 2010

Deaths			
Females			
Low- and Middle-Income Countries		*High-Income Countries*	
Rank	Cause	Rank	Cause
1	Stroke	1	Ischemic heart disease
2	Ischemic heart disease	2	Stroke
3	Lower respiratory infections	3	Lower respiratory infections
4	COPD	4	Alzheimer's disease
5	Diarrheal diseases	5	COPD
6	HIV/AIDS	6	Trachea, bronchus, and lung cancers
7	Diabetes	7	Breast cancer
8	Malaria	8	Colorectal cancer
9	Tuberculosis	9	Other cardiovascular and circulatory diseases
10	Preterm birth complications	10	Diabetes
DALYs			
Females			
Low- and Middle-Income Countries		*High-Income Countries*	
Rank	Cause	Rank	Cause
1	Lower respiratory infections	1	Ischemic Heart Disease
2	Diarrheal diseases	2	Low back pain
3	HIV/AIDS	3	Major depressive disorder
4	Malaria	4	Stroke
5	Stroke	5	Other musculoskeletal disorders
6	Ischemic heart disease	6	COPD
7	Preterm birth complications	7	Neck pain
8	Major depressive disorder	8	Alzheimer's disease
9	COPD	9	Breast cancer
10	Low back pain	10	Diabetes

(continues)

TABLE 2-9 Leading Causes of Deaths and DALYs by Sex, Low- and Middle-Income Countries and High-Income Countries, 2010 (*continued*)

Deaths			
Males			
Low- and Middle-Income Countries		*High-Income Countries*	
Rank	Cause	Rank	Cause
1	Ischemic heart disease	1	Ischemic heart disease
2	Stroke	2	Stroke
3	COPD	3	Trachea, bronchus, and lung cancers
4	Lower respiratory infections	4	COPD
5	Road injury	5	Lower respiratory infections
6	HIV/AIDS	6	Colorectal cancer
7	Tuberculosis	7	Prostate cancer
8	Diarrheal diseases	8	Alzheimer's disease
9	Malaria	9	Self-harm
10	Lung cancer	10	Cirrhosis
DALYs			
Male			
Low- and Middle-Income Countries		*High-Income Countries*	
Rank	Cause	Rank	Cause
1	Lower respiratory infections	1	Ischemic heart disease
2	Ischemic heart disease	2	Low back pain
3	Road injury	3	Lung, trachea, and bronchus cancers
4	Stroke	4	Stroke
5	Diarrheal diseases	5	COPD
6	Malaria	6	Road injury
7	Preterm birth complications	7	Self-harm
8	HIV/AIDS	8	Diabetes
9	COPD	9	Falls
10	Low back pain	10	Major depressive disorder

Note: Alzheimer's disease includes other dementias

Data from Institute for Health Metrics and Evaluation (IHME). (2013). GBD Heat map. Seattle, WA: IHME, University of Washington, 2013. Available from http://vizhub.healthdata.org/irank/heat.php. Accessed April 28, 2015.

causes of DALYs in high-income countries include low back pain, self-harm, falls, and major depressive disorder that are not among the leading causes of death in this group.[31]

The Burden of Deaths and Disease Within Countries

As you consider causes of death and the burden of disease globally and by region, age, and sex, it is also important to consider how deaths and DALYs would vary within countries, by gender, ethnicity, and socioeconomic status, among other things. In most low- and middle-income countries, the answer to this is relatively simple. Generally speaking:

- Rural people will be less healthy than urban people.
- Disadvantaged ethnic minorities will be less healthy than majority populations.
- Females will suffer a number of conditions that relate to their relatively weak social positions.
- Poor people will be less healthy than better-off people.
- Uneducated people will be less healthy than better-educated people.

In addition, people of lower socioeconomic status will have higher rates of communicable diseases, illness, and death related to maternal causes and malnutrition than will people of higher status. Lower socioeconomic status people will also suffer from a larger burden of disease related to smoking, alcohol, and diet than would be the case for better-off people. These points are fundamental to understanding global health.

RISK FACTORS

As we discuss the determinants of health and how health status is measured, there will be many references to *risk factors* for various health conditions. A risk factor is "an aspect or personal behavior or life-style, an environmental exposure, or an inborn or inherited characteristic, that, on the basis of epidemiologic evidence, is known to be associated with health-related condition(s) considered important to prevent."[17,p51] Risks that relate to health can also be thought of as "a probability of an adverse outcome, or a factor that raises this probability."[32,p7] We are all familiar with the notion of risk factors from our own lives and from encounters with health services. When we answer questions about our health history, for example, we are essentially helping to identify the most important risk factors that we face ourselves. Do our parents suffer from any health conditions that might affect our own health? Are we eating in a way that is conducive to good health? Do we get enough exercise and enough sleep? Do we smoke or drink alcohol excessively? Are there any special stresses in our life? Do we wear seat belts when we drive?

If we extend the idea of risk factors to poor people in low- and middle-income countries, then we might add some other questions that relate more to the ways that they live. Does the family have safe water to drink? Do their house and community have appropriate sanitation? Does the family cook indoors in a way that makes the house smoky? Do the father and mother work in places that are safe environmentally? We might also have to ask if there is war or conflict in the country, because they are also important risk factors for illness, death, and disability.

If we are to understand how the health status of people can be enhanced, then it is very important that we understand the risk factors to which their health problems relate. **Table 2-10** shows the relative importance of different risk factors to deaths and DALYs in low- and middle-income countries, compared to high-income countries. These are shown in the table in order of their importance by category of risk.

When we consider low- and middle-income countries, the most striking point is the extent to which matters related to nutrition are risk factors for deaths, including dietary risks, high blood pressure, high-fasting plasma glucose, high body mass index, physical inactivity, and high cholesterol. If we extended the list beyond the 10 leading risk factors, we would see that childhood underweight is the next most important risk factor. Smoking tobacco and indoor and outdoor air pollution are also in the top 10 risk factors for deaths. A similar pattern emerges for DALYs, but in this case childhood underweight, iron deficiency, and suboptimal breastfeeding are of increased importance compared to their association with deaths.[31]

When we look at the risk factors for deaths in high-income countries, the pattern of risks is similar in many ways to that for low- and middle-income countries. Most of the risk factors have to do with diet, physical activity, pollution, or smoking. However, lead also appears as an important risk factor. The risk factors for DALYs are similar to that for deaths but drug use is the 10th leading risk factor for DALYs in high-income countries and was not one of the top 10 risk factors for deaths.[31]

In high-income countries, there is little deficiency in protein, energy, or micronutrients, but there is a considerable amount of overweight and obesity. It is not surprising, therefore, that some of the most important risk factors for both deaths and DALYs in high-income countries are high body mass index, high blood pressure, high total cholesterol, high fasting blood glucose, and physical inactivity. Nor is it surprising that, despite important progress in reducing the prevalence of smoking in some countries, tobacco remains the leading risk factor for both deaths and DALYs in high-income countries.[31]

TABLE 2-10 Leading Risk Factors for Deaths and DALYs, Low- and Middle-Income Countries and High-Income Countries, 2010

Deaths			
Low- and Middle-Income Countries		*High-Income Countries*	
Rank	Risk Factor	Rank	Risk Factor
1	Dietary risks	1	Dietary risks
2	High blood pressure	2	High blood pressure
3	Smoking	3	Smoking
4	Household air pollution	4	High body-mass index
5	Ambient particulate matter pollution	5	Physical inactivity
6	High fasting plasma glucose	6	High fasting plasma glucose
7	Physical inactivity	7	High total cholesterol
8	High body-mass index	8	Ambient particulate matter pollution
9	Alcohol use	9	Alcohol use
10	High total cholesterol	10	Lead
DALYs			
Low- and Middle-Income Countries		*High-Income Countries*	
Rank	Cause	Rank	Cause
1	Dietary risks	1	Dietary risks
2	High blood pressure	2	Smoking
3	Smoking	3	High body-mass index
4	Household air pollution	4	High blood pressure
5	Childhood underweight	5	Physical inactivity
6	High fasting plasma glucose	6	High fasting plasma glucose
7	Ambient particulate matter pollution	7	Alcohol use
8	Alcohol use	8	High total cholesterol
9	Occupational risks	9	Ambient particulate matter pollution
10	High body-mass index	10	Drug use

Data from Institute for Health Metrics and Evaluation (IHME). (2013). *GBD heat map*. Seattle, WA: IHME, University of Washington. Retrieved April 28, 2015, from http://vizhub.healthdata.org/irank/heat.php.

DEMOGRAPHY AND HEALTH

There are a number of points related to population that are extremely important to people's health. Among the most important of these are:

- Population growth
- Population aging
- Urbanization
- The demographic divide
- The demographic transition

These are briefly discussed next, along with their implications for health. Other important matters related to population, such as the relationship between fertility and the health of women and children, are discussed in other chapters.

Population Growth

The population of the world is about 7.2 billion[33] and is still growing. As shown in **Figure 2-8**, it is estimated that by 2050 the population of the world will be about 9.2 billion. As also shown in the figure, the overwhelming majority of population growth in the future will occur in low- and middle-income countries.[4] This reflects the fact that fertility is falling slowly in many countries that have had high fertility rates historically, whereas many of the high-income countries already have very low fertility. At a minimum, we should expect that increasing population growth in low-income countries will put substantial pressure on the environment, with its attendant risks for health. It will also mean that infrastructure, such as water supply and sanitation, will have to be provided to an increasing number of people in the countries that have the largest service gaps and can least afford to expand such services. This could cause these countries to face substantial impacts on health as a result. Increasing population will also make it more difficult for low-income countries to provide education and health services, with additional consequences for the health of their people in the future.

Population Aging

As shown in **Table 2-11**, the population of the world is aging. This is especially true in high-income countries that have low fertility, but this is occurring in other countries as well. One impact of population aging is that it changes the ratio between the number of people that are 15–64 years of age, compared with the number that are 65 years of age or more. This is called the *elderly support ratio*. In Niger, with high fertility and a growing population, only 3 percent of the population is over 65 years of age, and there are 15 times more people between 15 and 65 than over 65. By contrast, in Japan, with very low fertility and a shrinking population, 24 percent of the population is over 65 and the number of people 15 to 65 is only about 2.5 times the number of people over 65.[4]

Population aging and the shift in the elderly support ratio have profound implications for the burden of disease and for health expenditures and how they will be financed.

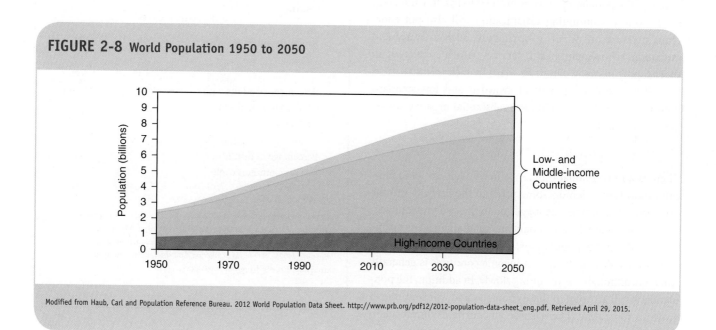

FIGURE 2-8 World Population 1950 to 2050

Modified from Haub, Carl and Population Reference Bureau. 2012 World Population Data Sheet. http://www.prb.org/pdf12/2012-population-data-sheet_eng.pdf. Retrieved April 29, 2015.

TABLE 2-11 Percentage of the Population Over 65 Years of Age

	2010	2050
High-income countries	15.9	26.2
Low- and middle-income countries	5.8	14.6

Adapted from Haub, C., & PRB. Data from United Nations Population Division. *World population prospects. The 2008 revision.* Retrieved December 4, 2010, from http://www.un.org/esa/population/publications /wpp2008/wpp2008_highlights.pdf. Data is shown only for the medium population variant of the UN.

In the simplest terms, people will live longer and spend more years with morbidities and disabilities related to noncommunicable diseases. This will raise the costs of health care. In addition, the large numbers of older adults for every working person will make it difficult for countries to finance that health care.

Urbanization

In the last decade, the majority of the world's population has lived in urban areas for the first time in world history. People are continuing to move from rural to urban areas, especially in low- and middle-income countries in which important shares of the population have continued to live in rural areas until recently. Continuing urbanization will also put enormous pressure on urban infrastructure, such as water and sanitation, schools, and health services, which are already in short supply in many countries. Gaps in such infrastructure, as well as the development of crowded and low-standard housing, for example, could have substantial negative consequences for health.

The Demographic Divide

There is an exceptional difference in the demographic indicators and future demographic paths of the best-off and the least-well-off countries, as suggested in the two previous sections. The highest income countries generally have very low fertility, declining populations, and aging populations. By contrast, fertility in the lowest income countries is generally still high, although it is declining slowly. In addition, the population is still growing in these countries and will continue to grow for some time. There is also an enormous difference in the health circumstances of the high- and low-income countries. **Table 2-12** portrays the demographic divide.

TABLE 2-12 The Demographic Divide: The Example of Nigeria and Japan

	Nigeria	Japan
Population 2012 (millions)	170.1	127.6
Population 2050 (millions)	402.4	95.5
Lifetime births per woman	5.6	1.4
Annual number of births (millions)	6.2	1.1
Births per 1,000 population	40	9
Percentage of population below age 15	44	13
Percentage of population age 65+	3	24
Life expectancy at birth	51	83
Infant deaths per 1,000 births	77	2.3
Annual number of infant deaths	465,000	2,900
Percentage of adults with HIV/AIDS, males/ females	2.9/4.4	< 0.1/< 0.1
Percentage of deaths due to noncommunicable diseases (2008)	27	80

Data from Population Reference Bureau. (2012). *2012 world population data sheet.* Retrieved September 16, 2013, from http://www.prb.org /pdf12/2012-population-data-sheet_eng.pdf; Population Reference Bureau. (2009). *2009 world population data sheet.* Retrieved April 9, 2011, from http://www.prb.org/pdf09/09wpds_eng.pdf.

The Demographic Transition[34]

One important demographic trend of importance is called the *demographic transition*. This is the shift from a pattern of high fertility and high mortality to low fertility and low mortality, with population growth occurring in between.

When we look back historically at the countries that are now high-income, we can see that they had long periods historically when fertility was high, mortality was high, and population growth was, therefore, relatively slow, or might even have declined in the face of epidemics. Beginning around the turn of the 19th century, however, mortality in those countries began to decline as hygiene and nutrition improved and the burden of infectious diseases became less. In most cases, this decline in mortality started before much decline in fertility. As mortality declined, the population increased and the share of the population of younger ages also increased. Later, fertility began to decline and, as births and deaths became more equal, population growth slowed.

As births and deaths stayed more equal, the share of the population that was of older ages increased.

The demographic transition is shown graphically in **Figure 2-9**.

The first population pyramid reflects a country with high fertility and high mortality. The second population pyramid is indicative of a country in which mortality has begun to decline but fertility remains high. This would be similar to the demographics one would find, for example, in a number of countries in sub-Saharan Africa that are undergoing demographic transition. The third pyramid looks more like a cylinder than a pyramid. This reflects a population in which fertility has been reduced for a substantial period of time and in which there is a much larger share of older people in the population than in the first and second pyramids. This would be similar to the demographics that one would find in a number of low-fertility, aging populations in Western Europe.

FIGURE 2-9 The Demographic Transition: (A) High Fertility/High Mortality, (B) Declining Mortality/High Fertility, (C) Reduced Fertility/Reduced Mortality

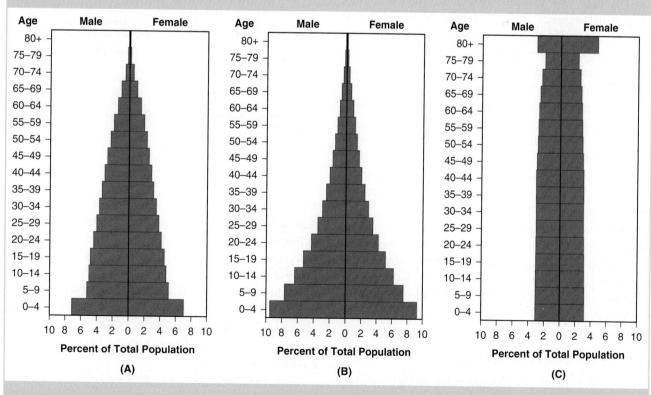

Reprinted from U.S. Census Bureau. International population reports WP/02. Global Population Profile: 2002. Washington, DC: U.S. Government Printing Office; 2004:35.

The Epidemiologic Transition[35]

The epidemiologic transition is closely related to the demographic transition, as suggested throughout the previous discussion. Historically there has been a shift in the patterns of disease that follows these trends:

- First, high and fluctuating mortality, related to very poor health conditions, epidemics, and famine
- Then, progressive declines in mortality as epidemics become less frequent
- Finally, further declines in mortality, increases in life expectancy, and the predominance of noncommunicable diseases

Figure 2-10 shows the distribution by cause group of deaths and the burden of disease for low- and middle-income countries and high-income countries.

You can see in Figure 2-10 how the pattern of deaths and DALYs differs between the low-, middle-, and high-income countries. You can also see the changes that will occur over time, as the burden of disease in low- and middle-income countries moves from one with a substantial share of communicable diseases to one in which noncommunicable diseases are very predominant.

The pace of the epidemiologic transition in different societies depends on a number of factors related to the determinants of health that were discussed earlier. In its early stages, the transition appears to depend primarily on improvements in hygiene, nutrition, education, and socioeconomic status. Some improvements also stem from advances in public health and in medicine, such as the development of new vaccines and antibiotics.[36]

Most of the countries that are now high-income went through epidemiologic transitions that were relatively slow, with the exception of Japan. Most low- and middle-income countries have already begun their transition; however, it is still far from complete in many of them.

In fact, most low-income countries are in an ongoing epidemiologic transition and many of them, therefore, face significant burdens of communicable and noncommunicable diseases and injuries at the same time. This strains the capacity of the health system of many of these countries. It is also expensive for countries that are resource poor to address a substantial burden of all three of these types of conditions simultaneously.

PROGRESS IN HEALTH STATUS

There has been substantial progress in improving health and raising life expectancy in many parts of the world. However, as also noted, those gains have not been uniform across regions. Rather, life expectancy in sub-Saharan Africa and

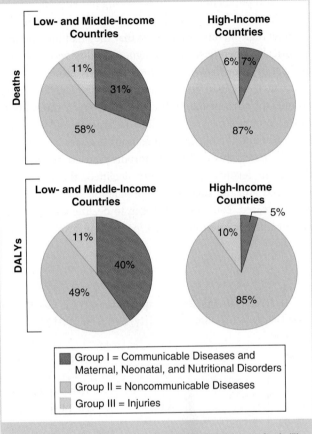

FIGURE 2-10 Deaths and DALYs by Group of Causes for Low- and Middle-Income and High-Income Countries, 2010

Group I = Communicable Diseases and Maternal, Neonatal, and Nutritional Disorders
Group II = Noncommunicable Diseases
Group III = Injuries

Data from Institute for Health Metrics and Evaluation (IHME). GBD Compare. Seattle, WA: IHME, University of Washington, 2013. http://vizhub.healthdata.org/gbd-compare. Accessed April 26, 2015.

South Asia continues to substantially lag behind that in other regions. In addition, for countries that had a life expectancy in 1960 of less than 50 years, the pace of improvements in life expectancy in sub-Saharan Africa has been much slower than in any other region.

Table 2-13 shows life expectancy in 1960, 1990, and 2013 by World Bank region, including for high-income countries. The table also shows the percentage gain in life expectancy over three different periods, 1960 to 2008, 1960 to 1990, and 1990 to 2013.

Life expectancy grew over each period in each region; however, the increases in Europe and Central Asia were very small in the period 1990–2013, largely reflecting the social and economic consequences of the breakup of the former

TABLE 2-13 Life Expectancy and Percentage Gain in Life Expectancy, by World Bank Region, 1960–2013

World Bank Region	Life Expectancy (Years)			Percentage Gain (1960–2013)	Percentage Gain (1960–1990)	Percentage Gain (1990–2013)
	1960	1990	2013			
East Asia and Pacific	46	67	75	63%	46%	12%
Europe and Central Asia	—	69	77	—	—	12%
Latin America and the Caribbean	56	68	75	34%	21%	10%
Middle East and North Africa	47	64	72	53%	36%	13%
South Asia	43	58	67	56%	35%	16%
Sub-Saharan Africa	41	50	57	39%	22%	14%
High-income	69	76	79	14%	10%	4%

Data from the World Bank. *World development indicators, data query.* Retrieved September 17, 2013, from http://databank.worldbank.org. No data for Europe and Central Asia for 1960.

Soviet Union and the impact of changes on the health system as well. The slow progress in improving life expectancy in sub-Saharan Africa between 1990 and 2013 mostly reflects the negative impact on life expectancy of the HIV/AIDS epidemic, as well as slow economic progress in some countries and political conflict. By contrast, the dramatic increases in life expectancy from 1960 to 2013 in the East Asia and Pacific region reflect the rapid pace of economic development in that region, usually accompanied by improvements in infrastructure, nutrition, education, and health. The region was also relatively free of conflict.

The factors that lead to improvements in health are complex, as suggested by the determinants of health that you reviewed earlier in this chapter. Additional comments are made at the end of this chapter about these factors, including the role, for example, of nutrition, education, political stability, and scientific improvements. Many other chapters also include comments on the progress in improving the health of women and children and in addressing particular causes of illness, disability, and death.

THE BURDEN OF DISEASE: LOOKING FORWARD

The burden of disease in the future will be influenced by a number of factors that will continue to change. Some of these will relate to the determinants of health discussed earlier in the chapter. Some will relate to the demographic forces just discussed, including population growth, population aging, and migration. The burden of disease in the future will also be driven, among other things, by:

- Economic development
- Scientific and technological change
- Climate change
- Political stability
- Emerging and reemerging infectious diseases
- Food security

These are discussed very briefly in the following sections.

Economic Development

The economies of low-income countries will need to grow if those countries are to generate the income they need to invest in improving people's health. The impact of economic development on health will depend partly on the extent to which economic growth is equitable across population groups. It will also depend on the extent to which countries are able—or choose—to use their increased income to invest in other areas that improve health, such as water, sanitation, hygiene, food security, and education. The extent and appropriateness of their investments in health, such as in low-cost, high-yielding efforts in health, will also be critical.

Scientific and Technological Change

Scientific and technological change has had an enormous impact on health and will continue to do so in the future. This is easy to understand, as one considers the development of vaccines or new drugs, such as antibiotics or antiretroviral therapy. The development of new diagnostics for TB, for example, would have an enormous impact on the health of the world, as would the development of a vaccine against HIV or malaria. The impact of scientific and technological change on the low-income countries of today will depend to a large extent on the pace at which they are able to effectively adopt any improvements when they are developed.

Climate Change

The impact of climate change on health is not clear; however, it is anticipated that climate change and its attendant impact on weather and rising sea levels could directly and indirectly have an important impact on health. On the indirect side, climate change could alter the nature of the food crops that can be grown in different places and lead to migration from some places to others that are deemed more habitable. On the more direct side, climate change could lead to weather changes and adverse weather that harm people's health. It could also lead to the disappearance of disease vectors in some places as the weather is no longer hospitable to them, while allowing the emergence or reemergence of disease vectors in other places.

Political Stability

In low-income countries, political stability appears to be necessary for achieving long-term gains in health. There is substantial evidence, for example, that the lack of political stability has been a major impediment to progress in achieving the Millennium Development Goals in a number of countries. It is not hard to imagine, for example, how conflicts that occurred in Liberia, Sierra Leone, and the Democratic Republic of the Congo could set back health status for many years. These conflicts led directly to substantial illness, disability, and death. In addition, by causing a breakdown in infrastructure, such as water, sanitation, and electricity, as well as the erosion of health services, they also had enormous indirect impacts on health.

Emerging and Reemerging Infectious Diseases

It is not possible to predict if and when new diseases will emerge or diseases already known will reemerge. It is also not possible to know how well individual countries and the world will do in recognizing any such problems and addressing them quickly and effectively. What is clear is that pandemic flu, for example, could have a major impact on future disease patterns. It is also clear, for example, that if the growth of drug resistance for, say, malaria, outpaced our ability to produce safe and effective drugs to fight malaria, this, too, could have a substantial impact on the burden of disease.

Projecting the Burden of Disease

Given the complex array of factors that influence health status and will drive future changes in the burden of disease, it is difficult to predict with any certainty how the burden of disease will evolve in different countries in the next 2 decades. Nonetheless, it is possible, using models, to project the future burden of disease, given assumptions about key health determinants and how they will evolve in different parts of the world.

The *Global Burden of Disease Study 2010* did not include projections of the future burden of disease. However, in 2008, WHO developed projections of the burden of disease, based on data that was collected in 2004. These projections included information on both deaths and DALYs. WHO more recently produced projections for 2030, but they only have data on deaths. The data that follows is from the earlier WHO projections since information about DALYs that this data uniquely contains is still enlightening and of more value, in many ways, than information solely on deaths.

Table 2-14 highlights the leading causes of the burden of disease in DALYs, as WHO projected them to 2030. These projections of percentage of total DALYs at that time are on the basis of data on the burden of disease from 2004. The data is presented by World Bank country income group for low-, lower-middle-, upper-middle-, and upper-income countries.

The main message of the table is clear: over the period to 2030, it is projected that there will be substantial changes in the burden of disease in all country income groups. In the simplest terms, low- and lower-middle-income countries will see a substantial shift away from communicable diseases and toward noncommunicable diseases and injuries. HIV/AIDS is projected to be the only communicable disease in the top 10 causes of DALYs in low-income countries, and no communicable diseases are predicted to be in the top 10 for lower-middle-income countries. Unipolar depressive disorders, ischemic heart disease, and cerebrovascular disease become more important causes of DALYs for both income groups. Some causes we associate with aging populations, such as hearing loss and refractive errors, also become more prominent, even in low-income countries. The projected growth of diabetes in all income groups is also evident in the table.

For the upper-middle-income countries, the burden would continue to shift in similar ways, as noted previously.

TABLE 2-14 Projections to 2030 for the 10 Leading Causes of the Burden of Disease by World Bank Income Group

Projected in 2030	Percentage of Total DALYs
Low-income countries	
1. Perinatal conditions	8.6
2. Unipolar depressive disorders	5.8
3. Road traffic accidents	5.5
4. Ischemic heart disease	5.2
5. Lower respiratory infections	5.0
6. Cerebrovascular disease	3.1
7. HIV/AIDS	3.1
8. Other unintentional injuries	3.1
9. Chronic obstructive pulmonary disease (COPD)	3.1
10. Hearing loss, adult onset	2.6
Lower- middle-income countries	
1. Unipolar depressive disorders	6.4
2. Cerebrovascular disease	6.0
3. COPD	5.9
4. Ischemic heart disease	5.2
5. Road traffic accidents	5.0
6. Refractive errors	3.3
7. Hearing loss, adult onset	3.1
8. Perinatal conditions	2.9
9. Diabetes	2.7
10. Alcohol use disorders	2.7

Projected in 2030	Percentage of Total DALYs
Upper-middle-income countries	
1. Ischemic heart disease	8.2
2. HIV/AIDS	6.2
3. Unipolar depressive disorders	6.0
4. Cerebrovascular disease	5.6
5. Diabetes	4.2
6. Interpersonal violence	3.9
7. Alcohol use disorders	3.1
8. Road injury	3.0
9. Hearing loss, adult onset	2.8
10. Osteoarthritis	2.3
High-income countries	
1. Unipolar depressive disorders	8.5
2. Ischemic heart disease	6.5
3. Alzheimer's and other dementias	5.5
4. Hearing loss, adult onset	4.1
5. Cerebrovascular disease	3.8
6. Alcohol use disorders	3.3
7. Osteoarthritis	2.8
8. Trachea, bronchus, and lung cancers	2.7
9. Refractive errors	2.4
10. Self-harm	2.4

Note: Perinatal conditions include prematurity and low birth weight; birth asphyxia and birth trauma; and neonatal infections and other conditions. Some cause definitions differ from the GBD heat map. In some cases, the GBD category was used for consistency. Please see source for more information on methods on how these projections were calculated and cause definitions.

Data from World Health Organization. Global Burden of Disease (GBD). Available at: http://www.who.int/healthinfo/global_burden_disease/en. Accessed September 14, 2010.

TB, which was the 11th leading cause of DALYs, would decline in relative importance, and no communicable disease would be in the top 10. Adult-onset hearing loss and arthritis, however, would join the top 10 leading causes of DALYs, clearly reflecting the aging populations in these countries.

The projected burden of disease in high-income countries also suggests an increase in burdens associated with aging, such as dementias, hearing loss, and refractive disorders.

Mental health issues are projected to increase in importance in all income groups over the period 2004 to 2030. The largest percentage increases will occur in low-income countries, probably reflecting the extent to which these issues arise as people lose connections with their families and their culture group, as often occurs in modernizing and globalizing economies in which people leave their native places to migrate to cities in search of employment. The neglected tropical diseases are not treated as a group in the burden of disease data, so each disease tends to be fairly low in rankings of DALYs. However, we should anticipate that the burden of these diseases will remain substantial for many years to come,

but that their burden will decline consistently between 2004 and 2030.

THE DEVELOPMENT CHALLENGE OF IMPROVING HEALTH

One of the key development challenges facing policymakers in low-income countries is how they can speed the demographic and epidemiologic transitions at the lowest possible cost. How can Niger, for example, improve its health status as rapidly as possible and at the least possible cost? Will it be possible for the people of Niger to enjoy the health status of a middle-income country, even if Niger remains a low-income country?

Figure 2-11 shows national income of a sample of countries, plotted against life expectancy at birth for females in those countries.

From this figure, one can see that, generally, the health of a country does increase as national income rises. However, one can also see that there are some countries, such as China, Costa Rica, Cuba, and Sri Lanka, that have achieved higher

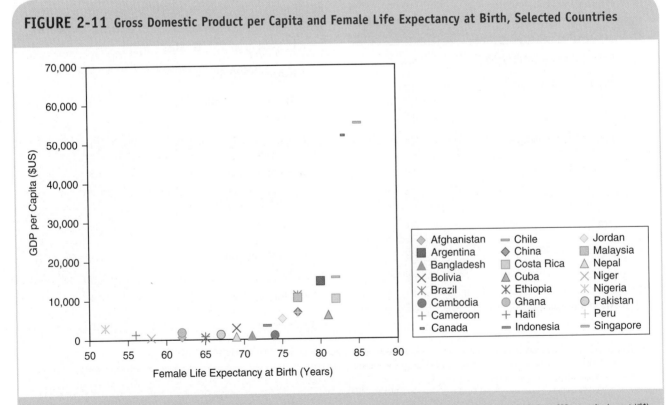

FIGURE 2-11 Gross Domestic Product per Capita and Female Life Expectancy at Birth, Selected Countries

Data from World Bank. Data: Life expectancy at birth (female). http://data.worldbank.org/indicator/SP.DYN.LE00.FE.IN. Accessed March 11, 2015; World Bank. Data: GDP per capita (current US$). http://data.worldbank.org/indicator/NY.GDP.PCAP.CD. Accessed March 21, 2015.

average life expectancies at birth than one would have predicted for countries at their level of income.

To a large extent, countries like those above achieved these important health gains as a result of:

- Focusing on investing in nutrition, health, and education, particularly of their poor people
- Improving people's knowledge of good hygiene
- Making selected investments in health services that at low cost could have a high impact on health status, such as vaccination programs for children and TB control

Indeed, in the long run, economic progress *will* help to bring down fertility, reduce mortality from communicable diseases, and help to produce a healthier population. However, at the present rates of progress in improving health in most low-income countries, these changes will take a very long time to occur. One great public policy challenge for these countries and their governments, therefore, is how they can short-circuit this process and reach reduced levels of fertility, lower mortality, and better health for their people, even as they remain relatively poor.

POLICY AND PROGRAM BRIEF

The Million Death Study on India

The Aims of the Study

The Centre for Global Health Research, at the University of Toronto, Canada, is carrying out the Million Death Study in India, in conjunction with the Registrar General of India. This study is one of the largest research efforts ever undertaken on the causes of premature mortality. Led by Professor Prabhat Jha, the study aims to help India improve the documentation of the underlying causes and risk factors of mortality, as a basis for enhancing investments in health, reducing premature death, and improving the health of India's people.[37]

Vital statistics, such as fertility and mortality data, are crucial for identifying major health issues, identifying new health problems as they arise, making cost-effective public health investments, and evaluating the progress of public health interventions. Yet, reliable mortality statistics are rare. A total of 75 percent of global deaths occur in low- and middle-income countries and the majority of these lack medical supervision and official certification of cause of death.[38] In India, for example, 70 percent of deaths go unreported or misclassified.[39] Previous mortality estimates for India were largely based on data from the limited spectrum of deaths that occur in hospitals and were consequently biased toward

causes of death that affect urban populations more than rural populations. They were also biased toward conditions that are more urgent and lead to hospitalization, rather than taking sufficient account of chronic health problems.[40] Moreover, in India and in many other middle- and low-income countries, there is a general dearth of knowledge around the causes of deaths, especially for middle-aged adults, and the corresponding risk factors leading to premature death.

The Study Approach

The Million Death Study seeks to assess the causes of death of one million people in India through monitoring 2.4 million households over two time periods: 1998–2003 and 2004–2014. The study is based on an approach called "verbal autopsy." The study uses India's Sample Registration System as its sampling framework. Twice a year trained surveyors conduct surveys in order to identify households in which a death occurred. They then interview household members about the deaths in their families and record information on the events leading to death and the symptoms of the deceased. The verbal autopsies are sent to two independent physicians to be analyzed and ascertain the underlying cause of those deaths.[37]

By early 2015, 600,000 deaths have been surveyed and 400,000 deaths have been fully coded. The study is expected in the next 2 to 3 years to have carried out all of the planned interviews and assessed all of the deaths it will consider. Nonetheless, the study authors believe that the emerging data already provides compelling information about mortality trends in India.[41]

Findings to Date

The study thus far has exposed some mortality estimates and trends that deviate from those previously recognized.[39] First, the study has suggested that the top four causes of death in India are cardiovascular disease, chronic respiratory disease, TB, and cancer. Second, one of the most striking findings is related to the effects of tobacco. The average Indian smoker starts smoking later in life than in many other countries and often smokes hand-rolled locally manufactured cigarettes called bidis, which have a lower concentration of cancer-causing agents than commercially manufactured cigarettes. Nonetheless, this study showed that in India smoking is as much a risk for premature death as in Europe and the United States. Moreover, study findings suggest that smoking is a risk factor for TB in India and that 40 percent of all TB deaths in middle-aged men in India can be attributed to smoking.[38] Third, the study suggests that some estimates of the burden of disease might be quite different from what was previously thought and that the burden of disease pattern varies greatly across the country. This study, for example, estimates that total malaria deaths are 10 times greater than the World Health Organization estimates, with over half of malaria deaths occurring in people 15–69 and the state of Odisha accounting for a quarter of India's annual malaria deaths.[38] On the other hand, the study suggests that mortality associated with HIV-related infections is lower than UNAIDS estimates, although the rural areas around Mumbai have a particularly high concentration of HIV-related deaths with an annual death rate of 56 per 100,000.[38,39]

Lessons of Experience

The Million Death Study may offer a model for improving mortality information that is reliable, high impact, low cost, and replicable in other countries. The ideal system to measure mortality would depend on a well-functioning system of vital registration. However, in the absence of such comprehensive registration programs, this study suggests that verbal autopsies can reduce inaccurate data by correctly classifying the underlying causes of 90 percent of the deaths occurring before age 70, an order of magnitude better than the limited cause of death data previously available.[40] This can help derive the probable cause of death when one has not been reported and help us to understand the leading causes of death.[37] Importantly, this approach has also been shown to be cost-effective. India added recording the causes of death and risk factors to a low-cost, preexisting sample registration system, at a cost of less than $2 per household.[41,42]

The long-term goal will always be universal civil registration of deaths with medical certification in order to best minimize misclassification and misrepresentation. However, approaches such as those applied in the Million Death Study offer an interim solution for better statistics on mortality for many low- and middle-income countries.

CASE STUDY

The State of Kerala

Having begun to review health status and how countries can speed improvements in health, it will be valuable to end this chapter by examining a well-known case of a place that improved health status considerably, even at relatively low levels of income. One of the best known of such success stories concerns Kerala State in India.

Introduction

Kerala is a coastal state in Southwestern India with a population of more than 33 million people.[43] Despite earlier slow rates of economic growth and a state per capita income lower than that of many other states in India, the health indicators for Kerala are the best in India and rival those in high-income countries. What approach did Kerala take historically to produce such high levels of health, even in the face of relatively low income? What factors contributed to improvements in health status? What lessons does the Kerala experience suggest for other countries and for other states within India?

The Kerala Approach

One of the primary reasons why people in Kerala have such high levels of health has been the emphasis that the state put on education and the exceptionally widespread access to education in Kerala. The state introduced free primary and secondary education in the early part of 20th century.[44] In addition, Kerala has always put important emphasis on the education of females.

Kerala also made an early commitment to widespread health services for its people. The state created, for example, an extensive network of primary healthcare centers. This provided its citizens, throughout the state, with access to free basic health care and free family planning services. This was coupled with programs to promote exclusive breastfeeding and the improved nutrition of infants, children, and pregnant women. The central government supported the family planning program, the maternal and child health program, and the universal immunization program in all of India, but they were implemented far more effectively and efficiently in Kerala than in most other states of India.[45]

The place of women in Kerala society also contributed to the uptake of education by females and improvements throughout Kerala in nutrition and health status. The role of women in many communities in Kerala differs from the roles ascribed to women in many other parts of India. In much of the rest of India, especially in parts of North India, women are regarded by families as liabilities rather than as assets. In most of India, this is partly represented in cultural terms by the fact that the family of a bride must pay a dowry to the family of the groom. In Kerala, however, women have been treated differently for over a century. They have been seen culturally as assets to families and could inherit and own land, giving them a financial independence and power that has been unrivalled among women elsewhere in India.[46]

It is also important to note that Kerala has historically been run by a government that has traditionally placed a premium on community mobilization on important social issues, such as education, greater empowerment of women, health, nutrition, and land reform. Many of these efforts were carried out in ways that raised social awareness about health and nutrition. In 1989, Kerala launched a total literacy campaign, for example, and by the start of the World Literacy

Year in 1990, Ernakulam district in Kerala was declared India's first totally literate district.[47]

Given widespread education in Kerala and the place of women in society, it is not surprising that Kerala went through the demographic transition quite early and well before other places in India. Women with more education are more likely to work and marry later and thus have wider choice in economic and social pursuits. They also have a better knowledge of and easier access to family planning methods and lower fertility than do women with less education.[48]

The Impact

What were the impacts on health status of the emphasis that Kerala placed on education, health, nutrition, and the empowerment of women? Although it is not possible to scientifically indicate which policy contributed what share of better health, we can say that for many years the people of Kerala have enjoyed the best educational attainment of any group within India. In the 2001 census, the literacy rates of people aged 7 years and above for India were about 65 percent on average, with about 76 percent for males and 54 percent for females. Kerala, however, had the highest literacy rate in the country, with about 91 percent overall and about 94 percent for males and 88 percent for females.[49] Kerala also boasted one of the highest newspaper readerships in the world, another feature that promotes the value of women, education, nutrition, and health. It also helps to raise political awareness and the demands of people for participation in and solutions to their concerns, such as education, health, and water.

Linked with this high level of education, especially of women, and the promotion of nutrition and health, infant mortality in Kerala in 2001 was 14 per 1,000, compared with 91 per 1,000 for low-income countries generally and 68 per 1,000 on average for India.[49] The national under-5 mortality rate for 1998–1999 was around 87 per 1,000 live births with a wide variation between states. In Kerala, however, the mortality of children under 5 years was the best in India with an impressive rate of only 19 such deaths per 1,000 births in 1998–1999.[50] In addition, maternal deaths in Kerala were much less common, at 87 per 100,000, than the Indian average of 407 per 100,000.[51] This partly reflects the extent to which deliveries take place in hospitals in Kerala. Indeed, Kerala's healthcare system garnered international acclaim when UNICEF and WHO designated it as the world's first baby-friendly state. This was in recognition of the fact that more than 95 percent of Keralite births are in hospitals.[52]

Finally, one should note that life expectancy for men and women in Kerala at the time of the 2001 census was 73 years. This was close to life expectancy in many high-income countries.[53]

Lessons Learned

Kerala has long been cited, along with China, Costa Rica, Cuba, and Sri Lanka, as a model of a country or state within a country that has achieved high levels of education and health for its people, before achieving high levels of income. It appears that Kerala achieved these impacts by politically supporting widespread access to education, nutrition, and health; mobilizing communities around the importance of these areas and of women's empowerment; and investing in low-cost but high-yielding areas of education, nutrition, and health. In a manner much like Sri Lanka, Kerala has also managed to achieve high levels of health status at relatively low cost.

Have the high levels of health and education in Kerala, however, been associated with high levels of growth of income in the state? The answer to that question, at least until recently, was no. The annual per capita gross domestic product (GDP) for the state in year 2001 was $469. This was close to the Indian average of $460.[54] It appears that the economic policies held by the state for many years did not yield high rates of economic growth or produced an environment in which domestic and foreign investors were prepared to work. Rather, the overall income of the state remained quite dependent on the money that workers from Kerala living abroad, especially in the Middle East, send back to their families in Kerala.[55]

What, then, are the messages to take away from Kerala in terms of the link between health and development? First, it is possible, even in the absence of high levels of income, to achieve high levels of health through political commitment, sound investments, and social mobilization. Second, however, in the absence of sound economic policies, the presence of a literate and healthy population alone will not be sufficient to promote rapid economic growth.

MAIN MESSAGES

To understand the most important global health issues, we must understand the determinants of health, how health status is measured, and the meaning of the demographic and epidemiologic transitions. There are a number of factors that influence health status, including genetic makeup, sex, and age. Social and cultural issues and health behaviors are also closely linked to health status. The determinants of health also include education, nutritional status, and socioeconomic status. The environment is also a powerful determinant of health, as is access to health services, and the policy approaches that countries take to their health sectors and to investments that could influence the health of their people.

Increasing attention is being paid to the social determinants of health.

There are a number of uses of health data including measuring health status, carrying out disease surveillance, making decisions about investments in health, and assessing the performance of health programs. Those working in health use a common set of indicators to measure health status, including life expectancy, infant and neonatal mortality, under-5 child mortality, and the maternal mortality ratio. They also use composite indices, such as DALYs, to measure the burden of disease. Vital registration systems are weak in low-income countries and need to be strengthened to improve the quality of health data.

There has been progress in all regions of the world in increasing life expectancy over the last several decades. In addition, the pace of those increases has been exceptionally rapid in East Asia and Pacific. However, it is clear that the basic health indicators are much worse in sub-Saharan Africa than in any other region and that these indicators also lag substantially in South Asia.

When considering the health status of a population, it is important to consider not only deaths, but also DALYs, which take account of premature death and years lived with disability. It is easy to understand this when examining causes of ill health that do not often lead to death but that, nonetheless, can lead to many years of disability, such as diabetes, depressive disorders, musculoskeletal disorders, and the neglected tropical diseases.

The leading cause of death worldwide for both sexes and all age groups is ischemic heart disease, followed by stroke. All of the other 10 leading causes, except lower respiratory infections, HIV/AIDS, and TB are noncommunicable diseases. The leading cause of DALYs for both sexes and all age groups globally is also ischemic heart disease when looking at both sexes combined and all age groups combined. However, the 10 leading causes of DALYs also include several diseases that especially affect large numbers of children in lower income countries, such as diarrhea and malaria. The leading causes of DALYs also include road traffic injuries and low back pain.

The burden of disease is predominantly noncommunicable in all regions of the world except sub-Saharan Africa, and South Asia also continues to have a substantial burden of communicable disease. Over the last several decades, the burden of disease within regions and globally has continued to shift more and more toward a pattern dominated by noncommunicable diseases. Projections suggest that this trend will continue, especially in the face of populations that are aging.

It is also important to understand the most important risk factors that are associated with deaths and DALYs. In the low-income countries, some of the most important risk factors include a range of nutritional issues, the lack of safe water or appropriate sanitation, indoor air pollution, and tobacco smoking. Poor diets that relate to obesity, high blood pressure, high cholesterol, and cardiovascular disease are becoming increasingly important problems as well, even in low-income countries. In the higher income countries, the key risk factors for deaths and DALYs are overwhelmingly behavioral and have to do with what people eat, their levels of physical activity, and if they smoke tobacco, engage in excessive alcohol use, and drive safely.

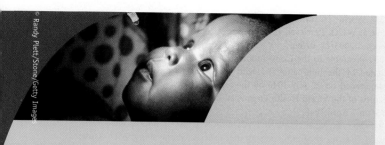

Study Questions

1. What are the main factors that determine your personal health?

2. What are the main factors that would determine the health of a poor person in a poor country?

3. If you could pick only one indicator to describe the health status of a poor country, which indicator would you use and why?

4. Why is it valuable to have composite indicators like DALYs to measure the burden of disease?

5. What is a HALE, and how does it differ from just measuring life expectancy at birth?

6. As countries develop economically, what are the most important changes that occur in their burden of disease?

7. Why do these changes occur?

8. In your own country, what population groups have the best health indicators and why?

9. In your country, what population groups have the worst health status and why?

10. How would the population pyramid of Italy differ from that of Nigeria and why?

11. How does the burden of disease differ from one region to another?

12. How will the burden of disease evolve in different regions over the next 20 years?

REFERENCES

1. World Health Organization. (2004). A global emergency: A combined response. In *The world health report 2004—Changing history* (pp. 1–10). Geneva: World Health Organization.

2. Population Reference Bureau. (2013). *2013 world population data sheet*. Retrieved April 26, 2015, from http://www.prb.org/pdf13/2013-population-data-sheet_eng.pdf.

3. Heleniak, T, (2002). Russia's Demographic Decline Continues. Population Reference Bureau. Retrieved June 14, 2015, from http://www.prb.org/Publications/Articles/2002/RussiasDemographicDeclineContinues.aspx.

4. Population Reference Bureau. (2012). *2012 world population data sheet*. Retrieved September 11, 2013, from http://www.prb.org/pdf12/2012-population-data-sheet_eng.pdf.

5. Public Health Agency of Canada. *What determines health*. Retrieved November 19, 2010, from http://www.phac-aspc.gc.ca/ph-sp/determinants/index-eng.php.

6. Centers for Disease Control and Prevention. *Social determinants of health: Definitions*. Retrieved September 13, 2013, http://www.cdc.gov/socialdeterminants/Definitions.html.

7. World Bank. (2011). *Social capital and health, nutrition and population*. Retrieved May 25, 2015, from http://go.worldbank.org/5DODHABMT0.

8. Hobcraft, J. (1993). Women's education, child welfare and child survival: A review of the evidence. *Health Transition Review*, 3(2), 159–173.

9. World Bank. (2006). *Repositioning nutrition as central to development—A strategy for large-scale action*. Washington, DC: The World Bank.

10. World Health Organization. (2008). *Commission on social determinants of health. Closing the gap in a generation*. Retrieved November 18, 2010, from http://www.who.int/social_determinants/thecommission/finalreport/en/index.html.

11. Basch, P. (2001). *Textbook of international health* (2nd ed.). New York: Oxford University Press.

12. Haupt, A., & Kane, T. T. (2004). *Population handbook*. Washington, DC: Population Reference Bureau.

13. World Health Organization. *Global Health Observatory Data Repository: Life expectancy*. Retrieved September 13, 2013, http://apps.who.int/gho/data/view.main.680?lang=en.

14. World Bank. (2015). *Mortality rate, infant (per 1,000 live births)*. Retrieved April 26, 2015, http://data.worldbank.org/indicator/SP.DYN.IMRT.IN.

15. World Bank. *Mortality rate, under-5 (per 1000)*. Retrieved September 13, 2013, from http://data.worldbank.org/indicator/SH.DYN.MORT.

16. World Bank. (2015). *Maternal mortality ratio (modeled estimate, per 100,00 live births)*. Retrieved April 27, 2015, from http://data.worldbank.org/indicator/SH.STA.MMRT.

17. Last, J. M. (2001). *A dictionary of epidemiology* (4th ed.). New York: Oxford University Press.

18. World Bank. (2015). *Prevalence of HIV, total (% of population ages 15–49)*. Retrieved April 27, 2015, from http://data.worldbank.org/indicator/SH.DYN.AIDS.ZS.

19. World Bank. (2015). *Incidence of tuberculosis (per 100,000 people)*. Retrieved April 27, 2015, from http://data.worldbank.org/indicator/SH.TBS.INCD/countries.

20. Lopez, A. D., Mathers, C. D., & Murray, C. J. L. (2006). The burden of disease and mortality by condition: Data, methods, and results for 2001. In A. D. Lopez, C. D. Mathers, M. Ezzati, D. T. Jamison, & C. J. L. Murray (Eds.), *Global burden of disease and risk factors* (pp. 45–240). New York: Oxford University Press.

21. Setel, P. W., Macfarlane, S. B., Szreter, S., et al. (2007). A scandal of invisibility: Making everyone count by counting everyone. *Lancet*, 370, 1569–1577.

22. World Health Organization. (2003). Address to WHO staff. Geneva: WHO. Retrieved June 16, 2015, from http://www.who.int/dg/lee/speeches/2003/21_07/en/.

23. Preamble to the Constitution of the World Health Organization as adopted by the International Health Conference, New York, 19-22 June, 1946; signed on 22 July 1946 by the representatives of 61 States (Official Records of the World Health Organization, no. 2, p. 100) and entered into force on 7 April 1948.

24. Merson, M. H., Black, R. E., & Mills, A. J. (2000). *International public health: Diseases, programs, systems, and policies*. Gaithersburg, MD: Aspen Publishers.

25. World Health Organization. *Global burden of disease*. Retrieved May 25, 2006, from www.who.int/trade/glossary/story036/en/.

26. Institute for Health Metrics and Evaluation. (2013). *The global burden of disease: Generating evidence, guiding policy*. Seattle, WA: Institute of Health Metrics and Evaluation. Retrieved July 2, 2015, from http://www.healthdata.org/sites/default/files/files/policy_report/2013/GBD_GeneratingEvidence/IHME_GBD_GeneratingEvidence_FullReport.pdf.

27. World Health Organization. (n.d.). *Health Status Statistics: Mortality. Healthy life expectancy (HALE)*. Retrieved June 16, 2015, from http://www.who.int/healthinfo/statistics/indhale/en/.

28. The Lancet. (2013). Global Burden of Disease Study 2010. Retrieved May 25, 2015, from http://www.elsevierdigital.com/The-Lancet/GBD/.

29. Lopez, A. D., Mathers, C. D., Ezzati, M., Jamison, D. T., & Murray, C. J. L. (2006). Measuring the global burden of disease and risk factors, 1990–2001. In A. D. Lopez, C. D. Mathers, M. Ezzati, D. T. Jamison, & C. J. L. Murray (Eds.), *Global burden of disease and risk factors* (pp. 1–13). New York: Oxford University Press.

30. Institute of Health Metrics and Evaluation. (2013). *GBD compare*. Retrieved April 27, 2015, from http://vizhub.healthdata.org/gbd-compare/.

31. Institute for Health Metrics and Evaluation. (2013). *GBD heat map*. Retrieved April 27, 2015, from http://vizhub.healthdata.org/irank/heat.php.

32. World Health Organization (WHO).(2002). *The world health report 2002: Reducing risks, promoting health life*. Retrieved June 14, 2015, from http://www.who.int/whr/2002/en/whr02_en.pdf.

33. Population Reference Bureau. (2014). *World population data sheet 2014*. Retrieved April 27, 2015, from http://www.prb.org/Publications/Datasheets/2014/2014-world-population-data-sheet.aspx.

34. Lee, R. (2003). The demographic transition: Three centuries of fundamental change. *Journal of Economic Perspectives*, 17(4), 167–190.

35. Omran, A. R. (2005). The epidemiologic transition: A theory of the epidemiology of population change. *Milbank Quarterly*, 83(4), 731–757.

36. Jamison, D. T. (2006). Investing in health. In D. T. Jamison, J. G. Breman, A. R. Measham, et al. (Eds.), *Disease control priorities in developing countries* (pp. 3–34). New York: Oxford University Press.

37. Jha, P., et al. (2005). Prospective study of one million deaths in India: Rationale, design, and validation results. *PLoS Medicine*, 3(2), e18. doi:10.1371/journal.pmed.0030018

38. Westly, E. (2013, December 4). Global health: One million deaths. *Nature*, 55, 22–23. doi:10.1038/504022a

39. Vyawahare, M. (2014, May 22). Door by door, India strives to know about death. *The New York Times*. Retrieved from http://www.nytimes.com/2014/05/23/world/asia/chasing-down-death-india-seeks-answers-on-premature-mortality.html?emc=edit_au_20140522&nl=afternoonupdate&nlid=54524785&_r=0.

40. Aleksandrowicz, L., Malhotra, V., Dikshit, R., Gupta, P. C., Kumar, R., Sheth, J., et al. (2014). Performance criteria for verbal autopsy-based systems to estimate national causes of death: Development and application to the Indian Million Death Study. *BMC Medicine*, 12(21). doi:10.1186/1741-7015-12-21

41. Jha, P. (2014). Reliable direct measurement of causes of death in low- and middle-income countries. *BMC Medicine, 12*(19). doi:10.1186/1741-7015-12-19

42. World Health Organization. (Interviewer) and Jha, P. (Interviewee). (2010). Save lives by counting the dead: Interview with Prabhat Jha. *Bulletin of the World Health Organization, 88*, 161–241. Retrieved from http://www.who.int/bulletin/volumes/88/3/10-040310/en/.

43. Government of Kerala. (n.d.). *Population 2011*. Retrieved June 16, 2015, from http://kerala.gov.in/index.php?option=com_content&view=article&id=4005&Itemid=3185.

44. Black, J. A. (1999). Kerala's demographic transition: Determinants and consequences. *BMJ, 318*(7200), 1771.

45. Zachariah, K. (1984). *The anomaly of the fertility decline in India's Kerala State*. Washington, DC: The World Bank.

46. Black, J. A. (1989). Family planning and Kerala. *National Medical Journal of India, 3*(4), 187–197.

47. Tharakan, P., & Navaneetham, K. (1999). *Population projection and policy implications for education: A discussion with reference to Kerala*. Kerala, India: Centre for Development Studies (Thiruvananthapuram).

48. Ratcliffe, J. (1978). Social justice and the demographic transition: Lessons from India's Kerala State. *International Journal of Health Services, 8*(1), 123–144.

49. United Nations Development Programme. *Kerala—Human development fact sheet*. Retrieved May 11, 2015, from http://www.in.undp.org/content/india/en/home/library/hdr/human-development-reports/State_Human_Development_Reports/Kerala.html.

50. International Institute for Population Sciences and OrcMacro. (2000). *National Family Health Survey (NFHS-2) 1998–1999*. Mumbai: International Institute for Population Sciences and OrcMacro.

51. United Nations Economic and Social Commission for Asia and the Pacific. *India: National population policy*. Retrieved July 21, 2006, from http://www.unescap.org/esid/psis/population/database/poplaws/law_india/indiaappend3.htm.

52. Kutty, V. R. (2000). Historical analysis of the development of health care facilities in Kerala State, India. *Health Policy and Planning, 15*(1), 103–109.

53. Centers for Disease Control and Prevention. *Life expectancy*. Retrieved May 11, 2015, from http://www.cdc.gov/nchs/fastats/life-expectancy.htm.

54. Tsai, K. S. (2006). Debating decentralized development: A reconsideration of the Wenzhou and Kerala models. *Indian Journal of Economics and Business (Special Issue China & India)*.

55. Joseph, K. (1988). *Migration and economic development of Kerala*. New Delhi: Mittal.

CHAPTER 3

Health, Education, Poverty, and the Economy

LEARNING OBJECTIVES

By the end of this chapter the reader will be able to:

- Describe the links between health and education
- Discuss the connections among health, productivity, and earnings
- Describe key relationships among health, the costs of illness, and the impact of health expenditure on poverty
- Discuss critical connections between health and equity
- Describe some relationships between expenditure on health and health outcomes
- Differentiate between public and private expenditures on health
- Understand the use of cost-effectiveness analysis as one tool for making investment choices in health
- Discuss the two-way relationship between health and development

VIGNETTES

Savitha lived in a poor village in south India. When she first became sick, she visited an unlicensed "doctor." She did not recover and then went to a practitioner of Indian Systems of Medicine. After another 2 weeks of illness, she went to the outpatient clinic of the main hospital. By the time Savitha had begun to recover, she had spent the equivalent of $20 on health services and transportation to get to them. She had also missed 2 weeks of work, during which she lost another $20 of income. The total cost of this illness was about 10 percent of Savitha's annual earnings.

Mohammed was in first grade in a small town in northern Nigeria. Mohammed's family was poor. Mohammed was very small and thin for his age and got sick more often than most children. Because of his poor health, Mohammed

was unable to attend school regularly and was forced to quit school after only 1 year. Unfortunately, he could not read or write, had little knowledge of how to work with figures, and was most likely destined for a life of limited job prospects at very low pay.

Birte was born in Denmark to a middle-class family. She was exclusively breastfed until she was 6 months old, when appropriate complementary foods were introduced in a hygienic manner. Her family took her regularly for "well baby" checkups, and she received all of her scheduled childhood immunizations. Her hearing and her eyesight were checked before she enrolled in school. Birte attended school regularly, was attentive in class, and performed well there. She was able to complete high school and medical school and today is a physician.

ABC company was looking for investments in forest products and examined in detail the possibility of investing in Africa. After carefully considering the potential costs and returns to such an investment, the company decided, however, not to invest in Africa but to invest instead in Asia. In the end, the company believed that they were unlikely to make an acceptable profit on any business in Africa because so many of their workers would be infected with HIV/AIDS and malaria.

INTRODUCTION

Health and economic matters are intimately linked in a number of ways. First, health is an important contributor to people's ability to be productive and to accumulate the knowledge and skills they need to be productive, known as "human capital." Second, health status is also a major determinant of one's enrollment in and success in school, which itself is an important contributor to future earnings. Third, the costs of health care are also extremely important to individuals, especially to poor people, because large out-of-pocket expenditures can have a major impact on their financial status and can push them into poverty. Fourth, the costs of health care are also very important because health is a major item of national expenditure in all countries. Finally, the approach that different countries take to the financing and carrying out of health services raises important issues of equity and inequality.[1]

The objective of this chapter is to introduce the two-way relationship between health and development. The chapter examines the connection between health and education. It then reviews the links between health and poverty and health, equity, and inequality. Lastly, the chapter explores the link between health and income at the level of individuals and the connections between health and development more broadly. As it reviews these themes, the chapter introduces some of the basic concepts of both global health and health economics.

HEALTH, EDUCATION, PRODUCTIVITY, AND POVERTY

Health and Education

Essentially, health and education are connected in three ways. First, there are intergenerational links: the health and education of parents affect the health and education of their children. Second, malnutrition and disease affect the cognitive development and school performance of children. Lastly, education enables people to better prevent and manage illness.

The global AIDS epidemic shows how the poor health of one generation can affect the schooling prospects and future earnings of the next generation. When mothers die of HIV/AIDS, for example, children are more likely to be poorly fed, malnourished, and in ill health. As a result, they are also less likely to attend school or to perform well there. During the period that a mother is sick with AIDS, it is also likely that one or more of her children will stay out of school to attend to the mother's health and the chores that the mother is no longer able to do.

Malnutrition and illness can limit schooling and school performance in a number of ways. First, families sometimes delay enrolling a sick or malnourished child in school. In addition, malnutrition and illness can reduce attendance at school and concentration when in school, thereby reducing student performance. Malnutrition and illness can also decrease cognitive development and ability. All of these

factors ultimately constrain children's ability to learn in school, decrease the number of years of schooling they complete, and thereby reduce future earnings.

However, there is also a powerful connection between health and education in the other direction—the impact of education on health. We already know that education and knowledge of appropriate health behaviors are important determinants of health and, indeed, that the education of a child's mother is an important predictor of the health of a child. The higher the level of education of a mother, the more likely she is to immunize her child, as further reflected in **Figure 3-1** for a number of countries.[2]

Another study done in the Philippines illustrated how better-educated mothers are able to keep their children healthy, even in locations without a safe water supply.[3] In a study of a large number of low- and middle-income countries, it was shown that every 10 percent increase in the level of education of mothers led to a reduction in the infant mortality rate by 4.1 deaths for every 1,000 live births.[3] In addition, education affects the extent to which people make use

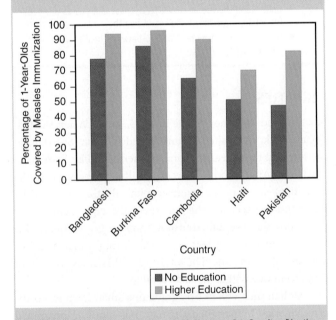

FIGURE 3-1 Percentage of 1-Year-Old Children Receiving Measles Immunization, by Mothers with No Education and Mothers with Higher Education, for Selected Countries, for Most Recent Year

Data from World Health Organization. Global Health Observatory Data Repository Education Data by country http://apps.who.int/gho/data/view.main.94190

of health services, and better education discourages people from engaging in unhealthy behaviors.

The most extensive studies of the links between education and health show that the education of women has a powerful impact on child survival. One key study showed that each additional year of schooling of a woman was associated with a 7–9 percent reduction in the mortality of her children under 5 years of age. That same study concluded that the mortality rate of children under 5 years of age was almost 60 percent lower for the children of mothers with at least 7 years of schooling, compared to the children of mothers with no schooling.[4]

A 2010 review of the available literature on the subject assessed the impact of the education of women on the mortality of children under 5 years of age over the period 1970 to 2009. That study also examined how the impact of a mother's education on child mortality compared with the impact of economic development on child mortality. The study focused on examining how many children died, compared to how many children would have died, if education and economic levels had stayed the same as they were in 1970. The study concluded that a little more than half of the 8.2 million deaths of children under 5 years of age that were averted over this period were attributable to higher educational attainment of women of reproductive age (15 to 44 years old). The study also concluded that economic development had an important association with averting child deaths. However, the association of increased educational attainment of women of reproductive ages with averting child deaths was greater than that of economic development.[5]

Health, Productivity, and Earnings

Health has an important impact on labor productivity and earnings, separate from its link with education. First, good health increases longevity and the longer one lives, the longer one can earn and the higher one's lifetime earnings will be. Second, a number of studies have shown that healthy workers are more productive than unhealthy workers. Among the most cited of such studies was one done on men who tapped rubber trees in Indonesia, many of whom were anemic due to hookworm infection. When the workers were treated for their infections, they became less anemic and their productivity increased by about 20 percent.[6] Third, many people when ill cannot go to work, and when they are absent from work, they often do not earn.

Health, the Costs of Illness, and Poverty

The costs of illness to individuals and their families can be high, can force them to lose or dispose of assets, and can cause them to fall into poverty. When people become ill in poor countries, as noted in the vignette about Savitha at the start of this chapter, they usually do seek health care and they often seek care of different types. They frequently have to pay for treatment and for drugs, the costs of which can be a very substantial share of their income. In addition, illness often leads to a decline in earnings, because people miss work. There are also other indirect costs that people bear when they are ill, such as the costs of transportation to and from a health service provider.

Beyond the costs of either a short-term or a chronic illness, we must also remember the cost to individuals of living with the disability that comes from different health conditions. Measles or meningitis, for example, could lead to severe disability. Polio can lead to paralysis, and leprosy can lead to deformity. A number of mental health conditions are associated with long-term disability. The number of people with diabetes is increasing in rich and poor countries alike, and diabetes is often associated with a variety of disabilities. Long-lasting disabilities generally require considerable expenditure on health services. In addition, they usually lead to a significant decline in the earnings of disabled persons, compared to what they could earn if they were not disabled.

The costs of illness can be devastating for poor families. A study done in Bangladesh, for example, showed that a Bangladeshi lost the equivalent of 4 months of income from being sick with tuberculosis.[7] A recent review of the literature on the financial costs of tuberculosis in low- and middle-income countries found that individuals lost on average 60 percent of their annual earnings due to being sick with tuberculosis and families lost almost 40 percent of their total household income due to such illnesses. These costs fell relatively harder on the poor and were often catastrophic.[8] Surveys done in India showed that hospitalization was a major contributor to people and families falling into poverty. Of the patients who were hospitalized at any point during a 1-year period that was studied, almost 25 percent of the people hospitalized were pushed below the official Indian poverty line because of the costs of their hospitalization, related expenditures, and lost wages. Moreover, more than 40 percent of those hospitalized borrowed money or sold assets to pay for their health care.[9]

In a study that was carried out in preparation for the 2000 World Development Report of the World Bank, poor people consistently noted the importance of maintaining good health. In addition, the report noted that ill health is an important contributor to poverty and to the economic vulnerability that is at the foundation of poverty.[10] Indeed, in many countries, people who do not have adequate health insurance are at risk for catastrophic healthcare costs that could drive them into poverty or bankruptcy.

HEALTH DISPARITIES

Health disparities are an important concern of public health. As we begin to explore this issue, therefore, it is important to review some of the key terms related to health disparities.

The first key term is "equity." The Nobel Laureate in Economics Amartya Sen has suggested that we should see health equity as multidimensional:

> It includes concerns about achievement of health and the capability to achieve good health, not just the distribution of health care. But it also includes the fairness of processes and thus must attach importance to non-discrimination in the delivery of health care.[11, p665]

Sen also suggested that health equity must be seen in the broader context of social justice issues, social structures within countries, and how countries choose to allocate their resources.[11]

A well-known British scholar of public health and the determinants of health, Margaret Whitehead, suggested another definition of equity that has been commonly used: "differences in health that are not only unnecessary and avoidable, but also unfair and unjust."[12]

Another important term is *inequality*. The World Health Organization (WHO) defines *health inequality* as "differences in health status or in the distribution of health determinants between different population groups."[13]

Health disparities is another very commonly used term in public health and global health. The U.S. Centers for Disease Control and Prevention define *health disparities* as "a type of difference in health that is closely linked with social or economic disadvantage."[14]

Although *equity* and *equality* are often used interchangeably when writing about health, in principle, *equity* concerns fairness whereas *equality* largely refers to outcomes. Obviously, the two concepts are closely related. If a health system treats minority people in inequitable ways, such as by offering them lower coverage of key health services than it offers to others, we would expect that the minority group would have poorer health outcomes. In this case, as well as in many other cases, *inequity* plays an important role in the *inequality* of outcomes and the creation of health disparities.

Equity, inequality, and health disparities are themes that run throughout this text. As the text covers these topics, it incorporates the thoughts noted previously of Amartya Sen and Margaret Whitehead, among others. However, the text does not examine in depth the processes by which different societies reach decisions about investing in health and the participation of different social groups in those processes.

It is essential to consider equity, inequality, and health disparities when discussing:

- Health status
- Access to health services
- Coverage of health services
- Protection from financial risks because of health costs
- The extent to which the approach to financing health is fair
- The distribution of health benefits

When thinking about these issues, one should consider the extent to which they vary across groups, why they vary, and what can be done to reduce inequity, inequality, and disparities.

In addition, when considering questions of access to and the coverage of health services, it will be important to consider such questions broadly. It has been suggested, for example, that one must take a multidimensional view of access that would include:[15]

- *Geographic availability*: Distance or travel time
- *Availability*: The extent to which needed services are offered in a convenient manner, by staff who are properly trained to deliver them
- *Financial accessibility*: The extent to which people are able or willing to pay for services and not fall into financial distress by doing so
- *Acceptability*: The extent to which services are in line with local cultural norms and expectations

When taking "an equity, inequality, and health disparity lens" to global health concerns, it is important to consider how they vary with:

- Social and economic status
- Health status and whether or not the person is disabled
- Ethnicity
- Gender
- Religion
- Location
- Occupation
- Social capital

It is also important to keep in mind differences in key health issues both *across* countries and *within* countries.

When proceeding through this book, one should understand that there is an enormous amount of inequity, inequality, and disparities in all of the areas noted here. To a large extent, the pattern of inequity, inequality, and disparities can be summarized relatively easily:

- Less well-off people, with less social and political power, will generally have worse health, poorer health services, and less fairness and protection in the financing of health services than those who are better off.
- These less well-off groups will generally include women, indigenous people, ethnic and religious minorities, the poor, those living in rural areas, those working in the informal sector of the economy, those with limited education, and those who have relatively lower levels of social capital. Generally, disabled people, people with mental illness, and lesbian, gay, bisexual, and transgender people will also face discrimination that leads to inequities, inequalities, and disparities in health.

The following section examines some examples of the most critical concerns about health disparities and their links with inequity and inequality.

Health Disparities Across Countries

World Bank data on some of the basic indicators of health status, including life expectancy, maternal mortality, and neonatal, infant, and under-5 child mortality, clearly portray the enormous variation across regions and countries. Life expectancy in the high-income Organisation for Economic Co-operation and Development (OECD) countries, for example, is about 30 percent higher than in sub-Saharan Africa.[16] The maternal mortality ratio in Sierra Leone, with the highest rate in the world at 1,100 per 100,000 live births, is 275 times higher than in Belarus, which has the lowest ratio in the world.[17] Infant mortality in sub-Saharan Africa is 15 times higher than in the high-income OECD countries, and in South Asia it is more than 10 times the rate in the high-income OECD countries.[18]

Some people see these differences largely as a reflection of the status of economic development in different parts of the world. They might also believe that inequitable relationships among countries are at least partly the cause of weak economic development in the poorer countries. These people would, therefore, see differences in health status at least partly as a reflection of inequity and injustice. However, some people might see health disparities both within and across countries as an indication of the political choices that are made in societies that lack concern for their less well-off people. They also believe this is inequitable and unjust.

Health Disparities Within Countries

Some countries have relatively little variation in health indicators across different population groups. This would generally be the case, for example, in Scandinavia and some of the other high-income countries of Europe. There are other countries, however, that have substantial variance in health indicators across population groups. These will tend to be high-income countries with disadvantaged ethnic minorities, such as the Australia, Canada, or the United States or they will be low- and middle-income countries. Life expectancy for a white American male in 2010, for example, was 76.5 years, whereas that for an African-American male was 71.8 years. This is a difference of about 10 percent.[19] Life expectancy for an aboriginal Australian or Torres Strait Islander female born between 2010 and 2012 was 73.7, compared to 83.1 for a nonindigenous female.[20]

Figure 3-2 shows the under-5 child mortality rate for a sample of five Indian states, including the state with the lowest rate and the state with the highest rate. Figure 3-3 shows the infant mortality rate for five states of Brazil, including the best and worst performing. The graphs show that the worst-performing Indian state has a child mortality rate about six times that of the best-performing state. At the time of this data, the worst-performing Brazilian state had an infant mortality rate almost four times that of Brazil's best performing state. These data are critical reminders of how important it is to look beyond *average* or *national* rates if one is to understand the health status of a country's people, particularly its poorer and more marginalized groups.

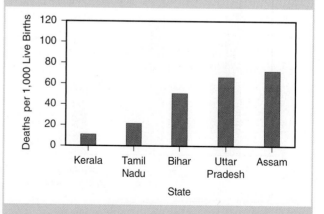

FIGURE 3-2 Projected Under-5 Mortality in Selected Indian States, 2015

Data from Infant and Child Mortality in India, Levels, trends, and determinants, Fact Sheet, Available at: http://www.unicef.org/india/FactsheetExperts.pdf, accessed December 7, 2014.

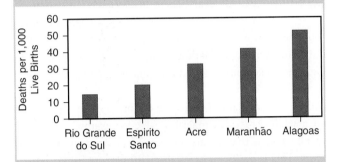

FIGURE 3-3 Infant Mortality Rates, for Selected States, Brazil, 2006

Data from Síntese de Indicadores Sociais: Uma Análise Das Condições de Vida. http://www.ibge.gov.br/home/estatistica/populacao/condicaodevida/indicadoresminimos/sinteseindicsociais2007/indic_sociais2007.pdf. Accessed May 25, 2015.

Health Disparities and Location

We should expect basic health indicators to vary by location, with urban dwellers generally enjoying better access to health services, coverage, and health status than rural dwellers. We would also expect the variation between urban and rural dwellers to be greater in low-income countries than in middle- and high-income countries.[21]

Figure 3-4 shows how the rate of stunting varied by location in three regions, Latin America and the Caribbean,

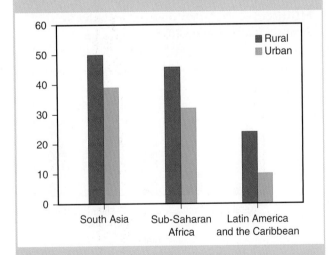

FIGURE 3-4 Percentage of Children, 0 to 5 Years, Who Are Stunted, by Location, for Selected Regions, Latest Data 2003–2009

Data from UNICEF. Progress for Children: Achieving the MDGs with Equity. Available at: http://www.unicef.org/media/files/Progress_for_Children-No.9_EN_081710.pdf. Accessed September 17, 2010.

South Asia, and sub-Saharan Africa. The gaps were most severe in Latin America and the Caribbean, with stunting of children under 5 years of age almost 2.5 times greater in rural areas than in urban ones. Rural children were about 33 percent more likely to be stunted in sub-Saharan Africa than urban children. In South Asia, rural children were about 25 percent more likely to be stunted than urban children. Although differences in health indicators between the lowest and highest income quintiles are often greater in poorer countries, it is important to note that the differences between the lowest and highest income quintiles for some health indicators will be greater in Latin America than elsewhere. This reflects the enormous gaps in some Latin American countries between the incomes of richer and poorer people.[21] These variances also reflect some of the substantial gaps in the way of life between indigenous and nonindigenous people in Central America and the Andean countries.

Figure 3-5 shows, in ascending order by region, how contraceptive use varied between rural and urban areas around the time UNICEF collected this data. In the East Asia and Pacific region, contraceptive prevalence rates were very high and about the same for urban and rural dwellers. In all other regions shown, however, there was a substantial gap in contraceptive prevalence between rural and urban dwellers, ranging from a more than 70 percent difference in sub-Saharan Africa to about a 10 percent difference in Latin America and the Caribbean.

We should expect there to be substantial variation in access, coverage, and health status between rural and urban

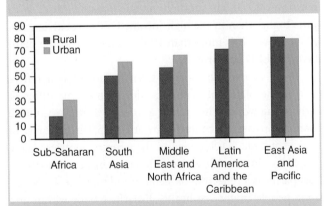

FIGURE 3-5 Percentage of Women 15–49, Married or in Union, Who Are Using Contraception, by Location, for Selected Regions

Data from UNICEF. Progress for Children: Achieving the MDGs with Equity. Available at: http://www.unicef.org/media/files/Progress_for_Children-No.9_EN_081710.pdf. Accessed September 17, 2010.

dwellers. Although many cities do contain large numbers of poor and slum-dwelling people, rural people generally will have lower incomes, less education, less access to health services and other health-related infrastructure, and less political voice than those who live in urban areas. Many ethnic minorities and indigenous people are also more likely to live in rural than in urban settings.

Health Disparities and Income

Much of the literature on health disparities and global health has focused on the relationship between those disparities and income. This literature has highlighted the sharp gaps in access, coverage, health status, fairness of financing, and health benefits between the less well-off and the better-off.[21] Much of this work examined the variation of different health indicators by income quintiles, meaning divisions of the population into five equal income groups from the least well-off to the best-off.

Figure 3-6 examines the extent to which births were attended by skilled personnel in South Asia and sub-Saharan Africa over the period 2003 to 2009. The figure reflects enormous gaps in both regions between the richest and the poorest income groups. In South Asia, the richest 20 percent of the population was four times more likely to have a birth attended by skilled personnel than the poorest 20 percent. In sub-Saharan Africa, the richest 20 percent were three times more likely than the poorest 20 percent to have their birth attended by skilled personnel.

Figure 3-7 looks at the percentage of children who were underweight by income group for South Asia and sub-Saharan Africa around the same time as the other UNICEF data cited previously. This figure reflects almost the same level of variation between the better-off and the least well-off as in the previous figure. Children under 5 from the lowest income group in South Asia were almost three times more likely to be underweight than children from the highest income group. Children under 5 from the lowest income group in sub-Saharan Africa were more than two times more likely to be underweight than those from the highest income group.

Figure 3-8 shows data from UNICEF on the coverage of measles immunization by income group in the UNICEF West and Central Africa and South Asia country groups in 2008. The rates of coverage in West and Central Africa were lower for each income group than in South Asia, and the gaps in immunization coverage between income groups were also greater in West and Central Africa. In West and Central Africa, the children of the richest 20 percent of the families were immunized against measles at more than two times the rate of the children from the poorest 20 percent of the families. In South Asia, the gap between the richest and poorest groups was slightly less than two times.

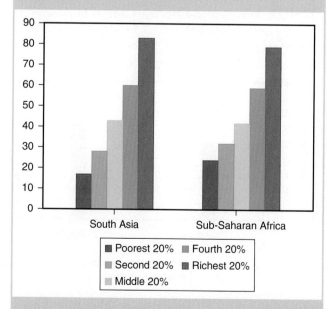

FIGURE 3-6 Percentage of Births Attended by Skilled Personnel, by Income Quintile, Latest Data 2003–2009, for Selected Regions

Data from UNICEF. Progress for Children: Achieving the MDGs with Equity. Available at: http://www.unicef.org/media/files/Progress_for_Children-No.9_EN_081710.pdf. Accessed September 17, 2010.

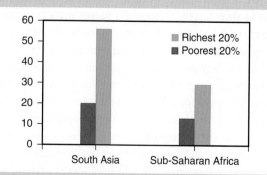

FIGURE 3-7 Percentage of Underweight Children, 0 to 5 Years of Age, by Income Quintile, Selected Regions, 2010

Data from UNICEF. Progress for Children: Achieving the MDGs with Equity. Available at: http://www.unicef.org/media/files/Progress_for_Children-No.9_EN_081710.pdf. Accessed September 17, 2010.

FIGURE 3-8 Coverage of Measles Immunization by Income Quintile, for Selected Regions, 2008

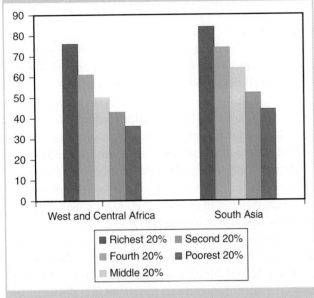

Data from UNICEF. Progress for Children: Achieving the MDGs with Equity. Available at: http://www.unicef.org/media/files/Progress_for_Children-No.9_EN_081710.pdf. Accessed September 17, 2010.

Although these differences by income may not be acceptable to us, they are not surprising. Income is associated with better education; better housing; better access to safe water, sanitation, hygiene, and health services; and safer work environments. It is also associated mostly with dominant ethnic groups, rather than indigenous people or other minorities, as in the Americas. Higher incomes are also associated with more political power and voice.

Health Disparities and Gender

Concerning the health of women, "being born female is dangerous to your health,"[22] especially in low-income countries. Women are discriminated against in many settings in ways that are harmful to their health. This starts with sex-selective abortion and female infanticide. In some settings, this discrimination is also evident in shorter duration of breastfeeding and less food for female children, lower enrollment of girls in school, and less attention to the healthcare needs of girls. There is also an exceptional amount of violence against women and neglect of the healthcare needs of adult women. In most settings, women will also have less power and voice than men. The main point to note here is the importance of keeping in mind the health concerns of women that relate to their diminished place and power in some societies.

Health Disparities and Ethnicity

There is a strong association in most countries between ethnicity and health status, access, and coverage. Examples were given previously of the large gaps between white people and African Americans in the United States and white people and Aboriginal people in Australia.

Figure 3-9 shows how maternal mortality ratios varied in Bolivia and Honduras in data published in 2008 between indigenous people and nonindigenous people, which is the most important ethnic difference in Central and South America that is associated with health. In Honduras, the maternal mortality ratio was about 60 percent higher among indigenous women than the national average. Indigenous women in Bolivia had a maternal mortality ratio that was more than twice the national average.[23]

Given the strong association between ethnicity and power, education, and income, it is not surprising to find such a strong association between ethnicity and health status.

Health Disparities and Other Marginalized Groups

Other marginalized groups also face inequity and health disparities. Some of these might be people who suffer social isolation because they engage in stigmatized occupations. Some might be people with disabilities or deformities, such as people with physical handicaps, blind people, or people with leprosy. Prisoners often lack access to appropriate health

FIGURE 3-9 Maternal Mortality Ratios in Honduras and Bolivia, for Indigenous People and National Averages, per 100,000 Live Births

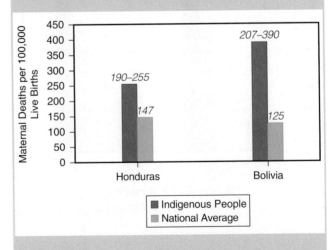

Data from Birdsall N, De La Torre A, Menezes R. Fair Growth: Economic Policies for Latin America's Poor and Middle-Income Majority. Washington DC: Center for Global Development & Inter-American Dialogue; 2008.

services, and prisons are often breeding grounds for communicable diseases. Other people whose behavior may seem to some people as not conforming to local mores, might also face inequity in health, such as lesbian, gay, bisexual, and transgendered people (LGBT), which is discussed further in a policy and program brief later in this chapter.

Financial Fairness

All high-income countries, except the United States, have some type of mandatory and universal health insurance system that is meant to ensure that access to health services is not dependent on income. The United States has recently adopted legislation moving in this direction, but it is not clear if these reforms will be maintained. Many middle-income countries also have such insurance systems. However, most low-income countries do not have formalized health insurance systems, outside of the free or low-cost provision of some health services by the public sector or nongovernmental sectors. Thus, the poor in many countries must bear substantial out-of-pocket costs for health, as discussed later. In addition, many low-income countries fail to protect their poor from potentially catastrophic health costs that higher-income individuals could afford. Moreover, the relative cost of those health services is much greater for the poor than for better-off people, which also raises important equity issues.

Another set of important equity concerns deals with the extent to which different income groups benefit from public subsidies for health services. This can be a complicated issue to assess.[9] Nonetheless, it is clear that there are many countries in which public subsidies for health are disproportionately received by better-off people, as shown in **Figure 3-10**, for India.

The data in this figure are not new, but they nonetheless point to an important issue that is quite common and often ignored even today. It is easy to imagine, for example, a country in which poor people use basic health services financed by the public sector that are relatively inexpensive, whereas better-off people in the urban areas disproportionately use publicly supported hospital services that are relatively expensive. Under these circumstances, better-off people, who will have higher rates of noncommunicable diseases, will get most of the expensive surgeries. Those surgeries will cost hundreds of times what basic health care costs, and the country would be providing a disproportionate share of public subsidies to the better off, rather than to the poor. There is no justification on clinical, economic, or equity grounds for this being the case.

Concluding Comments on Health Disparities

This section has only begun to introduce the many dimensions of equity, inequality, and health disparity issues in

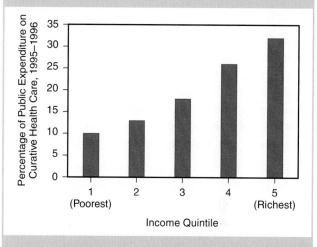

FIGURE 3-10 Percentage Distribution of Public Expenditure on Curative Health Care, India, by Income Quintile

Modified with permission from Peters DH, Preker AS, Yazbek AS, et al. Better Health Systems for India's Poor. Washington DC: World Bank; 2002:4.

global health. When engaging in global health activities, it is critical to:

- Keep equity, inequality, and disparities in mind at all times.
- Always consider the various dimensions of these issues.
- Be careful when using numbers that reflect averages for health indicators, because they may hide variation across and within groups.
- Examine how each piece of key data on health status, access, coverage, and financing relates to different population groups, especially the poor and marginalized.

As noted earlier, much of this text is oriented toward addressing the health concerns of the poor, especially in low- and middle-income countries. Different parts of the book will offer suggestions about how those health needs can be met as quickly as possible and at the lowest possible cost. One critical point in efforts to do this, which emerges partly from concerns for health disparities, is to ensure that the poor and other marginalized groups are involved in the design, development, monitoring, and evaluation of such efforts. It is also crucial to ensure that such activities pay particular attention to monitoring the benefits that accrue to them and the distribution of those benefits to various population groups. Without paying sufficient attention to these points, it is likely that health disparity issues will not be addressed satisfactorily and that it will be difficult to monitor the extent to which the desired benefits of an investment in health go to the intended beneficiaries.[15]

HEALTH EXPENDITURE AND HEALTH OUTCOMES

One of the reasons health is so important to countries is that they spend a lot of money on it. In addition, as noted earlier, they are also trying, in principle, to get the most for the money they spend, consistent with national values. **Figure 3-11** shows the relationship between gross domestic product (GDP) per capita and total health expenditure as a share of GDP.

The main themes that emerge from this figure are clear:

- Most high-income countries cluster around an expenditure of 9–12 percent of their national income on health.

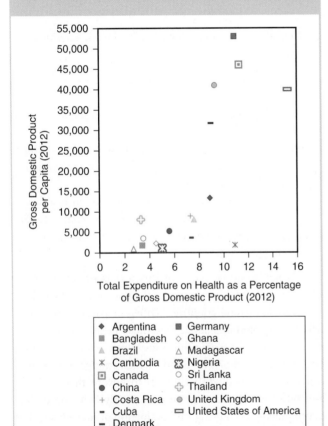

FIGURE 3-11 National Income and Total Health Expenditure, Selected Countries, 2012

Gross Domestic Product per Capita (2012)

Total Expenditure on Health as a Percentage of Gross Domestic Product (2012)

◆ Argentina	■ Germany
■ Bangladesh	◇ Ghana
▲ Brazil	△ Madagascar
✳ Cambodia	⊠ Nigeria
▣ Canada	○ Sri Lanka
● China	✛ Thailand
+ Costa Rica	● United Kingdom
– Cuba	▭ United States of America
– Denmark	

Data from World Bank. Core Development Indicators, 2014. Available at http://data .worldbank.org/indicator. Accessed December 8, 2014.

- Many low-income countries cluster around an expenditure of 3–6 percent of their national income on health. This can be seen for Bangladesh, Ghana, and Nigeria.
- Despite the clustering, there are countries that are outliers—they sit significantly away from the general relationship between income per capita and percentage of national income spent on health. The United States spends more than any other country on health as a share of GDP. Cambodia and Cuba spend relatively more than one would expect for countries at their level of income. Sri Lanka spends relatively less than one would expect.

Having seen what countries spend on health, it is now important to ask what they get in return for that expenditure. Do countries that spend higher shares of their national income on health have better health outcomes? **Figure 3-12** plots total health expenditure as a share of GDP against life expectancy for selected countries.

We can see from this figure that:

- Many low-income countries spend a relatively low share of their GDP on health and also have low life expectancy. This is seen in Ghana and Kenya.
- Some countries, such as Malawi, spend a relatively high share of their GDP on health but still have relatively short lives.
- Most high-income countries spend a relatively high share of their GDP on health and have high life expectancy. This can be seen in Germany and Iceland.
- Some low-income countries spend relatively little on health but still have relatively higher life expectancy than many countries that spend a higher share of GDP on health. This can be seen in China and Sri Lanka.
- Some high-income countries spend relatively high shares of GDP on health but still have lower life expectancy than countries that spend a lower share of GDP on health than they do. This is best shown by the United States, which is an outlier on this figure as well as on Figure 3-11, which portrays total expenditure on health as a share of GDP.

Why is it that some countries are outliers when considering their health outcomes related to health expenditure? First, we know that health status depends on a number of genetic, social, and economic factors, including the "social determinants of health," and those factors vary across countries. Second, health outcomes depend not only on how much countries spend per capita on health, but also on the particular investments they make with that money. In colloquial

FIGURE 3-12 Total Expenditure on Health as a Share of GDP, Compared to Life Expectancy, Selected Countries, 2012

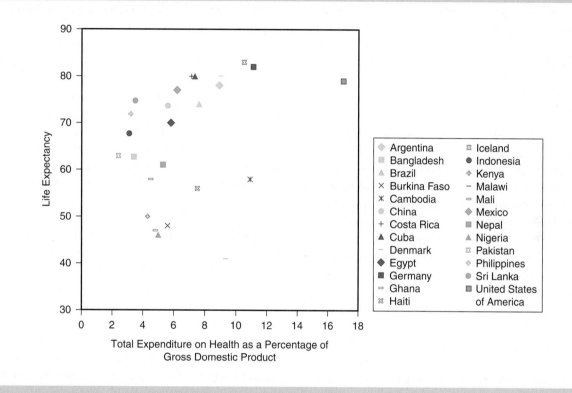

◆ Argentina		⊠ Iceland	
▪ Bangladesh		● Indonesia	
▲ Brazil		✢ Kenya	
✕ Burkina Faso		– Malawi	
✳ Cambodia		▭ Mali	
● China		◆ Mexico	
+ Costa Rica		▪ Nepal	
▲ Cuba		▲ Nigeria	
– Denmark		⊠ Pakistan	
◆ Egypt		✢ Philippines	
▪ Germany		● Sri Lanka	
▭ Ghana		▪ United States	
⊠ Haiti		of America	

Data from World Bank. Core Development Indicators, 2014. Available at http://data.worldbank.org/indicator. Accessed December 8, 2014.

terms we could say, "What you spend the money on is as important as how much you spend."

PUBLIC AND PRIVATE EXPENDITURE ON HEALTH

Another important concept is the distinction between public and private expenditures on health. Public expenditure refers to expenditure by any level of government or of a government agency. Expenditure by a city, state, or national government would be public expenditure. Expenditure on health by government agencies such as a social security system, as in many countries in Latin America; the national insurance agency, as in most countries in Western Europe; or of a specialized agency, such as a national commission on HIV/AIDS, would also be considered public expenditure.

Private expenditure is expenditure that comes from sources other than governments. One such source is the money that individuals spend on health. When this money is not covered or reimbursed by an insurance program, it is also called out-of-pocket expenditures on health. Other sources of private expenditure on health include expenditure by nongovernmental organizations (NGOs), such as by BRAC in Bangladesh or the Self Employed Women's Association (SEWA) in India. In addition, private expenditure on health includes expenditure by the private for-profit sector. Private sector firms, for example, might contribute to the cost of health insurance or health services for their employees. They might also make contributions to the health work of other organizations.

There is some debate about what are legitimate focuses of public expenditure on health.[24] However, there is widespread agreement that public expenditure on health is warranted when the investment benefits society as a whole, such as an immunization program; when health investments promote equity; and when such expenditure provides financial protection to the poor from expenditures on health that they cannot afford.[24]

THE COST-EFFECTIVENESS OF HEALTH INTERVENTIONS

Most governments have a limited amount of money for health, and that money is rarely enough to finance all of the health interventions that a country would like to carry out. Thus, governments have to decide what share of their total budget will go to health and how much of the health budget will be allocated to different health interventions. They also have to consider how those investments will be carried out. All governments have to set priorities for expenditure on health, just as they have to set priorities for expenditure in other sectors.

One important tool for setting priorities for public expenditure on health is cost-effectiveness analysis. This is a method for comparing the cost of an investment with the amount of health that can be purchased with that investment. The cost of the investment can be thought of as the price of the investment. The amount of health that can be purchased could be measured, for example, in deaths, life years saved, or disability-adjusted life years (DALYs). The cost-effectiveness of an investment in health will depend, among other things, on the incidence and prevalence of the health condition being considered; the cost of the intervention; the extent to which it can reduce morbidity, mortality, and disability; and how effectively it can be implemented.

One important example of the use of cost-effectiveness analysis is to set priorities among different ways of achieving the same health goal. Important studies were conducted, for example, on the cost-effectiveness of alternative approaches to treating tuberculosis. These studies examined the cost-effectiveness of 6 months of treatment with direct supervision of people taking their medicines, compared to treatment that was not supervised. The supervised method was more expensive than the unsupervised method. However, the supervised method led to a higher rate of people taking all of their medicine and being cured than the unsupervised approach. As a result, it proved to be more cost-effective than the traditional approach that had been used. These studies strengthened the case for the World Health Organization recommending the supervised approach to therapy, which continues to be the global standard of tuberculosis treatment.[25]

It is easy to imagine how important this type of cost-effectiveness analysis can be when considering different ways of delivering the same health services. In fact, there are many important issues in delivering health services in low-income countries in which such questions remain critical. In Haiti, for example, there is a program operated by Partners in Health. Those carrying out the program had to assess whether the services could be delivered as effectively by volunteer workers as they could be by workers who were paid for their efforts. Although it cost more to deliver the program when the workers were paid, the outcomes were superior to those when the workers were not paid, and Partners in Health has continued to use the approach of paid workers.[26] Another issue of great importance today is the extent to which antiretroviral drugs for HIV can be delivered effectively by nurses and community health workers instead of physicians, because physicians are in such short supply in many countries that have high rates of prevalence of HIV.

The second manner in which cost-effectiveness analysis is used is to compare the costs and the gains of different health interventions so that investment choices can be made among them. For every $100, for example, that a government spends on health, what allocation of government expenditure on health will buy the most DALYs averted? What is the cost per disability-adjusted life year saved from different interventions? In a relatively poor country, with a high burden of communicable diseases, such as tuberculosis and malaria, is it more cost-effective to invest public resources for health in communicable disease control or in coronary bypass surgery? In a richer country with little tuberculosis, will it be cost-effective to invest in vaccination against tuberculosis?

Even if we examine the first question in a somewhat exaggerated and simplistic manner, it will still help us to understand some of the value of cost-effectiveness analysis. Let us say, for example, that the cost of coronary bypass surgery in a low-income country is about $5,000. Let us also say that the costs of such surgery are covered completely by the public sector. This surgery would benefit one individual, who is aged 50 and will live an additional 20 years in perfectly good health because of the surgery. In the same country, we can assume an entire course of treatment for tuberculosis costs about $100. In addition, we can assume that people who get tuberculosis will all be 50 years of age and that they will live an additional 20 years in perfectly good health if they are treated for tuberculosis. What this means, in principle, is that if these were the only choices for the investment of $5,000 in health that a country faced and if this were the only type of analysis that would be done to assess investment choices, then the choice would be between spending the same amount of money to save 1 life or 50 lives. In addition, the choices would be between saving 20 additional years of healthy life of the coronary bypass patient or 1,000 additional healthy years of life of the 50 tuberculosis patients. **Figure 3-13** illustrates the cost-effectiveness of a selected number of health interventions. Although the data in this graphic are somewhat dated, they nicely reflect an important point about the relative cost-effectiveness of different investments in health.

The cost of avoiding ill health caused by tuberculosis, malaria, and hookworms, for example, is low, whereas the cost of saving a life through cancer treatment is high. It is very cost-effective to get people to use seat belts in cars, but much less cost-effective to save the lives of people after they have had car accidents. It is cost-effective to enhance the nutritional and health status of young children through supplementation with vitamin A. However, it is much less cost-effective in health centers and hospitals to deal with the additional morbidity and mortality that occur from measles and pneumonia for children who are deficient in vitamin A.[27]

It is important to note that cost-effectiveness analysis is rarely the sole means for determining choices among investments and generally should not be used in that way.[28]

However, it is one valuable tool in making such choices. It will always be important, however, to consider such analyses in light of a number of other factors, including:[28]

- Equity considerations
- The burden of disease
- The extent to which the investment serves society as a whole
- The extent to which the investment produces benefits in addition to its usual ones
- The impact of the intervention on the provision of insurance

In addition, those who set priorities for health investments will also have to take account of:[28]

- The capacity to deliver the proposed services
- The links between the proposed services and other important services
- The ability to change budget priorities in favor of the proposed investment
- Any transitional costs associated with making the proposed changes in priorities

In this book, most of the cost-effectiveness assessments are calculated using DALYs averted. This is because examining the cost of life years saved from death would fail to capture

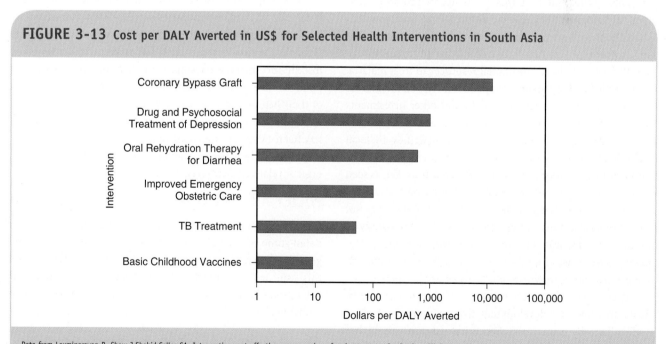

FIGURE 3-13 Cost per DALY Averted in US$ for Selected Health Interventions in South Asia

Data from Laxminarayan R, Chow J, Shahid-Salles SA. Intervention cost effectiveness: overview of main messages. In: Jamison DT, Breman JG, Measham AR, et al., eds. *Disease Control Priorities in Developing Countries*. Washington DC and New York: The World Bank and Oxford University Press; 2006:51.

reductions in morbidity and disability that are also important aims of health interventions. In addition, it is important to note that there is no unique cutoff below which interventions are considered "cost-effective" and above which they are not. WHO has, however, developed thresholds for cost-effectiveness. Using this approach, investments are "highly cost-effective" if the cost per DALY averted is less than GDP per capita, "cost-effective" if the cost per DALY averted is one to three times GDP per capita, and not cost-effective if the cost is more than three times GDP per capita. In any case, it is important to group the cost-effectiveness of different interventions into ranges and to use cost-effectiveness analysis to explore the relative extent to which various interventions will lead to DALYs averted and at what cost.

HEALTH AND DEVELOPMENT

An important question at the core of thinking about global health concerns the links between health and development at the individual, community, and societal levels. Does individual health produce more individual wealth and higher levels of economic development at the community and societal levels? Or are the effects in the opposite direction: Does more economic development at the societal level produce better health for individuals, communities, and societies? What we find when we examine these questions is that the effects of health and development go in both directions.

There is no question that good health promotes economic development at the societal level. First, we know that when countries have to spend money to address health problems, they cannot use that money for other purposes. Countries that have to spend substantial resources to treat malaria, for example, have less money to spend not only on other areas of health, but also on schools, roads, and other investments outside of the health sector that could spur economic growth.

In addition, investment in economic activities, by local and foreign investors, is an essential ingredient to the economic growth prospects of low-income countries. Yet, as seen in one of the vignettes that opened this chapter, countries that have high burdens of communicable diseases may not appear to be good investment choices. In fact, in a study of the impact of malaria on economic development that is frequently cited, it was found that a high prevalence of malaria reduces economic growth by about 1 percent per year.[29]

There is also growing evidence of the importance of health to economic development from a number of other studies done by economists. Some have shown that higher life expectancy at birth is associated with faster economic growth rates. These studies suggest that a country with a life expectancy at birth of 77 years would be expected to grow economically 1.6 percent faster each year than a country with a life expectancy at birth of 49 years.[29] Another study showed that poor health was an important contributor to the slow pace of economic growth of countries in Africa, compared to other countries with better health.[30] Another series of studies showed that improvements in nutritional status and related health status improvements were very important historically in boosting labor productivity and spurring economic growth in the United Kingdom and Europe.[31-34]

It is also true that higher levels of economic development do promote better health at the level of both individuals and society. In fact, studies on the impact of income on the health of different societies suggest that higher income is associated with better health and longer life expectancy.[34] However, more recent analyses of this question suggest that although income growth is associated with better health indicators for a country, the effect of income alone on health indicators is less significant than previously thought. Rather, these analyses suggest that a considerable share of the improvements in health indicators stem, as noted earlier, from progress in education; from technical progress such as the development of new vaccines or new drugs; or from simple life-saving approaches, such as the use of oral rehydration for young children with diarrhea.[35]

In this light, we should ask: Is income growth necessary or sufficient for enhancing health status at the individual, community, or societal levels? Over the long run, increases in income will improve health. However, they will not improve it fast enough in most settings to achieve the health status objectives that many countries have set for themselves or that are necessary to achieve the Millennium Development Goals in the time that has been set for them. What low- and middle-income countries must do, therefore, is adopt public policy choices that will allow them to speed the achievement of their health aims, even in the face of constrained income, as Kerala did. As indicated earlier, this is the approach that has been taken by the small number of countries that have been particularly successful in meeting their health aims, even at relatively low levels of income per capita.

POLICY AND PROGRAM BRIEF

One policy and program brief follows. It explores in greater detail some of the health equity issues that arise for lesbian, gay, bisexual, and transgender people. Although the data on this issue are not extensive, the brief will enable further consideration of this matter as one continues to study or work in global health.

Health Equity and Lesbian, Gay, Bisexual and Transgender People

There has been an increasing global awareness of the health disparities experienced by lesbian, gay, bisexual, and transgender (LGBT) individuals.[36] Conservative estimates suggest that there are 84 million individuals, or 1.2 percent of the world's population, who identify with a sexual orientation other than heterosexual, including LGBT people.[36] Stigma and discrimination often heighten the vulnerability of these populations to experiencing health disparities, as these populations are often subject to institutionalized prejudice, social stress, social exclusion, public hatred and violence, and consequently even possibly an internalized sense of shame about their sexuality.[37] In some low- and middle-income countries, these sociopolitical factors can be more pronounced because engaging in homosexual acts is considered a criminal offense.[38]

LGBT individuals can experience increased risk of certain health conditions because social factors such as stigma and discrimination can have a direct impact on an individual's health status. Negative social attitudes, perceived discrimination, and even violence can place stressors on the lives of these individuals that contribute to these observed health outcomes.[36] For example, lesbian, gay, and bisexual people (LGB) have a documented increased risk in mental disorders including depression, suicidal ideations, and substance dependence compared to heterosexuals in North America, Europe, and Canada.[36] Similarly, a meta-analysis of studies conducted in the United States and other high-income countries specifically found that over a period of one year, the risk of depression in LGB individuals was at least twice that of heterosexuals.[37] Overall, there is a lack of data on equity for LGB people in low- and middle-income countries, often because of cultural and political sensitivity. It is likely that these health inequities persist or are exacerbated in these contexts, and there is an urgent need to generate further evidence in order to better target interventions.

Recent literature has given light to the inequities faced by the global transgender community, which the United Nations Development Programme (UNDP) defines as "all people whose sense of their gender identity differs from the sex they were assigned at birth."[39] Many transgender people do not have access to the health care they need and deserve not only because of social stigma and discrimination, similar to the LGB community, but also because the appropriate services do not exist. A large-scale survey in the United Kingdom found that 17 percent of transgender people had been refused services by a doctor or nurse because of their gender identity.[39] Similar to LGB people, transgender people often have worse health outcomes because they lack access to the needed interventions. UNAIDS and WHO have noted that transgender women often experience HIV prevalence rates in excess of 60 percent but there are few targeted interventions for them and limited research on effective interventions.[39] Moreover, transgender people experience health conditions that do not fit into either men's or women's health areas, reflecting that healthcare services often fail to meet their needs or to have sufficiently sensitive healthcare workers.

Equity and MSM

Like LGBT people, men-who-have-sex-with men (MSM) often experience inequitable health outcomes because of their social status. For example, it is estimated that the HIV prevalence among MSM in southern Africa is 21.4 percent, compared to 10 percent for the general population.[40] MSM can experience an increased risk of certain diseases or conditions because of biological or behavioral factors that can become exacerbated in certain contexts when their marginalized status prevents them from receiving preventative interventions or appropriate treatment.[41] MSM have elevated risks for HIV infection, for example, because of higher probabilities of HIV transmission in receptive anal sex and because of their higher probability of engaging in risky behaviors such as extra-primary partnerships. Nonetheless, these risk factors can be mitigated with effective interventions such as targeted distribution of condoms and lubricant, as well as targeted pre-exposure prophylaxis. Yet, these interventions are currently lacking in most settings.[41,42]

Although most of the current literature on inequitable outcomes for MSM is on HIV, it has been suggested that these patterns affect MSM for other health conditions as well, especially those conditions associated with mental health, similar to LGBT community.[43] These differences may reflect a lack of healthcare access or fear of seeking health services for MSM. In general, research has shown that MSM who disclose their sexual orientation have better health outcomes than MSM who do not, but social stigma and discrimination often prevent this.[43] One study found that 17.6 percent of MSM in Malawi, 18.3 percent of MSM in Namibia, and 20.5 percent of MSM in Botswana were afraid to seek health services due to their sexual orientation.[44] In all three of these countries, prevention or treatment programs for this population did not exist before 2012 and remain limited in nature, as is the case for many other countries. The inequities in health outcomes for MSM will remain until interventions no longer neglect MSM or fail to acknowledge their unique needs.

Overall, there is a need for more comprehensive analyses of the inequities faced by LGBT people and MSM in low- and middle-income settings, if more effective health services are to be available to these groups. To achieve this, it will be essential to train healthcare workers to work with greater sensitivity to and respect for these groups.[40] It will also be important to educate society more broadly about the LGBT and MSM communities in order to help reduce stigma and discrimination against them.[45]

CASE STUDY

Having read about the high returns to some investments in health and the need to prioritize investments in health, it will be valuable to end this chapter with a case study of another public health success story. This one concerns Guinea worm. Those interested in more detail in the case should consult *Case Studies in Global Health: Millions Saved.*[46]

The Challenge of Guinea Worm in Asia and Sub-Saharan Africa

Background

Dracunculiasis, or Guinea worm disease, is an ancient scourge that once afflicted much of the world. Today, it is truly a disease of the poor, persisting only in some of the world's most remote and disadvantaged regions with limited access to potable water, despite being one of the most preventable parasitic diseases. In the 1980s, an estimated 3.5 million people in 20 countries in Africa and Asia were infected with Guinea worm disease, and an estimated 120 million were at risk of becoming infected.[47]

The disease is contracted by drinking stagnant water from a well or pond that is contaminated with tiny fleas that carry Guinea worm larvae. Once inside the human, the larvae can grow up to 3 feet long. After a year, the grown female worm rises to the skin in search of a water source to release her larvae. A painful blister forms, usually in the person's lower limbs. To ease the burning pain, infected individuals frequently submerge the blister in water, causing the blister's rupture and the release of more larvae into the water. This contaminated water, when it is drunk, perpetuates the cycle of reinfection. Worms, usually as wide as a match, can take up to 12 weeks to emerge from the blister. They are coaxed out by being slowly wound around a stick a few centimeters each day. Debilitating pain from this process can linger for as long as 18 months.

Although rarely fatal, the disease takes a heavy toll by causing low productivity that makes it both a symptom and perpetrator of poverty—in Mali, it is called the "disease of the empty granary." Because water in contaminated ponds is widely consumed during peak periods of cyclical harvesting and planting, an entire community can be left debilitated and unable to work during the busiest agricultural seasons. The economic damage is severe: annual economic loss in three rice-growing states in Nigeria was calculated at $20 million.[48] Although the disease afflicts all age groups, it particularly harms children.[48] School absenteeism rises when infected children are unable to walk to school and when children forgo school to take on the agricultural and household work

of sick adults. The likelihood of a child in Sudan being malnourished is more than three times higher when the adults in the child's home are infected with the disease.

The Intervention

In 1980, when the U.S. Centers for Disease Control and Prevention (CDC) first proposed an eradication campaign, the three interventions that would be required to address the disease effectively did not seem feasible: construction of expensive water sources, controlling the vector that spreads the disease through the use of larvicides in water sources, and health education campaigns promoting the filtration of water with a cloth filter, self-reporting of infections, and avoidance of recontamination of public water sources. The absence of a vaccine or cure made success seem even more improbable.

The International Drinking Water Supply and Sanitation Decade was launched the following year, however, and the CDC's D.A. Henderson seized the opportunity to include the eradication of Guinea worm disease as a subgoal of the Water Decade program. Nonetheless, progress against Guinea worm disease remained slow until 1986, when three key events occurred: WHO declared eradication of Guinea worm disease a goal, public health ministers from 14 African nations met to affirm their commitment to the eradication effort, and U.S. President Jimmy Carter became a powerful advocate, personally persuading many leaders to launch national eradication efforts. He also recruited the help of two former popular heads of state of Mali and Nigeria, General Amadou Toumani Touré and General Yakubu Gowon, respectively, thereby consolidating political commitment in Africa.

Meanwhile, technical and financial resources of the donor community were marshaled, and by 1995, eradication programs had been established in 20 countries. Water sources were provided, mainly through the construction of wells; in southeast Nigeria alone, village volunteers hand-dug more than 400 wells.[49] Larvicide was added to water sources to kill the fleas. People were taught to filter drinking water using a simple cloth filter. However, these filters were found to clog up and were used as decoration items instead.[48] A newly developed nylon cloth was then donated by the Carter Center, Precision Fabrics, and DuPont. Public education campaigns, including intensive efforts during so-called worm weeks, encouraged people to use the nylon filters, avoid recontaminating ponds, and report infections.[50] Most of the eradication staff were volunteers trained by the ministries of health, but they pioneered a monthly reporting system for tracking and monitoring that is now hailed as a model for disease surveillance.[51]

The Impact

The campaign led to a 99 percent drop in Guinea worm disease prevalence. In 2005, fewer than 11,000 cases were reported, compared with an estimated 3.5 million infected people in 1986. Most remaining cases were then in Sudan where civil conflict impeded progress against the disease over many years. By 1988, the campaign had already prevented between 9 million and 13 million cases of Guinea worm disease.[51] The Asian countries that were targeted–India, Pakistan, and Yemen–are now free of the disease.

Costs and Benefits

The total cost of the program between 1986 and 1998 was $87.5 million, with an estimated cost per case averted of $5 to $8.[51] The World Bank determined that the campaign has been highly cost-effective and cost-beneficial. In addition, the program had a very high economic rate of return, even when basing the calculation of economic benefits only on increases in agricultural productivity that accrued from people having avoided the disease.[51]

Lessons Learned

Success of the program has been attributed to three factors. The first is the exemplary coordination between major partners and donors. The second is the power of data, gathered through the monthly reporting system, to monitor national programs and to help keep countries focused and motivated on the program goals. The third is the high-level advocacy and political leadership from current and former heads of state, especially President Jimmy Carter and General Gowon, who visited and revisited villages in Nigeria to check on progress. The program drew on a truly global partnership among the CDC, UNICEF, WHO, the Carter Center, governments, NGOs, the private sector, and volunteers that was able to motivate changes in individual and community behaviors and successfully control a disease.

The Guinea Worm Eradication Campaign has continued to be successful and the world is nearing eradication of Guinea worm. Between January 1 and April 30 of 2015, there were only 3 reported cases of Guinea worm in the world.[52]

MAIN MESSAGES

The aim of this chapter was to introduce some of the basic concepts of economics as they relate to the global health arena. One important message of the chapter is that education and health are closely linked. Good health encourages school enrollment at the appropriate age, improves school attendance, enhances students' cognitive performance, and increases the completed years of schooling. Education and knowledge are consistently correlated with engagement in more appropriate health behaviors and living healthier lives compared to people with less schooling. Important progress in reducing child mortality, for example, is associated with increased educational attainment for women. In addition, education promotes greater opportunities for income earning, which itself is an important determinant of health.

We also learned that health is strongly associated with productivity and earnings. Healthier people can work harder, work more hours, and work over a longer lifetime than can those who are less healthy. Related to this in many ways, we also saw that health has an important relationship with poverty. If people work fewer hours because of ill health, then there is a risk that their income status will decline, perhaps below the poverty line. In addition, there is evidence from many countries that the direct and indirect costs to individuals of obtaining health services can push people into poverty.

Equity, inequality, and health disparities are important concerns of public health. It is essential to consider these factors when discussing health status, access to health services, coverage of services, protection from financial risk, the fairness of financing health, and the distribution of health benefits.

Health is an important subject for all countries for many reasons, among the most important of which is the amount of money they spend on health. Generally, high-income countries spend more money on health per capita and as a share of GDP than do low-income countries. However, health outcomes depend not just on how much money is spent, but also on how the money is used. One way that countries set priorities for health expenditure is by using cost-effectiveness analysis, a tool that is used in the health sector to compare how much health one can buy for a given level of expenditure. All countries, of course, face the question of how they can maximize the health of their population for the minimum cost.

There are also many strong relationships between the health of a population and the economic development of the society in which they live. Better health does promote wealth in a variety of ways, including enhancing labor productivity, reducing the amount countries have to spend on health, and enabling a more attractive investment climate. In addition, the negative impact of some diseases on economic development, such as tuberculosis, HIV/AIDS, and malaria, can be very significant. Economic development does improve health; however, many gains in health stem from educational and technological progress, such as on vaccines. Low-income countries have to develop approaches to improving population health faster than economic development alone will do.

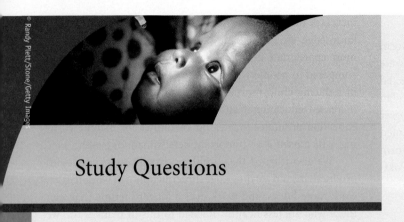

Study Questions

1. How does poor health status affect a person's income?

2. What is the relationship between health and the productivity of individuals?

3. What part does health play in promoting the education of a child?

4. What part does the education of a mother play in promoting the health of her children?

5. Why might the health of some culture groups be different from the health of others?

6. What is the relationship between a country's expenditure on health as a share of national income and its health status?

7. In your country, is expenditure on health from the public sector, private sector, or both?

8. In using cost-effectiveness analysis, why should you also take into account issues such as equity?

9. How could you ensure that public subsidies on health care appropriately benefit the poor?

10. Does "health make wealth," or does "wealth make health"?

11. What impact would the health status of a country have on the likelihood that people will invest in economic activity in that country?

12. Why did Guinea worm disease remain so prevalent for so long?

REFERENCES

1. Ruger, J. P., Jamison, D. T., & Bloom, D. E. (2001). Health and the economy. In M. H. Merson, R. E. Black, & A. J. Mills (Eds.), *International public health, diseases, programs, systems, and policies* (pp. 617–666). Gaithersburg, MD: Aspen.

2. Pebley, A., Goldman, N., & Rodriguez, G. (1996). Prenatal and delivery care and childhood immunization in Guatemala: Do family and community matter? *Demography, 33,* 197–210.

3. Glewwe, P. (1997). *How does schooling of mothers improve child health? Evidence from Morocco.* Washington, DC: World Bank.

4. Hobcraft, J. (1993). Women's education, child welfare and child survival: A review of the evidence. *Health Transition Review, 3*(2), 159–175.

5. Gakidou, E., Cowling, K., Lozana, R., & Murray, C. J. L. (2010). Increased educational attainment and its effect on child mortality in 175 countries between 1970 and 2009: A systematic analysis. *Lancet, 376*(9745), 959–974.

6. Basta, S. S., Soekirman, Karyadi, D., & Scrimshaw, N. S. (1979). Iron deficiency anemia and the productivity of adult males in Indonesia. *American Journal of Clinical Nutrition, 32*(4), 916–925.

7. Croft, R. A., & Croft, R. P. (1998). Expenditure and loss of income incurred by tuberculosis patients before reaching effective treatment in Bangladesh. *International Journal of Tuberculosis and Lung Disease, 2*(3), 252–254.

8. Tanimura, T., Jaramillo, E., Weil, D., Raviglione, M., & Lonnroth, K. (2014). Financial burden for tuberculosis patients in low- and middle-income countries: A systematic review. *European Respiratory Journal, 43*(6), 1763–1775.

9. Peters, D. H., Preker, A. S., Yazbek, A. S., et al. (2002). *Better health systems for India's poor.* Washington, DC: The World Bank.

10. World Bank. (2001). *World development report 2000/2001: Attacking poverty.* New York: Oxford University Press.

11. Sen, A. (2002). Why health equity? *Health Economics, 11*(8), 659–666.

12. Whitehead, M. (1992). The concepts and principles of equity and health. *International Journal of Health Services, 22,* 429–445.

13. World Health Organization. (n.d.). *Health impact assessment. Glossary of terms used.* Retrieved December 4, 2014, from http://www.who.int/hia/about/glos/en/index1.html.

14. Centers for Disease Control and Prevention. *Social determinants of health. Definitions.* Retrieved December 4, 2014, from http://www.cdc.gov/socialdeterminants/Definitions.html.

15. Peters, D. H., Garg, A., Bloom, G., Walker, D. G., Brieger, W. R., & Rahman, M. H. (2008, June). Poverty and access to health care in developing countries. *Annals of the New York Academy of Sciences, 1136,* 161–171.

16. World Bank. (n.d.). *Life expectancy at birth, total (years).* Retrieved November 13, 2014, from http://data.worldbank.org/indicator/SP.DYN.LE00.IN/countries/ZG-XS?display=graph.

17. World Bank. (n.d.). *Maternal mortality ratio (modeled estimate, per 100,00 live births).* Retrieved June 5, 2015, from http://data.worldbank.org/indicator/SH.STA.MMRT.

18. World Bank. (n.d.). *Infant mortality rate (per 1,000 live births).* Retrieved November 13, 2014, from http://data.worldbank.org/indicator/SP.DYN.IMRT.IN/countries/ZG-XS-8S?display=graph.

19. Centers for Disease Control and Prevention/National Center for Health Statistics. (2013). Table 18: Life expectancy at birth, at age 65, and at age 75, by sex, race, and Hispanic origin: United States, selected years 1900–2010. In *Health, United States, 2012.* Hyattsville, MD: Author. Retrieved October 25, 2013, from http://www.cdc.gov/nchs/data/hus/hus12.pdf#018.

20. Australian Institute of Health and Welfare. Life Expectancy. (2015). Retrieved February 10, 2015, from http://www.aihw.gov.au/deaths/life-expectancy/.

21. Gwatkin, D. R., Rutstein, S., Johnson, K., Suliman, E., Wagstaff, A., & Amouzou, A. (2007). *Socio-economic differences in health, nutrition, and population within developing countries.* Washington, DC: The World Bank.

22. Murphy, E. M. (2003). Being born female is dangerous to your health. *American Psychologist, 58*(3), 205–210.

23. Birdsall, N., De La Torre, A., & Menezes, R. (2008). *Fair growth: Economic policies for Latin America's poor and middle-income majority.* Washington, DC: Center for Global Development & Inter-American Dialogue.

24. Preker, A. S., & Harding, A. (2000). *The economics of public and private roles in health care.* Washington, DC: The World Bank.

25. Murray, C. J., DeJonghe, E., Chum, H. J., Nyangulu, D. S., Salomao, A., & Styblo, K. (1991). Cost effectiveness of chemotherapy for pulmonary tuberculosis in three sub-Saharan African countries. *Lancet, 338*(8778), 1305–1308.

26. Walton, D. A., Farmer, P. E., Lambert, W., Leandre, F., Koenig, S. P., & Mukherjee, J. S. (2004). Integrated HIV prevention and care strengthens primary health care: Lessons from rural Haiti. *Journal of Public Health Policy, 25*(2), 137–158.

27. Laxminarayan, R., Chow, J., & Shahid-Salles, S. A. (2006). Intervention cost effectiveness: Overview of main messages. In D. T. Jamison, J. G. Breman, A. R. Measham, et al. (Eds.), *Disease control priorities in developing countries.* New York: Oxford University Press.

28. Yazbeck, A. S. (2002). *An Idiot's Guide to Prioritization in the Health Sector.* The World Bank: Washington, DC.

29. Commission on Macroeconomics and Health. (2001). *Macroeconomics and health: Investing in health for economic development.* Geneva: World Health Organization.

30. Bloom, D. E., & Sachs, J. (1998). Geography, demography, and economic growth in Africa. *Brookings Papers on Economic Activity, 2,* 207–295.

31. Fogel, R. (1991). *New sources and new techniques for the study of secular trends in nutritional status, health, mortality and the process of aging* (NBER Historical Working Paper No. 26). Cambridge, MA: National Bureau of Economic Research.

32. Fogel, R. (1997). New findings on secular trends in nutrition and mortality: Some implications for population theory. In M. Rosenzweig & O. Stark, (Eds.), *Handbook of population and family economics* (Vol. 1a, pp. 433–481). Amsterdam: Elsevier Science.

33. Fogel, R. (2000). *The fourth great awakening and the future of egalitarianism.* Chicago and London: The University of Chicago Press.

34. Pritchett, L. H., & Summers, L. H. (1996). Wealthier is healthier. *Human Resources, 31*(4), 841–868.

35. Jamison, D. T., Sandbu, M., & Wang, J. (2004). *Why has infant mortality decreased at such different rates in different countries?* Bethesda, MD: Disease Control Priorities Project.

36. Logie, C. (2012). The case for the World Health Organization's commission on the social determinants of health to address sexual orientation. *American Journal of Public Health, 102*(7), 1243–1246. doi: 10.2105/AJPH.2011.300599.

37. King, M., Semlyen, J., Tai, S., Killaspy, H., Osborn, D., et al. (2008). A systematic review of mental disorder, suicide, and deliberate self harm in lesbian, gay and bisexual people. *BMC Psychiatry, 8,* 70.

38. Beyrer, C., & Baral, S. D. (2011, July 7–9). *MSM, HIV and the law: The case of gay, bisexual and other men who have sex with men (MSM),* Working Paper for the Third Meeting of the Technical Advisory Group of the Global Commission on HIV and the Law.

39. United Nations Development Programme. (2013). *Transgender health and human rights. Discussion paper.* Retrieved November 6, 2014, from http://www.undp.org/content/dam/undp/library/HIV-AIDS/Governance%20of%20HIV%20Responses/Trans%20Health%20&%20Human%20Rights.pdf.

40. Ryan, O., et al. (2013). *Achieving an AIDS-free generation for gay men and other MSM in southern Africa.* New York: AmfAR; Baltimore, MD: Johns Hopkins School of Public Health.

41. *Lancet special issue on HIV in men who have sex with men: Summary points for policy makers.* (2012, July). Retrieved October 21, 2014, from

http://www.amfar.org/uploadedFiles/_amfarorg/On_the_Hill/Summary PtsLancet2012.pdf.

42. Baral, S., Sifakis, F., Cleghorn, F., & Beyrer, C. (2007). Elevated risk for HIV infection among men who have sex with men in low- and middle-income countries 2000–2006: A systematic review. *PLoS Medicine, 4*(12), 1901–1911.

43. Centers for Disease Control and Prevention. (2010). *Gay and bisexual men's health.* Retrieved November 6, 2014, from http://www.cdc.gov/msmhealth/mental-health.htm.

44. Baral, S., Trapence, G., Motimedi, F., et al. (2009). HIV prevalence, risks for HIV infection, and human rights among men who have sex with men (MSM) in Malawi, Namibia, and Botswana. *PLoS ONE, 4,* e4997.

45. Reisser, W. (2014, September 26). Free and equal: Working with the United Nations to support LGBT rights. *Dipnote: U.S. Department of State official blog.* Retrieved November 6, 2014, from http://blogs.state.gov/stories/2014/09/26/free-and-equal-working-united-nations-support-lgbt-rights.

46. Levine, R., & What Works Working Group. (2007). *Case studies in global health: Millions saved.* Sudbury, MA: Jones & Bartlett.

47. Cairncross, S., Muller, R., & Zagaria, N. (2002). Dracunculiasis (Guinea worm disease) and the eradication initiative. *Clinical Microbiology Reviews, 15*(2), 223–246.

48. Hopkins, D. R. (1998). Perspectives from the dracunculiasis eradication programme. *Bulletin of the World Health Organization, 76*(Suppl 2), 38–41.

49. Hopkins, D. R., Ruiz-Tiben, E., Diallo, N., Withers, P. C., Jr., & Maguire, J. H. (2002). Dracunculiasis eradication: And now, Sudan. *American Journal of Tropical Medicine and Hygiene, 67*(4), 415–422.

50. Hopkins, D. R. (1998). The Guinea worm eradication effort: lessons for the future. *Emerging Infectious Diseases, 4*(3), 414–415.

51. Kim, A., Tandon, A., & Ruiz-Tiben, E. (1997). *Cost-benefit analysis of the global dracunculiasis eradication campaign.* Washington, DC: World Bank.

52. The Carter Center. Guinea Worm Disease: Worldwide Case Totals. Retrieved June 3, 2015 from: http://www.cartercenter.org/health/guinea_worm/case-totals.html.

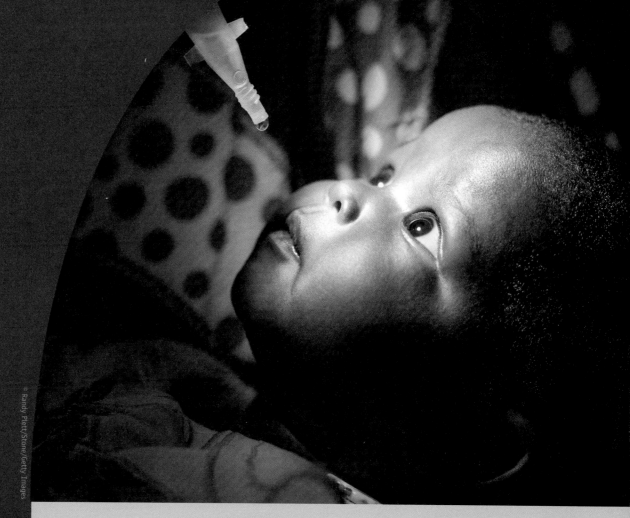

PART II

Cross-Cutting Global Health Themes

CHAPTER **4**

Ethical and Human Rights Concerns in Global Health[1]

VIGNETTES

Suraiya was a 21-year-old woman in Kabul, Afghanistan. Her sister recently died in childbirth at the age of 16. Suraiya took her sister to a health center when she was having trouble with her labor. However, the health center was 50 miles away from their house. In addition, partly because of the neglect of the last government and its discrimination against women, the health center was dilapidated. It had no equipment and the midwife there was unable to save Suraiya's sister. The baby died a few days later.

John Williams was a 32-year-old office clerk in a small country in sub-Saharan Africa. For three months he had experienced weight loss, continuous fever, and chronic fatigue. He finally got up the strength to visit the local hospital. When he got there, the staff was not welcoming. They did not treat him kindly. They did not offer to help him. They did not arrange for him to be seen by a doctor. They knew that he had HIV and did not want to treat him in their hospital.

A research team was conducting a study of malaria in villages in West Africa. When the doctors working for the study diagnosed children with severe malaria, they would provide treatment free of charge. However, sometimes the children in the study had other medical problems that needed attention. For example, many children presented with diarrheal diseases, parasitic infections, or pneumonia. Some of the doctors wanted to treat all these children, too. Other members of the team worried that their budget would not cover these extra costs. In any case, they said, the purpose of the study was to learn about malaria, not to provide clinical care.

The newly elected government of an Indian state won election on a pledge to increase investment in health care. The government plans to build new primary health clinics, but with the limited money available, only a few can be built and staffed. Some members of the government argue that the clinics should be located in the countryside. People there are poorer than in the cities and have less access to medical facilities. Others argue that the cities should get priority. An clinic in the urban slums serves more people than a rural clinic and is easier to staff and supply. Besides, they say, the party's electoral base is in the city, and if they want to be re-elected to continue their good work, it is important to keep their voters happy.

THE IMPORTANCE OF ETHICAL AND HUMAN RIGHTS ISSUES IN GLOBAL HEALTH

Painful ethical dilemmas arise in the pursuit of global health, whether planning healthcare provision, implementing public health measures, or conducting health research. It is important to address these issues, both for their own sake and because there is a strong complementarity between good ethical and human rights practices on the one hand and good health outcomes on the other.[2]

One set of important ethical issues that relate to global health concerns human rights. International conventions and treaties recognize access to health services and health information as human rights. Yet, there are remarkable gaps in many countries in access to health services. The poor and the disenfranchised suffer from those gaps the most.

The failure to respect human rights is often associated with harm to human health. This has often been the case, for example, with diseases that are highly stigmatized, such as leprosy, tuberculosis (TB), and HIV. If leprosy patients are not provided with the best care because some health workers are afraid to work with them, the leprosy patients cannot stop the progression of their disease. If TB patients are shunned by health workers, they may die, usually after infecting many other people.

Efforts to maintain public health while dealing with new and emerging diseases, such as SARS, a potential avian influenza, or the Ebola virus, raise another array of ethical and human rights issues. When we face a potential health threat, for example, what are the rights of individuals compared to the rights of society to protect its members from illness? Is it acceptable to quarantine a city? Is it fair to ban travel to and from certain places? These are real issues with which policymakers and health practitioners must wrestle.

Another set of ethical issues is associated with research with human subjects. Health research involving people is generally considered ethically challenging because, in contrast to clinical care, participants in research are put at risk for the sake of other people's health, rather than their own. An important part of the research that takes place in the pursuit of global health must also deal with further ethical concerns that arise when research is conducted with poor people who do not have access to satisfactory levels of health care outside of a research study.

Finally, it is important to ensure that health investments are fair and made in fair ways. Even in high-income countries, the resources available for health care are limited. In low- and middle-income countries, where there are fewer resources and greater needs, difficult decisions about which populations and disease groups should get priority must constantly be made.

This chapter provides an overview of some of the most important ethical issues pertaining to global health. It briefly reviews the most important charters and conventions that set the foundation for health-related human rights and shows some of the contexts in which human rights concerns arise. It summarizes some important cases and guidance documents pertaining to the ethics of international medical research and discusses how to evaluate the ethics of clinical research. It then lays out the principles that are often thought to underlie fair allocation decisions and some of the difficulties in applying them. The chapter concludes with comments on key challenges concerning ethics and human rights in global health activities.

THE FOUNDATIONS FOR HEALTH AND HUMAN RIGHTS

The cornerstone of human rights is the International Bill of Human Rights, which is made up of the Universal Declaration of Human Rights, the International Covenant on Civil and Political Rights, and the International Covenant on Economic, Social, and Cultural Rights. These documents place obligations on governments to *respect*, *protect*, and *fulfill* the rights they state; that is, to refrain from violating people's rights, to prevent others from violating them, and to actively promote the realization of people's rights.

The most significant international declaration on human rights is the Universal Declaration of Human Rights (UDHR), which was promulgated in 1948. The UDHR is generally regarded as the basis for most of the later treaties and documents pertaining to human rights. As a declaration, the UDHR does not have the force of law. However, it has moral force, it has influenced the development of a number of national constitutions, and its invocation by many states over the last 50 years has led some to argue that it has the status of customary international law—unwritten law that is nonetheless reflected in the practice of states.[3] With respect to health, the UDHR states in Article 25:

> (1) Everyone has the right to a standard of living adequate for the health and well-being of himself and of his family, including food, clothing, housing and medical care and necessary social services, and the right to security in the event of unemployment, sickness, disability, widowhood, old age or other lack of livelihood in circumstances beyond his control.
> (2) Motherhood and childhood are entitled to special care and assistance. All children, whether born in or out of wedlock, shall enjoy the same social protection.[4]

Since 1948, more than 20 multilateral treaties that are legally binding and relate to health have been formulated. In 1966, two important treaties were adopted—the International Covenant on Economic, Social, and Cultural Rights

(ICESCR) and the International Covenant on Civil and Political Rights (ICCPR).[5,6] These two covenants are legally binding on those states that have ratified them (155 countries in the case of the ICESCR and 160 in the case of the ICCPR). The ICCPR discusses rights of equality, liberty, and security, and freedom of movement, religion, expression, and association.[6] The ICESCR focuses on the well-being of individuals, including their right to work in safe conditions, receive fair wages, be free from hunger, get an education, and enjoy the highest attainable standard of physical and mental health.[5]

Although increasing attention is being paid to the links between health and human rights, there is no mechanism for holding countries accountable for ensuring that they honor or even try to honor the right to health. The international mechanism now in place for reviewing compliance with treaties and conventions that include the right to health is voluntary reporting by national governments. There are also provisions in human rights treaties and conventions that recognize that resource-poor countries will not be able to help all of their people to "achieve the highest standard of health possible."[7] Instead, states are required only to "take steps" toward the progressive realization of positive rights. There is also no clear definition of the meaning of the "right to health" or agreed indicators for measuring progress toward fulfilling it.[8] Although considerable attention is paid to the Millennium Development Goals (MDGs) and progress toward meeting them, the discussion about the MDGs frequently does not take human rights explicitly into account. It will be important to see the extent to which the Sustainable Development Goals that will be articulated in 2015 will make reference to human rights and the "right to health."

At least 115 countries have written a right to health or health care into their constitutions.[9] In recent years, several countries have seen litigation successfully result in access to previously unavailable treatment. For example, in Brazil there are thousands of court cases each year in which individual patients sue the government to receive drugs that they are not receiving through the public health system.[10] In South Africa, the Treatment Action Campaign successfully sued the national government over its failure to make the drug nevirapine widely available for HIV-infected pregnant women to prevent mother-to-child transmission.[11] In 1999, a court in Venezuela held that the Venezuelan government violated the constitutional right of its people to health by failing to guarantee access to antiretroviral therapy for people living with HIV/AIDS. The court ruled that this right is *both* part of the Venezuelan constitution and a part of the ICESCR, to which Venezuela is party.[12]

Women and children are especially vulnerable groups in many countries, and enhancing their health is central to improving the well-being of the poor. For these reasons, a number of international conventions focus on women and children.

The Convention on the Elimination of All Forms of Discrimination Against Women was adopted in 1979 by the United Nations General Assembly. It has been ratified by 83 countries. The convention commits states to legally promote equality between men and women and to eliminate discriminatory practices against women, and it affirms women's reproductive rights.[13]

Many international human rights documents, including the ICCPR, have specific clauses for protecting the rights of children. Most articles in the general human rights instruments also apply equally to both adults and children. The 1989 Convention on the Rights of the Child (CRC), however, is the first human rights document that focuses specifically on children. This document accords children—defined as "every human being below the age of 18 years"—the right to be free of discrimination, to health, and to education. In addition, it states that children must have a say in decisions affecting their lives and puts the rights of children on the same plane as the rights of adults.[14]

The CRC says the following concerning health:

> States Parties recognize the right of the child to the enjoyment of the highest attainable standard of health and to facilities for the treatment of illness and rehabilitation of health. States Parties shall strive to ensure that no child is deprived of his or her right of access to such health care services.[14]

SELECTED HUMAN RIGHTS ISSUES

There are many human rights issues relating to health that could be considered here. This section examines two overarching issues—the rights-based approach to health and limits to human rights—and then discusses some human rights issues related to HIV/AIDS, which illustrate many of the points previously made.

The Rights-Based Approach

Some scholars and global health advocates argue that we should adopt a human rights approach to global health. This approach builds upon the insight that the fulfillment of people's human rights is conducive to their health (and that the violation of human rights tends to be detrimental to health). For some human rights—such as the right to health or the right to an adequate standard of living—this is obvious. However, the importance of the social determinants of health, including relative social status, discrimination, and social exclusion, suggests that the fulfillment of civil and political rights may have an important relationship with population health.[15] Health and human rights are therefore inextricably linked.

In simple terms, if we were to apply the health and human rights approach to global health, this would mean that we would:

- Assess health policies, programs, and practices in terms of their impact on human rights
- Analyze and address the health impacts resulting from violations of human rights when considering ways to improve population health
- Prioritize the fulfillment of human rights

The health and human rights approach reminds us to take an inclusive view of what is needed to promote health: it is not just a matter of having sufficient doctors and drugs, but of addressing poverty, homelessness, education, discrimination, violence, and civil and political inclusion. Moreover, in the design and implementation of global health efforts, we should pay particular attention to factors such as the participation in program design of affected people and communities, equity across groups, and the empowerment of individuals over their own lives.

Limits to Human Rights

The importance of protecting human rights related to health is widely acknowledged. Yet, there are exceptional circumstances in which someone's rights may be temporarily suspended. For instance, in order to protect the interest of the public during an influenza epidemic or an outbreak of an emerging or reemerging infectious disease such as the Ebola virus, a government might suspend for a certain time the right of people to leave their homes, to go to work, to travel, or to participate in mass gatherings, such as sporting events. Few people would deny the obligation of governments to make laws that permit urgent action to protect public health. However, few would also deny the tendency of autocratic governments to use the excuse of public order or the public interest to consolidate power and squash political opposition. Consequently, any suspension of people's rights should be as narrow as possible, so that only those aspects of their rights that allow the government to achieve its legitimate goals are suspended. Furthermore, the suspension should be carried out with due process, rights should be monitored during the suspension period, and all efforts should be made to reinstate them as soon as possible.[16]

Human Rights and HIV/AIDS

As much as any health condition in history, HIV/AIDS raises a host of human rights issues. One reason for this is that HIV/AIDS is a health condition that is stigmatized and discriminated against in most cultures. For example, many people see HIV/AIDS as a disease that people bring on themselves by engaging in what they consider promiscuous behavior. This could be homosexual sex, injection drug use, having multiple sex partners, or commercial sex work. In addition, in places where people are not familiar with how the disease is spread, there is often great fear of catching the disease.

An important question that has arisen in many societies is how to protect the rights of people who are HIV-positive to employment, schooling, and participation in social activities. When the epidemic was first recognized, there was considerable discrimination in a number of countries against HIV-positive people, some of whom lost their jobs or were not allowed to enroll in school. Such discrimination continues in many places.

Another matter, as we saw in the opening vignette with John Williams, is the access of people with HIV to health care. In at least the early stages of the HIV/AIDS in many countries, most health workers were poorly informed about HIV, not aware of how it is spread, and were afraid to care for people who were HIV-positive. In fact, people living with HIV/AIDS have frequently been denied care or treated with discrimination when they did receive it.

HIV testing raises further questions related to protecting people's well-being while respecting human rights. For many years, a cardinal principle of work on HIV has been that testing for it should be voluntary and confidential. This is to ensure that people were not forced to get tested and then discriminated against if others find out that they were HIV-positive.

This point highlights the issues of confidentiality that also arise in the context of HIV/AIDS. Yet, the clinical settings in many resource-poor countries with high HIV prevalence are poorly organized, inefficient, and not accustomed to treating patients and patient records confidentially. They also may not have the physical space to treat people privately and confidentially.

Related to concerns about privacy are important questions about the disclosure of HIV status. Should the healthcare system notify spouses or sexual partners of the HIV status of patients? Should the patients do that? What are the risks? For example, if a husband is notified about the status of his wife, he may harm her, reject her, or his family might throw her out of the house.

As mentioned already, a constitutional right to health has been successfully invoked in several countries in order to get access to HIV/AIDS treatment. One of the reasons why this strategy has been adopted is the high market price of antiretroviral therapy (ART) in many settings. At present, patients with HIV/AIDS in low- and middle-income countries must be put on ART when their immune systems have deteriorated to a certain point and must then remain on ART for the rest of their lives. The majority of people living in these countries cannot afford the cost of such drugs.

The high market price of ART is, in part, a function of the patent system. Patents are intellectual property rights that allow the inventors of novel pharmaceutical products and medical technologies the right to exclude others from making, selling, or importing the invention for a fixed period (usually 20 years). The quasi-monopoly granted to the patent holder allows the setting of prices without regard to ordinary market forces and, therefore, allows higher prices than would be the case in the event of competition. Some countries historically refused to grant patents or granted only process patents on what they regarded as "essential drugs," because they believed that their people have a right to these drugs at affordable prices. However, recent international agreements have changed this picture. The World Trade Organization's (WTO's) 1994 Agreement on Trade-Related Aspects of Intellectual Property Rights (TRIPS), once fully implemented, will standardize intellectual property rights across WTO member states.

The basic principle behind granting intellectual property rights is to provide incentives for research, development, and use of new technologies. Some people believe that the possibility of getting a patent is essential to ensuring the continued search for new drugs. On the other hand, only 16 of the 1,393 new chemical entities marketed between 1975 and 1999 were to treat tropical diseases and tuberculosis,[17] a picture that does not appear to have greatly changed in the last decade.[18] This suggests that patents are not sufficient to encourage the development of drugs for low- and middle-income countries.[19] In the case of HIV/AIDS, the cost of antiretrovirals has dropped dramatically over the last decade or so, partly because of competition from generic manufacturers and partly because of extensive international activism and diplomacy.

In certain cases, intellectual property rights seem to be an impediment to the fulfillment of human rights, such as the right to health. The challenge with respect to patents for medicines is how to encourage scientific discovery of diagnostics, drugs, and vaccines while ensuring the affordability of medicines by poor people in poor countries. Those advocating a human rights approach to health, as well as others

concerned about the price of medicines, insist on safeguard mechanisms to ensure access to medicines by all who need them and on exceptions to intellectual property rights for least developed countries.[20]

Although these rights-related questions are particularly prominent when thinking about HIV/AIDS, many of them are relevant to global health more generally. For example, many vulnerable populations and disease groups are stigmatized or discriminated against. Likewise, all patients ought to be treated with respect and their medical records kept confidential. Finally, questions about the appropriate limits that can be placed on people's rights might arise even more dramatically with other communicable diseases. For example, the isolation or quarantine of people who have drug-resistant tuberculosis or the Ebola virus forcefully raises the question of how to balance individual liberty with the safety of the public.

RESEARCH ON HUMAN SUBJECTS

Research is essential for improving global health. Not only do new health interventions need to be developed to address the world's diseases, but ways to deliver existing interventions also need to be improved. However, health research generates some distinctive ethical problems. Eventually all new healthcare interventions must be tested with human beings, but most research studies are not designed to benefit the people who participate in them. Instead, they are designed to create knowledge that can help patients in the future. Medical research therefore raises special ethical concerns because research participants are put at risk for the sake of other people's health.

This section outlines some historically important cases in research ethics and surveys some of the ethical guidelines that emerged from them. It describes the current global system of review for research ethics. Finally, it considers how to go about the ethical evaluation of clinical research.

Key Human Research Cases

A number of historical cases of research on human subjects have raised ethical concerns and encouraged the development of guidelines for carrying out research ethically. Among the best known of these are the Nazi medical experiments, the Tuskegee Study in the United States, and the "short-course" trials for the drug zidovudine (AZT) in Africa and Asia.

The Nazi Medical Experiments

In 1931 the Reich Circular on Human Experimentation laid out German regulations for the conduct of research with human beings. With a strict requirement for the consent of the subject (or the subject's legal representative) and restrictions on the risks to which children could be exposed, these regulations were ahead of their time. But, just a few years later, German physicians and scientists perpetrated some of the worst medical atrocities in history.

Hitler's accession to the chancellorship in 1933 began a process of Nazification of the German state and German society. This included research institutions, universities, and the medical profession. It coincided with the rise in popularity of eugenics in many countries. With the Nazi emphasis on racial purity, this eventually led to widespread forced sterilization of "undesirable groups," such as people with disabilities, people with inherited mental and physical anomalies, and ethnic minorities, and eventually the "euthanasia" of hundreds of thousands of "incurables."[21] The views that justified these acts were supported by the research of anthropologists and geneticists.

German medical researchers conducted many experiments on euthanasia victims, prisoners of war, and the occupants of concentration camps. In support of the war effort, prisoners were deliberately infected with diseases like tuberculosis and malaria. Josef Mengele, as camp doctor at Auschwitz, studied around 900 children in his twin camp, where he conducted operations without anesthetic, killed children's siblings, and injected children with infective agents. Anthropologists collected body parts from prisoners of war and concentration camps for the study of comparative anatomy.

Following the end of World War II, amid widespread evidence of medical research abuses by the Nazis, the Allies set up an International Scientific Commission to investigate and document these abuses. Subsequently, 23 Nazi scientists were charged with war crimes and crimes against humanity at the Nuremberg Doctors' Trial. Sixteen were convicted, of whom seven were sentenced to death and hanged.

Most of the researchers who took part in medical research under the Nazis were not prosecuted. Indeed, many of them went on to scientific careers in postwar Germany, and until the 1990s, specimens taken from Holocaust and "euthanasia" victims were preserved in German medical institutes.[21] Debate continues over the use of the results of the Nazi medical research. Some commentators argue that most of the experiments were poorly designed and so the data are valueless. Others contend that the research does contain valuable data, but there is disagreement over whether it would be ethical to use it.[22]

The Tuskegee Study

In 1932, the U.S. Public Health Service (PHS), in collaboration with the Tuskegee Institute, began a study of syphilis in Macon County, Alabama. One of the study's original aims was to justify the creation of syphilis treatment programs for African Americans at a time of considerable racial discrimination.

Six hundred African American men took part in the study, 399 with syphilis and 201 without. The men were told by researchers that they were being treated for "bad blood," a term that was used locally to describe a number of ailments, including syphilis, anemia, and fatigue. Those participating in the study received aspirin and iron tonics to make them think that they were being treated, and their families were offered burial stipends if they agreed to autopsies.[23] In fact, the men were not being treated at all: the study's aim was simply to document the natural history of syphilis.

The Tuskegee Study of Untreated Syphilis in the Negro Male, though originally planned to last 6 months, went on for 40 years.[24] In its early years, the infected participants would not have received treatment outside of the study anyway, given the limited treatment options available for syphilis and their limited contact with doctors. However, during the late 1930s and the 1940s the PHS repeatedly intervened to prevent them from receiving effective treatment, even when penicillin became widely available after World War II.

In July 1972, a front-page article in the *New York Times* broke the story of the Tuskegee study. In response to the ensuing public outcry, the U.S. Assistant Secretary for Health and Scientific Affairs appointed an advisory panel to review the study, and it was swiftly brought to a close. In the summer of 1973, the National Association for the Advancement of Colored People (NAACP) filed a class-action lawsuit on behalf of the Tuskegee subjects. It was settled out of court. As part of the $9 million settlement, the U.S. government promised to give free medical and burial services to all living participants, as well as health services for wives, widows, and children who had been infected because of the study.

The impact of Tuskegee on human subjects research was profound. U.S. Senate hearings on human experimentation in 1973 focused further attention on the study. These hearings were followed by the creation of the National Commission for the Protection of Human Subjects of Biomedical and Behavioral Research, whose recommendations would eventually result in the U.S. regulations for the protection of human research subjects.[23]

The "Short-Course" AZT Trials

In 1994, a study conducted by the AIDS Clinical Trials Group demonstrated the effectiveness of the antiretroviral drug zidovudine (AZT) in preventing mother-to-child transmission of HIV. The complex "076 regimen," which started administering AZT in the second trimester of pregnancy and continued through to treatment of the infant, reduced HIV infection by two-thirds.[25] It immediately became the standard of care in high-income countries. In most low-income countries, however, the 076 regimen was thought to be too complicated and too expensive to implement. Such countries were exactly the places where the HIV epidemic was worst and where an effective preventive was needed. Consequently, there was great interest in developing a cheaper intervention that would be easier to implement.

Following a meeting organized by the World Health Organization (WHO), 15 trials were planned to take place in low- and middle-income countries, mostly in sub-Saharan Africa, including tests of simpler "short-course" AZT regimens. The trials provoked fierce criticism. Opponents of the trials noted that they would not be permitted to take place in high-income countries, where the 076 regimen was the standard of care. They therefore accused the sponsors of the short-course AZT trials of ethical double standards. Moreover, they claimed that the studies violated the restrictions on placebo use stated in the Declaration of Helsinki (which is discussed later in this chapter).[26] In 1997, Peter Lurie and Sidney Wolfe wrote in the *New England Journal of Medicine*:

> Residents of impoverished, postcolonial countries, the majority of whom are people of color, must be protected from potential exploitation in research. Otherwise, the abominable state of health care in these countries can be used to justify studies that could never pass ethical muster in the sponsoring country.[27]

Proponents of the trials defended their design. They noted that the results of the trials were likely to be valuable to the communities from which the participants were drawn. The trials were therefore not exploiting poor people for the gain of people in high-income countries. The 076 regimen would not, in any case, be available to the women enrolling in these trials, and so they were not being deprived of treatment. Finally, they argued that there were methodological reasons for using a placebo-controlled design. A study using the 076 regimen as an active control was quite likely to show that the short-course regimen was inferior. However, it would not show whether the short-course regimen was better than nothing at all. Furthermore, the background rate of mother-to-child transmission of HIV varied between populations, which meant that a comparison to placebo would be scientifically necessary.[28]

Unlike the Nazi experiments and the Tuskegee study, which were clearly unethical, the ethics of the short-course AZT trials remain controversial. Although some commentators remain convinced that they were unethical, many people think that trials like these are essential if we are to develop interventions that can help large numbers of people in low- and middle-income countries. The debate over these trials did highlight the existence of additional ethical issues concerning research conducted in low- and middle-income countries. Along with a framework for evaluating the ethics of human subjects research, these additional issues are outlined next.

RESEARCH ETHICS GUIDELINES

The Nuremberg Code

At the close of the Nuremberg Trial, the three presiding U.S. judges issued the Nuremberg Code (see **Table 4-1**). It was the first document to specify the ethical principles that should guide physicians engaged in human subjects research.[29] Among other principles, it states that the "voluntary consent of the human subject is absolutely essential," emphasizes

---

TABLE 4-1 The Standards of the Nuremberg Code

- Those who participate in the study must freely give their consent to do so. They must be given information on the "nature, duration, and purpose of the experiment." They should know how it will be conducted. They must not be forced or coerced in any way to participate in the experiment.
- The experiment must produce valuable benefits that cannot be gotten in other ways.
- The experiment should be based on animal studies and a knowledge of the natural history of the disease or condition being studied.
- The conduct of the research should avoid all unnecessary physical and mental suffering and injury.
- The degree of risk of the research should never exceed that related to the nature of the problem to be addressed.
- The research should be conducted in appropriate facilities that can protect research subjects from harm.
- The research must be conducted by a qualified team of researchers.
- The research subject should be able to end participation at any time.
- The study will be promptly stopped if adverse effects are seen.

Data from The Nuremberg Code. Available at: http://www.hhs.gov/ohrp/archive/nurcode.html. Accessed November 17, 2014.

that human subjects should only be involved in research if it is necessary for an important social good, and requires limits on and safeguards against risks to participants. The Nuremberg Code was foundational for later research ethics guidelines and national regulations.

The Declaration of Helsinki

In 1964, the World Medical Association (WMA) developed a set of ethical principles, the Declaration of Helsinki, to guide physicians conducting biomedical research with human subjects. Although the declaration targets physicians (the

members of the WMA), its principles are supposed to apply equally to nonphysicians. It is the most influential and most cited set of international research ethics guidelines. The Declaration of Helsinki was revised in 1975, 1983, 1989, 1996, 2000, 2008, and 2013.[30]

Some key principles from the Declaration of Helsinki are summarized in **Table 4-2**.

The Belmont Report

On July 12, 1974, the U.S. National Commission for the Protection of Human Subjects of Biomedical and Behavioral

---

TABLE 4-2 The Declaration of Helsinki: Key Principles

Scientific Validity
- Medical research involving human subjects must conform to generally accepted scientific principles and be based on a thorough knowledge of the scientific literature.

Fairness
- Groups that are underrepresented in medical research should be provided appropriate access to participation.
- Medical research with a vulnerable group is justified only if the research is responsive to the health needs or priorities of this group and the research cannot be carried out in a nonvulnerable group. In addition, this group should stand to benefit from the knowledge, practices or interventions that result from the research.
- In advance of a clinical trial, sponsors, researchers, and host country governments should make provisions for posttrial access for all participants who still need an intervention identified as beneficial in the trial.

Risks and Benefits
- The well-being of the individual research subject must take precedence over all other interests.
- The importance of the objective of a study must outweigh the risks to the research subjects.
- Physical, mental, and social risks must be minimized.

Placebos
- A new intervention must be tested against the best current proven intervention, except when:
  - No current proven intervention exists; or
  - Where for methodological reasons the use of placebo is necessary and subjects who receive placebo will not be subject to any risk of serious or irreversible harm.

Consent
- Potential subjects must give voluntary, informed consent.
- For a potential research subject who is incompetent, the physician must seek informed consent from a legally authorized representative.
- Where possible, the physician must seek the assent and respect the dissent of an incompetent potential research subject.

Oversight and Accountability
- The research protocol must be submitted to an independent research ethics committee before the study begins.
- Every clinical trial must be registered in a publicly accessible database before recruitment begins.
- Authors have a duty to make publicly available the results of their research, including negative and inconclusive results.

Modified from World Medical Association. Declaration of Helsinki. Available at: http://www.wma.net/en/30publications/10policies/b3/index.html. Accessed August 16, 2010.

Research was created via the U.S. National Research Act. The commission's mandate was to identify basic ethical principles for the conduct of biomedical and behavioral research with human subjects and to develop guidelines for researchers so that all human research would conform to the principles identified. The commission prepared what has come to be known as the Belmont Report.[31] The ethical principles of this report and their applications are outlined in **Table 4-3**.

EVALUATING THE ETHICS OF HUMAN SUBJECTS RESEARCH

The Nuremberg Code, the Declaration of Helsinki, and the Belmont Report all provide ethical principles that should be used to evaluate research protocols. But how should one carry out this evaluation? A simple framework, derived from the general principles enunciated in the Belmont Report, can help us systematically think through the ethics of many proposed clinical research studies. According to this framework, a clinical research protocol must satisfy at least six conditions: (1) social value, (2) scientific validity, (3) fair subject selection, (4) acceptable risk/benefit ratio, (5) informed consent, and (6) respect for enrolled subjects.[32]

In general, research is ethically justified only if it is socially beneficial; that is, if it generates knowledge that can help people. Otherwise, it exposes participants to risks and burdens for no good reason. A study can fail to be socially beneficial in two ways. First, if the scientific questions that the study seeks to answer are not important questions; for example, if the results of the study are known beforehand, then its data are not important. This gives rise to the requirement that research must have *social value*. Second, a study can fail to be socially beneficial, even if it is trying to answer important questions, if the study methodology is inadequate to answer those questions. For example, if a study will not enroll enough participants to generate a statistically significant result, then the methodology is inadequate. If a study cannot test its hypotheses, then no matter how important they are, it cannot result in social benefit. This gives rise to the requirement that research must be *scientifically valid*.

The third requirement, *fair subject selection*, concerns the equitable distribution of the benefits and burdens of research. When considering who will be asked to enroll in a study, researchers should make sure they do not enroll members of vulnerable populations in risky studies simply for

TABLE 4-3 The Belmont Report

Basic Ethical Principle	Application of the Principle
Respect for Persons: • Treat individuals as autonomous persons. • Protect individuals with diminished autonomy.	Informed Consent: • Individuals should be allowed to make an informed, voluntary decision about what happens to them. • Individuals whose capacity is limited should be given the opportunity to choose to the extent that they are able.
Beneficence: • Maximize possible benefits. • Minimize possible harms.	Assessment of Risks and Benefits: • A data-based risk/benefit assessment should be made. • Risks to subjects should be outweighed by the sum of the benefits to subjects and the benefit to society. The interests of the subjects should be given priority. • Risks should be reduced to those necessary to achieve the research objective.
Justice: • The benefits and burdens of research must be distributed fairly.	Selection of Subjects: • There must be fair procedures and outcomes in the selection of those participating in the research.

Data from U.S. National Institutes of Health, Office of Human Subjects Research. *The Belmont Report: Ethical Principles and Guidelines for the Protection of Human Subjects of Research.* Available at: http://www.hhs.gov/ohrp/humansubjects/guidance/belmont.html. Accessed November 17, 2014.

reasons of convenience. Similarly, privileged people should not be preferred for participation in research that promises to be beneficial. Sometimes enrollment criteria are explicit; for example, a study may exclude children or people with certain comorbidities. Other times they are more subtle; for example, a study that requires extended visits to a hospital may exclude people who cannot take time away from work or family responsibilities, and a study that advertises for participants online will exclude people who do not have access to the Internet.

The requirement for an *acceptable risk/benefit ratio* combines several concerns. First, the risks to participants should be minimized as much as possible consistent with meeting the scientific objectives of the study. Second, there is a limit to the level of risk to which participants may be exposed. We do not, for example, think that people should be asked to risk their lives for the cause of science. Finally, the risks to participants must be balanced by the possible benefits to the participants and to society. Thus, the social value of a study is a vital part of the assessment of whether the risk/benefit ratio is acceptable.

Obtaining competent people's *informed consent* to research participation respects them by letting them choose what happens to them. Valid informed consent consists of several elements, including that potential participants must understand key elements of the research and that they must make a voluntary choice to participate. Some individuals, such as children, are unable to give their own consent. They are respected by having a surrogate decision maker give permission for research enrollment on their behalf and by being involved in the decision as far as they are able.

In some cultures, there are people with the authority to make decisions on behalf of other competent adults. For example, it may be considered normal for a village elder to make decisions on behalf of the people living in the village or for a husband to make decisions on behalf of his wife. It is important that research be conducted in culturally sensitive ways. However, this does not imply that any competent adult may be enrolled in research against his or her will. The individual's informed consent should always be obtained.

Researchers still have a number of ethical duties once participants are enrolled. For example, they must respect participants' rights to withdraw from research, protect their confidentiality, and so on. These duties fall under the umbrella of *respect for enrolled subjects*.

Going through these principles in order is a helpful way to systematically evaluate the ethics of a proposed research study. However, they are not the only considerations that are ethically relevant, and the framework does not tell us how

to balance conflicting principles against one another. For example, how should we decide when it is permissible to use a study design that exposes subjects to a slightly greater risk of harm in order to collect more valuable data? Thus, the framework does not constitute a checklist, but simply a guide to some of the most important ethical considerations and an order in which to consider them.

Research in Low- and Middle-Income Countries

The short-course AZT trials controversy put a spotlight on the ethics of clinical research conducted in low- and middle-income countries. Such research is frequently sponsored by institutions or companies based in high-income countries, and it draws on a pool of potential participants who are likely to be poor, undereducated, and without access to good quality medical care outside of research participation. Consequently, some ethical issues arise much more frequently in this research. Three of the most important issues are summarized here: (1) the standard of care, (2) posttrial benefits, and (3) ancillary care.

The "standard of care" discussion centers on questions concerning what level of medical care should be provided to participants in controlled clinical trials. These trials give an experimental intervention, say a new drug, to members of one group of participants and compare their symptoms with a similar group of people who do not receive the intervention. Sometimes the comparison group, or *arm*, receives an established treatment, sometimes an inactive substance (placebo), and sometimes nothing at all. Much debate has focused on when it is permissible to give participants a placebo when an effective treatment already exists for the condition being studied. This was the question at the heart of the dispute over the short-course AZT trials. However, similar questions can arise whenever the standard of care offered in any arm of the trial is less than the standard available to patients in high-income countries with universal health care.[28] At present, there is some consensus that a lower standard of care may be offered when this is both scientifically necessary to answer a socially valuable question and participants receiving a lower standard of care will not be at risk of serious harm. Other cases remain controversial.

The issue of posttrial benefits arises both with respect to participants and with respect to the community or society they come from. When research participants are also patients, they may receive treatment during a trial. But at the end of the trial their condition may not be cured. For example, participants in HIV/AIDS treatment trials may be treated with antiretroviral therapy during the trial. However, if they do not continue this treatment after the trial, their condition will start to deteriorate again. In high-income countries with universal health care this is not a problem, because participants will leave the trial and then receive continuing treatment in their communities. However, in low- and middle-income countries this may not be an option for the majority of participants. It is widely recognized that posttrial benefits to participants is an important ethical issue. Nonetheless, what benefits should be provided and by whom has not been decided in a definitive manner. [33,34]

Concerns have also been raised about whether other members of the communities hosting research will benefit. For example, a pharmaceutical company might test a new drug for schizophrenia on patients in Peru, but either not market the drug in Peru or price it out of the reach of most of Peru's population. To some commentators, such trials seem exploitative. They argue that research should not be permitted unless the communities that host it will have access to successful interventions that result.[35,36] Other commentators argue for a broader understanding of how exploitation can be avoided. They think that communities that host research should receive a fair level of benefits from the research, but this need not be in the form of posttrial access to interventions.[37] So, for example, the provision of other medical care or investment into health-care facilities might be acceptable community benefits.

Ancillary care is medical care that is given to study participants but that is not required by the scientific design of the study. In the vignette at the beginning of this chapter, malaria researchers were conflicted about whether they should provide ancillary care to the children in their study, including treatment for malaria, diarrhea, parasitic infections, and pneumonia. Such dilemmas are common for researchers who are working in environments where many people lack access to health care. The researchers may be trained clinicians who could provide much-needed care. However, time and resources spent on medical care take away from those that can be spent on conducting research. There is no established way to work out how much ancillary care researchers ought to provide to participants. However, there is agreement that researchers have *at least* the following duties:

- First, researchers, like other people, have a duty to provide life-saving medical care when they can do so at a relatively low cost.
- Second, if participants are harmed by research procedures and do not have access to health care outside the trial, they should be treated for those harms.
- Third, ancillary care should be incorporated into the planning for research studies conducted in poor populations.

Some bioethicists have also tried to work out further ancillary care responsibilities on the basis of the contribution participants make and the relationship that develops between researchers and participants.[38]

Human Subjects Research Oversight Today

In the majority of countries today, it is a legal requirement for most clinical research with human subjects to undergo independent ethical review by a research ethics committee (REC). Also called a research ethics board, an institutional review board, or an independent ethics committee, the REC is intended to provide a safeguard against the exploitation of human subjects in research. Many countries also have a national ethics committee, which may oversee the local RECs, review certain studies, or promulgate guidelines for research.

The regulations that govern REC review of research vary from country to country. Some RECs are regionally based, so they are responsible for all the human subjects research taking place in a particular area of the country. For example, Sweden has six regional boards for research ethics. Others are institutionally based, so they review research that is conducted by that particular institution, as well as research by other bodies that do not have their own REC. This is the situation in South Africa, for example. The U.S. system requires ethical review for research that is funded by the federal government or regulated by the U.S. Food and Drug Administration (FDA). This is important when research sponsored by the U.S. government is carried out in another country, because the research is then subject to both the U.S. and the host country regulations.

ETHICAL ISSUES IN MAKING INVESTMENT CHOICES IN HEALTH

As noted earlier, one central issue in global health is the need to make choices among investments that can enhance the health of a population. This is necessary, especially in low- and middle-income countries, because resources will always be fewer than needed to meet everyone's health needs. Sometimes a single type of scarce resource needs to be distributed. For example, there may be a limited number of kidneys or a limited amount of blood for transfusion. More commonly, government ministries have tight budgets and must decide how to allocate their funds among many options, ranging from the purchase of medicines to investments in infrastructure. These investment choices will get made, one way or another. It is better that they be made according to explicit, publicly justified criteria, than in secret or without serious consideration of the ethical reasons for different distributions.

Cost-effectiveness analysis is one important tool for making decisions about health investments; however, it is rarely a sufficient approach to deciding what to do. Decision makers must still make value judgments about what use to make of a cost-effectiveness analysis. Consider the vignette about the Indian state discussed at the beginning of this chapter. Investing in urban clinics would likely have the greatest total impact on health—it would avert the most disability-adjusted life years (DALYs). But the poorer people in the countryside might still, quite reasonably, think that they were being unfairly treated. After all, they were already worse off than the city folks, so why should they lose out again? Health economics, although indispensable for making health investment choices, cannot replace hard decisions about what is fair.

Principles for Distributing Scarce Resources

Various ways to distribute scarce resources have been suggested. Take the problem of allocating live organs for transplant. One way to allocate organs is to have a waiting list, so that those people who are diagnosed as needing a transplant first are also the people who receive an organ first. This would be a "first come, first served" principle. Alternatively, some sort of lottery might seem fair, so that everyone diagnosed as needing an organ would have the same chance of receiving one. Lotteries might not be equal in this way, however. It might be thought that someone whose lifestyle choices made her illness more likely, such as an alcoholic who develops liver failure, is less deserving of a transplant. It might alternatively be thought that people who have better prognoses should receive some sort of priority. A weighted lottery could incorporate these considerations, giving smaller or larger chances to members of particular populations. Similar, but more complex, systems could be developed for allocating different types of resources within a healthcare system.

Some ways to allocate scarce resources are obviously unfair. Preferring certain people's health needs over others because they are of a particular ethnic group or sexual orientation is unethical. But there are various alternative ways to allocate resources that may seem more reasonable. The justification underlying most plausible allocation proposals is one or more of four basic ethical principles:

- Health maximization
- Equality
- Priority to the worst off
- Personal responsibility

Methods for allocating resources, like lotteries or queues, are ways to put these principles into practice. Decision makers

should be aware of possible unintended effects, where the method for allocating resources does not result in the desired pattern of allocation. For example, the "first come, first served" system might accidentally favor the well-connected or people who already have access to good quality medical care and so are likely to get an early diagnosis.[39]

The principle of *health maximization* tells us that we should allocate healthcare resources in such a way that the total beneficial impact on health is as large as possible. For example, if someone proposed allocating kidneys based on the criterion of best prognosis for the recipient, this would be a form of health maximization. If health maximization were the only principle used, then people making health investments might simply look at the DALYs averted by different allocations of interventions and choose the most cost-effective way to avert DALYs.

Health maximization has obvious appeal: it means producing the greatest benefit that we can. However, it also has drawbacks. One important drawback is illustrated by the vignette at the beginning of this chapter. Sometimes a given amount of money could do the greatest good if it is spent helping people who are already well off. For example, if a government wants a new clinic to vaccinate the greatest number of children possible, it should locate the clinic in a city, not in the countryside. But people living in cities are usually better off already than people living in the country—they are likely to make more money, have better education, and have improved water supplies and sanitation. So, just focusing on helping people in cities looks unfair. The principles of equality and priority to the worst off seek to address this unfairness.

There are several ways to interpret the principle of *equality*. One interpretation is that we should try to ensure that everyone has an equal chance at receiving a scarce resource or having access to health care. In this case, people are treated equally by treating them the same. Giving *priority to the worst off* takes existing health disparities even more seriously. When we adopt this principle we make decisions about providing health care on the basis of who is already badly off, rather than on the basis of who would benefit the most (as maximization would dictate). This principle works well when the worst off can be helped relatively easily. It works less well when helping the worst off would be a severe drain on resources, for example, when terminally ill patients require continuous expensive therapies. There is also the question of how to identify the worst off. Are they the people who are sickest now? Those who have the worst health over a lifetime? Those who are poorest, even if their health is not the worst?

Each of these three principles has some plausibility. In general, if each is taken to an extreme, it would justify allocations of resources that seem unfair. Most people therefore think that some balance of maximizing benefits, giving equal chances, and prioritizing the worst off is the best way to decide how to invest resources in health. Exactly how to balance these principles in any particular case is difficult.

Finally, some people cite *personal responsibility* as a principle that can be used in combination with other principles to make decisions about health investments. Those who think that personal responsibility can be a basis for allocation decisions argue that when spending society's resources, lower priority should be given to people whose health problems may relate to their own health behaviors. Why, they may ask, should the tax money of responsible citizens be spent treating lung cancer in smokers, providing methadone and clean needles to heroin addicts, or providing ICU beds to motorcycle riders who refuse to wear helmets? Alternatively, it may be proposed that people who contribute to society should be thanked by giving them greater priority. For example, organ donors might be given greater priority to be organ recipients.

Doctors' decisions about whether to treat are traditionally based only on need and not on actions that have led to that need. Generally, those analyzing these decisions believe that it would only be fair to give a lower priority to the care of people whose behaviors appear to have caused the need for care under the following conditions:

> [T]he needs must have been caused by the behavior; the behavior must have been voluntary; the persons must have known that the behavior would cause the health needs and that if they engaged in it their health needs would receive lower priority.[40]

At present, these conditions are rarely, if ever, met.

Fair Processes

Whatever the content of a decision about health investments, there are better and worse ways to make the decision. If an unelected civil servant in a ministry of health were to unilaterally decide which medicines would be provided in the public healthcare system, this would be troubling. Justice is not just a matter of the result, but of the process, too. The idea of fair process is accorded great importance in contemporary democracies. For example, people accused of crimes are supposed to get a fair trial, and political leaders are supposed to be fairly elected. The proper processes for making health investment decisions have not been completely worked out. However, it seems clear that a fair process will involve at least transparency about how decisions are made and representation from stakeholders affected by the results of the process.

The National Institute for Health and Clinical Excellence (NICE) in the United Kingdom, which makes recommendations for how the National Health Service should provide treatments and procedures, is one example of an institution that has attempted to combine fair processes for making recommendations about health spending with an appropriate use of scientific data and medical expertise.[41]

In cases where disagreement about principles of distribution seems intractable, the introduction of a fair process has been proposed as a way to resolve the disagreement.[42] The idea here is that even if people cannot agree, for example, on how their state should spend its tax revenue on health and welfare, they may still be able to agree on a process for making such decisions. By analogy, a divorcing couple might not be able to agree between themselves how to divide up their possessions; however, they might be able to agree on a process of mediation by a third party, which would lead to a division that they would both accept. This may be one solution to disagreements. However, it has its own potential problems. First, there may be similarly intractable disagreement about what counts as a fair process. Second, the fact that people agree on a process does not guarantee that either the process or its results are fair.

This overview has only scratched the surface of the ethical problems involved in deciding how to allocate resources for health. Many other questions arise when considering investment choices in health and the use of cost-effectiveness analysis. One concerns the way that cost-effectiveness analyses are conducted; for example, measuring health benefits in DALYs may seem to discriminate against disabled people, because the methodology for DALYs inherently values a condition of disability less highly than a condition of good health. Another important question is how to balance present benefits against future benefits. Should governments give greater priority to giving people vital medications now, or should they equally focus on training doctors, building infrastructure, and conducting medical research to help future patients? One could consider these and other related issues at great length. The important point of this section, however, is that, when considering investment choices and the tools one will use to make decisions about them, it is necessary to critically assess the value judgments that are implicit in them.

CHALLENGES FOR THE FUTURE

Efforts to incorporate ethical and human rights concerns into global health work face a number of challenges. Some of these are briefly explained here.

First, many students of public health and global health get insufficient exposure in their training to ethical and human rights issues. Normally, they do have to understand the core concepts of research on human subjects and how an institutional review board functions. However, they may have few opportunities to take courses that cover broader issues of human rights and health or give them the tools to think systematically through the ethical aspects of research and policymaking. This chapter is a small attempt to correct that gap.

Second, there are deficits in implementation. As noted earlier, compliance with human rights norms is self-reported by countries. There are really no indicators for measuring such compliance, and no enforcement mechanisms either. Perhaps the movement to focus attention on global health needs can serve as a platform for having civil society hold countries more accountable for fulfilling the right of their people to health.

The governance of human subjects research has been more successful. In most countries there are systems for ethics review. However, these remain patchy—there is still a shortage of trained personnel for reviewing research; research ethics committees are understaffed, underfunded, and often undervalued; and it is not known how effective even established review systems are at protecting research participants.

There is a lack of explicit review of the fairness of many of the investment choices that are made, both by countries and by the development assistance agencies with which they work. If one reviews the documents that relate to investments in health in low- and middle-income countries, attention is generally paid to ensuring that project benefits go to disadvantaged people. However, it is rare that there are explicit reviews or articulation of how investment choices are made and the ethical choices that are a part of them. With respect to HIV/AIDS, for example, what criteria will be used to allocate drugs if there are more people clinically eligible for drugs than the amount of drugs available? Will it be access to the health center, so that there is a greater likelihood that the person will comply with treatment? Will it be pregnancy, so that one can reduce mother-to-child transmission?[43] If there were greater pressure to articulate these choices openly, then these decisions might be made more fairly.

Third, there are many unsolved ethical problems for people working in global health. For example, if human rights are going to guide decisions about global health interventions, we need to know exactly what those rights include. How do we work out what is included in the right to health and what is not? The discussion of the ethics of research in low- and middle-income countries indicated a number of unanswered questions about what is owed to research participants and poor communities in which researchers work.

Those studying global health or working in the global health field are encouraged to think carefully about their answers to the ethical questions that this chapter has left open and to articulate the reasons that justify their answers.

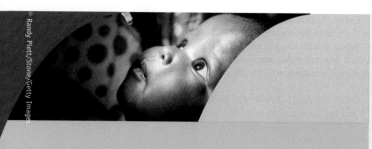

Study Questions

1. The chapter begins with four vignettes. Briefly explain what ethical or human rights issue each vignette reveals.

2. What do the human rights documents mentioned in this chapter say about health?

3. Consider a disease other than HIV/AIDS, such as tuberculosis. How might public health efforts with respect to this disease raise human rights concerns?

4. How do intellectual property laws affect the development and pricing of medicines?

5. Explain the three ethical principles stated in the Belmont Report. Give an example of a research study and show how the three principles apply to it.

6. What are the most important ethical concerns that arise when research is conducted with people in low- and middle-income countries?

7. Do you think the short-course AZT trials were ethical? Give reasons why or why not.

8. What principles might be used to justify a decision about how to allocate scarce resources for health care?

9. Why should we pay attention to the process by which health investment decisions are made?

10. How do you think cost-effectiveness analysis should be used by a government making an ethical decision about allocating a scarce healthcare resource, such as antiretroviral therapy for HIV/AIDS?

REFERENCES

1. This chapter is coauthored by Joseph Millum and Richard Skolnik. Joseph Millum is a bioethicist who serves as a staff scientist at the Clinical Center Department of Bioethics and the Fogarty International Center, U.S. National Institutes of Health. The opinions expressed are the authors' own. They do not reflect any position or policy of the National Institutes of Health, U.S. Public Health Service, or Department of Health and Human Services.

2. Mann, J., Gostin, L., Gruskin, S., Brennan, T., Lazzarini, Z., & Fineberg, H. (1994). Health and human rights. *Health and Human Rights, 1*(1), 6–23.

3. Hannum, H. (1998). The UDHR in national and international law. *Health and Human Rights, 3*(2), 144–158.

4. United Nations General Assembly. *Universal Declaration of Human Rights.* Reprinted with the permission of the United Nations. Retrieved September 10, 2006, from http://www.un.org/Overview/rights.html.

5. Office of the United Nations High Commissioner for Human Rights. *International Covenant on Economic, Social and Cultural Rights.* Retrieved November 17, 2014, from http://www.ohchr.org/en/professionalinterest/pages/cescr.aspx.

6. Office of the United Nations High Commissioner for Human Rights. *International Covenant on Civil and Political Rights.* Retrieved November 17, 2014, from http://www.ohchr.org/en/professionalinterest/pages/ccpr.aspx.

7. Gruskin, S., & Tarantola, D. (2004). Health and human rights. In S. Gruskin, M. A. Grodin, G. J. Annas, & S. P. Marks (Eds.), *Perspectives on health and human rights* (pp. 3–58). New York: Routledge.

8. Mokhiber, C. G. (2005). Toward a measure of dignity: indicators for rights-based development. In S. Gruskin, M. A. Grodin, G. J. Annas, & S. P. Marks (Eds.), *Perspectives on health and human rights* (pp. 383–392). New York: Routledge.

9. Office of the United Nations High Commissioner for Human Rights, World Health Organization. (2008, June). *The right to health.* Fact sheet No 31. Retrieved August 20, 2010, from http://www.ohchr.org/documents/publications/factsheet31.pdf.

10. Biehl, J. et al. (2009). Judicialisation of the right to health in Brazil. *Lancet, 373*(9682), 2182–2184.

11. Annas, G. J. (2003). The right to health and the nevirapine case in South Africa. *New England Journal of Medicine, 348*(24), 2470–2471.

12. Torres, M. A. (2005). The human right to health, national courts, and access to HIV/AIDS treatment: a case study from Venezuela. In S. Gruskin, M. A. Grodin, G. J. Annas, & S. P. Marks (Eds.), *Perspectives on health and human rights* (pp. 507–516). New York: Routledge.

13. United Nations. *Convention on the Elimination of All Forms of Discrimination Against Women.* Retrieved September 8, 2010, from http://www.un.org/womenwatch/daw/cedaw/text/econvention.htm.

14. Office of the United Nations High Commissioner for Human Rights. *Convention on the Rights of the Child.* Reprinted with the permission of the United Nations. Retrieved November 17, 2014, from http://www.ohchr.org/en/professionalinterest/pages/crc.aspx.

15. Wilkinson, R., & Marmot, M. (2003). *Social determinants of health: The solid facts.* Geneva: World Health Organization. Retrieved September 10, 2010, from http://www.euro.who.int/__data/assets/pdf_file/0005/98438/e81384.pdf.

16. Easley, C. E., Marks, S. P., & Morgan, R. E., Jr. (2005). The challenge and place of international human rights in public health. In S. Gruskin, M. A. Grodin, G. J. Annas, & S. P. Marks (Eds.), *Perspectives on health and human rights* (pp. 519–526). New York: Routledge.

17. Trouiller, P., Olliaro, P., Torreele, E., et al. (2002). Drug development for neglected diseases: a deficient market and a public-health policy failure. *Lancet, 359*(9324), 2188–2194.

18. Cohen, J., Dibner, M. S., & Wilson, A. (2010). Development of and access to products for neglected diseases. *PLoS ONE, 5*(5), e10610.

19. World Health Organization. (2006). *Public health, innovation, and intellectual property rights.* Retrieved September 8, 2010, from http://www.who.int/intellectualproperty/documents/thereport/ENPublicHealthReport.pdf.

20. Cullet, P. (2005). Patents and medicines: the relationship between TRIPS and the human right to health. In S. Gruskin, M. A. Grodin, G. J. Annas,, & S. P. Marks (Eds.), *Perspectives on health and human rights* (pp. 179–202). New York: Routledge.

21. Weindling, P. J. The Nazi medical experiments. In E. Emanuel, C. Grady, R. A. Crouch, et al. (Eds.), *The Oxford textbook of clinical research ethics* (pp. 18–30). Oxford: Oxford University Press.

22. Moe, K. (1984). Should the Nazi research data be cited? *Hastings Center Report, 14*(6), 5–7.

23. Jones, J. H. (2008). The Tuskegee syphilis experiment. In E. Emanuel, C. Grady, R. A. Crouch, et al. (Eds.), *The Oxford textbook of clinical research ethics* (pp. 86–96). Oxford: Oxford University Press.

24. Centers for Disease Control and Prevention. *The Tuskegee timeline.* Retrieved November 17, 2014, from http://www.cdc.gov/tuskegee/timeline.htm.

25. Connor, E. M., Sperling, R. S., Gelber, R., et al. (1994). Reduction of maternal-infant transmission of human immunodeficiency virus type 1 with zidovudine treatment. *New England Journal of Medicine, 331*, 1173–1180.

26. Angell, M. (1997). The ethics of clinical research in the third world. *New England Journal of Medicine, 337*, 847–849.

27. Lurie, P., & Wolfe, S. M. (1997). Unethical trials of interventions to reduce perinatal transmission of the human immunodeficiency virus in developing countries. *New England Journal of Medicine, 337*(12), 853–856.

28. Wendler, D., Emanuel, E., & Lie, R. (2004). The standard of care debate: can research in developing countries be both ethical and responsive to those countries' health needs? *American Journal of Public Health, 94*(6), 923–928.

29. U.S. National Institutes of Health. *The Nuremberg Code.* Retrieved November 17, 2014, from http://history.nih.gov/about/timelines/nuremberg.html.

30. World Medical Association. *Declaration of Helsinki.* Retrieved August 16, 2010, from http://www.wma.net/en/30publications/10policies/b3/index.html.

31. U.S. National Institutes of Health Office of the Secretary. *The Belmont Report.* Retrieved November 17, 2014, from http://science.education.nih.gov/supplements/nih9/bioethics/guide/teacher/Mod5_Belmont.pdf.

32. Emanuel, E. J., Wendler, D., & Grady, C. (2000). What makes clinical research ethical? *JAMA, 283*(20), 2701–2711.

33. Millum, J. (2011). Post-trial access to antiretrovirals: who owes what to whom? *Bioethics, 25*(3), 145–154.

34. Slack, C. et al. (2005). Provision of HIV treatment in HIV prevention trials: A developing country perspective. *Social Science & Medicine, 60*, 1197–1208.

35. Glantz, L. H., Annas, G. J., Grodin, M. A., et al. (1998). Research in developing countries: taking "benefit" seriously. *Hastings Center Report, 28*(6), 38–42.

36. Council for International Organizations of Medical Sciences. (2002). *International ethical guidelines for biomedical research involving human subjects* (2nd ed.). Geneva: CIOMS.

37. Participants in the 2001 Conference on Ethical Aspects of Research in Developing Countries. (2004). Moral standards for research in developing countries: from "reasonable availability" to "fair benefits." *Hastings Center Report, 34*(3), 17–27.

38. Richardson, H. S., & Belsky, L. (2004). The ancillary-care responsibilities of medical researchers: an ethical framework for thinking about the clinical care that researchers owe their subjects. *Hastings Center Report*, *34*(1), 25–33.

39. Persad, G., Wertheimer, A., & Emanuel, E. J. (2009). Principles for allocation of scarce medical interventions. *Lancet*, *373*(9661), 423–431.

40. Brock, D., & Wikler, D. (2006). Ethical issues in research allocation, research and new product development. In D. T. Jamison, J. G. Breman, A. R. Measham, et al. (Eds.), *Disease control priorities in developing countries* (2nd ed., pp. 259–270). New York: Oxford University Press.

41. National Institute for Health and Clinical Excellence. *What we do*. Retrieved November 17, 2014, from http://www.nice.org.uk/about/what-we-do.

42. Daniels, N., & Sabin, J. E. (2002). *Setting limits fairly: Can we learn to share medical resources?* New York: Oxford University Press.

43. Macklin, R. (2004). *Ethics and equity in access to HIV treatment—3 by 5 initiative*. Geneva: World Health Organization.

CHAPTER **5**

An Introduction to Health Systems

VIGNETTES

Uchenna lived in Nigeria. She had a high fever and suspected she had malaria. Her family took her to the local health clinic. When they arrived at 11:00 in the morning, the clinic was not open. In addition, the community health worker who staffed the clinic was nowhere to be found. Uchenna's family knew that the clinic rarely operated as it was supposed to, so they took her instead to the district hospital. She waited 6 hours to be seen, but was finally examined by a doctor and given medicine for malaria.

Sajitha lived in a small village in northern India. She woke up with a rash that covered the upper half of her body. Her family lived quite far from the government health center and had little faith in the quality of the staff there. Thus, they took Sajitha to a local medical practitioner. He came from the village, was always polite to people, could be paid in cash or in kind, and seemed to have a good record in curing people of their ills. He examined Sajitha, gave her an injection of vitamin B_1, and told her she would be fine. He used the same needle on Sajitha that he had used on several other people that day.

Melissa lived in the state of Virginia in the United States. She had been unemployed for some time, had little money, and had no health insurance. She also had cancer. She was thousands of dollars in debt to doctors and hospitals for the tests and treatment she had received so far; however, she needed more treatment, more drugs, and additional surgery. Several physicians would not take her as a patient because she had no health insurance. Eventually, after she became sicker, she found a physician who would do the surgery for very low cost. Unfortunately, she was so ill by the time she got the operation that she died a few months later from the cancer.

Cesar lived in San José, the capital of Costa Rica, and had been ill for some time. He visited his local health center, where he was referred to the national hospital because it appeared that he might have cancer. The hospital confirmed the diagnosis of cancer and then treated him with drugs and surgery. He stayed several weeks in the hospital during his recovery. The national health insurance program of Costa Rica covered the cost of Cesar's care.

INTRODUCTION

This chapter is about health systems. It introduces the definition of a health system, the functions of a health system, and how health systems are organized. The chapter also examines some aspects of how health systems are financed. The chapter briefly reviews some examples of health systems in different countries, before turning to critical issues which health systems in low- and middle-income countries face and how they are being addressed. The chapter concludes with a series of policy and program briefs and case studies that are meant to illustrate the key themes of this chapter.

It is especially important for several reasons to learn about health systems early in one's study of global health:

- Health systems are the vehicle through which health services are delivered.
- The health of individuals has an important relationship with the effectiveness of health systems.
- Most countries spend a substantial share of national income on their health system, often with major gaps in effectiveness and efficiency.
- Individuals in many countries spend an important share of their family income on health.
- Global forces such as population aging are exerting pressure on the costs of health systems.
- Achieving the best population health at the lowest possible cost is an important goal for individual countries.
- Developing and sustaining an effective and efficient health system is a goal for every country and an

especially challenging one for countries with limited financial and human resources.

This chapter focuses mainly on health services, which is only one important aspect of a health system. When reading this chapter, keep in mind the following questions:

- To what extent do different health systems value the "right to health?"
- What is the role in various health systems of individuals, and of the public, private, and nongovernmental organization (NGO) sectors?
- What is the extent to which different actors in the system are engaged in the financing and provision of health services?
- How are different health systems organized and managed?
- What are key issues constraining the effectiveness and efficiency of health systems in different settings?
- How can those constraints best be addressed?

Before reading this chapter, it will be valuable to review some key terms that will be used, which are shown in **Table 5-1**.

TABLE 5-1 Definitions of Key Terms

Term	Definition
Health System Organization and Management	
Brain Drain	The migration of health personnel in search of the better standard of living and quality of life, higher salaries, access to advanced technology, and more stable political conditions in different places worldwide.
Governance	The actions and means adopted by a society to organize itself in the promotion and protection of the health of its population.
Health System	The sum of organizations, institutions, and resources whose primary purpose is to improve health.
Primary Care	The provision of first contact, person-focused, ongoing care over time that meets the health-related needs of people, referring (to hospital) only those problems too uncommon to maintain competence and coordinates care when people receive services at other levels of care.
Responsiveness to the Expectations of the Population	How the system performs relative to nonhealth aspects, meeting or not meeting a population's expectations of how it should be treated by providers of prevention, care, or nonpersonal services.
Secondary Care	Medical care provided by a specialist or facility upon referral by a primary care physician.

TABLE 5-1 Definitions of Key Terms (*continued*)

Term	Definition
Stewardship	The wide range of functions carried out by governments as they seek to achieve national health policy objectives/The careful and responsible management of something entrusted to one's care.
Task Shifting	The rational redistribution of tasks among health workforce teams. Specific tasks are moved, where appropriate, from highly qualified health workers to health workers with shorter training and fewer qualifications in order to make more efficient use of the available human resources for health.
Tertiary Care	Specialized consultative care, usually on referral from primary or secondary medical care personnel, by specialists working in a center that has personnel and facilities for special investigation and treatment.
Financing Health Systems	
Conditional Cash Transfers	Programs that provide cash payments to poor households that meet certain behavioral requirements, generally related to children's health care and education.
Contracting In (Health Services)	One level of government or a public institution contracts with a lower level of government facility—such as, a district, a province, or another facility to deliver services.
Contracting Out (Health Services)	A financing agency (government, insurance entity, or development partner), also known as a "purchaser," provides resources to a nonstate provider (NSP, such as a nongovernmental organization [NGO] or private sector firm), also known as a "contractor," to provide a specified set of services, in a specified location, with specified objectives.
Fairness of Financial Contribution	The risks each household faces due to the costs of the health system are distributed according to ability to pay rather than to the risk of illness.
Financial Protection	Financing health care in a way that does not cause people to be denied access to health care or to become impoverished because of their inability to pay for health services.
Out-of-Pocket Health Expenditure	Any direct outlay by households, including gratuities and in-kind payments, to health practitioners and suppliers of pharmaceuticals, therapeutic appliances, and other goods and services whose primary intent is to contribute to the restoration or enhancement of the health status of individuals or population groups. It is a part of private health expenditure.
Private Health Expenditure	The sum of total expenditure on health by private entities, notably commercial insurance, nonprofit institutions, and households including out-of-pocket health expenditure, patient copayments, private health insurance premiums, and health expenditures by nongovernmental organizations.
Public Health Expenditure	The sum of outlays by government entities to purchase healthcare services and goods, notably by ministries of health and social security agencies. The revenue base may comprise multiple sources, including external funds.

(continues)

TABLE 5-1 Definitions of Key Terms (*continued*)

Term	Definition
Results Based Financing	Any program that rewards the delivery of one or more outputs or outcomes by one or more incentives, financial or otherwise, after the principal has verified that the agent has delivered the agreed-upon results.
Right to Health	The highest attainable standard of health is a fundamental right of every human being including access to timely, acceptable, and affordable health care of appropriate quality.
Risk-pooling	Those who are healthy subsidize those who are sick, and those who are rich subsidize those who are poor.
Total Expenditure on Health	The sum of general government expenditure on health (commonly called public expenditure on health) and private expenditure on health.
Universal Health Coverage	Ensuring that all people can use the promotive, preventive, curative, rehabilitative and palliative health services they need, of sufficient quality to be effective, while also ensuring that the use of these services does not expose the user to financial hardship.
User Fees	Charges levied at the point of use for any aspect of health services. For example, registration fees, consultation fees, fees for drugs and medical supplies, or charges for any health service rendered, such as outpatient or inpatient care.

Dodani, S., & LaPorte, R. E. (2005). Brain drain from developing countries: How can brain drain be converted into wisdom gain? *Journal of the Royal Society of Medicine*, *98*(11), 487–491.

Dodgson, R., Lee, K., & Drager, N. (2002). *Global health governance: A conceptual review* (Discussion Paper 1). London: Centre on Global Change & Health, London School of Hygiene & Tropical Medicine; Geneva: Department of Health & Development, World Health Organization.

Q&As: Health systems. Retrieved May 29, 2015, from http://www.who.int/topics/health_systems/qa/en/.

Starfield, B., Shi, L., & Macinko, J. (2005). Contribution of primary care to health systems and health. *Milbank Quarterly*, *83*, 457–502.

World Health Organization. (2000). *The world health report 2000*. Geneva: World Health Organization.

Definition of secondary care. Merriam-Webster Dictionary. Retrieved January 16, 2015, from http://www.merriam-webster.com/dictionary/secondary%20care.

World Health Organization. *Stewardship*. Retrieved January 14, 2015, from http://www.who.int/healthsystems/stewardship/en/.

World Health Organization. (2008). *Task shifting: Global recommendations and guidelines*. Geneva: WHO. Retrieved January 15, 2015, from http://www.who.int/healthsystems/TTR-TaskShifting.pdf?ua=1.

Johns Hopkins Medicine. *Tertiary care definition*. Retrieved January 16, 2015, from http://www.hopkinsmedicine.org/patient_care/pay_bill/insurance_footnotes.html.

World Bank. *Conditional cash transfers*. Retrieved January 15, 2015, from http://go.worldbank.org/BWUC1CMXM0.

Abramson, W. (2004). *Contracting for health service delivery: A manual for policy makers*. Boston, MA: John Snow Inc. Retrieved January 15, 2015, from http://www.jsi.com/JSIInternet/Inc/Common/_download_pub.cfm?id=10351&lid=3.

Loevinsohn, B. (2008). *Performance-based contracting for health services in developing countries: A toolkit*. Geneva: The World Bank.

World Health Organization. (2000). *The world health report 2000*. Geneva: World Health Organization.

World Health Organization. (2000). *The world health report 2000*. Geneva: World Health Organization.

World Bank. *Out-of-pocket health expenditure*. Retrieved January 16, 2015, from http://data.worldbank.org/indicator/SH.XPD.OOPC.ZS.

World Health Organization. *Definition of terms*. Retrieved January 14, 2015, from https://web.archive.org/web/20110303183810/http://www.wpro.who.int/NR/rdonlyres/45B45060-A38E-496F-B2C1-BD2DC6C04C52/0/44Definitionofterms2009.pdf.

World Health Organization. *Definition of terms*. Retrieved January 14, 2015, from https://web.archive.org/web/20110303183810/http://www.wpro.who.int/NR/rdonlyres/45B45060-A38E-496F-B2C1-BD2DC6C04C52/0/44Definitionofterms2009.pdf.

Musgrove, P. (2011). *Rewards for good performance or results: A short glossary*. Washington, DC: World Bank. Retrieved January 15, 2015, from https://www.rbfhealth.org/sites/rbf/files/documents/Rewards%20for%20Good%20Performance%20or%20Results%20-%20Short%20Glossary.pdf.

World Health Organization. (2013). *The right to health*. Retrieved January 14, 2015, from http://www.who.int/mediacentre/factsheets/fs323/en/.

World Health Organization. (2000). *The world health report 2000*. Geneva: World Health Organization.

World Health Organization. *Definition of terms*. Retrieved January 14, 2015, from https://web.archive.org/web/20110303183810/ http://www.wpro.who.int/NR/rdonlyres/45B45060-A38E-496F-B2C1-BD2DC6C04C52/0/44Definitionofterms2009.pdf.

World Health Organization. What is universal health coverage? Retrieved January 14, 2015, from http://www.who.int/health_financing/universal_coverage_definition/en/.

Lagarde, M., & Palmer, N. (2011). The impact of user fees on access to health services in low- and middle-income countries. Cochrane Database of Systematic Reviews, Issue 4. doi: 10.1002/14651858.CD009094

WHAT IS A HEALTH SYSTEM?

The World Health Organization (WHO) defines a health system as "all actors, institutions and resources that undertake health actions—where a health action is one where the primary intent is to improve health."[1] A related definition of a health system is "the combination of resources, organization, and management that culminate in the delivery of health services to the population."[2]

Another way to put this would be to see the health system as:[3]

- Agencies that plan, fund, and regulate health care
- The money that finances health care
- Those who provide preventive health services
- Those who provide clinical services
- Those who provide specialized inputs into health care, such as the education of healthcare professionals and the production of drugs and medical devices

It is important to remember when considering health systems that they are composed of a set of interdependent parts. The organizations, money, and people that compose health systems may be public, private, for-profit, or private, not-for-profit.

THE FUNCTIONS OF A HEALTH SYSTEM

The *World Health Report 2000*, produced by WHO, focused entirely on health systems.[4] That report has been widely read and has been the basis for considerable analysis of the goals of health systems, their functions, how they are organized, and how well they perform.

The *World Health Report 2000* suggests that there are three goals for every health system:[5]

- Good health
- Responsiveness to the expectations of the population
- Fairness of financial contribution

The report further suggests that if these are the goals of health systems, then each health system has four functions to play:[5]

- Provide health services
- Raise money that can be spent on health, referred to as "resource generation"
- Pay for health services, referred to as "financing"
- Govern and regulate the health system, referred to as "stewardship"

Elaborating somewhat on those ideas, one could say that all health systems should do the following:[6]

- Provide access to a comprehensive range of health services, including prevention, diagnosis, treatment, and rehabilitation
- Protect the sick and their families against the financial costs of ill health and disability through the establishment and operation of some type of insurance scheme
- Improve the health of populations through appropriate governance of the health system, regulation of that system, promotion of good health, and the carrying out of key public health functions, such as surveillance, the operation of public health laboratories, and food and drug regulation.

The World Health Organization has also developed a framework for considering the different parts of health systems and the roles they play in health system performance.[7] This framework includes the six building blocks of a health system, depicted in **Figure 5-1**.

WHO defines the health system building blocks in the following ways:

- *Good health services* deliver safe and effective health interventions to people where and when they need them, in an efficient manner.
- A *health workforce* performs well when it has an appropriate number of trained staff, in the right fields, in the places they are needed, and they perform their work as effectively and efficiently as possible.
- A *health information system* functions well when it delivers the information needed for monitoring health status and health system performance in a reliable and timely manner.
- A health system should ideally provide equitable access to *medical products, vaccines, and technologies* that are safe, of appropriate quality, have been procured at the best available prices, and can be used in cost-effective ways.
- An effective *health financing system* is one that raises enough money to fund an agreed-upon health program and protect individuals from financial harm due to the costs of health services.
- *Leadership and governance* concern the management, oversight, and regulation of health systems in open, participatory, and accountable ways, that seek to maximize health for the money spent.

The WHO framework suggests that if countries combine these building blocks with attention to ensuring quality, safety, and universality of coverage, then the services are most

FIGURE 5-1 Health System Building Blocks

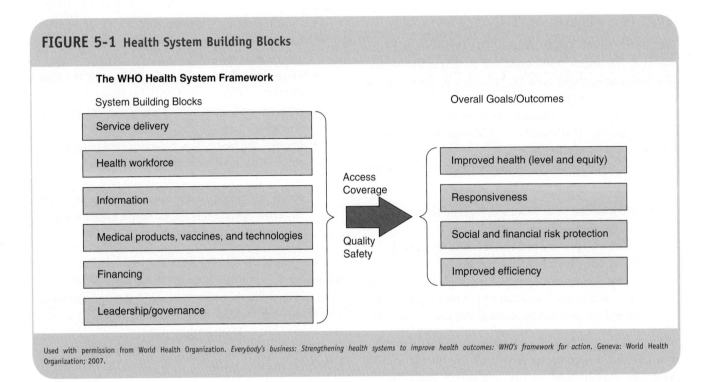

Used with permission from World Health Organization. *Everybody's business: Strengthening health systems to improve health outcomes: WHO's framework for action.* Geneva: World Health Organization; 2007.

likely to improve health in equitable ways that are responsive to the needs of individuals, protect them from financial risk, and get as much health for the money spent as possible.

HOW ARE HEALTH SERVICES ORGANIZED?

Categorizing Health Services

The manner in which health systems are organized is related to the history, politics, and values of individual countries. To a large extent, countries spend more money per capita on health as their incomes rise. At the same time, as countries become better-off, they generally focus greater attention on trying to ensure universal access to a basic package of health services and universal coverage of health insurance. As they develop economically, they also pay increasing attention to improving the effectiveness, efficiency, and equity of their health systems. Of course, one goal of low- and middle-income countries must be to address these aims, as far as possible, even before their incomes have risen to substantially higher levels.

There is no ideal way of categorizing healthcare systems because they are so varied and so complex. However, **Table 5-2** reflects one way of thinking about how health systems are organized to address several key health sector issues.[8] Nonetheless, keep in mind that the table represents a dramatic oversimplification of a very complicated subject.

In this table, health systems are organized into three types:

- Systems that include a national health insurance scheme, such as in Canada, France, Germany, and Japan. These systems, in principle, offer health insurance to all people for an agreed package of services. Some systems include a number of different insurance providers who cover similar or identical service packages. In other systems, insurance is generally provided through a government entity or entities, as in Canada.
- Systems organized around a national health service, in which, outside of a relatively small private health sector, the government is the sole payer for health care and owns most of the healthcare facilities. This is the case, for example, in the constituent parts of the United Kingdom. In this case, some, but not all, healthcare providers are essentially state employees.
- Pluralistic systems, such as those in the United States, India, and Nigeria, in which the public sector, private for-profit sector, and private not-for-profit sectors play important roles. In some of these systems, the private sector has a predominant place in the system. In all of them it plays a large role.

TABLE 5-2 Simplified Categorization of Approaches to Selected Health System Issues

	National Health Service	National Health Insurance	Pluralistic
Health as a Right	Fundamental	Fundamental	Health as a personal good
Ownership of Facilities	Overwhelmingly public	Vast majority public and private, not-for-profit	Public, private, for-profit, and private, not-for-profit
Employment of Providers	The health service and private	Largely private	Largely private
Form of Insurance	Overwhelmingly public insurance linked to the health service	Largely government single payers and firms working with government schemes	Public insurance and private, for-profit and private, not-for-profit insurers, with substantial numbers lacking insurance
Financing of Insurance	Overwhelmingly tax-based	Some based on individual premiums; others based on employee and employer payroll taxes; some are tax-based	Taxes, employer and employee insurance contributions, individual purchase of insurance, and out-of-pocket
Country Examples	United Kingdom	France, Canada, Japan, Germany	India, Nigeria, United States

Data from Birn, A.-E., Pillay, Y., & Holtz, T. H. (2009). *Textbook of international health*. New York: Oxford University Press.

It is also worth noting that in Cuba today, essentially all health services, facilities, and personnel are part of a government-operated healthcare system. Such systems were also the case in the former Soviet Union.

Table 5-2 first examines the approach of each type of health system to providing universal coverage of an insured basic package of health services as a "right." Most high-income countries do have such an approach, except the United States, which has recently taken some steps in that direction. Most middle-income countries have accepted the principle of "universal health care" as a right, but not all of them have attained it. A few low-income countries, such as Ghana and Rwanda, are striving to implement universal health care as a right. However, most low-income countries have not yet moved very far toward implementing such an approach, even if it is sometimes enshrined in the laws of the country.

The table also examines who owns health facilities. In the health systems of most high-income countries, facilities are generally owned by the public sector or by private, not-for-profit organizations. In more pluralistic systems, however, including both the United States and a number of low- and middle-income countries, facilities could be owned by the public sector, private for-profit sector, or private not-for-profit sector.

Table 5-2 also examines the manner in which insurance is operated in different healthcare systems. In the national health insurance models like those in some high-income countries, a number of private firms, which could be for-profit or nonprofit, provide insurance for a package of services that is agreed upon with the government. The price of the insurance is generally the same across all insurers. In the United Kingdom model, the public insurance scheme is inherent to and linked with the National Health Service. In pluralistic systems, insurance can come in many forms and many people may lack insurance. The public sector may operate some insurance schemes. In addition, people may purchase insurance from private, for-profit insurers and from private, not-for-profit insurers.

Another dimension for examining health systems is the manner in which they finance their insurance schemes. The constituent parts of the National Health Service of the United Kingdom raise their funds through general taxes. The Canadian government and provincial governments also raise money for their health insurance schemes through general taxes. In some of the other countries with national insurance schemes, such as Germany, however, most of the funding for health insurance comes from payroll tax contributions from employers and employees. In national health insurance schemes, governments usually use funds from general taxes to purchase insurance for those who are not able to make contributions to the insurance scheme, such as the unemployed. In more pluralistic settings, the government may finance health insurance for special groups, such as the disabled, poor, and aged, through general and earmarked taxes. In addition, individuals and employers generally contribute to the purchase of insurance. In these systems, significant numbers of people may be without insurance, and such systems usually feature substantial out-of-pocket expenditures.

Most low-income countries have very fragmented and pluralistic health systems that include both public and private providers. Many of these countries have a publicly supported and provided health system and a range of private providers and facilities. They often have publicly organized insurance programs for government employees and relatively small private insurance markets. They may also have a number of community-based insurance schemes. Private out-of-pocket payments represent a substantial share of the costs of health in low-income countries.

Many of the middle-income countries, particularly in Latin America, have organized a substantial part of their health system around a national health insurance scheme or schemes. Many of them are also working to expand the schemes to be universal in coverage, as noted later in this chapter. Private out-of-pocket expenditures are generally lower in these countries than in many other low- and middle-income countries and are concentrated in those individuals who are not covered by the insurance schemes.

Finally, it is valuable to keep the financing and provision of healthcare services conceptually separate and to examine whether the public or private sector delivers healthcare services in settings with varying financing arrangements. Again, the reader is reminded of the extent to which these comments are oversimplified.

- Cuba is the only country today in which the public sector essentially finances and delivers all healthcare services.

- In many low- and middle-income countries in which the private healthcare sector is not well developed, most formal healthcare services will be provided by the public sector. They will generally be financed through a combination of public funds and private payments for some services.
- The National Health Service (or its related entities) finances most healthcare services in the United Kingdom. It owns most healthcare facilities. The National Health Service can purchase services from providers it does not employ.
- There are many countries, such as Canada, Thailand, and New Zealand, in which the private sector delivers services, but the public sector is responsible for healthcare financing.
- There are also countries in which most healthcare services are in the private sector, with some of those services being paid for through public financing schemes and some through privately financed schemes. Such countries usually also contain a substantial establishment of government-owned healthcare services, which are generally financed through the public sector and through private payments for services. Such countries would include, for example, the United States and a number of low- and middle-income countries, such as India and Nigeria.

Levels of Care

Health systems are generally organized into three levels of care that are referred to as primary, secondary, and tertiary. In most high-income countries, primary care is provided by a physician who is the first point of contact with the patient. In many systems, nonemergency patients must see a primary care provider before they can be treated by a specialist, and such providers are often referred to as "gatekeepers." Secondary care is usually provided by specialist physicians and general hospitals, which are generally located in towns and cities. At these physician services and hospitals, one would get treatment for certain illnesses and conditions, including medical procedures and surgery that primary-level providers cannot do. Tertiary care is provided in specialized hospitals that are generally located only in cities. In principle, these specialized hospitals are staffed with a wide range of physicians and can address a diverse array of illnesses with high-level diagnostics, treatments, and surgeries.

Many low- and middle-income countries have established primary, secondary, and tertiary level facilities by geographic area, depending on the size of the population. These

TABLE 5-3 Selected Examples of Health Services by Level in a Low-Income Country

Primary Level
Family planning
Maternal health care
Well baby care
Diagnosis and treatment of simple childhood ailments
Diagnosis and treatment of simple adult ailments and injuries
Diagnosis and treatment of malaria and TB

Secondary Level
As above, plus:
Emergency obstetric care
Diagnosis and treatment of sick children
Diagnosis and treatment of adult illness
Basic surgical services
Some emergency care

Tertiary Level
As above, plus:
Treatment of complicated pediatric cases
Treatment of complicated adult cases
Specialist surgical services
Advanced emergency care

countries, for example, might have a center for primary care for every 5,000 to 10,000 people, a secondary hospital in each district, and a tertiary hospital in large cities. In many low-income countries, medical assistants, nurses, or nurse-midwives would staff the lowest level of the system. The first level at which there might be a trained physician would be in large primary healthcare centers or district hospitals. Table 5-3 shows the types of services that one might typically expect to find at the different service levels in a low-income country.

PRIMARY HEALTH CARE, FROM ALMA-ATA TO THE PRESENT

At the core of ideas about health systems in low- and middle-income countries is the notion of "primary health care," which springs partly from a historic conference in 1978 in Alma-Ata, (now called Almaty), in Kazakhstan in the former USSR. This was one of the most important meetings in the history of global health, and it produced the Declaration of Alma-Ata.[9]

To a large extent, the declaration discusses two matters. First, it speaks of health as a human right. These parts of the declaration note the right to health, the unacceptable levels of health disparities, and the need for social and economic development to enable better health, as better health would promote social and economic development. It also speaks about people's right to participate in the planning and implementation of health care. In addition, it set a goal of ensuring that there would be health for all by the year 2000, in a manner that would help people to enjoy the health needed to fulfill their capabilities.

The document also outlines the concept of "primary health care." This is care that is essential and socially acceptable. It must also be based on evidence and made universally available. It would address the needs of the community and be affordable. It would provide preventive, promotive, curative, and rehabilitative services. Personnel who are sensitive to the needs of the community would staff primary health-care services. Primary health care would be linked to other levels of health services through a referral system. It would also be linked to action on the key determinants of health, including health education, water supply and sanitation, and nutrition. The approach to primary health care would promote self-reliance in the community. It would pay particular attention to infectious diseases and other common causes of morbidity and mortality, family planning, immunization, and the provision of essential drugs.

This notion of primary health care that was articulated at Alma-Ata remains an important one. Many countries—at all income levels, but especially low- and middle-income countries—continue to work toward a model of primary health care that is effective and efficient. It is important to be familiar with the concept of primary health care and the efforts under way to achieve it, and to not confuse it with *primary care*, which is the first level of health services. Approaches to primary health care are discussed further later in this chapter.

THE ROLES OF THE PUBLIC, PRIVATE, AND NGO SECTORS

It is important to distinguish among the different actors that participate in health systems and the different functions they play. The public sector is the first actor in most health systems. The involvement of the public sector could be at the national, state, or municipal level, depending on the country. The public sector is responsible for the stewardship of the system, meaning its governance, policy setting, rule making, and enforcement of rules. The public sector is also responsible for raising the funds for the health system, making decisions about allocating those funds, and establishing approaches to health insurance—often referred to as "financial protection" from health costs. In addition, the public sector is responsible for managing and financing key public health functions, such as setting public health policies, enforcing laws related to health, disease surveillance, and food and drug regulations. In some countries, as noted later, the public sector provides health services through facilities that it owns and operates. However, the public sector can also purchase health services from the private, for-profit or private, not-for-profit sectors.

Although some people believe that health is a right that should not be "for sale," the private, for-profit sector is involved in the provision and financing of health systems in all countries. There are many types of private health service providers that go beyond those involved in formal health services. Especially in low- and middle-income countries, people often buy health services from medicine men, shamans, healers, and bonesetters. There is also a range of nonlicensed medical practitioners who operate in many settings, including traditional birth attendants. In addition, many people get medical advice from drug vendors that operate small kiosks or mobile drug stores, or from pharmacies and pharmacists. Many people also seek care from practitioners of traditional forms of medicine, such as those in China and India. When considering the ways in which health systems function and how they can be made more effective and efficient, it is essential to keep in mind where people get their health services, the role those providers play in the health system, and how people pay for these different kinds of services.[10]

In some countries, physicians operate in the private, for-profit sector. In some countries, the private sector may also operate health clinics, hospitals, and health services. Private sector health insurers are also involved in health in many countries. The private sector might also operate laboratories. The private, for-profit sector can operate on its own financing, sell selected services to the government, or operate under contract to the government for a range of services. The private, for-profit sector can play a very important role for those people who are willing and able to pay for it, or whose care is paid for by others, such as employers or by insurance.

When one thinks about the private, not-for-profit sector, particularly in low- and middle-income countries, one is often thinking about nongovernmental organizations, or NGOs. Broadly defined, an NGO is:

> A not-for-profit group, principally independent from government, which is organized on a local, national or international level to address

issues in support of the public good. Task-oriented and made up of people with a common interest, NGOs perform a variety of services and humanitarian functions, bring public concerns to governments, monitor policy and programme implementation, and encourage participation of civil society stakeholders at the community level. Some are organized around specific issues, such as human rights.[11]

NGOs may be large or small, may be local, national, or international, and may work in one area of activity or many. Some examples of NGOs are given in **Table 5-4**.

NGOs are actively involved in many areas of health in a large number of countries. Typical examples would be in community-based efforts to promote better health through health education and improved water supply and sanitation. NGOs are also very involved in carrying out various health services. Like the private, for-profit sector, NGOs can operate with their own financing or they can work under contract to the government, the private sector, or the philanthropic sector.

A critical issue in designing and operating health systems is the roles that ought to be assigned to the public, private for-profit, private not-for-profit, and NGO sectors and how those roles should be paid for. It is particularly important to carefully consider the extent to which the public sector should provide services, compared to the extent to which it would be more cost-efficient for the public sector to buy certain services from the private for-profit, private not-for-profit, and NGO sectors. It could be the case that public sector health services at the primary level are not as effective and efficient as similar services operated by the NGO sector. As Afghanistan engaged in reconstruction after its civil war, for

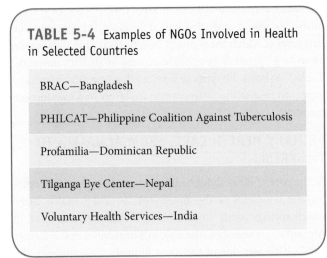

TABLE 5-4 Examples of NGOs Involved in Health in Selected Countries

BRAC—Bangladesh

PHILCAT—Philippine Coalition Against Tuberculosis

Profamilia—Dominican Republic

Tilganga Eye Center—Nepal

Voluntary Health Services—India

example, it contracted out a package of primary healthcare services to the NGO sector.[12] In Bangladesh, BRAC, a large NGO with a significant presence throughout the country, has carried out a number of nutrition programs under contract to the government of Bangladesh.[13] Contracting out for services is reviewed in one of the policy and program briefs at the end of the chapter.

HEALTH SECTOR EXPENDITURE

The health sector is an important part of the economy in all countries and a matter on which government and private individuals spend a substantial amount of resources. **Table 5-5**

shows the total expenditure on health as a share of gross domestic product (GDP) for selected countries organized by level of total health expenditure as a percentage of GDP. The table also shows the share of total expenditure that is private.

Table 5-5 highlights a number of important points. First, total health expenditure as a share of GDP varies substantially across countries. It is around 3 to 4 percent in a number of countries, such as Indonesia, Pakistan, and Bangladesh. A number of lower- and middle-income countries spend about 4 to 7 percent of their GDP on health. Most of the higher-income countries spend between 7 and 12 percent of their GDP on health. However, the United States spends almost

TABLE 5-5 Total Health Expenditure as a Percentage of GDP and Private Expenditure on Health as a Percentage of Total Expenditure on Health, Selected Countries, 2012

Country	Total Health Expenditure as Percentage of GDP	Private Health Expenditure as Percentage of Total Health Expenditure
Indonesia	3.0	60.4
Pakistan	3.1	68.6
Sri Lanka	3.1	60.2
Bangladesh	3.6	65.6
Thailand	3.9	23.6
India	4.0	66.9
Philippines	4.4	62.3
Kenya	4.7	61.9
Egypt	5.0	61.0
Cameroon	5.1	66.5
Peru	5.1	41.1
Ghana	5.2	42.9
Cambodia	5.4	75.3
China	5.4	44.0

continues

TABLE 5-5 Total Health Expenditure as a Percentage of GDP and Private Expenditure on Health as a Percentage of Total Expenditure on Health, Selected Countries, 2012 (*continued*)

Country	Total Health Expenditure as Percentage of GDP	Private Health Expenditure as Percentage of Total Health Expenditure
Dominican Republic	5.4	49.1
Nepal	5.5	60.5
Nigeria	6.1	68.9
Haiti	6.4	77.2
Vietnam	6.6	57.4
South Sudan	7.2	61.3
Israel	7.5	38.3
Ireland	8.1	35.6
Afghanistan	8.6	79.2
Cuba	8.6	5.8
South Africa	8.8	52.1
Australia	9.1	33.1
Brazil	9.3	53.6
Jordan	9.8	36.9
Costa Rica	10.1	25.4
Denmark	11.2	14.5
France	11.7	23.1
United States	17.9	53.6

Data from The World Bank. (2015). Health expenditure, total (% of GDP). Retrieved June 22, 2015, from http://data.worldbank.org/indicator/SH.XPD.TOTL.ZS.

18 percent of its GDP on health. In addition, there are some countries that spend a substantially higher share of GDP on health than one might anticipate given their income level, including Afghanistan, Costa Rica, Cuba, and Haiti.

We can also see a very wide range in the share of total expenditure on health that is private sector expenditure. Only about 15–25 percent of total expenditure on health is private sector expenditure in a number of high-income countries that have substantial health insurance programs, such as Denmark and France. In some other high-income countries, such as Ireland and Israel, private sector expenditure as a share of total expenditure on health is between 35 and 40 percent. On the other hand, in a number of poorer countries such as Bangladesh, India, Kenya, and Pakistan, which lack widespread coverage with formal insurance, private sector expenditure on health as a share of total expenditure on health is around 60–70 percent.[14]

In some respects, these data are contrary to what one might expect: poorer countries, in which people can least afford to spend for health out-of-pocket, have the highest private expenditure. Better-off countries, in which people can most afford out-of-pocket expenditure, spend relatively less out-of-pocket, because their insurance schemes are very well-developed. Among high-income countries, only the United States spends more than 50 percent of total expenditure in the private sector.[14]

SELECTED EXAMPLES OF HEALTH SYSTEMS

The section that follows provides very brief and stylized comments on the main features of a small number of health systems in low-, middle-, and high-income countries. It is important to note the common approaches of some of the countries to selected issues. However, it is also important to remember that each country has its own health system, built from its unique historical experience.

High-Income Countries

Germany

Germany was the first country in the world to have a universal program of health insurance, which started in the 1880s.[15] The federal and state governments have established a legal environment for health services but are not engaged in the direct provision of medical services. The German system is based on the notion of universal health coverage. Those people earning less than 4,350 Euros per month are required to be covered by statutory health insurance. Others, including the self-employed and those earning more than this amount, may opt for a voluntary private health insurance scheme. These schemes also cover the dependents of the enrolled person.[16]

The insurance carriers for the mandatory insurance in Germany are 134 sickness funds. These are not-for-profit insurance funds that are financed by contributions from employers and employees. In 2013, employees and pensioners paid 8.3 percent of their wages or pension up to an agreed limit and employers paid 7.3 percent. Various arrangements are made to pay for the health insurance contributions for people who are disabled or unemployed. Those participating

in the statutory health insurance scheme have small copayments for certain medicines, inpatient hospital stays, and medical aides. The private health insurance schemes are underwritten by 43 companies, of which 24 are for-profit companies. The sickness funds cover about 90 percent of the population. About 10 percent of the population has private insurance.[16] The statutory health insurance package of benefits covers a wide range of medical, dental, and eye care services. It also covers prescription medicines, medical aids, and physical therapy. The package includes a range of preventive services, such as well-baby checkups, immunizations, some cancer screenings, and dental checkups.[16]

In the German healthcare system, sickness funds contract physician associations to provide care to people who do not require hospitalization. Most physicians work in their own private practices. The sickness funds also make arrangements for hospital services for the people they insure by entering into agreements with hospitals about how many services they will be able to render at a certain price that the sickness fund will pay. Generally, individuals can choose the general practitioner, specialist, or hospital that they want to use.[16]

The United Kingdom

The United Kingdom (UK) established a system of universal healthcare coverage in 1946, following World War II.[15] It aimed to provide a comprehensive set of health services to all people in the UK, without regard to their ability to pay for such services. The National Health Service (NHS) is that part of the health system that is responsible for health services and related insurance.

The Parliament, the Secretary of State for Health, and the Department of Health are responsible for the NHS, which is now overseen by the NHS Commissioning Board. The NHS is universal in coverage. Essentially, the NHS covers a wide range of preventive and therapeutic services, mental health care, physical therapy, some palliative care, and dental and eye care. People can buy supplementary voluntary private insurance if they would like, which they mostly use to reduce waiting times for services that are not urgent. About 11 percent of the population has such insurance.[17]

Three quarters of NHS funding comes from general taxes, and the rest mostly from a payroll tax. The system requires minimal copayments for drugs prescribed outside a hospital and for dental services. The system offers a safety net of exemptions from copayments for certain groups who may be financially unable to make the required payments.[17]

The NHS purchases primary healthcare services from groups of physicians who are trained as general practitioners and work as private independent contractors to the NHS. Specialist physicians overwhelmingly work in hospitals for the NHS. In principle, people can choose their general practitioners, who do play a gatekeeping role in the NHS system. NHS-affiliated hospitals are owned and managed by NHS Trusts.[17]

The United States

The United States has a complex and very fragmented healthcare system. The federal government oversees and operates some programs, such as the military's medical services, the Department of Veterans Affairs, and the Indian Health Services. The federal government oversees and works with state governments on a number of other programs such as Medicaid, which provides insurance to the indigent, and Medicare, which provides insurance to the elderly. State governments regulate health insurance. With the recent adoption of the Affordable Care Act, the United States has moved toward insuring more of its people, but it has not yet made a commitment to universal health coverage.[18]

Fifty-six percent of the U.S. population had private voluntary health insurance in 2011. About half of them received it through their employer, and the remainder bought it themselves. In addition, almost 30 percent of the population was covered by Medicare (15 percent), Medicaid (12 percent), and insurance for the military (1 percent). About 15 percent of the population in 2011 did not have health insurance. In addition, it was estimated that about 30 million people had policies offering them only limited coverage.[18]

There is no standard package of insurance benefits in the United States, although the Affordable Care Act, if fully implemented, would move the United States closer to insured people having at least a minimum package of services. Today, different insurers offer different insurance packages, with substantial variation in what is covered and what copayments and deductibles apply. The typical policy, however, covers both physicians' services and hospitalization. Many policies and Medicare also cover prescription drugs, and some cover dental and eye care, which some people can also purchase separately.[18]

The U.S. government finances about half of all healthcare expenditure in the United States, mostly through the public programs noted previously. About half of all expenditure is private. Those who get insurance through their employer generally share the cost of the insurance with their employer, through tax-exempt premiums. It was estimated that in 2011 about 11 percent of all healthcare expenditure, or almost $1000 per capita, was out-of-pocket payments.[18]

The overwhelming majority of U.S. physicians work as private practitioners, either on their own or in group practices. Patients are usually free to choose the doctor or hospital they wish to use, unless they are part of an insurance plan that limits providers to those who are preferred. In most cases, primary care physicians in the United States are not formally charged with being gatekeepers, although some insurance plans do require referral from a primary care physician.[18]

About 70 percent of the hospitals in the United States operate on a nonprofit basis. Another 15 percent are public hospitals, and the final 15 percent are for profit. Most payments to physicians and hospitals are on a fee-for-service basis.

Upper Middle-Income Countries

Brazil

The Brazilian healthcare system is referred to as the SUS—Sistema Única de Saúde (Unified Health System). SUS is essentially composed of three parts:

- Services funded and provided by SUS itself.
- Private healthcare services, made up of for-profit and not-for-profit organizations and providers, from which the SUS and the private insurance system contract services.
- A private insurance system, the Supplementary Health System, which includes over 1,500 private insurers, and which supports the purchase of services by the insured from either SUS providers or private providers.[19,20]

In principle, the Brazilian healthcare system seeks to promote universal coverage through a decentralized system in which the federal and state governments provide oversight and financing and the municipalities provide or manage services.

The public system is based partly on a model of integrated primary care, called the Family Health Program (PSF). About 70 percent of the population is covered by PSF. The remainder purchase private insurance, sometimes with the support of their employer. The PSF has a health team for every 600 to 1,000 people, composed of a doctor, a nurse, an auxiliary nurse, and six community health workers. In 2010, Brazil had about 33,000 PSF teams.[21]

Most of the nonhospital services are operated by the SUS. However, about 75 percent of the hospital beds, more than 80 percent of the clinics, and 40 percent of the specialty diagnostic and therapeutic centers are in the private sector.[19]

The SUS is funded from general tax contributions from the federal, state, and municipal levels and from social insurance contributions. SUS services are free, although copayments are required for pharmaceuticals.[20] Public spending on health in Brazil in 2012 was about 46 percent of total health expenditure, and private spending was about 54 percent of total expenditure on health.[22]

Costa Rica[23]

Costa Rica has had a commitment to universal health coverage for many years. Costa Rica is also a country that is well-known for having achieved high levels of health outcomes even before it had achieved a relatively high level of national income per capita.

The health system of Costa Rica resembles the health systems of many Latin American countries in some ways; it also resembles the National Health Service of the United Kingdom. The most important part of the health system is the Costa Rican Social Security Administration (Caja Costaricense de Seguro Social—CCSS). The CCSS is both a financier and a provider of health services.

The CCSS has three main parts: Illness and Maternal Health; Disability, Old Age, and Death; and the noncontributive regime. People who work in the formal sector of the economy are obliged to participate in the CCSS. Informal sector workers may also join the CCSS, with fees that depend on their income. More than 90 percent of the financing of the CCSS comes from employer and employee taxes, with the remainder coming from government. The government has a mechanism, related to the noncontributive regime, to cover the costs of insurance of those unable to pay into the system. Participants in the CCSS receive most services for free, but do have copayments for some services as well.

Somewhat like Brazil, Costa Rica has established a national system of primary care that is community-oriented. The government has divided the country into health regions and 105 health areas, each of which has 30,000 to 60,000 people. The basic unit of health coverage is 950 "health teams for integrated primary care" (EBAIS), which each serves 3,500 to 4,000 people.[23]

Lower-Middle-Income Countries

India[24]

The health system in India bears many resemblances to the health system in the United States. First, India has moved increasingly toward accepting the principle of universal health coverage, but it still has a significant distance to go to achieve it. Second, India's health system is highly fragmented, with a range of public and private financiers and providers. Third, India is a federal system; health is largely under state jurisdiction, but the federal government nevertheless plays an important role in many aspects of the system. This federal role focuses in principle on public goods such as family planning and the control of communicable diseases.

One part of the Indian healthcare system is a publicly financed and provided set of healthcare services. For this, India has a tiered network of health services in the public sector. At the lowest level is a health subcenter, which serves 3,000 to 5,000 people, depending on whether it is in a difficult geographic area or serves tribal people. Subcenters are staffed by one female and one male multipurpose worker. India has almost 150,000 subcenters. Primary health centers serve 20,000 to 30,000 people and are staffed with a physician, a nurse, a female multipurpose worker, a health educator, a laboratory technician, and assistant-level staff. India has almost 25,000 primary healthcare centers. Community health centers (CHC) serve 80,000 to 120,000 people and are staffed with a physician, a pediatrician, a gynecologist, and a surgeon, as well as a number of paramedical staff. Each operates as a small hospital with 30 beds and a laboratory and x-ray facilities. India has about 4,500 CHCs.

At the top of the Indian publicly provided healthcare system are hospitals of varying sizes and complexities. These hospitals are at the district, regional, and national levels, with the latter able to treat very complicated cases and with a full range of staff.

In addition to having an extensive array of public facilities, India also has a very large private healthcare sector. This ranges from unlicensed medical practitioners, to practitioners of Indian systems of medicine, to very well-trained practitioners of allopathic medicine. In addition, there is an equally wide variety of private healthcare facilities, from simple nursing homes to the most sophisticated hospitals. The private sector treats almost 80 percent of outpatients and 60 percent of inpatients.

India is just beginning to develop more extensive approaches to insurance. It previously had schemes for the military and government workers. However, it has more recently developed a scheme, RSBY, which is intended to insure people living below the poverty line. About 300 million people in India, or about 30 percent of the population, are now covered by health insurance, with about 250 million in public schemes and 50 million in private schemes.

The lack of insurance, coupled with the extensive use of private sector services by all socioeconomic classes, has led to about 80 percent of all healthcare expenditure being private and much of that being out-of-pocket.

Ghana

The health system is Ghana is moving from one that was overwhelmingly dependent on publicly funded and provided services to a system that would be based on everyone having access to insurance that would allow them to purchase service from a variety of providers. Ghana is among the first African countries to commit to universal coverage, and as a result it is important to learn from Ghana's experience.[25]

Until recently Ghana's health system was largely publicly financed and provided. Like the foundation of the Indian system and the systems in many other low- and middle-income countries, Ghana has had a public system that is a pyramid of services at different levels, following population-based norms. In addition to the public system, Ghana has had services provided by NGOs, other nonprofits, and the for-profit private sector.[26]

Although the government largely financed the public system, it also required that those using the system pay user fees for the services they received. In Ghana, this became known as the "cash and carry system," which has been shown to be an important constraint to the demand for and use of health services by the poor.[26]

In 2003 Ghana established the National Health Insurance System, which was financed by a value-added tax. NHIS is meant to be universal in coverage. Prior to the launching of the NHIS, less than 1 percent of the population was insured.[26]

Some estimates suggest that Ghana has made substantial progress in enrolling people in the NHIS, perhaps enrolling 30 percent of the population. In addition, it has been estimated that the use of healthcare services among the insured has risen dramatically and that out-of-pocket payments for this group have substantially declined.

Other views of the NHIS, however, have been more critical. An assessment of the NHIS carried out by Oxfam, for example, concluded that enrollment has only reached about 18 percent of the population, that the rich are enrolling at much higher rates than the poor, and that many people continue to pay for health services they cannot afford through the cash and carry system.[27]

Ghana is one of the first low-income countries to commit to universal health coverage and to take steps to achieve it. The lessons that emerge from Ghana's experience, which will hopefully be based on rigorous and independent assessment, will be very important for other low-income countries that are planning to move to universal health coverage.

KEY HEALTH SECTOR ISSUES

When we consider the extent to which various health systems meet the criteria WHO has set for measuring health system performance, it is clear that some health systems produce better outcomes than others. **Table 5-6** indicates how a selected group of countries fared in the 2000 WHO ranking

of health systems performance. Although these rankings are not current and they were a source of considerable controversy, they are nonetheless useful.

The WHO ranking suggests that health systems in high-income countries generally perform better than health systems in low- and middle-income countries. However, the ranking also confirms a point noted earlier: the health systems of a small group of middle-income countries, such as Costa Rica and Morocco, rate higher in the WHO ranking than a number of countries with higher incomes. Cuba ranked almost as high as many countries with higher incomes.[28]

As we explore health systems in greater detail, however, it becomes clear that all systems wrestle with a variety of challenges and constraints. Some of the most important challenges are related to changing epidemiologic and demographic patterns, governance of the health sector, having an appropriate number and placement of healthcare personnel, the financing of health care, and the role of the private sector in the overall health system. Other important issues include the quality of care, how to finance services so that people are protected from their costs, and the extent to which people have access to and get covered by the most appropriate health services for their needs. As discussed earlier, the health systems in many countries also face critical issues of equity and financial protection. Finally, health systems face a number of problems concerning their design and the overall achievement of health outcomes, some of which have been the subject of health sector reform efforts and some of which will relate to the growing need to address noncommunicable diseases. These themes are explored briefly here.

Demographic and Epidemiologic Change

Demographic and epidemiologic changes raise critical challenges for the health systems of most countries. In high-income countries and in many low- and middle-income countries, people are living longer. As they do so, societies face higher burdens of noncommunicable diseases. Many of these conditions are chronic, and the cost of treating them is high compared to acute bouts of communicable diseases or conditions that occur at younger ages. As a result, relatively poor countries, with few resources to spend on health and weak institutions to address health issues, face a triple burden of disease simultaneously—the burdens of noncommunicable disease, communicable disease, and injuries.[29]

Stewardship

The quality of governance is an important determinant of outcomes in the health sector, as well as in many other sectors. In high-income countries, the health sector will tend to

TABLE 5-6 Overall Health System Performance Ranking, Selected Countries, 2000

Country	Overall Performance Ranking	Country	Overall Performance Ranking
France	1	Bangladesh	88
Germany	25	India	112
Morocco	29	Pakistan	122
Canada	30	Bolivia	126
Denmark	34	Peru	129
Costa Rica	36	Ghana	135
United States of America	37	Haiti	138
Cuba	39	China	144
Dominican Republic	51	Nepal	150
Philippines	60	Vietnam	160
Mexico	61	Niger	170
Egypt	63	Afghanistan	173
Turkey	70	Cambodia	174
Argentina	75	South Africa	175
Sri Lanka	76	Cameroon	164
Jordan	83	Zambia	182

Data from WHO. *The world health report 2000*. Geneva: WHO; 2000:Annex Table.

be governed in relatively open and transparent ways. These countries will usually have clear rules and regulations for the management and operation of the health sector, and high-income countries can enforce those regulations. There is usually relatively little corruption in the health sectors of high-income countries.

Unfortunately, however, there are major problems of governance in many low- and middle-income countries. These problems often affect the performance of the healthcare system and penalize poor people more than other people, because the poor have fewer choices about where they can go for their health care and have less power in dealing with healthcare personnel. Governance in these settings will tend to be weak across most sectors, and governments in low- and middle-income countries are often unable to enforce health sector rules and regulations. This may be especially true with respect to the inability of the health sector to oversee the work of the private healthcare sector.[30]

The management of human resource matters is often especially weak, with staff sometimes being recruited by virtue of their connections, rather than their merit or fit with existing hiring rules. In addition, some staff that are recruited have to pay off the people who are recruiting them by giving them an upfront payment for their post or a percentage of their salary each month. Healthcare personnel are often absent from their jobs without sanction. When health services procure goods or construct facilities, they frequently do not get the best prices available, because they are engaging in corrupt practices with the providers of those goods or because they do not have the capacity to engage in sound procurement practices. In many countries, healthcare personnel arrange to get payments from patients for services that are intended to be free.[30]

Human Resource Issues

The most severe human resource issues in better-off countries will tend to be imbalances in the number of certain types of healthcare personnel. Some countries do not produce enough physicians. Others do not produce enough nurses, and they tend to make up these shortages through the recruitment of healthcare personnel from other countries, particularly low- and middle-income countries. This greatly contributes to the problem of "brain drain" in the healthcare sector of low- and middle-income countries, as discussed later in the chapter.[31]

The human resource issues in many low-income countries are considerable and consistent. The very poorest countries, especially in sub-Saharan Africa, will not have enough healthcare personnel to operate a health system effectively. They will face shortages of physicians, midwives, nurses, and laboratory and other technicians. Despite their needs for better stewardship, they will also face important gaps in qualified health service managers, both clinical and nonclinical. In addition, the quality of training, knowledge, and skills of many of their healthcare staff will be deficient. Those staff who are well-trained will usually be clustered in major cities, and there are often important shortages of appropriately trained healthcare personnel everywhere else in the country, especially in rural and poor areas. Public sector salaries of staff will be very low compared to salaries in the private sector and overseas. As a result, many staff lack the incentive to perform their jobs properly, often practice in both the private and public sectors even if this is not allowed, and are frequently absent from work. In the face of poor salaries and working conditions in which they often lack the facilities, equipment, and materials needed to perform their work well, many healthcare personnel move to other countries, particularly higher-income countries, in which salaries and working conditions are much better.[31,32]

Quality of Care

The United States Institute of Medicine (IOM) defines quality as "the degree to which health services for individuals and populations increase the likelihood of desired health outcomes and are consistent with current professional knowledge."[33,p3] According to the IOM approach, health services need to be:[33]

- Safe
- Effective
- Patient-centered
- Timely
- Efficient
- Equitable

There is good evidence from low-, middle-, and high-income countries that many health systems suffer from important problems of quality, and that quality varies considerably within health systems. Studies in the United States, for example, showed that "physicians complied with evidence based guidelines for at least 80 percent of patients in only 8 of 306 U.S. hospital regions."[34,p1295] In a study in Papua New Guinea, a low-income country with rampant malaria, only 24 percent of health workers could indicate the correct treatment for malaria.[35] In a similar study in Pakistan, only 35 percent of the health workers could indicate the proper treatment for a certain type of diarrhea.[36] In another study of clinical practices in seven low- and middle-income countries, 76 percent of the cases were not adequately diagnosed, treated, or monitored, and inappropriate treatment with antibiotics, fluids, feeding, or oxygen occurred for 61 percent of the patients.[37]

A study that further reflects the depth of quality issues was published in 2015. This examined how health practitioners in rural India treat childhood diarrhea and pneumonia. This was assessed by seeing how the practitioners responded both to vignettes and to standardized patients. Only 3.5 percent of those given a diarrhea vignette offered oral rehydration for diarrhea, despite this being the standard of care and it being available locally. None of those given a standard patient offered the correct care for diarrhea, but 13 percent of them offered the correct treatment for pneumonia. Seventy-two percent of those given the standard patient prescribed potentially harmful treatments for diarrhea.[38]

There are many causes of poor-quality health services in low- and middle-income countries, including poor management, a lack of financial resources, poorly trained and inappropriately deployed staff, a failure of staff to do their work as intended, and unempowered patients, as discussed throughout this chapter. Many health systems also provide very little supervision of healthcare personnel and have only weak systems for monitoring the performance of their health system.[34]

The Financing of Health Systems

The health systems in many countries battle continuously for sufficient financing to meet their highest priorities in effective and efficient ways. Many countries, especially better-off ones, face issues of rising costs because of aging populations and the ever-increasing demands for the use of new technologies and new drugs. In addition, all health systems ration health services to some extent. In many high-income countries, a critical issue is how to find the funding that is needed, even with increased efficiency, to reduce the waiting times for certain medical procedures that are financed through the national insurance program. This has been a highlight of the healthcare debates in the United Kingdom and Canada, for example. A few of the high-income countries, such as Switzerland and the United States, also face important questions about the share of their total GDP that they are devoting to health and the implications of this for the rest of the economy.

As one might expect, the financing issue in most low- and middle-income countries often revolves around the absolute lack of public sector financial resources for health. It is true that many low-income countries do not spend effectively or efficiently the financial resources that they do have for health. However, it is also true that many countries do not provide the health sector with the public funds needed to ensure that an appropriate basic package of health services is available to all people without respect to their ability to pay. The costs of such a basic package were estimated in 2006 to range in the low-income countries between the equivalent of $12 and $50 per person.[39] We have already seen, however, that the very poorest countries allocate from public funds only between 1 and 3 percent of their GDP for health, which would give them only about $3 to $10 per person annually to finance such a basic package.[40]

Financial Protection and the Provision of Universal Coverage

As also discussed earlier, one measure of the performance of a health system is fairness of financial contribution, as WHO calls it. This refers to financing health care in a way that does not cause people to be denied access to health care or to become impoverished because of their inability to pay for health services.[4]

The capacity of people to pay for health services *is* a barrier to their access to health care, and catastrophic health costs impoverish people in many settings. In most high-income countries, this is not a significant problem because they have social insurance schemes and essentially offer health insurance to all of their people. However, this is a common problem in poorer countries. Studies in India have shown, for example, that expenditure on health is a leading cause of families falling below the poverty line and a major cause of families selling assets to pay their bills for health care.[41] Although the evidence is of poor quality and mixed, some studies have shown a decline in the use of tuberculosis medicines and hospital deliveries of babies when charges were levied on these services.[42]

Access and Equity

Health disparities are an important feature of many health systems. It is always important to assess health status, the provision of health services, and health outcomes by sex, age, ethnicity, income, education, and location. In low- and middle-income countries, disparities in access to services and in equity are often reflected in the following ways, among others:

- A lack of coverage of basic health services in areas where poor, rural, and minority people live
- Service coverage with a lower level of inputs in the areas previously noted, compared to other areas, such as fewer trained personnel and less equipment and drugs
- Service coverage that varies, such as already illustrated for immunization programs, with income and education levels, as well as by location, with urban dwellers getting preference
- Better-off people getting access to relatively expensive services that are generally less available to the lower-income and socially marginalized groups

It is very important as we assess the performance of health systems that we examine the coverage of health programs for different types of people. It is also important that we examine how accessible services are to lower-income and other disadvantaged groups compared to the services available to higher-income and other advantaged groups.

ADDRESSING KEY HEALTH SECTOR CONCERNS

There are few easy answers to effectively addressing the most critical health sector issues, particularly in low-income countries. Nevertheless, there is an increasing body of evidence about measures that can be taken to deal with some of the specific problems noted above and to design and manage health systems more effectively and efficiently. These are discussed briefly here.

Demographic and Epidemiologic Change

The very poorest countries can take only a limited number of steps at once to deal with the multiple burdens of communicable and noncommunicable diseases and injuries. Yet most of these countries will face an increasing burden from noncommunicable disease, particularly cardiovascular disease, and road traffic accidents.

Perhaps the single most important step that low- and middle-income countries can take today to reduce the future burden of cardiovascular disease is to reduce the disease burden that is related to tobacco use. There is very good evidence that even in low-income settings, measures to make it harder and more expensive to buy cigarettes can reduce tobacco smoking.[43] Even with their limited financial resources and management capacity, low-income countries need to start to take these steps now. They can also take other measures to begin to reduce road traffic accidents, including better engineering of roads, safer cars, and more traffic enforcement.[44]

The way in which health systems are organized and operated in many low- and middle-income countries will need to be strengthened to address the growing burden of noncommunicable diseases related to economic, demographic, and epidemiologic change. These countries will need to pay increasing attention to these problems, even as they continue to confront the problems of communicable diseases and undernutrition. To an important extent, countries will need to assess the six building blocks of health systems from the perspective of managing prevention, treatment, and care related to noncommunicable diseases. Addressing chronic noncommunicable diseases requires prolonged and frequent contacts with patients, unlike care for most communicable diseases, with the exception of HIV treatment. Countries will need to develop or adopt models of care that can sustain more frequent contacts with patients over a longer period of time than they have had to do thus far.[45]

Stewardship

It will also be difficult to improve health system governance in countries in which overall governance is weak and corruption is high. Nonetheless, a number of measures are proving to be useful in addressing key governance issues in health. Corruption has been reduced, for example, in countries like Poland that have launched national anticorruption programs with strong political backing. In addition, reforming procurement systems and making them more open and transparent has been associated with reducing corruption in contracting in countries such as Chile and Argentina. Increasing audits

of the health system and enforcing penalties to deal with adverse findings have assisted Madagascar in reducing corruption. There is an increasing number of efforts at reducing corruption and enhancing management through oversight by communities. In a number of cases, such as in Uganda, the Philippines, and Bolivia, community boards were provided more information about the money and services that the community should have received and the authority to provide oversight of these resources in a way that could lead to the firing of corrupt officials. Contracting out some services, carrying out customer satisfaction surveys among the users of the health system, and letting communities provide services with "citizen report cards" are also proving to be helpful to enhancing governance in some settings.[30]

Human Resources

The problems of human resources for health relate largely to a lack of staff, a maldistribution of staff, the inadequate training and quality of personnel, and the poor environment in which many of them have to carry out their work. An international group examining human resources for health has suggested that there needs to be more shared global responsibility for these resources, given the extent to which health workers migrate in search of better pay and working conditions. In addition, they suggested that countries need to have much more explicit strategies for workforce development that would focus on coverage, motivation, and competence. They also highlighted the need for countries and their development partners to provide greater support for education and training of health personnel and to develop better policies and programs for retaining personnel.[46]

Even as they seek to address these problems in more comprehensive ways, some countries have taken steps to deal with human resource issues. Countries might be able to reduce the share of their health workers who are migrating, for example, by training them so they gain needed skills but do not get credentials for those skills that would be recognized by other countries.[32] Moreover, lower-level health personnel can be trained to carry out a number of functions often reserved for higher-level staff, a strategy known as "task shifting." In Malawi, where there is an acute shortage of doctors, nurses were trained to perform caesarean sections.[32] As antiretroviral therapy is being scaled up for HIV/AIDS, community-based workers are being taught how to dispense drugs for patients who have been doing well on treatment and to recognize when the patients are having problems and need to be referred for more specialized care. These are tasks reserved for doctors in some HIV/AIDS treatment programs. A number of mental health programs in places where there are very few mental health professionals are training healthcare workers at the primary level or community health workers to be the front line in the diagnosis and treatment of mental health issues.

A number of countries also use financial incentives to encourage better performance of healthcare personnel. These might include better salaries, additional payments for serving in hard-to-reach areas, bonus payments for meeting certain health service or health outcome objectives, providing housing for people who work in those areas, or special allowances for training. There is also good evidence that the productivity of health workers is higher when their pay is tied to services provided per patient that they actually perform, rather than just paying them a salary. The design of incentives and provider payment mechanisms, of course, has to take account of what one is trying to achieve and of the local culture. Incentives might be different, for example, if one were trying to reduce migration, trying to get staff to serve in rural areas, or just trying to get staff to come to work in a timely way.[32] One of the policy and program briefs later in the chapter discusses results-based financing.

Financing Health Services

The scope for very low-income countries to raise additional resources for health is limited, given the overall scarcity of resources. Nevertheless, there is some scope for shifting resources from other areas of the economy in some countries, given the potentially high returns to investments in health. Some of the low-income countries, however, will require development assistance for health for some time in order to boost expenditure on health and more effectively address some of their key health goals, such as HIV.[47]

As shown in the case study on Tanzania at the end of this chapter, however, there is also some scope for enhancing health outcomes by shifting expenditure within the health sector. By focusing expenditure on a selected group of low-cost investments that are known to be effective if managed properly, even very poor countries may be able to improve health outcomes of their poorest people.[4,39] To assist in raising and managing resources for health more effectively, many countries will need to enhance the data they have on health expenditure and also monitor health investments and expenditures more carefully.

Many countries also have substantial room for improving the efficiency of the resources they spend on health. WHO has estimated that between 20 and 40 percent of the expenditures on health in low-income countries are wasted by spending that is not effective or efficient. Improvements in the efficiency of expenditures could help to free resources for high-priority expenditures. In addition, the better management of financial resources by ministries of health will strengthen any arguments they make to ministries of finance about the need for additional financing for health and their ability to use it wisely.[7]

Financial Protection and Universal Coverage

WHO has suggested that countries need to take a number of steps to enhance people's protection from the burden of health expenditure and to achieve universal coverage with a basic package of health services. These measures would include raising additional revenue for health, improving the efficiency of health sector expenditure, reducing dependence on out-of-pocket expenditures, and enhancing equity. Although efforts to achieve universal coverage were once generally considered possible only in middle- and high-income countries, a number of low- and middle-income countries in the last decade have made substantial progress toward providing universal coverage, including Brazil, Ghana, Mexico, Rwanda, and Thailand.[7] Ghana was discussed briefly earlier. The policy and program briefs section of this chapter includes additional briefs on the efforts to achieve universal coverage.

As countries move toward universal coverage, in what probably has to be a phased manner, they can take a number of measures to reduce out-of-pocket expenditures. Greater financial protection would be offered to the poor, for example, if governments allocated a larger amount of funding to a basic package of free primary health care and targeted that to those places and people most in need. Governments could couple this with subsidies for selected hospital services for the poor, as well, although these schemes are often difficult to manage. Second, governments could also contract a package of primary healthcare services from NGOs and the private sector and subsidize that package for the poor. This has been done with some success in Afghanistan and Cambodia. Third, governments could encourage NGOs to provide services from their own resources, as selected local and international NGOs have the resources to do. BRAC, which will be discussed later, is one such NGO, with a long record of involvement in primary health care for the poor. Fourth, there is some evidence that schemes in which communities raise funds for an insurance pool and purchase health services with those funds might enhance the availability of health services to communities.[4,40,48]

Access and Equity

Improving access to and equity of services is largely a question of political will and health systems planning. Many countries have not focused sufficient attention on the health of their disadvantaged people and have not been sufficiently aware of the kinds of gaps in health coverage and health status that these people face. There is increasing evidence, however, like that cited earlier, that the coverage of health services is inequitable and often leaves out those living in difficult regions and those with less income, less education, and less empowerment. Countries need to use the data they get from national surveys, such as the Demographic and Health Surveys,[49] to identify gaps in health status and health coverage. They then need to specifically target health resources to the places and people most in need. Very substantial gains could be made in health status within many countries, for example, if the coverage of effective programs for at least childhood vaccination, tuberculosis, and malaria were increased among the poor. The enhancements in health would be even greater if carried out in conjunction with improvements in water supply, sanitation, nutrition, and overall hygiene and health-caring behaviors. This can be partly accomplished through improvements in knowledge that also need to be at the core of efforts to improve the health of the poor.

Quality

Low-quality health services waste money and are dangerous to people's health. Although most of us probably believe that low quality is primarily a reflection of inadequate financial resources, there is good evidence that quality can be enhanced in a number of ways even in the absence of additional resources.

It is very important, first, that health systems carry out assessments that will help them to understand the quality gaps in their programs. Second, there is evidence that better professional oversight, supervision, and continuing training can enhance the quality of care provided by health service providers. Third, the use of clear guidelines, protocols, and algorithms for services can also improve quality, particularly where health workers are not well-educated or trained. Fourth, when contracting services to the private and NGO sectors, governments can link their payments with performance against specific goals and can independently verify that they have been achieved. This can also be done through results-based financing schemes in the public sector, as discussed in the policy brief later in this chapter. Finally, focusing some health staff on becoming very proficient at a small number of services is consistently associated with better quality of care.[50]

There is also evidence that total quality management approaches can enhance the quality of care, even in low-income countries. In this approach, groups of health providers define goals, measure how the system is doing in achieving them, together decide how they might best address the gaps in their program, and then evaluate whether their proposed improvements are working. Even in the poorest areas of North India, this kind of effort, coupled with standard guidelines for managing certain services, has produced improvements in the quality of care. The safety of anesthesia has been enhanced in Malaysia in similar ways.[50]

Delivering Primary Health Care

In the end, of course, trying to enhance health outcomes for the poor through better health services in low- and middle-income countries is not just a question of addressing the specific issues discussed previously. Rather, it is also a question of the overall orientation of the health system and how it will carry out the services that can potentially have the biggest impact on improving health outcomes for disadvantaged groups.

There is a broad consensus that a number of measures are needed to achieve this aim. First, services should be focused on the most important burdens of disease. Second, health outcomes can only be achieved if the health system is strengthened to deliver those services effectively, efficiently, and at an appropriate level of quality. Third, the core of activities to meet these goals should be through primary health care and the district hospital.[51]

There have been a number of very important declarations, studies, and reports that have suggested what the basic healthcare package should contain. The most important elements of what a primary healthcare package might contain are noted in **Table 5-7**.

Although there are differences in the exact content of the suggested package, there is consensus around most of the elements it might contain. To a large extent, it is recommended that countries deliver the services listed in **Table 5-8** as close to where people live as possible, through close collaboration between primary healthcare services and the district hospital. The hospital would help to supervise the work in primary health care as well as serve as the referral service for activities that cannot be handled adequately at the primary level, such as complications of pregnancy. The components of the package are outlined in Table 5-8.[51] It is important to note that services like those outlined in Table 5-8 need to be provided regardless of whether countries organize their health system along public or private provision of services.

Ideally, these services would be delivered in an integrated manner. However, because of weaknesses in the health systems of many countries, especially low-income ones, a substantial number of countries have established "vertical" programs to address some of these health problems. These have historically been used to deal with diseases such as smallpox, malaria, neglected tropical diseases, and

TABLE 5-7 Model Primary Care Package of Essential Health Services Interventions

Maternity-related interventions	**Childhood disease-related interventions (treatment)**	**HIV prevention**
Prenatal care	Acute respiratory infections early diagnosis and treatment	Youth-focused interventions
Tetanus vaccine	Diarrhea—oral rehydration with zinc	Interventions with sex workers and clients and interventions for other most at risk populations, such as men who have sex with men
Skilled attendant at delivery	Causes of fever—early diagnosis and treatment	Condom social marketing and distribution
Treatment of complications during pregnancy	Undernutrition—measures to enhance protein, energy and needed micronutrients, including iron, iodine, vitamin A and zinc	Workplace interventions
Emergency obstetric care		Strengthening of blood transfusion systems
Postpartum care	Feeding and breastfeeding counseling	Voluntary counseling and testing
Family planning	**Malaria prevention**	Prevention of mother-to-child transmission
Childhood disease-related interventions (prevention)	Insecticide-treated nets	Treatment for sexually transmitted infections
Bacillus Calmette-Guérin vaccination for tuberculosis	Residual indoor spraying	**HIV care**
Polio vaccination	Intermittent treatment of pregnant women	Palliative care
Diphtheria-pertussis-tetanus vaccination	**Malaria treatment**	Clinical management of opportunistic illnesses
Measles vaccination	Early diagnosis and treatment with Artemisinin-based combination therapy	Prevention of opportunistic illnesses
Hepatitis B vaccination		Home-based care
Haemophilus influenza type B vaccination	**Tuberculosis treatment**	Provision of highly active antiretroviral therapy (HAART) for HIV
Rotavirus vaccination	Directly Observed Therapy, Short-Course (DOTS)	**Tobacco control program**—taxes, ban smoking in public places, ban advertising, ban sales to minors, health education, nicotine replacement)
Pnumococcal vaccination		
Vitamin A supplementation		**Alcohol control program**—taxes, ban advertising, ban sales to minors, laws against drunk driving, short counseling sessions
Anthelmintic treatment		
School health program (incorporating micronutrient supplementation, school meals, anthelmintic treatment, and health education)		

Data used with permission from Tollman, S., Doherty, J., & Mulligan, J.-A. (2006). General primary care. In D. T. Jamison, J. G. Breman, A. R. Measham, et al. (Eds.), *Disease Control Priorities in developing countries* 2nd ed. Washington, DC and New York: The World Bank and Oxford University Press, 1193–1209.

tuberculosis, for example, for which governments set up separate management, financing, procurement, staffing, and reporting in parallel with the regular health programs of the government.

Although in principle this vertical approach may not be the most efficient and effective manner in which to operate health services, in practice it has sometimes been seen as the only way to accomplish urgent goals in weak health systems. There is an increasing consensus that if such approaches are going to be taken, then they should be linked with efforts to improve related aspects of the health system. The polio eradication program, for example, can be used to strengthen laboratories, surveillance, and the management of the cold chain for some medicines and vaccines. In any case, there is now a growing effort globally to focus on health systems strengthening and to try to ensure that countries increasingly take more integrated approaches to their health systems.[52]

POLICY AND PROGRAM BRIEFS

Seven policy and program briefs follow to illustrate some of the concepts that were discussed in this chapter. The first discusses the concept of *universal health coverage* and the progress toward this goal in an increasing number of countries. The second examines the efforts of Rwanda to

TABLE 5-8 Selected Essential Healthcare Interventions by Level of Service in a Close to the Client System

Level of Care	Tuberculosis	Malaria	HIV	Childhood Diseases	Maternal/ Perinatal	Smoking
Outreach services		Epidemic planning and response Indoor residual spraying	Peer education for vulnerable groups Needle exchange	Specific immunization campaign Outreach for integrated management of childhood illness (IMCI): home management of fever Outreach for micronutrients and deworming		
Health center/ health post	DOTS	Treatment of uncomplicated malaria Intermittent treatment of pregnant women for malaria	Antiretrovirals Prevention of opportunistic infections (OIs) and treatment of uncomplicated OIs Voluntary counseling and testing (VCT) Treatment of sexually transmitted infections (STIs)	IMCI Immunization Treatment of severe anemia	Skilled birth attendants Antenatal and postnatal care Family planning postpartum	Cessation advice Pharmacological therapies for smoking
Hospital	DOTS for complicated tuberculosis cases	Treatment of complicated malaria	Blood transfusion for HIV HAART treatment of severe OI for AIDS Palliative care	IMCI: severe cases	Emergency obstetric care	

Modified with permission from Jha, P., & Mills, A. (2002). *Improving health outcomes for the poor: Report of Working Group 5 of the Commission on Macroeconomics and Health*. Geneva: WHO 52.

provide insurance for its poorest people through community-based insurance schemes. The third brief reviews Thailand's experience in trying to achieve universal coverage of health services, in conjunction with the development of a national health insurance scheme. The fourth brief discusses efforts to improve access to and the effectiveness and efficiency of services by contracting out services to the private and NGO sectors. The fifth brief addresses efforts to improve the demand for health services and the supply of better-quality and more effective and efficient services through results-based financing. The sixth brief discusses the important place of pharmaceuticals in healthcare systems. The last brief reviews the need for countries to enhance their capacity for essential surgery and how countries might achieve this in high quality and cost-efficient ways.

Universal Health Coverage

As noted earlier, WHO defines *universal coverage* or *universal health coverage* (UHC) as:

> ensuring that all people can use the promotive, preventive, curative, rehabilitative and palliative health services they need, of sufficient quality to be effective, while also ensuring that the use of these services does not expose the user to financial hardship.[53]

According to WHO, the aim of universal health coverage is to ensure "that people get the health services they need, without suffering financial hardship when paying for them."[54] WHO also suggests that this aim reflects three fundamental concerns:[54]

- Fairness of access to services, regardless of people's ability to pay for them
- That services should be of appropriate quality
- That the financial arrangements for such services should protect people from suffering financial hardship

In the simplest terms, *universal health coverage* can be seen as ensuring that all people have access to an agreed set of at least basic healthcare services either free or at such low cost that it does not constrain access or cause hardship.

The importance of universal health coverage should be clear, in light of the comments earlier in the text on equity and on the financing of health care. The costs of care are an important barrier to many people seeking health services. In addition, in general, the poorer the country, the larger the share of health costs that are met by out-of-pocket costs—and these costs often lead to temporary or even permanent impoverishment. Moreover, as the Nobel Laureate Amartya Sen has recently written, universal health coverage is a foundation for better health, and better health is a foundation for social well-being and economic prosperity at the level of individuals, families, and societies.[55]

In principle, the achievement of universal health coverage requires, first of all, a health system that works. Building on the WHO health systems framework described earlier in the chapter, this would ideally mean a system that:[53]

- Offers an integrated package of basic services for maternal and child health, noncommunicable diseases, and the control of key communicable diseases, such as HIV, TB, malaria, and neglected tropical diseases (NTDs)
- Is affordable
- Offers fair access to essential medicine and medical technologies
- Has a well-trained and highly motivated workforce

Of course, these inputs must also be managed effectively if a health system is to function properly and achieve desired outcomes at a reasonable cost.

Although countries can provide financial protection in a number of ways, most have chosen to do so by pooling risks across part or all of the population through insurance. As countries seek to develop an insurance scheme, they face a number of key questions. Among the most fundamental, of course, are:[56]

- Who should be covered?
- What services should be covered?
- What share of the costs should the insurance scheme pay?

At the same time, countries, especially low-income ones, must wrestle with how they will finance the provision of insurance. Generally, countries may finance insurance through some combination of payroll taxes on employers and employees, general taxes, and contributions from the insured in the form of premiums. The options for financing, however, are constrained in countries that have only a small formal sector of the economy and a large informal sector. In these countries, the people who pay taxes are a relatively small share of the population. In addition, trying to collect contributions from participants who are largely rural and poor can be challenging and costly.[56]

As countries establish programs for UHC, they must also assess the most efficient and effective ways to pay the healthcare providers from whom the insurance system will buy services. Should this be on a fee-for-service basis, a fixed fee per person covered per year (capitation), or paying for the achievement of certain health goals or the successful completion of certain procedures?[56]

It will also be important for some countries, as they seek to achieve universal health care, to increase the financial resources available to the health sector. Although this will not happen quickly, many countries do have the capacity to increase the efficiency of tax collection, orient more public resources toward health, and improve the effectiveness and efficiency of existing healthcare expenditure.[56]

Countries must also wrestle with questions concerning how they will organize their risk pooling—insurance—arrangements. Should they have a single national insurance scheme, many schemes operated by different groups, or many schemes based on different kinds of beneficiaries?[56]

The operation of insurance schemes also requires careful attention to deciding how those schemes will finance the purchase of services. Should insurance cover the costs of public sector services, private sector services, or both? Will it be fair, effective, or efficient if the public sector continues to offer free or nearly free but often low-quality services to mostly poor people, whereas other people are able to purchase insurance and buy services in the private sector?[56,57] For many years, there was enormous skepticism about the possibility that some countries, especially low-income ones, could achieve universal health coverage. Today, however, there is a global movement around ensuring that all countries have universal health coverage.

There are also a number of countries that have made important progress toward achieving universal coverage, including some countries that continue to have very low per capita income. In the last decade or so, Mexico has made enormous progress in achieving universal health coverage through a health reform effort that has been the subject of substantial and careful study. In Africa, Ghana, Nigeria, and Rwanda have moved in important ways toward UHC. Korea, Singapore, and Taiwan have had universal health coverage for some time. In addition, Thailand and the Philippines have made important progress toward UHC over the last decade, and other countries, such as China, Indonesia, and Vietnam, are now also moving toward UHC. Countries in South Asia are also making progress toward UHC, such as India's implementation of an insurance program for the poor.[57-60]

Moving toward UHC is a highly political matter, and achieving it will not come quickly or easily in most settings. This suggests that many countries may wish to take a phased approach, such as Mexico did, by phasing in both the coverage of an increasing number of people and an increasing number of services.[60] At the same time, as countries move forward, they will want to take account of the accumulating body of evidence about what works in efforts to achieve UHC. It will also be essential to focus on the achievement of

the goals of UHC through research and rigorous data collection on the impacts and outcomes of UHC. It appears that the establishment of UHC does increase the use of health services. However, in the absence of other measures to improve the quality of services, it is not clear that access alone will lead to better health at a reasonable cost.[57]

Rwanda—Reducing Financial Barriers to Care and Improving the Coverage and Quality of Health Services

Background

Rwanda has made great strides since the 1994 genocide toward social and economic reform, especially in the health sector. From 1999 to 2014, GDP per capita increased from $231 to $620.[61] In 1999, Rwanda also began to implement a health insurance scheme to reduce barriers to health care. In 2007, Rwanda established a system of results-based financing (RBF) of healthcare services, aimed at further improving the coverage and quality of care. Today, many global health researchers and practitioners believe the Rwandan experience with community-based health insurance and RBF is an important one, with many lessons for other countries.

Mutuelles de Santé

Prior to 1999, many government and private health facilities in Rwanda were underused, partly because the majority of citizens could not afford health care. To reduce financial barriers to health care, the government in 1999 began a pilot health insurance program in three districts.[62] Under the pilot program, individuals joined prepayment schemes (PPS), which are community-based health associations called "mutuelles" run by the members themselves. Each PPS was partnered with three health centers. For roughly $2 annually, each individual living in the three villages received annual health insurance. This insurance provided for services both at local health centers and district hospitals. All citizens enrolled in this plan received a minimum package of services at local health centers, such as child growth monitoring, vaccinations, and chronic care management; and complementary packages at district hospitals, including surgical emergencies, specialty appointments, and family planning services.

Evaluations of the pilot program found that PPS had enrolled 88,303 members within the first year itself, more than 20 percent of the target populations in the pilot districts. The overall use of preventative health services was five times higher for members who had PPS, especially for prenatal care and immunization services. By the end of the first year, PPS members had lower unit costs for drugs and personnel per healthcare visit, making the schemes financially sustainable for health centers. This was because members sought treatment earlier than individuals not enrolled in PPS. Given the improvements in preventative care and financial sustainability of health centers, the central government decided to expand PPS nationwide. Now known as *Mutuelles de Santé*, or *Mutuelles* for short, Rwanda's community-based health insurance scheme has now become a critical component of the national health strategy.[63]

Scaling Up Mutuelles

By 2004, the government had standardized the benefits package, enrollment fees, subsidy mechanisms, and organization of the *Mutuelles* health insurance policy. Since then, citizens have paid annual member premiums of 1,000 Rwandan Francs (roughly equal to $2 per year) to fund 50 percent of the scheme.[62] The other half of Mutuelles' funding comes from NGOs, multilateral agencies, and the government of Rwanda.

Although the central government establishes national guidelines, such as annual premiums and benefits covered by the scheme, the implementation of these policies happens on a community level. Community representatives and local healthcare providers organize and run *Mutuelles*. All annual premiums are also paid to the local *Mutuelles*.[64]

Impact of the Mutuelles

Rwanda has significantly expanded healthcare coverage since the introduction of the *Mutuelles* and related investments in results-based financing to improve the quality of health services. Since April 2008, every Rwandan has been obligated to have some form of health insurance, and by 2008, 85 percent of the population was covered under the national *Mutuelles* scheme.

In fact, between 2000 and 2005, the use of health services increased by 50 percent in the general population, and by almost 63 percent among the poorest quintile. Use of insecticide-treated bed nets increased from 6 percent to almost 60 percent among children under 5 years of age, assisted birth deliveries increased from 27 percent to 52 percent, and the number of antenatal care appointments and immunizations also increased across the country.

At the same time, Rwanda was also making reforms to its healthcare system other than the creation of *Mutuelles*, including results-based financing, which could also have contributed to the greater use of health services and health impact. Nevertheless, studies conducted in 2005 found that populations with health insurance were twice as likely to seek medical care as those without health insurance.[65]

Lessons Learned

Rwanda's progress in the health sector over the last 15 years is promising. With a heavy emphasis on making health care affordable, the central government applied a series of innovative strategies to reduce financial barriers and improve the coverage and quality of health care. As of February 2013, 91 percent of Rwandans were insured.

Nonetheless, challenges persist.[66] Annual premium rates are the same for all income quintiles, meaning that some individuals in the lowest income quintile are still unable to afford the program because premium rates are not income-dependent. Furthermore, although financial barriers have been reduced, many Rwandan citizens must still travel long distances to reach health centers, leaving indirect costs as a barrier to care.

Despite these persistent issues, Rwanda may provide some valuable lessons for other low-income countries working to make health care more affordable and accessible. The community-based *Mutuelles* provided a platform for both insurance and greater use of health services. In addition, by expanding health insurance schemes, making health care a priority for low-income individuals, decentralizing healthcare delivery, and providing a set of incentives for performance, Rwanda is quickly approaching universal health coverage for a set of interventions increasingly being delivered at an acceptable level of quality.

Universalizing Insurance Coverage in Thailand

Thailand introduced a reform of its health system more than a decade ago, with the goal of achieving universal health coverage. The Thai experience has a number of useful lessons for other countries.

Despite increases in health expenditure in Thailand from 3.82 percent of GDP in 1980 to 6.21 percent in 1998, nearly 30 percent of the country's population remained uninsured. In addition, the cost of health care rose during that period, creating important financial constraints that affected people's ability to access appropriate health care.

In 2001, the Thai Ministry of Public Health (MoPH) announced its desire to provide universal health care. The approach to universalizing health care would have four important objectives, each of which would seek to remedy a critical deficiency of the existing health system. First, they sought to promote equal sharing of health expenditure and equitable access to high-quality services regardless of income. Second, the new system should facilitate the efficient allocation of resources by trained and experienced administrative and management officials. Third, the system should allow citizens to choose what health services they wish to receive, rather than distribute services uniformly. Finally, universal coverage was intended to promote good health for all through the provision of preventive and health-promoting services, as well as treatment and care.[67]

With these aims in mind, the Thai government introduced the "30 baht health policy" in 2001. The cornerstone of the policy was a public insurance scheme that provided services within a standardized benefit package for a small copayment of 30 baht ($0.80). Registered members of the health plan received a gold card permitting them access to treatment in their health district. Patients could also be referred to specialists from other districts for more complicated cases. Under this system, elderly people, children, and poor people were entitled to a free registration card for the insurance scheme. Prescription drugs under this plan were limited to those included on a national list, which later expanded to include antiretroviral therapy and other high-cost drugs. Accident and emergency care was also included in the basic benefit package.[68]

The 30 baht policy had some important early successes. Prior to the introduction of the policy, nearly a fifth of the population was covered under the health card scheme, which provided treatment for families within a defined benefit scheme for 500 baht ($13.30) per year. Public servants and the poor were also covered through several different government policies, although these programs collectively provided coverage to only 20 percent of the population. However, between 2001 and 2004, after the introduction of the 30 baht policy, Thailand's insured population increased from 25 million to more than 59 million. This increase was mainly due to the new scheme.[68]

Health reforms increased public health expenditure from 66.25 billion baht in 2000–2001 to 72.78 billion baht in 2004–2005. In order to efficiently coordinate this increased funding, the 30 baht program relied on two major changes in the existing system for allocating health resources. First, a purchaser–provider system was created; it established the National Health Security Office (NHSO) as the primary purchasing agency for health services financed by the 30 baht scheme. In addition, the majority of the system's finances would be funneled through contracting units for primary care (CUPs), primary care providers responsible for managing the treatment of their registered population. In theory, the advantage of this approach was increased responsiveness of the provider due to the proximity of the CUP to the patient, as well as increased cost control and accountability.[68] Second, a funding system was created that would reflect the demographics of the population and reduce geographic spending inequalities. Under this scheme, 1,404 baht per capita per year was paid to healthcare facilities from government tax revenues.[67]

Despite some widely regarded successes, the 30 baht program has been criticized for several reasons. The quality of care under this scheme was initially viewed with skepticism. To some patients, the provision of services was seen as substandard and worse than the care they had previously been receiving. To address this concern, the government requested that all hospitals participate in the Hospital Accreditation Program to provide standardized and high quality care.[67] Further criticism focused on the way finances were allocated within the local health systems. CUPs in rural areas were commonly pressured by the directors of community hospitals to distribute resources in the way they saw fit. This often led to funds being tied up in community hospital projects. Critics also noted that funding on a per-patient basis led to deficits among larger hospitals, which have to deal with health problems that are more complicated and expensive than those faced by other parts of the system. This problem was addressed when the Ministry of Public Health introduced the central contingency fund in 2002, which guaranteed funding for hospitals by disbursing the salary budget at the national level.[68]

Lessons Learned

The establishment of universal healthcare insurance in Thailand suggests a number of lessons for other countries. First, it demonstrates that universal health insurance, a goal once viewed as unachievable for low- and middle-income countries, is within reach for many middle-income countries. Thailand's experience also demonstrates that although reforms may quickly expand coverage, they require a sustained political and financial commitment on the part of the government in order to be successful in the long term. Financing reforms take time and could require a series of changes that place large burdens on state funding.

Despite several shortcomings in how Thailand achieved a rapid increase in coverage, the importance of primary care in the healthcare financing system may also be instructive for other countries. Other valuable areas for assessment include the problems the Thais faced after the initial reforms, the purchaser–provider split, the creation of the CUPs, and the risks of creating competing responsibilities between agencies that can lead to tensions, as was seen with the National Health Security Office and the Ministry of Public Health in Thailand.[68] It will also be important for Thailand and other countries to examine the functioning of the Thai hospitals to determine their effectiveness and efficiency in the face of Thailand's changing demographics, growing burden of noncommunicable diseases, and relatively low expenditure on health.

Contracting Out Health Services

As noted earlier in this chapter, countries have taken a number of steps to try to improve access, coverage, effectiveness, and efficiency of their health systems. One approach has been to contract out services. This refers to governments making contracts with health service providers in the private and NGO sectors for health service delivery. In this case, the government becomes the purchaser and financer, rather than the provider, of services. Generally, it is recommended that the government finance services against a clearly defined set of achievements that the contracted party should attain, and that those achievements be independently verified before the government pays for such services.

The premise behind contracting out to the private or NGO sector is that they can provide the desired services more effectively and more efficiently than the government can, particularly in low-income countries with very weak health systems. Both Afghanistan and Cambodia, for example, made important use of contracting out as they sought to rebuild their health systems after periods of conflict, at a time when their health systems were barely functional.

Individual evaluations have been conducted of many of the contracting-out schemes that have been implemented. However, questions remain about the extent to which such schemes have met their aims. In this light, two researchers conducted a review in 2008 of all of the evaluations of contracting out that had been done up to that point, to further understand if contracting out had been successful in increasing access to health services, improving equity in services, and enhancing the quality and efficiency of services.[69]

This review of 13 projects found that contracting out to private providers was associated with improved access to health services. The study further concluded that improvements in access to the services purchased by the government through contracting out did not lead to decreases in the use of other desirable services or have other negative consequences on the health system.[69]

Of the 13 projects the study reviewed, only two focused on improving the equity of health services for the poor. The first was a project in Bangladesh that targeted a poor urban slum population. The second was a project in Cambodia that resulted in a decrease in out-of-pocket expenditures by the poor. The researchers concluded that these two projects were associated with an increase in the access of the poor to health services, by reducing the costs of services to the poor. They also concluded that contracting out projects does have the potential to increase equity in health care.[69]

The majority of the 13 projects that were studied focused on improving the quality of health care. However, it was difficult for the study authors to determine if contracted-out projects were able to increase the quality of services provided compared to the public sector, because of the manner in which quality was defined in the evaluations and the lack of clear indicators for measuring quality. The study highlighted the importance of clearly defining quality and indicators for measuring quality if rigorous assessments are to be made of the impact of contracting out on quality. This would also have to be coupled with an understanding of how much the contracted-out services are used. Additionally, indicators need to take into account how much the government pays providers for their services to see if there is a relationship between cost and quality.[69]

Five of the 13 studies addressed improved efficiency in health services. The researchers found that in some cases, healthcare costs were lower among contracted-out projects than public services, but in other cases, health-related costs were higher in contracted-out projects than in government schemes. The study acknowledged that contracted-out projects could lead to lower health costs; however, they were not able to conclude that these projects have increased the efficiency of healthcare systems.[69]

Overall, based on the assessments of contracting-out schemes carried out to date, the study concluded that contracted-out projects are able to increase access to services and equity in health care. However, the study also concluded that the effects of these projects on quality and efficiency are difficult to determine, and further research is necessary on these points.

Results-Based Financing

Results-based financing (RBF), also known as performance-based incentives (PBI), is an umbrella term that encompasses many different financing approaches that create incentives for healthy outcomes. RBF can be defined as "a cash payment or non-monetary transfer made to a national or sub-national government, manager, provider, payer or consumer of health services after predefined results have been attained and verified. Payment is conditional on measurable actions being undertaken."[70,p1] In simple terms, RBF is the provision of cash or in-kind incentives for measurable results, upon verification by a third party.

RBF tries to address health system problems through incentives. These rewards and penalties seek to improve health-related behaviors and ultimately health outcomes. The RBF approach reflects a move away from investing in inputs, such as drugs and equipment, and a renewed focus on outputs, such as deliveries in a facility, or outcomes, such as a decrease in maternal mortality.

In recent years, individual countries and the development community have shown a growing interest in RBF for health because of its potential to increase the impact of health investments. RBF is now being used in a number of different countries to help carry out national health plans and try to accelerate progress toward achievement of the Millennium Development Goals (MDGs).

RBF can create incentives on the supply side, to improve the quantity and/or quality of health services delivered, or on the demand side, to increase use of health services. RBF can also be applied simultaneously to both the supply and demand side. RBF incentives can function at many levels, including at the "level of health facilities (or networks of facilities), the individual provider, the household decision makers, and the patients."[71,p6]

In a supply-side scheme, for example, a health worker or facility may receive a cash incentive for every fully vaccinated child, a curative consultation, or an attended delivery. In a demand-side scheme, a woman might, for example, receive a transport voucher to deliver in a facility or receive a cash transfer based on certain conditions, such as bringing her child in for growth monitoring. Ideally, barriers on both the supply and demand side will be addressed to ensure that the quantity and quality of health services can be improved and that there will be the desired demand for such services. To encourage institutional deliveries, for example, a project with an RBF approach might provide cash incentives to health workers attending deliveries, and transport vouchers to pregnant women who deliver in a facility.

At the core of RBF is a performance contract that specifies what is to be paid for and under what conditions.[70] That contract can be written between many different parties. A few examples follow of how incentives might be structured in different RBF approaches, one concerning development assistance; a second, government efforts to improve the quality and quantity of services; and the third, with respect to government incentives to individuals to participate in selected health schemes:[72]

- *Cash on delivery (COD):* Transfers are made from donor aid agencies to governments.
- *Performance-based contracting (PBC) and performance-based financing (PBF):* Transfers are made from payers to providers.
- *Conditional cash transfers (CCTs):* Transfers are made from governments to their citizens.

RBF approaches can be categorized by the following key elements:[73]

- Who gets paid the incentive?
- What are the actions, outputs, and outcomes for which they get paid?
- How are these things measured and verified?
- What is the nature of the incentive? How big is it? Is it monetary or nonmonetary? What can people do with it?

RBF emphasizes transferring autonomy and flexibility to the local level, thereby encouraging local creativity and innovation in devising solutions to improve health. In addition, the necessity of monitoring results and payments and third-party verification means that RBF can strengthen health management information systems by "improving the timeliness, credibility and accuracy of national reporting and monitoring."[74]

Only a small number of impact evaluations have been done on RBF schemes broadly. Some evidence shows that "positive effects have been demonstrated when only a modest sum was used as the reward (or penalty) and that incentives do appear to be effective ways to achieve important improvements in health."[71,p7]

On the other hand, other data from a review of 13 RBF schemes suggest that RBF schemes may be linked with better improvement in healthcare supply and coverage than other types of health investments. However, it was not clear from this data that these outcomes were linked to the results based approach, rather than to just additional funding. Moreover, this data was insufficient to show a link between the RBF schemes and improved quality of services or improved effectiveness and efficiency of services.[75]

Several CCT programs, however, have been widely recognized for their innovative approach to poverty reduction and for their impressive results. Brazil's Bolsa Família, for example, is a family stipend program aimed at reducing poverty for 11 million families. The program has shown positive results in child health, nutrition, and empowerment of women, and is credited with helping achieve an 81 percent drop in poverty.[76] Mexico's Oportunidades CCT program resulted in households with more income, more children in school, and improved health and nutrition for participants of all ages.[77]

In addition, an RBF model in Rwanda, which provides supply-side incentives through a fee-for-service model that is conditional on quality of care at the health center level, has also shown promising results. According to an evaluation published in 2010, the scheme was already associated with:[78]

- A 21 percent increase in institutional deliveries
- A 64 percent increase in preventative visits for children less than 2 years of age

- A 133 percent increase in visits for children between ages 2 and 5
- Improved quality of prenatal care

The impact evaluation also showed that these results would not have occurred if financing were not conditional on performance. It is important to note, however, that perverse effects can potentially occur if RBF programs are not carefully designed and implemented. These effects include corruption, trying to maximize benefits, and failure to carry out the desired behaviors in the absence of incentives. In addition, paying for some services and not others may discourage the provision or use of some important services.[79]

Concerns about the sustainability of RBF have also been raised. RBF projects are complex and can take 12–18 months to design.[80] In addition, they require a substantial amount of technical expertise to get off the ground, and there is a limited number of experts in the field. Furthermore, financial sustainability must be considered. Although inputs and transaction costs vary depending on the approach, RBF can cost as much as $4.82 per capita per year, as in the USAID REACH Program in Afghanistan.[81] This is a substantial sum for low-income countries that spend little per capita per year on health.

Limited studies have been carried out so far about the cost-effectiveness of RBF approaches, which has also been questioned.[82] One systematic review, for example, showed that although "the evidence suggests that conditional cash transfer programs are effective in increasing the use of preventive services and sometimes improving health status . . . further research is needed to clarify the cost effectiveness of conditional cash transfer programs and better understand which components play a critical role."[83,p1900] Another systematic review of nine RBF schemes, which was published in 2012, suggested that the quality of the evidence was weak and that it was difficult to draw any conclusions about the effectiveness of such schemes.[84] Among other things, more information is needed on the cost-effectiveness of supply-side schemes, especially in comparison with demand-side approaches, and more research must be done to assess the appropriate size of cash transfers.[85] An increasing amount of research is also being done on whether or not unconditional cash transfer programs are as cost-effective as conditional cash transfers.

The RBF agenda faces a number of challenges besides cost-effectiveness and sustainability. Decentralizing public health systems so that health centers are given true financial autonomy to carry out RBF schemes is a major obstacle. To ensure autonomy, local capacity must be developed, including health management information systems (HMIS), financial management, and training.

Pharmaceuticals

The Importance of Pharmaceuticals

Pharmaceuticals play an essential role in the health systems of all countries. They are essential for the care of many health conditions, and people can spend a significant part of their income on medicines. Additionally, many countries spend an important part of their health budgets on pharmaceuticals. It has been estimated, for example, that expenditure on pharmaceuticals as a share of total health expenditure ranges from approximately 20% in high-income countries to 30% in low-income countries.[86]

In the simplest terms, countries should ensure that they can procure in a timely manner drugs of appropriate quality for key health conditions faced by their people. They must also ensure that the drugs are affordable by those who need them. In addition, of course, they need to be able to transport the drugs so they can get where they are needed and be able to safely store them. They must also ensure that they are prescribed, dispensed and used properly, for the appropriate health conditions.

This section briefly explores some of the key questions concerning the role of pharmaceuticals in health systems, critical issues in procuring appropriate medicines at reasonable prices, and selective issues in the appropriate management and use of those medicines.

Procuring the Right Drugs

Countries need to manage their drug supplies effectively and efficiently. Historically, many countries have purchased a wide array of drugs, not always consistent with clinical needs. In addition, many countries failed to procure those drugs at the lowest cost.

To assist in getting more appropriate medicines at better prices, WHO has helped countries improve the effectiveness and efficiency of their procurement of medicines by producing lists of essential medicines. The broader focus of this effort has been to help countries and their public health systems to procure the medicines that are most needed, in the most effective and efficient ways, in order to get better prices than would otherwise be possible. This effort began in 1977, and many countries have been able to achieve better outcomes at lower cost through the use of the essential medicines approach.[87]

Medications that are procured, of course, need to have certain quality standards. Low-quality medicines cannot provide the intended therapeutic benefit; they can also cause harm. In addition, the purchase of low-quality medicines is a waste of money by individuals and by health systems.

To ensure that medicines sold in their country are safe and effective, countries need to have a competent regulatory authority. The U.S. Food and Drug Administration (FDA) is one such regulatory body, and there are similar bodies in Australia, the European Union, India, and Japan. However, many low- and middle-income countries do not have the resources necessary to establish competent organizations for ensuring the quality of medicines.

Partly related to these institutional gaps in some countries, a widespread problem in pharmaceutical quality is counterfeit or fake medicines. Fake medicines often look, taste, and are packaged exactly like real medications. However, they have none, too little, or too much of the active ingredients. The U.S. FDA estimates that around 10 to 15 percent of all medicines on the global market are fake medicines. In some low- and middle-income countries, this number is estimated to exceed 50 percent.[88]

Another major source of counterfeit medicines is Internet pharmacies. Over 50 percent of medicines sold on Internet pharmacies are counterfeit. The main driver for these counterfeit medicines is financial gain, as global sales of counterfeit medications were estimated at $75 billion worldwide in 2010.[89] This is despite the fact that the distribution of counterfeit or falsely labeled medicines is universally considered a crime.[90]

In 2010, in fact, WHO established a working group on spurious, falsely labeled, fake, or counterfeit medicines (SFFC). This group has worked to collect data and information about SFFCs around the world. Some of their findings, for example, show surprising amounts of counterfeit medicines in major global markets:[91]

- In 2009, two deaths and nine hospitalizations occurred in China from a traditional medicine for diabetes containing six times the normal dosage.
- In 2011, 3,000 Kenyan HIV patients received a false batch of the antiretroviral Zidolam-N.
- In 2012, 19 U.S. medical facilities found that they were using a counterfeit version of Avastin, a widely-used cancer therapy.

The SFFC Working Group has continued to monitor and make recommendations regarding regulatory systems to prevent counterfeit medicines from entering the market. These recommendations build upon the findings of an earlier working group, IMPACT (International Medical Products Anti-Counterfeiting Taskforce) and include:[92]

- Proper political will and enforcement of criminal offenses for distribution of these counterfeit products
- Administrative and operational tools to handle offenses and enforcement
- Creating awareness among healthcare providers and consumers about the dangers of purchasing medicines outside regulated markets.

A collaboration of nongovernmental organizations, pharmaceutical companies, healthcare providers, legitimate Internet pharmacy organizations and patient advocacy organizations have also worked together in a campaign called Fight the Fakes.[93] This group works across borders to raise public awareness about the dangers of shopping outside of regulated markets, as well to educate governmental and other leaders about the issue of counterfeit medicines.[93] The partnership is working with new mobile technologies to increase reporting of counterfeit medicines. The campaign has noted that antibiotics are some of the most counterfeited medications, which has serious implications for the issue of antimicrobial resistance.

Procuring Drugs at the Right Price

Pharmaceutical companies are mostly for-profit businesses that design, produce, and market medications. These medications can incur high investment costs, from discovery of basic molecules to clinical trials for safety and efficacy. The cost to bring a single medicine through this process can be as much as $1.5 billion.[94] The costs for research and development can be a large barrier for new medicines to make it to market, as well as a contributor to high prices for medicines.

Moreover, since pharmaceutical companies are businesses, they have to make a profit to continue to exist. In order to incentivize the development and sale of new medicines, governments grant temporary monopolies on them called patents. A patented medicine is under the sole ownership and control of the patent holder.[95] While patents may inspire innovation, they also contribute to medicine prices that may be unaffordable for low- and middle-income countries.

Beyond the essential medicines approach, a number of measures have also been taken to make these medicines more affordable in low- and middle-income countries. Many pharmaceutical companies, for example, sell medicines at reduced prices in some resource-poor settings. Pharmaceutical companies also donate drugs to countries and to global health campaigns and a number of companies have made long-term commitments to donate drugs to address the neglected tropical diseases.

Companies also engage in tiered pricing. Under this mechanism, companies sell medicines at different prices, depending on the income level of the country involved. However, tiered pricing is often criticized as providing only a temporary solution to a permanent problem, as well as not lowering the cost of the medicine to an affordable price for individuals.[96]

Low- and middle-income countries can also gain access to quality medicines at affordable prices through procurement programs set up in partnership with a range of organizations. The Global Drug Facility,[97] the Global Fund,[98] and the Supply Chain Management System that works with PEPFAR,[99] UNITAID,[100] and the Clinton Foundation,[101] among others, have helped negotiate reduced prices for some medicines, such as HIV drugs needed by low- and middle-income countries.

Some international trade agreements, including the Trade-Related Aspects of Intellectual Property Rights (TRIPS) Agreement, have been criticized as being significant constraints to access to affordable medicines by low- and middle-income countries. However, under these arrangements, countries can issue a "compulsory license" which allows outside parties, such as generic manufacturers, to produce and distribute patented drugs without the drug company's consent in order to meet public health needs or help deal with a public health emergency.[102] For example, in 2007 Thailand used compulsory licenses for the heart disease drug Plavix. With this approach, the government predicted a decrease in costs for Plavix from $2 to $0.20 per pill.[103] Compulsory licensing has also been used for HIV drugs in Brazil, South Africa, and Malaysia, among others.[104]

The "patent pool" funded by UNITAID is another approach that is now used to enable the production of generic medicines. The patent pool is a collection of HIV drug patents for which the patent holders voluntarily allow the manufacture of generics for low- and middle-income countries.

Procuring Drugs at the Right Time

A country must have an effective supply chain in order to ensure that medicines reach the patients who need them, in a timely manner and at an affordable price. An interruption in the supply chain can have serious or even disastrous effects. For example, interruption in treatment for tuberculosis, among other diseases, can breed drug-resistant strains and cause the death of patients who are lacking necessary medications.

A supply chain for medicines includes multiple actors:[105]

- Manufacturers who produce the raw materials and medicines required
- Procurement agents such as ministries of health, government procurement offices, public organizations that assist countries with procurement of medicines, such as UNICEF, or private organizations that also do this, such as IDA or Crown Agents

- Distributors to transport medicines at national, regional, and district levels
- Warehouses at each level of the system to safely store medicines
- Service providers who order and dispense medicines

Unfortunately, many low- and middle-income countries lack the capacity to manage an effective supply chain for essential medicines. They may lack staff trained in logistics or an appropriate logistical management system that can keep inventory, track the medicines given out, and ensure that orders for new medicines are placed in a timely manner. Many countries also lack appropriate storage facilities for medicines or vaccines, some of which have to be kept cold. Vaccines for polio, influenza, and hepatitis for example, require storage temperatures between 2°C and 8°C.[106]

Many low- and middle-income countries, however, have taken steps to improve supply chain management for pharmaceuticals. They have established supply chain organizations, trained staff, and improved the legal environment for procurement. Some countries have also sought innovative approaches to enhancing their supply chain management.

The Tanzanian Medical Supplies Department and the Coca-Cola Company, for example, began working with the Global Fund in 2010[107] to strengthen the supply chain for essential medicines in Tanzania. In 2011, staff of Yale University joined this effort, which has been called Project Last Mile. This effort seeks to build on the strong supply chain of Coca-Cola and the company's knowledge of supply chain management to ensure that the Tanzanian government can get pharmaceuticals to the right place at the right time and at affordable prices. Based on the successes of the Tanzania collaboration, Project Last Mile will be expanded to 10 African countries by 2019.[108]

Procuring Drugs for the Right People

Even if countries can get the right drugs to the right place, at the right time, and at the right price, countries still have to ensure that the right people take them in the appropriate manner. In fact, it has been estimated that around half of all prescribed medicines are dispensed incorrectly. Moreover, even when distributed adequately, only half of all patients take them correctly.[109]

Another global effort, therefore, has focused on the rational use of medicines. WHO has emphasized several measures to promote rational use:[109]

- Establishing regulatory bodies to set rules for medicine use
- Following clinical guidelines from WHO and other authorities

- Developing national lists of essential medicines
- Creating local committees in hospitals and districts to monitor medicine use and distribution
- Improving medical training to include problem-based curricula
- Requiring continued medical education on medicines for healthcare providers
- Ensuring supervision of medicine use, audits of facilities, and feedback reviews
- Using information about medicines from sources outside the company creating them
- Rolling out public education on medicine use
- Avoiding the use of financial incentives for drug usage
- Enforcing appropriate regulations on medication use
- Ensuring adequate numbers of human resources and medicines needed for the system

There are significant challenges to rational use in all countries, but achieving more rational use of medicines can be especially challenging in low- and middle-income countries. This is due to the poor quality of some care, including misdiagnosis, prescribing the wrong medicines, and overprescribing, for medical and financial reasons; patient demands for medicines, even if they are not needed; and the failure of patients to adhere to treatment regimens, some of which can be long and have unpleasant side effects.

Measures to improve the use of medicines can yield high returns. Correct diagnostic tests and rational use of antimalarial artemisinin combination therapy (ACT), for example, were vital to successfully reducing malaria in Senegal.[109] In 2007, Senegal moved from primarily clinical assessment for malaria to rapid diagnostic tests, which are low-cost and accurate.[109] As a result, ACT has been used only for confirmed cases, curbing the overuse of ACT and reducing unnecessary costs of malaria control.

The Antibiotics Smart Use program in Thailand decreased the use of antibiotics while maintaining high treatment success rates between 2007 and 2012.[109] The Thailand Food and Drug Administration trained medical staff on rational antibiotic use and educating patients through easy-to-read brochures.[109] As a result, there was an 18–23 percent decrease in antibiotic use in community hospitals, with a decrease in primary hospitals as high as 46 percent.[109,110]

Essential Surgery

The Relative Neglect of Essential Surgery

A number of health conditions, including injuries, malignancies, congenital anomalies, obstetrical complications, cataracts, glaucoma, and perinatal conditions, require surgery to be addressed. However, these surgeries are often not available in a timely or appropriate way in low- and lower-middle-income countries. Moreover, until recently, relatively little attention was paid to surgical needs in these settings, as countries and their partners focused most of their attention on women and children's health and the control of communicable diseases.

In the last decade or so, however, increasing attention has been paid to the role that surgery can play in low- and lower-middle-income settings in averting deaths and disability in cost-effective ways. An important work published in 2006, *Disease Control Priorities in Developing Countries, Second Edition* (DCP2), included a chapter on essential surgery. The third edition of that work, *Disease Control Priorities in Developing Countries, Third Edition* (DCP3), builds upon the earlier work and further examines the needs for essential surgery, the cost-effectiveness of such surgeries, and measures that low- and lower-middle-income countries can take to improve access to, the quality of, and outcomes from such surgery. In addition, the *Lancet* has recently established a commission on global surgery.

This policy and program brief outlines the findings of the essential surgery volume of DCP3, as they were recently summarized in an article in the *Lancet*.

What Is Essential Surgery?[111]

The term *essential surgery* is not commonly used and it is important to define it:

> Essential surgical disorders can be defined as those that are mainly or extensively treated by surgery (procedures and other surgical care), have a large health burden, and can be successfully treated by a surgical procedure (and other surgical care) that is cost-effective and feasible to promote globally.[111,p2210]

It is especially important to note that the term *surgical care* includes preoperative care, including assessment of whether or not to perform surgery, safe anesthesia, and postsurgical care.

Table 5-9 indicates a proposed package of essential surgical interventions and the level of the health system at which low- and lower-middle income countries should aim to carry out such surgeries.

The Burden of Disease

It has been estimated that about 6.5 percent of all deaths in low- and lower-middle-income countries could be averted if the package of essential surgery noted previously could be made universally available in those countries.

TABLE 5-9 An Essential Surgery Package

	DELIVERY PLATFORM		
	Community Facility and Primary Health Centers	First-Level Hospitals	Referral and Specialised Hospitals
Dental procedures	Extraction Drainage of dental abscess Treatment for caries		
Obstetric, gynecological, and family planning	Normal delivery	Caesarean birth Vacuum extraction or forceps delivery Ectopic pregnancy Manual vacuum aspiration and dilation and curettage Tubal ligation Vasectomy Hysterectomy for uterine rupture or intractable postpartum hemorrhage Visual inspection with acetic acid and cryotherapy for precancerous cervical lesions	Repair obstetric fistula
General surgical	Drainage of superficial abscess Male circumcision	Repair of perforations (perforated peptic ulcer, typhoid ileal perforation, etc.) Appendectomy Bowel obstruction Colostomy Gallbladder disease (including emergency surgery for acute cholecystitis) Hernia (including incarceration) Hydrocelectomy Relief of urinary obstruction; catheterization or suprapubic cystostomy (tube into bladder through skin)	
Injury	Resuscitation with basic life support measures Suturing laceration Management of non-displaced fractures	Resuscitation with advanced life support measures, including surgical airway Tube thoracostomy (chest drain) Trauma laparotomy Fracture reduction	

continues

TABLE 5-9 An Essential Surgery Package (*continued*)

	DELIVERY PLATFORM		
	Community Facility and Primary Health Centers	First-Level Hospitals	Referral and Specialised Hospitals
		Irrigation and debridement of open fractures Placement of external fixator, use of traction Escharotomy or fasciotomy (cutting of constricting tissue to relieve pressure from swelling) Trauma-related amputations Skin grafting Burr hole	
Congenital			Cleft lip and palate repair Club foot repair Shunt for hydrocephalus Repair of anorectal malformations and Hirschsprung's disease
Visual impairment			Cataract extraction and insertion of intraocular lens Eyelid surgery for trachoma
Nontrauma orthopedic		Drainage of septic arthritis Debridement of osteomyelitis	

Reproduced from Debas, H. T., P. Donkor, A. Gawande, D. T. Jamison, M. E. Kruck, and C. N. Mock, editors. 2015. Essential Surgery. Disease Control Priorities, third edition, volume 1. Washington, DC: World Bank. doi: 10.1596/978-1-4648-0346. License: Creative Commons Attribution CC BY 3.0 IGO

It should also be noted, however, that there are substantial gaps in the data on this point. In addition, the proportion of deaths that are avertable through the application of this package will be very sensitive to the share of the population that lacks access to such services.

Gaps in Access to Essential Surgery of Good Quality

In fact, only about 3.5 percent of all surgeries take place in low- and lower-middle income countries, which are home to about 35 percent of the world's population. This discrepancy should not be a surprise and reflects, among other things, the lack of skilled human resources in such countries, the lack of facilities, and the lack of equipment and supplies. The United

States, for example, has more than 60 times the number of general surgeons per 100,000 population and more than 100 times the number of anesthesiologists per 100,000 population than some of the lowest income countries. The United States has about 6 times more general surgeons per 100,000 population and more than 2 times the number of anesthesiologists per 100,000 population than even the better-off of the lower-middle-income countries. In addition, the United States has more than 10 times more operating rooms (theaters) per 100,000 people than the countries of sub-Saharan Africa and South Asia.

There are also major gaps in the quality of surgical care in many countries. The risk of a complication or death from caesarean section is 6 to 10 times greater in South Asia than in Sweden and 100 times higher in sub-Saharan Africa than in Sweden. The deaths related to complication from anesthesia are more than five times higher in low- and middle-income countries than in high-income countries.

Closing the Gaps in Access and Quality

In the long run, it would be valuable if low- and lower-middle-income countries could train the highly skilled surgeons needed to effectively and universally implement a package of essential surgery. Indeed, some countries, such as Ghana, have made important strides in increasing the number of trained surgeons.

Nonetheless, it is clear that it will be many years before the poorest countries will have the number of licensed surgeons they need to implement a package of essential surgical interventions. Thus, they will for some time need to engage in task shifting for an important part of that work. This would include training general practitioners and nonphysician clinical personnel to carry out such work. There is good evidence from a number of countries, including Burkina Faso, Mozambique and Tanzania, that these staff can be more cost-effective than surgeons in doing procedures such as cataract surgeries and caesarean surgeries.

Some countries, such as Vietnam, have also made progress in improving their equipment and supplies for essential surgery, often following guidelines produced by WHO on the infrastructure needed for surgical care at first-level hospitals and for emergency and essential surgery care.

More and more countries are moving toward programs of universal health coverage. Access to a package of essential surgery would be enhanced if countries include such a package in their programs for universal health coverage.

Addressing issues of the quality of care will not be easy in countries that lack many of the inputs needed to implement a package of essential surgical interventions and that have such large gaps in quality compared to the standard of care in better-off countries. However, a number of models for quality improvement have shown excellent and sustainable results. These approaches are also uncomplicated and inexpensive. Such measures could include, for example, implementing the WHO 19-point checklist on surgical safety, the use of which has improved outcomes in low-, middle-, and high-income countries for both elective and emergency surgery.

Many higher-income countries have made substantial progress in reducing complications from anesthesia by adopting standards of care and careful monitoring of patients' breathing, level of oxygen saturation, and flow of blood to the capillaries. This has been helped in these countries by the use of certain medical equipment, such as the pulse oximeter, which monitors the patient's level of oxygen saturation. As countries begin to make progress in improving the quality and safety of anesthesia, it would be helpful if lower cost versions of key equipment, like the pulse oximeter, could be developed and made available to them. Work is ongoing in this direction.

Essential Surgery Is Cost-Effective

The evidence suggests that essential surgery is a cost-effective investment. In fact, some of the procedures that are part of the essential surgery package are as cost-effective, in terms of dollars per DALY averted, as almost any other of the best buys in global health. Surgical repair of a cleft lip or inguinal hernia, cataract surgery, and caesarean section, for example, appear to be as cost-effective or almost as cost-effective as vitamin A supplementation and more cost-effective than oral rehydration therapy or antiretroviral therapy for HIV.

Studies have also shown that these basic and essential surgeries are cost-effective at first-, second-, or third-level hospitals. However, the studies also show that these surgeries are more cost-effective when done at first-level hospitals.

Conclusion

Low- and lower-middle-income countries should implement a package of essential surgery. In the long run, they should aim to have such surgeries performed by fully trained personnel. For now, however, countries can engage in task shifting coupled with the use of WHO guidelines on equipment and materials and the quality and safety of care, to produce good outcomes in highly cost-efficient ways. As countries increase the coverage of such programs, they can avert a substantial burden of deaths and DALYs at reasonable costs. Like the tropical diseases that had previously been neglected but now get more attention, it is important that countries increasingly understand the burden of surgical needs and act to address it.

CASE STUDIES

Many countries have undertaken efforts to address the key health sector challenges discussed earlier. One consistent theme that arises when looking at successful efforts is the importance of community-based approaches to health services at the lowest level. Three cases are discussed here. The first is a very well-known case about the work of BRAC in helping Bangladesh to reduce mortality from diarrhea. The intervention started by BRAC has been shown to be replicable in other countries and has provided the world with a number of very important lessons about improving health services for the poor in low- and middle-income countries. The second and third cases in this section discuss some interesting efforts in Africa to enhance the effectiveness and efficiency of health systems. They were small in size when the cases were prepared and had not been fully and independently evaluated. However, at the time, they did suggest opportunities for expansion of their approaches that could become important.

The case on vitamin A and onchocerciasis reviews the attempts by a number of African countries to provide services in more effective and efficient ways by combining the delivery of several programs. The third case discusses a pilot project in Tanzania that sought to improve health outcomes by explicitly targeting a larger share of health expenditure for the diseases that most affect the poor.

Combating Diarrheal Disease in Bangladesh

Introduction

In Bangladesh, diarrhea is a major cause of morbidity and mortality for young children. Children under the age of 2 have the highest rate of diarrhea and are prone to severe illness and mortality. Diarrhea results in the loss of water and electrolytes, which causes dehydration and subsequent morbidity and mortality. Therefore, it is essential that fluids and electrolytes be replaced.

The Intervention

BRAC is an important nongovernmental organization that is active in health and community development in Bangladesh. In 1980, BRAC began to implement a large-scale intervention to make oral rehydration therapy widely available and easy to administer by nonprofessionals without special equipment. As part of this effort, BRAC taught mothers to prepare oral saline and to treat their children with it. However, because about 80 percent of the population was illiterate, there was concern that mothers would not be able to prepare the solution accurately and that this could result in their children having high blood sodium rather than overcoming their diarrhea.

Through its Oral Rehydration Teaching Program, BRAC communicated a 10-point health message, including how to prepare the oral rehydration solution (ORS) using local ingredients and accurate measurements. ORS was prepared with a three-finger pinch of common table salt and one fistful of unrefined brown sugar in half a local container (467 cc) of water and was stirred well. The salt–sugar solution was simple to make, cheap, safe, and effective, and the ingredients were readily available.[112]

Female health workers, or oral rehydration workers (ORWs) as they were called, were trained in the preparation of the solution. The ORWs worked in teams to visit every household in each village. One woman/mother in every household was taught the 10 critical points using a flip chart with pictorial representations of ORS preparation and diarrhea management. Questions asked on each of the points ensured that the messages were understood before the workers left. Most importantly, the mother had to prepare the solution under the direct supervision of the ORW. The ORWs ensured that the women accurately measured the right amount of water. The process of accurate measurement was reviewed and the women were asked to repeat the preparation process. The team moved from one location to another approximately every two weeks.

The Impact

Oral rehydration workers visited all the villages in Bangladesh, except for a few tribal districts. Twelve million households received supervised teaching, and often more than one woman in a household was taught to prepare the ORS. When tested later, over 90 percent of the women knew of and could prepare the solution, and about 90 percent of the solutions they prepared were safe and effective. In addition, prior to BRAC's initiation of this program, there was very little knowledge of oral rehydration in Bangladesh, and ORS packets were not available in rural Bangladesh. However, from the mid-1980s, the sale of these packets increased. If all types of diarrhea, mild or moderate, watery or nonwatery, are included, then about half the diarrhea episodes in the following decade were treated with oral rehydration therapy.[113] Furthermore, another study done in the mid-1990s showed that treatment of diarrhea by oral rehydration therapy was known to over 70 percent of children who were 11 to 12 years of age in Bangladesh, 10 to 15 years after their mothers were taught this method.

The Costs and Benefits

In addition to using its own funds, BRAC also received financial support for this effort from Oxfam, the government of the United Kingdom, the Swedish Free Church Aid, the aid agency of the Swiss government, and the United Nations Children's Fund (UNICEF). The total value of this assistance was about $9.3 million. The cost of teaching one household about oral rehydration therapy was a one-time investment of $0.75.

Lessons Learned

BRAC's intervention in Bangladesh shows that mothers, regardless of their literacy level, can learn to improve health behaviors when provided with the right kind of training. When BRAC started the pilot, the general opinion was that illiterate women would not be able to learn how to measure and mix the ingredients. The strategy chosen by BRAC was not new or unknown to the women—BRAC simply built on their knowledge of cooking and feeding their children. The training was also done in familiar surroundings with ingredients that they use on a daily basis. The women were also taught in groups and found it easier to learn from each other than learning on their own.

Evaluation of the program indicated some of the characteristics that made scaling up oral rehydration therapy possible. The intervention was relatively simple, requiring no assistance once the method was taught. It was also inexpensive, requiring no household expenses, except for the purchase of the salt and sugar. The training and messages were built on existing knowledge and skills, such as childcare and cooking, and were also culturally acceptable. The performance of the ORWs was measured through the knowledge acquired by mothers. Though the program was large, an administrative structure of checks and balances could be put into place along with rigorous supervision. Lastly, there was a clear goal with a specific outcome and an institutional commitment to the process.[113]

NGOs often focus on small populations, which are not representative, and on pilot projects that do not get scaled up. BRAC's effort showed that NGOs are capable of taking to scale pilot or demonstration projects. To do so, however, required strong supervision, supervisor accountability, and local-level flexibility and autonomy. In addition, however, experience with the incentive salary system used by BRAC shows that this approach can be used only when employees who are not effective can be dismissed and not reassigned to any other position or job, as is usually the case for government workers. It is also important that there be tangible and quantifiable outcomes that are relatively easy to measure, and an independent monitoring unit is necessary. Finally, the strategic use of male and female workers allowed female workers to access households and gain the confidence of women, while male workers talked to the men in places where men congregate.

Integrating Services at the Grassroots Level

Introduction

All health systems face the question of how they can most effectively and efficiently provide health services, particularly in difficult-to-reach areas. Often these programs are carried out in a vertical manner. In this case, the program is operated parallel to other programs and may have its own management, staff, financing, and procurement arrangements. It might even have its own facilities. In some settings, vertical programs are undertaken because of extreme weaknesses in the overall health system. However, it would be much more efficient if programs could be carried out in an integrated

fashion, as they are performed in the health systems of most high-income countries. This case study discusses efforts to integrate the delivery of vitamin A and drugs for onchocerciasis (river blindness) in a number of countries in Africa, in hopes of improving the effectiveness and efficiency of the vitamin A program, the onchocerciasis program, and the overall health system.

Vitamin A deficiency is a leading risk factor for under-5 childhood mortality,[114] childhood blindness, and infectious disease in many low- and middle-income countries worldwide. In 2001, 140 million preschool children and more than 7 million pregnant women suffered from vitamin A deficiency. Vitamin A supplementation has proven effective in combating vitamin A deficiency and has therefore become a key intervention to improve child survival. At the time this program was started, more than 40 percent of the children in sub-Saharan Africa were at risk for vitamin A deficiency. Estimates indicated that correcting vitamin A deficiency would avert more than 645,000 child deaths per year in sub-Saharan Africa.[115]

Onchocerciasis is the second-leading infectious cause of blindness in the world and is endemic throughout much of sub-Saharan Africa. It is caused by a parasite, the filaria *Onchocerca volvulus*. The transmission of this parasite to humans takes place through the bite of the blackfly (*Simulium* genus). According to 2005 estimates,[116] about 37 million people were infected with the disease in Africa. Approximately 270,000 people were then blind due to onchocerciasis. However, it is more than a blinding disease; it can also cause disfiguring skin changes, musculoskeletal problems, weight loss, immune system changes, and in some cases epilepsy and growth arrest. Onchocerciasis is commonly found in remote regions where government health services are unavailable.

Ivermectin is the frontline drug used to treat onchocerciasis and is usually delivered through community-directed treatment. This strategy trains community volunteers to educate other community members about the disease and its treatment and to organize campaigns to distribute ivermectin to eligible members of a community once a year for 15 to 20 years.

The Intervention

As progress was made against polio in sub-Saharan Africa, some governments began to phase out National Immunization Days (NID). This policy change left a gap in the delivery of vitamin A supplementation to children younger than 5 years, which was previously included in NID campaigns. Nigeria and Cameroon sought, with the assistance of an NGO called Helen Keller International, to bridge this gap by combining vitamin A supplementation with community-directed treatment with ivermectin for river blindness. Both countries had high vitamin A deficiency among young children at the time this program was developed. In Nigeria, 25 percent of the children were vitamin A deficient,[117] and in Cameroon about 40 percent of the children were vitamin A deficient.[118]

Integrating the two treatments seemed logical for a number of reasons. First, both are relatively easy to deliver by trained community volunteers. Second, they target complementary beneficiary groups, thereby providing something for both young children and women who have recently delivered babies. In addition, both rely on similar supply systems and support from ministries of health. It was estimated that combining the treatments had the potential to supplement over 11 million children at least once per year with high doses of vitamin A.[118]

To test the integration, pilot studies were conducted in Nigeria, beginning in 2001, and in Cameroon, beginning in 2003, where community-directed treatment with ivermectin was well-established. Careful planning was undertaken with community representatives and Ministry of Health personnel, and training modules and materials were adapted to include vitamin A information and messages. Community volunteers were trained to discuss the practical aspects of how to integrate the two interventions in their village. Volunteers then explained to village residents the importance of vitamin A for child survival and that vitamin A doses would be given only to children from 6 to 59 months of age and to women who had given birth within the last two months, during the campaign period. They also discussed the need for a second vitamin A dose for children in six months, and the importance of exclusive breastfeeding to protect young children from malnutrition.

The Impact

A program evaluation of the Cameroon pilot showed good results, with high vitamin A supplementation and high ivermectin coverage maintained in all pilot communities. As the project was scaled up in a two-month campaign, from one health district covering under 50,000 people to 15 health districts covering over 642,000 people, vitamin A supplementation coverage was 77 percent among children from 6 to 59 months of age and 90 percent among women who had given birth in the last two months. In addition, ivermectin coverage increased from 70.3 percent in 2003 to 74 percent in 2004 in the 15 districts studied.

In Nigeria, the integrated program was tested in two states, reaching more than 300,000 children from 6 to 59 months of age and about 72,000 postpartum women. By 2003 and 2004, the strategy was replicated in an additional four states supported by the State Onchocerciasis Control Programs with assistance from UNICEF, Sight Savers International, and the Mission to Save the Helpless. During the scaling-up phase, the pilot program provided supplements to about 950,000 children from 6 to 59 months of age with 80 percent coverage and to about 117,000 women within six weeks of giving birth, with 60 percent coverage. Ivermectin coverage did not decline in these areas, but rather was maintained at over 80 percent of the total population, indicating again that community volunteers were able to provide both interventions together.

Costs and Benefits

The cost of integrating vitamin A supplementation into community-directed treatment with ivermectin was minimal compared to implementing two separate interventions. The cost of undertaking key community-directed treatment activities, including training, supervision, distribution, and reporting, was cost-shared among the Ministry of Health, NGOs, communities, and donors, including the African Program for Onchocerciasis Control. Ivermectin was donated by Merck and Co. Inc., through the Mectizan Donation Program to governments.

A World Health Organization cost-effectiveness study[119] found that the average cost of one ivermectin treatment is $0.58, without volunteer time included, and $0.78 if volunteer time was included. In Nigeria, the study found that integrating vitamin A supplementation and ivermectin treatment cost an extra $0.18 per vitamin A treatment but decreased to $0.15 per treatment when scaled up to six states. At the national level, the cost of integrating the two treatments at the time would have been $0.10 per vitamin A treatment.

Lessons Learned

The program suggested a number of lessons, including:

- Integration means expanding partnerships to include all stakeholders at each level.
- Advocacy is essential to ensure that governments are willing to bring in relevant partners and commit funding to an integrated approach.
- To scale up, a strategy must be fully tested and well-planned.
- Ongoing supervision, monitoring, and evaluation are critical during scale-ups to improve program results across a more diverse cultural and geographic area.

Based on this experience, a number of other countries adopted similar approaches.

Enhancing Community Health Services in Tanzania[120]

Introduction

Tanzania is a low-income country in sub-Saharan Africa. Most people in Tanzania live in rural areas. The burden of disease in Tanzania is typical of that for a low-income African country, with high rates of infant and child mortality, maternal mortality, and high prevalence of malaria, tuberculosis, and HIV. At the end of the last decade, the government of Tanzania was spending about $8 per person each year on health.

The Intervention

The International Development Research Center (IDRC) of Canada and the government of Tanzania established a joint program to determine if health outcomes of poor people in rural areas could be improved by aligning health expenditure more closely with the burden of disease and increasing expenditure on selected health conditions. This effort was called the Tanzania Essential Health Interventions Project and took place in two rural districts with a total population of about 700,000 people.

The program started by trying to map the burden of disease. Given the poor database with which they had to work, this was done by a door-to-door survey of the involved communities to see what people said were the causes of ill health, disability, and death. The program team then calculated the burden of disease and reviewed government expenditure to see if it was being allocated in accordance with that burden.

What they found was substantial gaps between the two. Only 5 percent of the budget went for malaria, although it caused 30 percent of the disability-adjusted life years (DALYs). Only 13 percent went to the leading causes of DALYs in children, despite the fact that they were responsible for 28 percent of the disease burden. In addition, some diseases received more funding than seemed reasonable, given their contributions to the burden of disease and the cost of addressing them.

An additional $2 was allocated to the two pilot communities per person to spend on areas of high disease burden. In addition, the communities began to use simple algorithms for diagnosing and treating common diseases in a standardized way, such as diarrhea, pneumonia, and malaria. The health districts also began to order drugs more in line with their needs, rather than just using a common package of drugs sent by the government that did not always meet their needs. Finally, health education was undertaken to convince members of the community to use insecticide-treated bed nets when they slept to reduce the likelihood of contracting malaria.

The Outcome

Studies showed that in one of the districts, the infant mortality rate decreased from 100 deaths per 1,000 live births in 1999 to 72 deaths per 1,000 live births in 2000, which was a decrease of 28 percent. The under-5 child mortality rate decreased from 140 per 1,000 live births to 120 per 1,000 live births over the same period, which was a drop of 14 percent. It appears that the second district had similar results to the first. Comparable communities that did not participate in this pilot did not see drops in infant and child mortality like those experienced by the pilot communities. People in the involved communities also decided to build their own health centers so that they had to travel less distance for health services.

Costs

The communities did not use all of the $2 that was allocated for the program. Rather, to achieve the outcomes noted, they used only about $0.80, which was a 10 percent increase in public expenditure per person on health in these two areas.

Lessons Learned

The success of this pilot program appears to have depended on a number of factors. First, the project was carefully planned. Second, the communities were involved in the planning, designing, and execution of the program. Third, the approach of the project was based on solid data and evidence about the burden of disease. Fourth, the program focused on implementing low-cost interventions that are known to be highly effective and that targeted health conditions of importance. Finally, the program reflects an important point: The manner in which countries spend money on health is as important, or more important, than how much they spend. These lessons are consistent with the lessons learned from a variety of other important health programs over the last several decades.

MAIN MESSAGES

A health system is "the combination of resources, organization, and management that culminate in the delivery of health services to the population."[2,p31] The main functions of a health system are to raise money for health services, provide health services, pay for health services, and engage in governance and regulation of health activities. In line with this, health systems provide prevention, diagnosis, treatment, and rehabilitative services; protect the sick and their families against the cost of ill health; and carry out key public health functions, such as surveillance, the operation of public health laboratories, and food and drug regulation. Health systems are important parts of all economies.

Health systems have three levels of health care: primary, secondary, and tertiary. Depending on the country, the public, private, and nongovernmental sectors participate in different parts of the health system. A critical issue in the design of health systems is the roles that each of these sectors should play. There is agreement that governments must regulate and provide oversight of the health system. However, there is also a growing view that the government does not need to provide all services but should instead consider how they might most effectively be provided, which could mean government contracting the private or NGO sectors for some services.

The notion of primary health care, as developed at the Alma-Ata Conference in 1978, remains very important. Many countries continue to try to provide essential and socially acceptable health services close to the people who need them most. They also seek to embody preventive, promotive, curative, and rehabilitative services in their primary healthcare programs and to link them with higher levels of the health system. Achieving such programs, however, has remained a challenge for many countries, especially low-income countries.

Health systems reflect the unique history and culture of each country. They are also diverse, complex, and very difficult to categorize. One very simplified approach to thinking about health systems, however, considers those that are based on a national health service model, like the United Kingdom; those that have national health insurance programs, such as Canada, Japan, and Germany; and those that have pluralistic systems like the United States, India, or Nigeria. When thinking about different approaches to health systems, it is valuable to consider the roles different actors play in the regulation, financing, and provision of services. It is also important to consider the extent to which these systems offer financial protection through insurance, how such insurance is organized, and how insurance is financed.

Countries spend a wide range of their GDP on health, from about 3 percent in Indonesia to about 18 percent in the United States. Most of the high-income countries have health systems that provide a universal package of insured health benefits. In low-income countries that lack national health insurance, most expenditure on health is private and out of pocket. In general, the health systems of high-income countries are more effective at meeting health system aims than are the systems in low- and middle-income countries.

The health systems of all countries, but especially those in low- and middle-income countries, face a number of important challenges, including:

- How to cope with an aging population and increasing amounts of noncommunicable disease
- Quality of governance
- Number, quality, and distribution of healthcare personnel
- Mobilization of sufficient financial resources for the health sector
- How to provide health care at an appropriate level of quality
- How to ensure access to and equitable provision of services
- Creation of mechanisms to provide the poor with protection from the costs of health services

Governance is a difficult issue to address because governance issues are generally problems across all sectors, and not just the health sector. Nonetheless, by giving communities more control over health sector resources, having them openly monitor their use, enhancing the capacity of the health sector to engage in procurement functions, and contracting out services that can most effectively and efficiently be delivered by the private or NGO sectors, governance can be improved.

Ensuring that countries have the right number of trained health personnel in the right places will continue to be difficult. However, there is evidence that different kinds of incentives, such as housing, additional pay, and greater access to training, can encourage health personnel to serve in underserved areas. The productivity of health providers can also be encouraged through appropriate incentives.

It will continue to be difficult for low-income countries to raise the resources they need to finance a cost-effective package of health services. However, given the potential returns to investments in health, even very poor countries must consider allocating a larger share of their overall resources to health. In addition, existing expenditure on health is very inefficient in many countries, and some financial savings can be generated from improving the efficiency of existing expenditure and by allocating a higher share of resources to areas that will yield the highest returns.

The quality of services can be improved, even in low-income settings. Accreditation of services is potentially promising, but not yet a proven way of improving health outcomes. Oversight by senior health staff in structured ways has improved outcomes in some settings. Providing health personnel with clear guidelines, protocols, and algorithms for treatment of patients can also improve the quality of care. There is also increasing evidence that total quality management activities can improve health outcomes, even in very low-income settings. Efforts at improving quality through results-based financing are also becoming more prominent.

Greater attention needs to be paid in most countries to enhancing the coverage by the health system of poor and marginalized populations. One way to do this is to engage these communities in the planning and design of health system interventions. Improving services for the poor and ensuring that these services do not hurt families financially will also require that greater attention be paid to various insurance schemes.

In addition, low- and middle-income countries can help enhance the health of their poor by moving in the previously noted directions, achieving universal health coverage, and then focusing expenditure on a package of services that at relatively low cost will have the highest impact on preventing illness among the poor and on treating the illnesses that most affect them. This would include:

- Promoting access to safe water and enhanced sanitation and encouraging improved hygiene

- Enhancing people's food habits and providing selective nutrition supplementation
- Providing a basic package of reproductive health services, including emergency obstetric care
- Providing a basic package of neonatal health services
- Vaccinating and deworming young children, providing oral rehydration for diarrhea, and treating of pneumonia and malaria in a timely and appropriate way
- Preventing and treating, as appropriate, HIV, tuberculosis, and malaria
- Preventing tobacco use and reducing salt consumption
- Treating hypertension and high cholesterol, aspirin for heart attacks, and community-based mental health services

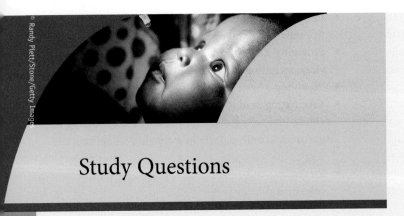

Study Questions

1. What is a health system?

2. What are the primary functions of a health system?

3. What are primary, secondary, and tertiary health care, and what services are generally rendered at each level?

4. How might one compare and contrast the organization of the healthcare systems of the United Kingdom, Germany, and the United States?

5. What is the range of public expenditure on health as a share of their GDP that countries spend on health? Why is there such a wide range?

6. Which types of countries tend to have a larger share of private expenditure on health than public expenditure on health? Why is this so, compared to countries that have health systems that are mostly publicly funded?

7. What are some of the significant issues that arise in trying to govern health systems in low- and middle-income countries?

8. What are some of the key human resource challenges that low- and middle-income countries face in staffing and operating their health systems?

9. What are the most important epidemiologic and demographic issues that face health systems, and what are the implications of those issues for healthcare costs?

10. What are some of the most important steps that can be taken to improve the effectiveness and efficiency of weaker health systems in low- and middle-income countries?

REFERENCES

1. World Health Organization. (2005). *What is a health system?* Retrieved March 9, 2015 from http://www.who.int/features/qa/28/en/.

2. Roemer, M. (1991). *National health systems of the world* (Vol. 1: The Countries). Oxford, England: Oxford University Press.

3. Roberts, M. J., et al. (2004). *Getting health reform right: A guide to improving performance and equity.* New York: Oxford University Press.

4. World Health Organization (WHO). (2000). *The world health report 2000.* Geneva: World Health Organization.

5. World Health Organization (WHO). (2000). Overview. *The world health report 2000.* Geneva: World Health Organization.

6. Southby, R. (2004). Presentation at George Washington University.

7. World Health Organization. (2007). *Everybody's business: Strengthening health systems to improve health outcomes: WHO's framework for action.* Geneva: World Health Organization.

8. Birn, A.-E., Pillay, Y., & Holtz, T. H. (2009). *Textbook of international health.* New York: Oxford University Press.

9. World Health Organization. (1978). *Declaration of Alma-Ata.* International Conference on Primary Health Care, September 6–12, 1978, Alma Ata, USSR. Geneva: World Health Organization.

10. Bloom, G., Champion, C., Lucas, H., et al. (2008). Health markets and future health systems: innovation for equity. *Global forum update on research for health, 5,* 30–33.

11. United Nations Rule of Law. (n.d.). *Non-governmental organizations.* Retrieved June 22, 2015, from http://www.unrol.org/article.aspx?article_id=23.

12. World Bank. (2003). *Afghanistan health sector and emergency reconstruction and development project.* Washington, DC: World Bank.

13. World Bank. (1995). *Bangladesh integrated nutrition project.* Washington, DC: World Bank.

14. World Health Organization. Global Health Observatory. Health expenditure ratios. Retrieved December 28, 2010, from http://apps.who.int/gho/data/node.main.75.

15. Basch, P. (2001). *Textbook of international health* (2nd ed.). New York: Oxford University Press.

16. Blumel, M. (2013). The German health care system, 2013. In S. Thomson, R. Osborn, D. Squires, & M. Jun (Eds.), *International profiles of health care systems, 2013* (pp. 57–66). New York: The Commonwealth Fund.

17. Harrison, A. (2013). The English health care system, 2013. In S. Thomson, R. Osborn, D. Squires, & M. Jun (Eds.), *International profiles of health care systems, 2013* (pp. 37–45). New York: The Commonwealth Fund.

18. The Commonwealth Fund. (2013). The U.S. health care system, 2013. In S. Thomson, R. Osborn, D. Squires, & M. Jun (Eds.), *International profiles of health care systems, 2013* (pp. 128–135). New York: The Commonwealth Fund.

19. BrazilWorks. (2012). *Brazil's healthcare system: Towards reform.* Washington, DC: BrazilWorks.

20. World Bank. (2014). *Health financing profile—Brazil.*

21. Dugan, B., Hsiao, W., Roberts, M., Sinclair, M., & Noronha, J. (2013). *Brazil's national health system.* Boston, MA: Harvard School of Public Health and Harvard Kennedy School.

22. World Bank. (n.d.). Data Health expenditure, public (as % of total health expenditure). Retrieved March 9, 2015, from http://data.worldbank.org/indicator/SH.XPD.PUBL.

23. Torres, F. M. (2013). *Costa Rica case study: Primary health care achievements and challenges in the framework of social health insurance.* Washington, DC: The World Bank; and Saenz, M. dR., Bermudez, J. L., & Acosta, M. (2010). *Universal coverage in a middle-income country: Costa Rica.* Geneva: World Health Organization.

24. Swedish Agency for Growth Policy Analysis. (2013). *India's healthcare system—overview and quality improvement.* Stockholm: Swedish Agency for Growth Policy Analysis.

25. Saleh, K. (2013). *The health sector in Ghana.* Washington, DC: The World Bank.

26. Gajate-Garrido, G., & Owusua, R. (2013). *The national health insurance scheme in Ghana.* Washington, DC: IFPRI.

27. Apoya, P., & Marriott, A. (2011). *Achieving a shared goal: Universal health care in Ghana.* London: Oxfam International.

28. World Health Organization (WHO). (2000). Statistical annex. *The world health report 2000.* Geneva: World Health Organization.

29. Mathers, C. D., Lopez, A. D., & Murray, C. J. L. (2006). The burden of disease and mortality by condition: data, methods, and results for 2001. In A. D. Lopez, C. D. Mathers, M. Ezzati, D. T. Jamison, & C. J. L. Murray (Eds.), *Global burden of disease and risk factors* (pp. 45–93). New York: Oxford University Press.

30. Lewis, M. (2006). *Tackling healthcare corruption and governance woes in developing countries* (Working Paper 78). Washington, DC: Center for Global Development.

31. Physicians for Human Rights. (2004). *An action plan to prevent brain drain: Building equitable health systems in Africa.* Retrieved February 5, 2015, from http://physiciansforhumanrights.org/library/reports/action-plan-to-prevent-brain-drain-africa-2004.html.

32. Hongoro, C., & Normand, C. (2006). Health workers: Building and motivating the workforce. In D. T. Jamison, J. G. Breman, A. R. Measham, et al. (Eds.), *Disease control priorities in developing countries* (2nd ed., pp. 1309–1322). New York: Oxford University Press.

33. Institute of Medicine. (1999). *Measuring the quality of health care.* Washington, DC: IOM.

34. Peabody, J. W., Taguiwalo, M. M., Robalino, D. A., & Frenk, J. (2006). Improving the quality of care in developing countries. In D. T. Jamison, J. G. Breman, A. R. Measham, et al. (Eds.), *Disease control priorities in developing countries* (2nd ed., pp. 1293–1307). New York: Oxford University Press.

35. Beracochea, E., Dickenson, R., Freemand, P., & Thomason, J. (1995). Case management quality assessment in rural areas of Papua New Guinea. *Tropical Doctor, 25*(2), 69–74.

36. Thaver, I. H., Harpham, T., McPake, B., & Garner, P. (1998). Private practitioners in the slums of Karachi: what quality of care do they offer? *Social Science & Medicine, 46*(11), 1441–1449.

37. Nolan, T., Angos, P., Cunha, A. J., et al. (2001). Quality of hospital care for seriously ill children in less-developed countries. *Lancet, 357*(9250), 106–110.

38. Mohanan, M., Vera-Hernandez, M., Das, V., et al. (2015). The know-do gap in quality of health care for childhood diarrhea and pneumonia in rural india. *JAMA Pediatrics.* February 16, 2015.

39. Jamison, D. T., Breman, J. G., Measham, A. R., et al. (Eds.), (2006). *Priorities in health.* Washington, DC: World Bank.

40. Schieber, G., Baeza, C., Kress, D., & Maier, M. (2006). Financing health systems in the 21st century. In D. T. Jamison, J. G. Breman, A. R. Measham, et al. (Eds.), *Disease control priorities in developing countries* (2nd ed., pp. 225–242). New York: Oxford University Press.

41. Peters, D. H., Preker, A. S., Yazbek, A. S., et al. *Better health systems for India's poor.* Washington, DC: The World Bank.

42. Lagarde, M., & Palmer, N. (2011). *The impact of user fees on access to health services in low- and middle-income countries* (Review). Hoboken, NJ: The Cochrane Collaboration.

43. Jha, P., Chaloupka, F. J., Moore, J., et al. (2006). Tobacco addiction. In D. T. Jamison, J. G. Breman, A. R. Measham, et al. (Eds.), *Disease control priorities in developing countries* (2nd ed., pp. 869–885). New York: Oxford University Press.

44. Norton, R., Hyder, A. A., Bishai, D., & Peden, M. (2006). Unintentional injuries. In D. T. Jamison, J. G. Breman, A. R. Measham, et al. (Eds.), *Disease control priorities in developing countries* (2nd ed., pp. 737–753). New York: Oxford University Press.

45. Samb, B., Desai, N., Nishtar, S., et al. (2010). Prevention and management of chronic disease: A litmus test for health-systems strengthening in low-income and middle-income countries. *Lancet, 376,* 1785–1797.

46. Joint Learning Initiative. (2004). *Human resources for health: Overcoming the crisis.* Cambridge, MA: Joint Learning Initiative.

47. Resch, S., Ryckman, T., & Hecht, R. (2015). Funding AIDS programmes in the era of shared responsibility: An analysis of domestic spending in 12 low-income and middle-income countries. *Lancet Global Health*, 3, e52–e61.

48. Mills, A., Rasheed, F., & Tollman, S. (2006). Strengthening health systems. In D. T. Jamison, J. G. Breman, A. R. Measham, et al. (Eds.), *Disease control priorities in developing countries* (2nd ed., pp. 87–102). New York: Oxford University Press.

49. USAID. Demographic and health surveys. Retrieved February 5, 2015, from http://dhsprogram.com/.

50. Peabody, J. W., Taguiwalo, M. M., Robalino, D. A., & Frenk, J. (2006). Improving the quality of care in developing countries. In D. T. Jamison, J. G. Breman, A. R. Measham, et al. (Eds.), *Disease control priorities in developing countries* (2nd ed., pp. 1293–1307). New York: Oxford University Press.

51. Tollman, S., Doherty, J., & Mulligan, J.-A. (2006). General primary care. In D. T. Jamison, J. G. Breman, A. R. Measham, et al. (Eds.), *Disease control priorities in developing countries* (2nd ed., pp. 1193–1210). New York: Oxford University Press.

52. Sepulveda, J., Bustreo, F., Tapia, R., et al. (2006, December 2). The improvement of child survival in Mexico: The diagonal approach. *Lancet*, 368(9551), 2017–2027.

53. World Health Organization. (2014). What is universal health coverage? Retrieved January 19, 2015, from http://www.who.int/features/qa/universal_health_coverage/en/.

54. World Health Organization. (2014). Health financing for universal coverage. Retrieved January 19, 2015, from http://www.who.int/health_financing/universal_coverage_definition/en/.

55. Sen, A. (2015, January 6). Universal healthcare: The affordable dream. *The Guardian*. Retrieved June 22, 2015, from http://www.theguardian.com/society/2015/jan/06/-sp-universal-healthcare-the-affordable-dream-amartya-sen.

56. World Health Organization. (2010). *World health report 2010*. Geneva: World Health Organization.

57. Langomarsino, G., Gabarant, A., Adyas, A., Muga, R., & Otoo, N. (2012, September 8). Moving towards universal health coverage: Health insurance reforms in nine developing countries in Africa and Asia. *Lancet*, 380, 933–943.

58. Patcharanarumol, E., Ir, P., et al. (2011, January 25). Health financing reforms in southeast Asia: Challenges in achieving universal coverage. *Lancet*, 377, 863–873.

59. Kumar, A. K. S., Chen, L. C., Choudhury, M., et al. (2011, January 12). India: Towards universal health coverage 6—Financing health care for all: Challenges and opportunities. *Lancet*, 377, 668–679.

60. Atun, R., Andrade, L. O., Md. Almeida, G., Cotlear, D., et al. (2014, October 16). Universal health coverage in Latin America 1—Health system reform and universal coverage in Latin America. *Lancet*. doi:dx.doi.org/10.1016/S0140-6736(14)61646-9.

61. World Bank. *GDP per capita (current US$)*. Retrieved from http://data.worldbank.org/indicator/NY.GDP.PCAP.CD.

62. Twahirwa, A. (2008). Sharing the burden of sickness: Mutual health insurance in Rwanda. *Bulletin of the World Health Organization*, 86(11), 823–824. Retrieved from http://www.pubmedcentral.nih.gov/articlerender.fcgi?artid=2649549&tool=pmcentrez&rendertype=abstract.

63. Sekabaraga, C., Diop, F., Martin, G., & Soucat, A. (2011). Innovative financing for health in Rwanda: A report of successful reforms. In P. Chuhan-Pole & M. Angwafo (Eds.), *Yes, Africa can* (pp. 403–416). Washington, DC: The World Bank. doi:10.1596/978-0-8213-8745-0.

64. Schneider, P., & Hanson, K. (2007). The impact of micro health insurance on Rwandan health centre costs. *Health Policy and Planning*, 22(1), 40–48. doi:10.1093/heapol/czl030.

65. Sekabaraga, C., Diop, F., & Soucat, A. (2011). Can innovative health financing policies increase access to MDG-related services? Evidence from Rwanda. *Health Policy and Planning*, 26(Suppl 2), ii52–ii62. doi:10.1093/heapol/czr070.

66. Partners in Health. (n.d.). *Infographic: Health care in Rwanda improves dramatically*. Retrieved October 8, 2014, from http://www.pih.org/blog/health-care-in-rwanda-improves-dramatically.

67. Sreshthaputra, N., & Kawmthong, I. (2001). *The universal coverage policy of Thailand: An introduction*. A paper prepared for Asia-Pacific Health Economics Network (APHEN), July 19, 2001. Retrieved from http://www.unescap.org/aphen/thailand_universal_coverage.htm.

68. Hughes, D., & Songkramachai, L. (2007). Universal coverage in the land of smiles: Lessons from Thailand's 30 baht reforms. *Health Affairs*, 26(4), 999–1008.

69. Liu, X., Hotchkiss, D. R., & Bose, S. (2008). The effectiveness of contracting-out primary health care services in developing countries: A review of the evidence. *Health Policy and Planning*, 23, 1–13.

70. Musgrove, P. (2011). *Financial and other rewards for good performance or results: A guided tour of concepts and terms and a short glossary*. Washington, DC: The World Bank. Retrieved February 5, 2015, from http://www.rbfhealth.org/sites/rbf/files/RBFglossarylongrevised_0.pdf.

71. Center for Global Development. (2009). *Performance incentives for global health: Potential and pitfalls*. Washington, DC: Author. Retrieved January 4, 2010, from http://www.cgdev.org/doc/books/PBI/00_CGD_Eichler_Levine-FM.pdf.

72. Glassman, A. (2010). Comments presented at The Alphabet Soup of Results-Based Financing (RBF), September 14, 2010, World Bank, Washington, DC. Retrieved January 4, 2010, from http://www.rbfhealth.org/rbfhealth/library/doc/392/alphabet-soup-results-based-financing-rbf.

73. Loevinsohn, B. (2010). Comments presented at The Alphabet Soup of Results-Based Financing (RBF), September 14, 2010, World Bank, Washington, DC. Retrieved January 4, 2010, from http://www.rbfhealth.org/rbfhealth/library/doc/392/alphabet-soup-results-based-financing-rbf.

74. Morgan, L. Results-based financing for health: Performance incentives in global health: Potential and pitfalls. The World Bank. Retrieved June 1, 2015, from https://www.rbfhealth.org/sites/rbf/files/RBF_FEATURE_PerfIncentivesGlobalHealth.pdf.

75. Grittner, A. M. (2013). *Evidence from performance-based financing in the health sector*. Bonn: German Development Institute.

76. The World Bank. Results-Based Financing for Health (RBF). Brazil: Results-based financing (rbf) helps achieve decline in family poverty. Washington, DC: World Bank. Retrieved November 30, 2010, from http://www.rbfhealth.org/rbfhealth/news/item/320/brazil-results-based-financing-rbf-helps-achieve-decline-family-poverty.

77. The World Bank. Results-based financing for health (RBF). *Mexico's model conditional cash transfer (CCT) program for fighting poverty*. Washington, DC: World Bank. Retrieved February 6, 2015, from http://www.rbfhealth.org/resource/mexico%E2%80%99s-model-conditional-cash-transfer-cct-program-fighting-poverty.

78. Basinga, P., Gertler, P. J., Binagwaho, A., Soucat, A. L. B., Sturdy, J. R. & Vermeersch, C. M. J. (2010). *Paying primary health care centers for performance in Rwanda*. Washington, DC: World Bank. Retrieved January 4, 2010, from http://siteresources.worldbank.org/EXTDEVDIALOGUE/Images/537296-1238422761932/5968067-1269375819845/Rwanda_P4P.pdf.

79. The World Bank. Results-based financing (RBF) for health. *Cure, curse, or mixed blessing?* Washington, DC: World Bank. Retrieved February 6, 2015, from http://www.rbfhealth.org/resource/cure-curse-or-mixed-blessing.

80. USAID. (2010). *Performance-based incentives primer for USAID missions*. Washington, DC: Author. Retrieved February 6, 2015, from http://pdf.usaid.gov/pdf_docs/PNADX747.pdf.

81. Canavan, A., Toonen, J., & Elovainio, R. (2008). *Performance based financing: An international review of the literature*. Amsterdam: KIT Development Policy and Practice. Retrieved February 6, 2015, from http://www.kit.nl/health/wp-content/uploads/publications/1533_PBF%20literature%20review_December%202008.pdf.

82. Brenzel, L. (2010). *Evaluating the cost and financial impact of RBF schemes*. Presentation, Results Based Financing for Health Impact

Evaluation Workshop, Tunis, Tunisia. Retrieved February 6, 2015, from https://rbfhealth.org/sites/rbf/files/1_Tools%20for%20Impact%20Analysis%20Costing%20and%20Cost%20effectiveness_Brenzel_ENG_0.pdf.

83. Lagarde, M., Haines, A., & Palmer, N. (2007). Conditional cash transfers for improving uptake of health interventions in low- and middle-income countries: A systematic review. *JAMA, 298*, 1900–1910.

84. Witter, S., Freithem, A., Kessy, F., & Lindahl, A. (2012). *Paying for performance to improve the delivery of health interventions in low and middle-income countries (Review).* New York: The Cochrane Review.

85. Pantoja, T. (2008). *Do conditional cash transfers improve the uptake of health interventions in low and middle-income countries? Summary of a systematic review.* SUPPORT. Retrieved January 4, 2010, from http://apps.who.int/rhl/effective_practice_and_organizing_care/SUPPORT_cash_transfers.pdf.

86. Lu, Y., Hernandez, P., Abegunde, D., & Edejer, T. (2011). The World Health Organization. The World Medicines Situation 2011. Retrieved March 2015, from http://www.who.int/health-accounts/documentation/world_medicine_situation.pdf.

87. World Health Organization. (2012). The pursuit of responsible use medicines: Sharing and learning from country experiences. Retrieved July 2014, from http://apps.who.int/iris/bitstream/10665/75828/1/WHO_EMP_MAR_2012.3_eng.pdf?ua=1.

88. Cockburn, R., Newton, P. N., Agyarko, E. K., Akunyili, D., & White, N. J. (2005). The global threat of counterfeit drugs: Why industry and governments must communicate the dangers. *PLOS Medicine.* Retrieved June 22, 2015, from http://journals.plos.org/plosmedicine/article?id=10.1371/journal.pmed.0020100.

89. World Health Organization. (2010). Growing threat from counterfeit medications. Retrieved March 2015, from http://www.who.int/bulletin/volumes/88/4/10-020410/en/.

90. World Health Organization. (2012). The pursuit of responsible use medicines: Sharing and learning from country experiences. Retrieved July 2014, from http://apps.who.int/iris/bitstream/10665/75828/1/WHO_EMP_MAR_2012.3_eng.pdf?ua=1.

91. World Health Organization. (2012). Medicines: Spurious/falsely-labelled/falsified/counterfeit (SFFC) medicines. Retrieved March 2015, from http://www.who.int/mediacentre/factsheets/fs275/en/.

92. IMPACT. (2010). The handbook. Retrieved March 2015, from http://www.who.int/impact/handbook_impact.pdf?ua=1.

93. Fight the Fakes Campaign. (2014). Fight the Fakes Campaign joint statement. Retrieved July 2014, from http://fightthefakes.org/wp-content/uploads/2014/06/Joint-statement-_Fight-the-Fakes-Campaign-06022014.pdf.

94. Levine, D. S. (2012). New estimates of drug development pegs total at $1.5 billion. The Burrill Report: Drug Development. Retrieved from http://www.burrillreport.com/article-new_estimate_of_drug_development_costs_pegs_total_at_1_5_billion.html.

95. Hoen, E. (2009). *The global politics of pharmaceutical monopoly power: Drug patents, access, innovation, and the application of the WTO Doha Declaration on TRIPS and public health.* AMB.

96. Moon, S., Jambert, E., Childs, M., & von Schoen-Angerer, T. (2011). A win-win solution? A critical analysis of tiered pricing to improve access to medicines in developing countries. *Globalization and Health, 7*, 39.

97. STOP TB Partnership. (2015). What is the GDF? Retrieved March 2015, from http://www.stoptb.org/gdf/whatis/default.asp.

98. The Global Fund. (2015). Procurement support services. Retrieved March 2015, from http://www.theglobalfund.org/en/procurement/vpp/.

99. Supply Chain Management System. About us. Retrieved March 2015, from http://scms.pfscm.org/scms/about.

100. UNITAID. (2015). About UNITAID. Retrieved March 2015, from http://www.unitaid.eu/en/who/about-unitaid.

101. Clinton Health Access Initiative. (2015). About CHAI. Retrieved March 2015, from http://www.clintonhealthaccess.org/about.

102. Doha WTO Ministerial 2001: TRIPS. (2001). Declaration on the TRIPS agreement and public health. Retrieved 2014.

103. Savoie, B. (2007). Thailand's test: Compulsory licensing in an era of epidemiologic transition. *Virginia Journal of International Law, 48*, 212–246.

104. Beall, R., & Kuhn, R. (2012). Trends in compulsory licensing of pharmaceuticals since the doha declaration: A database analysis. PLOS ONE. Retrieved March 2015, from http://journals.plos.org/plosmedicine/article?id=10.1371/journal.pmed.1001154.

105. Raja, S., & Mohammad, N. (2005). National HIV/AIDS programs: A handbook on supply chain management for HIV/AIDS medical commodities. World Bank.

106. Centers for Disease Control and Prevention. (2012). Appendix C: Vaccine storage & handling. Retrieved March 2015, from http://www.cdc.gov/vaccines/pubs/pinkbook/downloads/appendices/appdx-full-c.pdf.

107. The Global Fund, Coca-Cola, Bill and Melinda Gates Foundation, Accenture, MSD, and Yale Global Health Leadership Institute. (2012). An innovative public-private partnership.

108. Coca-Cola Company. (2014). "Project Last Mile" expands to improve availability of life-saving medications in additional regions of Africa. Retrieved March 2015, from http://www.coca-colacompany.com/press-center/press-releases/%20project-last-mile-expands-in-africa.

109. World Health Organization. (2012). The pursuit of responsible use medicines: sharing and learning from country experiences. Retrieved July 2014, from http://apps.who.int/iris/bitstream/10665/75828/1/WHO_EMP_MAR_2012.3_eng.pdf?ua=1.

110. So, A., & Woodhouse, W. (2014). Medicines in Health Systems: Advancing access, affordability and appropriate use. Thailand's Antibiotic Smart Use Initiative. Alliance for Health Policy and Systems Research Flagship Report 2014. Retrieved March 2015, from http://www.who.int/alliance-hpsr/resources/FR_Ch5_Annex3a.pdf.

111. Mock, C. N., Donkor, P., Gawande, A., Jamison, D. T., Kruk, M. E., Debas, H. T. for the DCP3 Essential Surgery Author Group. (2015). *Essential surgery: Key messages from Disease Control Priorities* (3rd ed.). *Lancet, 385,* 2209–2219.

112. Chowdhury, S. *Educating mothers for health—Output based incentives for teaching oral rehydration in Bangladesh.* Retrieved January 22, 2007, from http://documents.worldbank.org/curated/en/2001/08/16253103/educating-health-using-incentive-based-salaries-teach-oral-rehydration-therapy.

113. Chowdhury, A., & Cash, R. (1996). *A simple solution: Teaching millions to treat diarrhea at home.* Dhaka: University Press.

114. Beaton, G. H., Martorell, R., Aronson, K. J., et al. (1993). *Effectiveness of VAS in the control of young children morbidity and mortality in developing countries* (ACC/SSN nutrition policy discussion paper 13). Geneva: World Health Organization.

115. Aguayo, V., & Baker, S. (2005). Vitamin A deficiency and child survival in sub-Saharan Africa: A reappraisal of challenges and opportunities. *Food and Nutrition Bulletin, 26*(4), 348–355.

116. World Health Organization. (2005). *Report of the Joint Action Forum of the African Program for Onchocerciasis Control.* Geneva: World Health Organization.

117. Maziya-Dixon, B., Akinyele, I. O., Oguntona, E. B., Nokoe, S., Sanusi, R. A., & Harris, E. (2004). *Nigeria food consumption and nutrition survey 2001–2003: Summary.* Ibadan, Nigeria: International Institute of Tropical Agriculture. Retrieved June 22, 2015, from http://pdf.usaid.gov/pdf_docs/PNADC880.pdf.

118. Haselow, N., Obadiah, M., & Akame, J. (2004). *The integration of vitamin A supplementation into community-directed treatment with ivermectin: A practical guide for Africa.* New York: Helen Keller International. Retrieved February 6, 2015, from http://www.coregroup.org/storage/documents/Diffusion_of_Innovation/How_To_Guide_English.pdf.

119. McFarland, D., et al. (2005). *Study of cost per treatment with ivermectin using CDTI strategy.* Geneva: WHO/APOC.

120. For 80 cents more: Even a tiny health budget, if spent well, can make a difference. (2002, August 15). *Economist.* Retrieved May 20, 2011, from http://www.economist.com/node/1280587?story_id=1280587.

CHAPTER 6

Culture and Health

VIGNETTES

Joshua was 1 year old and lived in eastern Zimbabwe. His mother could tell that he had a fever. She wondered what caused it. Was it the food that he ate? Was it the mixing of the "hot" foods and the "cold" foods? Or was it possible that they had done something to offend local custom? If the fever did not get better by the next day, then she would take Joshua to the local healer.

Siu-Hong was 80 years old and lived in Hong Kong. He had a severe toothache for more than a week. His children repeatedly encouraged him to go to the dentist, but he would not go. He did not like dentists or "Western medicine." In addition, he would have to wait in line to be seen at the dentist's office and would miss work at the clothes market. His children finally convinced him to go to the dentist by giving

him a present of $25 and offering to take him to "dim sum," the traditional South Chinese brunch.

Dorji lived in Bhutan, just outside the capital city of Thimpu. He felt tired, weak, and dizzy for some time but had no fever. After another week of feeling this way, Dorji went to visit his local health clinic. Each clinic in Bhutan had two medical practitioners, one who practiced the indigenous system of medicine and the other who practiced "Western biomedical medicine."[1] In light of Dorji's symptoms, he visited the indigenous practitioner inside the clinic. The "doctor" gave him some herbs that he thought would help his condition. However, he also thought Dorji had an underlying infection and took him across the hall to the "other doctor" who prescribed antibiotics for him.

Arathi was a young mother in southeast India. She and the other women in her village were participating in the Tamil Nadu Nutrition Project. They were all young mothers, many of whose babies were underweight for their age. Arathi nursed her baby as she had learned to do from her mother. She also gave the baby some other foods as she had learned from her mother and grandmother. Despite this, her baby was quite small for her age. As part of the project, the community nutrition workers taught all the women and children in the village songs about proper feeding and about the vitamins the children needed. They also sponsored weekly weighing parties, in which all of the babies of the village were weighed and the mothers together decided if the baby was growing properly and what could be done to make the baby healthier. They also helped the mothers to make a food supplement for the babies who were "too small."

THE IMPORTANCE OF CULTURE TO HEALTH

Culture is an important determinant of health in a number of ways. First, culture is related to health behaviors. People's attitudes toward foods and what they eat, for example, are closely related to culture. The food that pregnant women eat, birthing practices, and how long women breastfeed are also linked to their cultural backgrounds. Hygiene practices are closely tied to culture, as well. Second, culture is an important determinant of people's perceptions of illness. Different cultural groups may have different beliefs about what constitutes good health and what constitutes illness. Third, the extent to which people use health services is also very closely linked with culture. Some groups may use health services as soon as they feel ill. Others, however, may visit health practitioners only when they are very sick. Fourth, different cultures have different practices concerning health and medical treatment. Chinese and Indian cultures have well-defined systems of medicine. There is a long history in many other societies, as well, of local systems of medicine that include notions of illness, various types of practitioners of medicine, and different kinds of medicines.

The purpose of this chapter is to introduce you to the most important links between health and culture, particularly as they relate to global health and people in low- and middle-income countries. The chapter begins by introducing you to the concept of *culture*. It then examines how views of health, illness, the use of health services, and the role of different health providers vary by culture. The chapter also reviews some of the theories of behavior change that relate to enhancing people's health. The chapter concludes with four policy and program briefs that reflect some of the critical relationships between culture and health and how they need to be taken into account in efforts to improve health.

As you review this chapter, it is important to note that some cultural values enhance health. A culture, for example, that puts a strong emphasis on monogamy in marriage should have lower rates of HIV/AIDS than cultures in which having concurrent sexual partners is more tolerated. However, some cultural values do not enhance health. A cultural preference for heaviness in people, for example, as a sign of prosperity or wealth, may be harmful to health, because it would encourage cardiovascular disease and diabetes. Some cultures have food taboos that prevent pregnant women from getting all of the nutrients they need in pregnancy. This chapter aims to help you to understand the relationship between culture and health, identify practices helpful and hurtful to good health, and learn about approaches to promoting healthier behaviors.

THE CONCEPT OF CULTURE

Anthropologists developed the concept of culture at the end of the 19th century. There have been many definitions of culture. An early definition suggested that culture was:

> that complex whole which includes knowledge, beliefs, art, law, morals, custom and any other capabilities and habits acquired by man [sic] as a member of society.[2,p43]

A relatively modern definition states that culture is "a set of rules or standards shared by members of a society, which when acted upon by the members, produce behavior that falls within a range of variation the members consider proper and acceptable."[3,p30] In the simplest terms, one may call culture "behavior and beliefs that are learned and shared."[4]

Cultures operate in a variety of domains, including:[4]

- The family
- Social groups beyond the actor's family
- Individual growth and development
- Communication
- Religion
- Art
- Music
- Politics and law
- The economy

As one thinks about the links between culture and health, it is also important to understand the term *society*, which refers to "a group of people who occupy a specific locality and share the same cultural traditions."[3] Societies have social structures that are the "relationships of groups within society that hold it together."[3,p31] In addition, we must note that there is heterogeneity within all cultures. Sometimes this is reflected in what people call subcultures. There are many shared aspects, for example, of Chinese culture. However, China is a very large country, and even among the Han Chinese, there are important variations as one moves across China in language, food, wedding customs, and music, among other things. The same would be true of North India. People across North India have much in common. Yet, there are variations of North Indian culture in different places, such as in the state of West Bengal, on the one hand, and Rajasthan, on the other. This can be seen, again, in language, music, art, and food.

When thinking about the links between culture and health, one also needs to consider that some cultural practices may be well adapted to some settings but poorly adapted to others. Alternatively, they may be well adapted to the way people have been living, but less well adapted to the way people live after important changes or developments in their communities.[3,p46] The culture of nomadic people, for example, may be well suited to their nomadic lifestyle. However, their culture may be very ill equipped to deal with a lifestyle after societal change that would cause them to be more sedentary.

As we consider the relationship between culture and health, we should be aware of the ways in which a culture is viewed by people from outside that culture group. This helps us to understand the difference between looking at another culture from our perspective and looking at it from the perspective of those who live within that culture.

Especially in the early days of anthropology, those who studied cultures other than their own often viewed them solely through the prism of their own society and judged much of what they saw to be lacking. This view is called ethnocentrism. Contrary to this view is cultural relativism, or the idea that "because cultures are unique, they can be evaluated only according to their own standards and values."[3,p51]

The approach that will guide the rest of this chapter and, indeed, the book as a whole, is the question: "How well does a given culture satisfy the physical and psychological needs of those whose behavior it guides?"[3,p51] For example, is female circumcision, also called female genital mutilation, a health-enhancing procedure or a harmful procedure? Is it good or bad for the health of a newborn to be given sugar water? How should one see cultural practices that discriminate against women and cause them to eat less well than men or are associated with the disproportionate abortion of female fetuses, as in India and China? How should one see cultural practices that discriminate against sexual minorities, that drive them underground, and that therefore may contribute to less healthy sexual practices? On the other hand, what about cultures that encourage exclusive breastfeeding for 6 months? What about male circumcision, which is associated with reduced transmission of HIV?

You will realize as you make your way through the text that those responsible for guiding health policies and programs in different countries must have a good understanding of the cultures with which they are working if they are to be helpful in enhancing health for the members of those societies. This is also true of outsiders, including development assistance agencies. They must be very sensitive to local cultures, while simultaneously considering with their government partners and with insiders to the culture what behavior changes may be needed to enhance individual and population health in a particular setting.[1,p56]

HEALTH BELIEFS AND PRACTICES

Different cultures vary in their perceptions of the body and their views of what is illness, what causes illness, and what should be done about it. They have different views on how to prevent health problems, what health care they should seek, and the types of remedies that health providers might offer.[4] This section highlights selected aspects of belief systems about health that one would see most in low- and middle-income countries and in immigrant populations in high-income countries.

Perceptions of Illness

Perceptions of illness vary considerably across culture groups. What one culture may view as entirely normal, for example, another culture may see as an affliction. Worms are so common among children in some cultures that people do not see infection with worms as an illness. Malaria is so common in much of sub-Saharan Africa that many families see it as normal. In much of South Asia, back pain among women is very common and is also seen as just a normal part of being a woman.[5] Schistosomiasis is very common in Egypt. It causes blood in the urine, which is referred to in Egypt as "male menstruation," and it is often considered normal because it is so widespread.[1,p57]

Perceptions of Disease

Medical anthropologists, among others, define disease as the "malfunctioning or maladaptation of biologic and psycho-physiologic processes in the individual."[6,p252] Pneumonia is a disease. HIV is a disease. Polio is a disease. Illness, however, is different from disease. "Illness represents personal, interpersonal, and cultural reactions to disease or discomfort."[6] People may feel like they have an illness. They can describe it and its symptoms. They may have a name in their culture for this problem. However, they may not have a "disease," which is a physiological condition. This is a very important point, because different cultures may have very different perceptions of the causes of illness.

Most people in high-income countries follow the "Western medical paradigm" in explaining the causes of disease. This will be familiar to you. You get influenza and colds from viruses. You get diabetes as an adult from an inability to control your blood sugar, although there may be a genetic component to it. You get heart disease from smoking, from being obese, or from having cholesterol that is too high.

On the other hand, many people, especially those in or from low- and middle-income countries and more traditional societies, often see illness as being caused by factors other than disease, as defined in the biomedical model. There are many cultures, for example, that believe the body being "out of balance" brings on illness. Among the most common of these concepts is the notion of "hot" and "cold." In this case, the body may get out of balance if one engages in certain unhealthy practices. In certain cultures, some foods are regarded as "hot" and some foods are regarded as "cold" and people are supposed to achieve a balance between these foods to avoid illness.

Many people also believe that illness has supernatural origins. A study done among people in the United States of Caribbean and African descent showed that many people believed that the symptoms of illness stem from supernatural causes.[7] There are many cultures in which people believe that illness comes from being affected by "the evil eye," being bewitched or possessed, losing their soul, or offending gods.[1] Some First Nations people in Canada have a belief that "illness is not necessarily a bad thing, but instead a sign sent by the Creator to help people re-evaluate their lives."[8,p81] A study of the cultural perceptions of illness among Yoruba people in Nigeria found that illness could be "traced to enemies, including witchcraft, sorcery, gods, ancestors, natural illnesses, or hereditary illness."[9,p328]

Emotional stresses are also seen in different cultures as causes of illness. This could come about as a result of being stressed or extremely frightened. Being too envious is also viewed as a cause of illness.[1] Sexual matters are seen as causes of illness in some cultures as well. In several cultures, for example, frequent sexual relations are believed to weaken men by taking away their blood.[1] These beliefs are quite common in parts of India.

Folk Illnesses

Many cultures also have what are called "folk illnesses." These are local cultural interpretations of physical states that people perceive to be illnesses without a physiologic cause. *Empacho* is an illness that is commonly described in a number of Latin American cultures. This is often described as a condition caused by food that "gets stuck to the walls of the stomach or intestines, causing an obstruction."[10,p693] Empacho is said to be caused by any of a variety of inappropriate food practices, and in children it is said to produce a number of gastrointestinal symptoms, including bloating, diarrhea, and a stomachache.

To cure empacho, families may, for example, limit some foods or give abdominal massages with warm oil. They will also often consult a local healer, such as the *santiguadora* in the Puerto Rican community and *sobadora* in the Mexican community. Some Mexican communities in both the United States and Mexico also treat this "illness" with medicinal powders.

To understand health problems in low- and middle-income countries, it is very important to understand the existence of folk illnesses such as empacho. It may be that the condition described by communities as empacho has no known or real biomedical basis. However, even if this condition has no biomedical basis, if people believe it is an important illness, any efforts to improve the health of the community will have to consider such beliefs.[10] **Table 6-1** lists some of the culturally defined causes of illness.

TABLE 6-1 Selected Examples of Cultural Explanations of Disease

Body Balances	Emotional	Supernatural	Sexual
Temperature	Fright	Bewitching	Sex with forbidden person
Energy	Sorrow	Demons	Overindulgence in sex
Blood	Envy	Spirit possession	
Dislocation	Stress	Evil eye	
Problems with organs		Offending God or gods	
Incompatibility of horoscopes		Soul loss	

Modified from Scrimshaw, S. C. (2006). Culture, behavior, and health. In M. H. Merson, R. E. Black, & A. Mills (Eds.), *International public health: Diseases, programs, systems, and policies* (pp. 53–78). Sudbury, MA: Jones and Bartlett.

The Prevention of Illness

Given the wide range of views on what causes illness, it is not surprising that there are many different cultural practices that concern avoiding illness. Many cultures, for example, have taboos, or behaviors and practices that they forbid people to engage in if they are to stay healthy. A large number of taboos concern what not to eat during pregnancy, as was suggested in a study of traditional beliefs in Western Malaysia, including avoiding certain important sources of protein.[11] A study in southern Nigeria about traditional beliefs concerning eating in pregnancy found widespread belief that pregnant women must avoid:[12]

- Sweet foods, so the baby would not be weak
- Eggs, so the baby would not grow up to be a thief
- Snails, so the baby would not be dull, would not salivate excessively, or would develop speech properly

A study in Brazil suggested that women should not eat game meat and fish during pregnancy, although both could be good sources of protein.[13] A study of poor women in South India showed that the intake of fruits and legumes was affected by taboos and legumes are among the most important sources of protein for many Indian women.[14]

There is also a wide array of ritual practices that people undergo to avoid illness. Related to this, there are traditions in some cultures to get rid of bad spirits or evil forces to ensure that one does not fall ill. There are beliefs among the Yoruba people in Nigeria, for example, that charms, amulets, scarification, or some oral potions can prevent illness that is caused by one's enemies.[9] Some tribal groups in Rajasthan, India, put charms at certain crossings to inflict harm on others, to avoid harm to themselves, to appease an evil spirit, or to leave their affliction there with the spirit.[15] In rural Senegal, a special ritual is performed for women who have lost two children, had two miscarriages, or appear to be infertile. The ritual is intended to prevent the causes of child death and infertility.[16]

The Diagnosis and Treatment of Illness and the Use of Health Services

In many cultures, when people are ill, it is common that they first try to care for the illness themselves or with the help of family members, using home remedies. This is often followed by a visit to some type of local healer and the use of indigenous medicines from that healer. Only if the illness does not resolve after that will families seek the help of a "Western doctor." Even then, it is quite common for people to use modern medicines and indigenous medicines at the same time.

The manner in which people and families care for illnesses is called "patterns of resort." People seek help from different healthcare providers at different times for a number of reasons.[1] One important concern is the cost of services, both direct, such as fees, and indirect, such as the cost of transportation, time en route, or waiting. Another concern is the means of payment. People with little cash may prefer to visit a healer or doctor who takes payment in kind, rather than in cash. This could be in small gifts or payment in farm products such as fruits, vegetables, or poultry. People are also driven by the reputation of the provider. They will go to a provider who is reputed in their community to have good results over a provider who does not enjoy this type of reputation.

The manner in which the provider treats them socially is also an important determinant of the use of services. People generally prefer to go to a provider who is from their community, speaks their language, is known to them, and treats them with respect, rather than an outsider who may be disrespectful. It is interesting to note that people tend to treat folk illnesses at home and then go to a local healer. As a last resort, they may go to a physician, even if they understand that the physician does not treat this condition.[10]

It is also very important to understand the extent to which a large share of the treatment of illness in most cultures takes place first at home. People in high-income countries may take some aspirin, drink plenty of water, eat a certain soup, and try to rest when they first develop symptoms. They may also take a variety of different types of herbal products or vitamins. Only if people do not feel better by a certain time will they try to see a health provider. People in more traditional societies have analogous patterns of behavior when they believe themselves to be ill. Understanding these patterns, of course, is central to any efforts to enhance their health.

Health Providers

There are also many different types of health service providers. Some of these are shown in **Table 6-2**. As you can see in the table, some of the providers are practitioners of indigenous systems of medicine, such as ayurvedic practitioners in India and practitioners of Chinese systems of medicine like herbalists and acupuncturists. Other practitioners will be part of a wide array of local health providers. These include, for example, traditional birth attendants, priests, herbalists, and bonesetters. The types of practitioners of Western medicine will depend on the size and location of the place in which they work, and could include, for example, community

TABLE 6-2 Selected Examples of Health Service Providers

Indigenous	Western Biomedical	Other Medical Systems
Midwives	Pharmacists	Chinese medical system
Shamans	Nurse–midwives	• Practitioners
Curers	Nurses	• Chemists/herbalists
Spiritualists	Nurse–practitioners	• Acupuncturists
Witches	Physicians	Ayurvedic practitioners
Sorcerers	Dentists	
Priests		
Diviners		
Herbalists		
Bonesetters		

Modified from Scrimshaw, S. C. (2006). Culture, behavior, and health. In M. H. Merson, R. E. Black, & A. Mills (Eds.), *International public health: Diseases, programs, systems, and policies* (pp. 53–78). Sudbury, MA: Jones and Bartlett.

health workers, nurses, midwives, nurse–midwives, physicians, and dentists. You should also be aware that in many low- and middle-income countries, pharmacists or stores that sell drugs also frequently dispense both drugs and medical advice. Although prescriptions for drugs may be legally required, many low- and middle-income countries are unable or unwilling to enforce this requirement. It is also important to note that many healthcare providers will combine indigenous health practices with Western medicine.[1]

HEALTH BEHAVIORS AND BEHAVIOR CHANGE

The leading causes of death in low- and middle-income countries for all age groups and both sexes in 2010 were stroke, ischemic heart disease, chronic obstructive pulmonary disease, lower respiratory infections, and diarrhea. HIV/AIDS, malaria, road injury, tuberculosis (TB), and diabetes were among the top 10 causes of death in these countries.[17] The most important risk factors for these diseases and conditions include nutritional concerns, including both undernutrition and obesity, tobacco use, indoor and outdoor air pollution, unsafe sex, and unsafe water and sanitation.[17] There are many behaviors that *are* conducive to good health. However, what is the extent to which behavior is a contributing factor to the leading risk factors for illness and premature death in low- and middle-income countries? A number of examples are discussed next.

An infant's being underweight for age is among the most important risk factors for premature death in low-income countries. Although income and education are closely linked with nutritional status of both mother and child, cultural variables are also important determinants of their nutrition. As noted earlier, many cultures have food taboos for pregnant women that are not helpful to birth outcomes, and other cultures encourage pregnant women to eat less rather than more. In addition, how much women breastfeed their babies is closely linked with culture, as is the timing for the introduction of complementary foods. Undernutrition also stems from other eating practices that are also closely tied to culture. Can behaviors be changed so that pregnant women will eat the most nutritious foods they can, given their level of income, and exclusively breastfeed their babies for 6 months?

Unsafe sex is the major risk factor for HIV in low-, middle-, and high-income countries. Some people, such as commercial sex workers, may not have the bargaining power with their clients to negotiate sex with a condom. The same will often be true of women who are forced into unsafe sex by their husbands and boyfriends or because of their own economic position. However, many people who engage in unsafe sex do have control over whether or not to use a condom. What would it take to ensure that they do so?

Hygiene is another area that closely relates to health behaviors, and the lack of safe water and sanitation is a major risk factor for diarrheal disease. In many low- and middle-income countries, hygiene may be low, and families need to learn to use water safely, dispose of human waste in sanitary ways, and wash their hands with soap and water after defecating. Behaviors regarding hygiene, of course, are intimately linked with culture. How can they be changed?

As you will read about later, indoor air pollution is a major risk factor for respiratory infections. This relates largely to the fact that families in many cultures cook indoors with biomass fuels without appropriate ventilation. Some families may not be able to afford an improved stove. However, other families cook as they do because of tradition and the lack of knowledge of the health impacts of indoor air pollution. How could the way people cook be changed?

Tobacco smoking is a leading risk factor for cardiovascular disease and cancer. Most people who smoke cigarettes start smoking as adolescents. Are there measures that can be taken to change these behaviors? How would the efforts to change behavior have to differ if one tried to stop adolescents from taking up smoking, compared to helping adult smokers to quit?

Of course, behaviors are closely linked with culture and health not only in low- and middle-income countries but also in high-income countries. Moreover, in high-income, as well as in low- and middle-income countries, there is a wide array of behaviors that do not promote good health. In the high-income countries, for example, an increasing number of people are obese and have diabetes. Many people also continue to smoke, even though smoking is a major risk factor for both cardiovascular disease and cancer. Despite the widespread availability of seat belts in cars, some people still do not use them. What needs to be done to get people to change these behaviors to ones that are healthier?

Improving Health Behaviors

There are a number of models or theories that explain why people engage in certain health behaviors and what can be done to encourage changes in those behaviors. Those interested in greater detail in health behaviors can review *The Essentials of Health Behavior*, another book in this series.[18] Some of the most important concepts about health behavior and models about behavior change, however, are examined very briefly here.

The Ecological Perspective

As one considers the factors that influence behaviors that relate to health, it is important to take what is called an ecological perspective. This is a concept that suggests that the factors influencing health behaviors occur at several levels. These are noted in **Table 6-3**.

The basic precepts concerning the ecological approach are:

- "Health related behaviors are affected by, and affect, multiple levels of influence: intrapersonal or individual factors, interpersonal factors, institutional factors, community factors, and public policy factors."[19,p4]
- "Behavior both influences and is influenced by the social environments in which it occurs."[19,p5]

TABLE 6-3 The Ecological Perspective

Factors	Definition
Individual	Individual characteristics that influence behavior such as knowledge, attitudes, beliefs, and personality traits
Interpersonal	Interpersonal processes, and primary groups including family, friends, and peers
Institutional	Rules, regulations, policies, and informal structures
Community	Social networks and norms or standards that exist formally or informally among individuals, groups, and organizations
Public policy	Local, state, and federal policies and laws that regulate or support healthy actions and practices for disease prevention, early detection, control, and management

Modified with permission from Murphy, E. (2005). *Promoting healthy behavior. Health bulletin 2*. Washington, DC: Population Reference Bureau.

You can try to imagine, for example, whether or not an adolescent male will take up smoking. This will depend on how he feels about smoking, what he thinks others think of his smoking, the setting in which he operates, how expensive it is to buy cigarettes, and how easy it is to buy them. Of course, if he does start smoking, some of his own peer group may follow.

The Health Belief Model

The Health Belief model was the first effort to articulate a coherent understanding of the factors that enter into health behaviors. It was developed by the U.S. Public Health Service as it tried to understand why people did or did not avail themselves of the opportunity to get chest x-rays for tuberculosis.[20] The premises of this model are that people's health behaviors depend on their perceptions of:

- Their likelihood of getting the illness
- The severity of the illness if they get it
- The benefits of engaging in behavior that will prevent the illness
- The barriers to engaging in preventive behavior

In this model, people's health behavior also depends on whether or not people feel that they could actually carry out the appropriate behavior if they tried, which is called *self-efficacy*.[19]

One could think about how this model pertains to engaging in safe sex. The extent to which a young man uses a condom will be influenced by his fear of getting HIV, how serious a disease he believes it to be, the extent to which a condom can prevent HIV, and how easy it is to buy a condom and get a partner to agree to use it. The young man must also feel that he will buy the condom and use it.

Stages of Change Model

The Stages of Change model was developed in the 1990s in the United States in conjunction with work on alcohol and drug abuse.[19] The premise behind this model is that change in behavior is a process and that different people are at different stages of readiness for change. The stages of change are outlined in **Table 6-4**.

It is easy to see how this model might apply to alcohol and drug abuse. You can imagine an excessive drinker who is not aware of his problem or who will not face it and needs help in doing so. Other people, who are aware of their problem and willing to do something about it, may need help to stop. Still others, who have already broken their addictions, need positive reinforcement to maintain their health.[19]

TABLE 6-4 The Stages of Change Model

Stages
Precontemplation
Contemplation
Decision/Determination
Action
Maintenance

Reprinted with permission from Murphy, E. (2005). *Promoting healthy behavior. Health bulletin 2.* Washington, DC: Population Reference Bureau.

The Diffusion of Innovations Model

The Diffusion of Innovations model had its origins in work that was done on promoting agricultural change in the United States. In this model, "an innovation is an idea, practice, service, or other object that is perceived as new by the individual or group."[1,p66] This model is based on the notion that communication is needed to promote social change and that "diffusion" is the process by which innovations are communicated over time among members of different groups and societies.[21] This model focuses on how people adopt and can be encouraged to adopt innovations, but does not get involved with how they might maintain what they have adopted.

Table 6-5 outlines the stages that have to be undertaken to try to diffuse a health innovation.

This model also suggests that as the innovation begins to be diffused, people will fall into six groups:[1,21]

- Innovators
- Early adopters
- Early majority
- Late majority
- Late adopters
- Laggards

In addition, the model also indicates that the pace of adoption will be influenced by:[1,21]

- The gains people think they will get by adopting the innovation
- How much the innovation fits in with their existing culture and values
- How easy it is to try out the innovation
- Whether or not there are role models who are already trying out the innovation

TABLE 6-5 Diffusions of Health Innovations Model

Stages of Diffusion

Recognition of a problem or need

Conduct of basic and applied research to address the specific problem

Development of strategies and materials that will put the innovative concept into a form that will meet the needs of the target population

Commercialization of the innovation, which will involve production, marketing, and distribution efforts

Diffusion and adoption of the innovation

Consequences associated with adoption of the innovation

Modified from Scrimshaw, S. C. (2006). Culture, behavior, and health. In M. H. Merson, R. E. Black, & A. Mills (Eds.), *International public health: Diseases, programs, systems, and policies* (pp. 53–78). Sudbury, MA: Jones and Bartlett.

- The extent to which potential adopters see the innovation as cost-efficient and not taking too much of their time, energy, or money

One can imagine how the Diffusion of Innovations model may apply to efforts to change diets in high-income countries away from certain fats and toward more fruits and vegetables, fewer processed foods, and more whole grains. Some people change their diets relatively quickly. Others in the community make these shifts only as they can overcome some of their long-held dietary patterns. Some people shift as they learn more from their friends, some of whom become role models for change. The relatively high costs of some of the organic and other healthy foods may be a constraint to adoption of change by some people. Others may simply not be willing or able to change the way they and their families have always eaten.

UNDERSTANDING AND ENGENDERING BEHAVIOR CHANGE

As you can clearly see, in many instances, improving health requires that the behaviors of individuals, families, and communities be changed. You also see, however, that behaviors are intimately connected to culture, which is inherently difficult to change. Under these circumstances, what can be done, first to understand what behaviors need to be changed and, second, to change them? These questions are answered briefly here.

Understanding Behaviors

A first step in trying to promote behavior change must be to gain a good understanding of the behaviors that are taking place. This requires a careful assessment of:

- The behaviors that are taking place
- The extent to which they are helpful or harmful to health
- The underlying motivation for these behaviors
- The likely responses to different approaches to changing the unhealthy behaviors

By taking a look at breastfeeding, for example, we can get a sense of how one would carry out such an assessment. One can consider how infant deaths might be reduced. As part of this effort, it is important to get a better sense of the extent to which any nutritional issues are harmful to infant health and how they might be improved. One important part of this effort would be to examine breastfeeding practices. In doing so, we would try to answer the following questions, among others:

- When do women start breastfeeding?
- Do they feed on schedule or on demand?
- Do they feed male and female children the same way?
- For how long do they breastfeed exclusively?
- At what age do they introduce complementary foods?
- Until what age do they continue to breastfeed, even while the children are getting complementary foods?
- Why do they engage in these practices?
- Why do some women not breastfeed?
- Who breastfeeds and who does not?
- Who has influence over their breastfeeding practices?

The answers to these questions, of course, will vary by culture group; however, once we get answers to them, we can begin to formulate a plan for behavior change that is built on the cultural values and approaches of the people. Without understanding current practices, the rationale for them, and who has influence over them, it will be impossible to promote behavior change in the appropriate directions. When we do have a sense of the existing practices and why they take place, what can be done to change behaviors?

Changing Health Behaviors

There are many different approaches to changing health behaviors. Some operate at the level of the individual, some at the level of the community, and some at the level of society as a whole. Generally, they include some combination of communication through the mass media and more personal communication. Several approaches to behavior change are discussed briefly here.

Community Mobilization

One very important way to encourage change in health behaviors is to engage in community mobilization. In this case, the effort focuses on getting an entire community to engage in the effort of promoting more healthy behaviors. This requires considerable efforts aimed at helping people across the community identify the problems they face, find potential solutions to the problems, and then work together to implement those solutions. Generally, it also requires that the leaders within the community are mobilized, willing to be champions for the needed change, and then willing to promote that change.[19] You will read more later, for example, about the Tamil Nadu Nutrition Project, which was noted in one of the vignettes at the opening of this chapter, and the manner in which the affected communities were involved in promoting a variety of innovations. The innovations included weighing babies together, identifying together the babies who were not thriving, and working together to make supplementary food for their children. In addition, all of the community was involved in learning about appropriate foods and needed micronutrients. You will also read later about a variety of community-based activities, including efforts to address diarrheal disease through oral rehydration in Egypt and polio campaigns in Latin America.

Mass Media

The mass media is often used to promote change in health behaviors. Most people in low- and middle-income countries have access to radio, which is often used for this purpose. Increasingly, however, those engaged in promoting better health are using a tool referred to as "entertainment-education." Many of these efforts have focused on soap opera series in which the characters bring out the main messages about healthy behaviors. The British Broadcasting Company has a group, for example, that works with low- and middle-income countries to produce soap operas on health topics of importance such as HIV/AIDS. Such a series was done on HIV/AIDS in India and Nigeria. The government of Myanmar had a soap opera about leprosy that featured Myanmar's best-known actress. The aims of the soap opera were to help destigmatize leprosy, let people know how to diagnose leprosy, inform them that it could be treated completely if treated early, and get people to come forward for treatment at an early stage. The Population Media Center's radio serial drama, *Yeken Kignit*, in Ethiopia reached nearly half of the population and addressed reproductive health and gender equality. After 2 1/2 years of the show being broadcast, demand for contraceptives increased by 157 percent and listeners were five times more likely than those who did not listen to the show to know three or more family planning methods. Additionally, male listeners requested HIV tests four times the rate of male nonlisteners.[22]

Social Marketing

Social marketing is the application of the tools of commercial marketing to try to promote behavior change and the uptake of important health actions or products. This has been used widely in family planning work. It is also being used in other fields, such as in selling bednets for malaria control. In social marketing, a local brand of a product is often created, such as a condom, a contraceptive pill, or an insecticide-treated bednet. Mass media and other forms of communication are then used to promote the brand and the behaviors related to the product. Of course, successful marketing depends on very careful market research and a good understanding of the local culture, values, and behaviors. It also depends on what is called "the four Ps" in social marketing:[19]

- Attractive product
- Affordable price
- Convenient places to buy the product
- Persuasive promotion

Often the products being marketed through social marketing are sold through commercial channels but the government subsidizes their price.

Health Education

Health education is something with which every reader of this text will be familiar. It comes in many forms, such as in the classroom, in the news media, on the radio and television, and on the Internet. Successful health education programs that were aimed at sex education have several features in common that hold lessons for other efforts at making health education effective:[19]

- They focused on risky behaviors and were clear about abstinence and consistent condom use
- They provided accurate information
- They addressed how to deal with social pressures
- They selected teachers and peer educators who believed in the program

- They geared the content of the program to the age, sexual experience, and culture of the students

Conditional Cash Transfers

A number of countries are turning increasingly to the use of economic incentives to encourage behavior change in health and help reduce poverty, as discussed in the policy and program brief on the *Oportunidades* (Opportunities) program in Mexico near the end of this chapter. These incentives are called *conditional cash transfers*. In this case, a government program offers a payment to families on an agreed-upon time frame, provided that the family engages in agreed-upon nutrition, health, or education behaviors. The desired behaviors could include activities such as giving birth in a hospital; engaging in regular well-baby care like immunizations; participating in a nutrition program that checks on the nutritional status of a child and offers food supplements, as needed; or sending female children to school on a regular basis.

Achieving Success in Health Promotion

The previous section refers to specific types of health promotion that can be used to encourage a change in health behaviors or the adoption of healthy behaviors. There are a number of lessons that have emerged both about these approaches and when looking broadly at what constitutes an effective health promotion effort. These are noted in **Table 6-6**.

SOCIAL ASSESSMENT

Concerning the links between health and culture, *social assessment* or *social impact assessment* must also be addressed. A social impact assessment is "a process for assessing the social impacts of planned interventions or events and for developing strategies for the ongoing monitoring and management of those impacts."[23,p2] In more expansive terms,

> Social impact assessment includes the processes of analyzing, monitoring, and managing the intended and unintended social consequences, both positive and negative, of planned interventions (policies, programs, plans, projects) and any social change processes invoked by those interventions. Its primary purpose is to bring about a more sustainable and equitable biophysical and human environment.[23,p2]

The social impact assessment looks at a variety of domains that go beyond health. These include impact on historical artifacts and buildings, communities, demography, gender, minority groups, culture, and health. The

TABLE 6-6 Selected Factors for Success in Health Promotion

Identify specific health problems, related behaviors, and key stakeholders.

Know and use sound behavioral theories.

Research motivations and constraints to change, considering biologic, environmental, cultural, and other contextual factors.

Use participatory assessment tools and include relevant stakeholders in the design, implementation, and evaluation of the intervention.

Plan and budget carefully.

Identify people who exhibit healthy behaviors that differ from the social norm.

Create an environment that enables behavior change through policy dialogue, advocacy, and capacity building.

Organize an intervention that addresses both specific behaviors and contextual factors.

Work to ensure sustainability.

Evaluate from the beginning.

Form partnerships to scale up and/or adapt the most successful interventions for implementation in other settings.

Modified with permission from Murphy, E. (2005). *Promoting healthy behavior. Health bulletin 2.* Washington, DC: Population Reference Bureau.

assessment should be carried out in a way that builds on local processes, engages the community fully, and proactively tries to maximize the potential good that can come from the proposed investment. It "promotes community development and empowerment, builds capacity, and develops social capital."[23,p2] The detailed approach of a social impact assessment is outlined in **Table 6-7**.

Many readers will be familiar with environmental assessment of proposed investment schemes, and many countries require such assessments be done before any major physical investment. In some respects, a social assessment is the social analogue to an environmental assessment. In this case, let us suppose that a development agency and a government are going to collaborate to develop a series of health centers in a particular region of a country. First, the country would carry out a social assessment to set the foundation for the project design. The affected communities should participate in this

TABLE 6-7 Selected Focuses of Social Impact Assessment

Identifies interested and affected peoples

Facilitates and coordinates the participation of stakeholders

Analyzes the local setting of the planned intervention to assess likely impacts to it

Collects baseline data to allow for evaluation of the impact of the intervention

Gives a picture of the local cultural context, and develops an understanding of local community values, particularly how they relate to the planned intervention

Identifies and describes the activities that are likely to cause impacts

Predicts likely impacts and how different stakeholders are likely to respond

Assists in evaluating and selecting alternatives

Recommends measures to mitigate any likely negative impacts

Assists in the evaluation process and provides suggestions about compensation for affected peoples

Describes potential conflicts between stakeholders and advises on resolution processes

Develops coping strategies for dealing with residual and nonmitigatable impacts

Contributes to skill development and capacity building in the community

Assists in devising and implementing monitoring and management programs

Modified from Vanclay, F. (2003). International principles for social impact assessment. *Impact Assessment and Project Appraisal, 21*(1), 5–11.

assessment. The country would also ensure that the design took account of the needs of various groups in the community and was based on their culture and values, and it would keep in mind how programs need to be tailored to address them. The assessment would seek to identify any negative consequences that might emerge from the investment and how those consequences might be mitigated. The plan emerging from the assessment would also include a scheme for monitoring and evaluating the social impacts of the project and if the program design really is consistent with local values and the underlying needs of the community.

Some years ago, very little attention was paid in some development assistance agencies and in some governments to social assessment. Little effort was spent on examining the social and cultural issues involved in designing appropriate interventions in health. In addition, little attention was paid to the potential impact on health or on other social areas of investments in sectors outside of health. Although the quality of social assessment may vary both within and across some agencies and governments, social assessments are now done more frequently for major development projects.

POLICY AND PROGRAM BRIEFS

Six policy and program briefs follow. They are largely based on published reports and literature from peer-reviewed journals. They are meant to illustrate some of the key issues concerning the relationship between culture and health and how some of those issues can be addressed in trying to engender better health through behavior change.

The first case examines breastfeeding practices in Burundi and the barriers to exclusive breastfeeding for 6 months, as WHO recommends. The second case reviews some of the cultural issues related to efforts to eradicate polio in India and how communications programs have been enhanced to address them. The third reviews a program that was established in the Andean region of Peru to encourage women, by building on local cultural practices, to give birth in hospitals with trained birth attendants. The fourth case reviews the *Oportunidades* program in Mexico, which provides conditional cash transfers to the poor to promote better nutrition, health, and education behaviors. The fifth case reviews the experience with CARE Groups, which are peer-based efforts at health promotion. The last case examines some of the key linkages between cultural practices and the spread of the Ebola virus.

Breastfeeding in Burundi[24]

There is substantial evidence that giving only breast milk to an infant for the first 6 months of life is a critical health-promoting practice. This is called *exclusive breastfeeding (EBF)*. Nonetheless, data from 2011 indicate that the rate of exclusive breastfeeding in low-income countries was only 39 percent.[25] In order to promote exclusive breastfeeding and enhance the health of young children, it is critical to understand why many women do not engage in EBF at higher rates.

An examination of the factors that motivate the duration of EBF was carried out in December 2009 in Burundi, a low-income country in Africa. In Burundi, the rate of EBF for the first 4 months was then about 74 percent. However, many women stopped this practice after the fourth month, and the rate of EBF for 6 months was only 45 percent.

The study focused on breastfeeding practices in families in two provinces, Cancuzo and Ruyigi. Given the importance of cultural beliefs to health behaviors, the study aimed at understanding how certain beliefs affected whether a woman chose to breastfeed exclusively for 6 months. The goal of the study was to understand barriers to EBF in order to develop an effective EBF promotion program.

The study was based on an approach called *barrier analysis*, which focuses on trying to understand barriers to the adoption of positive health behaviors so that more effective behavior change communication messages and support activities can be developed.[26] This methodology has been used for work not only on breastfeeding, but also on other nutrition practices, the use of latrines, and the use of bednets. With respect to exclusive breastfeeding, the study set out to gain a better understanding of the extent to which a mother believes:

- People important to her would approve of EBF
- God would approve of EBF
- She has sufficient knowledge, capacities, and resources to successfully perform EBF
- Malnutrition is a serious problem
- Her child could become malnourished
- EBF is effective in preventing malnutrition
- She can remember to practice EBF
- In certain negative or positive attributes of practicing EBF

Following barrier analysis methods, 45 women with children under 1 year of age who had exclusively breastfed their children were interviewed. Forty-nine women who had not exclusively breastfed their children under 1 year of age were also interviewed. The questions they were asked included:

- Do you think that exclusive breastfeeding until the age of 6 months could help your child avoid becoming malnourished?
- Do you think that God approves of mothers exclusively breastfeeding their children until the age of 6 months?
- In your opinion, would most of the people you know approve of your exclusively breastfeeding your child?
- Who are the people who would approve of your breastfeeding your child?
- With your current knowledge and abilities, do you think you would be able to exclusively breastfeed your next child until the age of 6 months?
- What are the disadvantages of exclusively breastfeeding your child?

- If you wanted to exclusively breastfeed your child until the age of 6 months, would it be difficult to remember to not give your child other foods or liquids other than breast milk?

A number of statistically significant findings emerged from the research:

- Those who exclusively breastfed were 21 times more likely than those who did not to say that a child who does not exclusively breastfeed will become malnourished.
- Those who did not exclusively breastfeed were 17.6 times more likely than those who did to say that God does not approve of exclusive breastfeeding.
- Those who exclusively breastfed were many times (10.4, 6.5, 5.9, 3.8 times) more likely than those who did not to say that mothers-in-law, husbands, cousins, and mothers, respectively, approved of exclusive breastfeeding.
- Those who exclusively breastfed were 8 times more likely than those who did not to say that they had the knowledge and abilities to practice exclusive breastfeeding.
- Those who did not exclusively breastfeed were 7 times more likely than those who did to believe that exclusive breastfeeding would lead to babies always being hungry.
- Those who exclusively breastfed were 6.3 times more likely to say that it is not difficult at all to remember to practice EBF.

Among these findings, three stood out as especially significant in terms of designing a breastfeeding promotion program. These included the extent to which women believed: (1) that a child who is not exclusively breastfed can become malnourished, (2) God approved of exclusive breastfeeding, and (3) persons important to them approved of exclusive breastfeeding.

With these findings in mind, the study authors and local staff made a number of recommendations for strengthening the promotion of breastfeeding in these two provinces. These included:

- Track and expose to the communities positive deviants who faithfully practice EBF and who also have healthy, well-nourished babies.
- Provide peer-based lactation counseling to help women understand the importance of EBF in combating malnutrition.
- Educate health promotion trainers on how to effectively demonstrate the link between EBF and good nutrition.

- Mobilize spiritual leaders to show support for EBF.
- Give pastors and priests sermon guidelines related to breastfeeding practices and good nutrition.
- Use radio broadcasts featuring mothers-in-law, husbands, cousins, and mothers who support EBF.
- Train some of these mothers-in-law, female cousins, and mothers to be "Leader Mothers," the community-level cadre of health promoters in the project.

Polio Vaccination in India

In early 2014, India was declared polio free, having gone three consecutive years without a single case of polio. India has become a success story, from once having the highest burden of polio in the world to celebrating zero cases.[27]

In 1988, India launched its Polio Eradication Initiative. India's polio eradication program is a part of the Global Polio Eradication Initiative and includes a social mobilization and communication component.[28] This is meant to encourage universal immunization by providing accurate information about the vaccine, mobilizing demand for vaccination, and countering popular beliefs and behaviors that might constrain vaccination against polio.

India's polio program is a collaborative effort of national and international partners. These include India's national and local governments, via the Ministries of Health and Family Welfare, UNICEF, the World Health Organization National Polio Surveillance Project, Rotary International, the United States Centers for Disease Control and Prevention, and numerous nongovernmental organizations.[29,30]

India is the second largest country in the world and has a population over 1 billion. The country is divided into 29 states and has a very diverse population.[31] As would be expected, health beliefs vary across India and among different social groups.

Until recently, India was one of the last four countries in the world with endemic polio.[32] In addition, there were periodic outbreaks of polio in India in the last 15 years, with the annual number of cases jumping to 1,600 in 2002 and 874 in 2007, from considerably lower levels in most other years.[32] The more recent polio outbreaks occurred primarily in the states of Uttar Pradesh and Bihar.[33]

These outbreaks were attributed to a variety of biological, social, political, and programmatic factors. Biological factors contributing to persistent polio outbreaks included high population density, poor sanitation, and pervasive poverty in certain regions. The primary social forces that contributed to the outbreaks were resistance to immunization among minority communities, as well as difficulty in vaccinating the children of the great numbers of people who migrate for work. Political forces that inhibited the polio program were rooted in tensions between Muslim minorities and the Hindu-dominated government. Programmatic challenges, such as low coverage of immunization activities and falsification of data, also affected some regions of India.[33]

Certain communities and social groups, primarily marginalized Muslim minority groups, have been resistant to giving oral polio vaccine to their children. This has been attributed partly to a failure of the parents to understand the need for repeated vaccinations. It has also been due to misinformation that has circulated in some communities that the vaccine was ineffective, causes illness in children, causes infertility, or is part of a plot to curb the population growth of Muslims.[34] The strength of these rumors may be exacerbated by the fact that most health professionals and community health workers tend to be Hindu.

In the face of these difficulties, public health leaders in India and from key international organizations have collaborated to enhance the health communication and social mobilization aspects of India's polio program. Greater focus has been put on reaching those resistant to vaccination and convincing them both to immunize their children and to continue vaccinating them with the appropriate number of doses.[34] In addition, efforts at communication and social mobilization have been decentralized to the district, block, and village level, which has allowed them to be more closely tailored to local mores. The program has also enlisted community members in communication efforts to a greater extent than earlier.[29,35] These measures are intended to ensure that families receive information about the program from respected community members with whom they already have a relationship and trust.[35]

Some of the major steps that have been taken to support this approach have included:

- The establishment of a social mobilization network that extended to the village level.
- The linking of the social mobilization network, including community mobilization coordinators, with vaccination teams. These teams work in booths on immunization days and then go house to house to immunize children who were missed on those days.
- Greater involvement of community and religious leaders in mobilizing members of their communities to be vaccinated.
- More use of intensive, house-to-house, interpersonal communications to ensure families would vaccinate their children.

- Greater engagement of well-known celebrities for mass media advertisements to support the polio program.
- Greater involvement in the program of professional associations, such as the Pediatric Association.

The evidence suggests that communities in which these social mobilization and communications activities have taken place have higher rates of immunization coverage than other communities.[34] These measures have also been associated with the decreasing number of new polio cases. In the first 9 months of 2010, for example, as these measures were implemented, India had 37 new cases of polio, compared to 367 during the same period in 2009.[32]

The implementation of the polio eradication program in India suggests that health communication efforts must pay particular attention to cultural context as well as epidemiologic factors and the political environment. The polio program in India has also highlighted the importance of:[34]

- Engaging more effectively with marginalized communities
- Ensuring messages reach the village level
- The need in some settings for intensive interpersonal communications from respected people with influence who are seen as members of the community
- The power of involving religious leaders in programs, as well

Birthing Services in Peru

As discussed earlier in the chapter, cultural values can have an immense bearing on where and how people give birth, who attends the delivery, and their willingness to address complications that do arise with emergency obstetric care, if available. As noted, however, other factors, such as a lack of empowerment and discrimination, may also influence health-seeking behavior.

In the Andean region of Peru, both of these factors have been at play. Women in some settings have traditionally given birth at home, without the help of a skilled birth attendant. They have done this not only for cultural reasons, but also because they did not always feel welcome in healthcare settings in which health providers may not speak their language, may not treat them respectfully, and often insist that they give birth in a manner different from their traditional ways.

These factors, combined with poverty and low educational levels, especially among women, contributed in the late 1990s to very high maternal mortality ratios in some places in the Peruvian Andes. In Ayacucho, for example, maternal mortality ratios were six times the rates in Lima, the capital of Peru.

If women are not comfortable with available birthing services, they are less likely to use them. This is of critical concern when most obstetric complications occur during or immediately after delivery and cannot be predicted. It is therefore crucial that women, especially high-risk groups such as the indigenous women around Ayacucho, deliver with a skilled birth attendant.[36] In an effort to address these concerns, the international nongovernmental organization Health Unlimited teamed up with Salud Sín Límites Perú (Health Without Limits Peru) to create a model for birthing services that is more responsive to the needs of indigenous communities in the Santillana district in Ayacucho.

The new model of care was planned in stages, with the participation of all key stakeholders.[36]

- A survey was done to understand local birthing practices. Men and women in the community were surveyed, as well as traditional birth attendants and trained health professionals.
- The stakeholders then designed the new model over a series of meetings. The aim of these meetings was to design a model that would respect local beliefs and practices as much as possible, but still ensure better outcomes for pregnant women.
- The model was rolled out over a nearly 2-year period and promoted through a variety of communication efforts in the local language, Quechua.
- The new model was then evaluated and refinements were made to the model, based on what was learned in the evaluation.
- A long-run evaluation of the model was set up on a continuous basis.

During the planning stages of the program, a number of barriers were identified by women giving birth in government health centers, including:

- Health professionals spoke only Spanish, although most indigenous women in this region speak Quechua.
- The husband, family, and traditional birth attendant were not permitted in the delivery room, although the women prefer their participation in the delivery.
- There was no option to use traditional medicines such as herbs and oils during the delivery process.
- Women were required to deliver in a horizontal position on a gynecological bed, although they prefer a traditional, vertical, squatting position.

- The umbilical cord could not be cut by a family member, following their tradition.
- The placenta was thrown away, so it could not be buried according to tradition.

Solutions to these barriers, as well as others identified during the interviews, were proposed and incorporated into a new healthcare model for birthing services in the Santillana district. This new model combines certain aspects of Andean "traditional" medicine with "modern" medicine to ensure that indigenous women will be comfortable with the birthing services and receive high-quality care.

Some features of the new model include Quechua language training for health professionals, the option to include the husband and traditional birth attendant in the labor and delivery process, use of traditional medicines, delivery in the vertical squatting position or on a normal bed, and return of the placenta to the family for proper burial. Although these and other aspects of traditional birthing were incorporated into the new model, there were certain things that the program managers felt could not be compromised if high-quality care was to be ensured. For example, in the new model the umbilical cord must still be cut by a health professional, despite the tradition of having this done by a family member.

Women in the Ayacucho region appear to have been receptive to the new model for birthing services. Between 1999 and 2007, the proportion of deliveries in a health facility with a skilled birth attendant increased from 6 percent to 83 percent in the Santillana district in Ayacucho. At the time the study of this approach was carried out, data were still being collected to allow for more extensive evaluation of the impact of the new model on maternal mortality.[36]

Programs such as this one highlight the importance of trying to improve the health of poor and marginalized people by understanding and building on their cultural practices rather than asking them to change their behaviors in ways that may seem contrary to their traditions. This work in Peru also highlights the importance of careful planning, implementation, and evaluation of programs in ways that engage all key stakeholders and give them a stake in the program's success.

Conditional Cash Transfers in Mexico

The poor are often unable to purchase sufficient foods to ensure that their children are well nourished and healthy. In addition, the poor often have difficulty accessing health services, even when they are available in principle, because of the direct and indirect costs, such as transportation, the time spent using these services, and payment for services. The poor also underinvest in the education of their children,

not only because of their poverty, but also because the family may depend on income from working children.

One of the approaches that governments have adopted to try to reduce poverty and enhance the future prospects of poor families and their children is the conditional cash transfer (CCT). A CCT is a cash payment to a household for meeting specific requirements, primarily related to preventive health care and children's education. CCT programs generally try to enhance the income available to the poor so they can increase food consumption. They also try to increase the demand of the poor for health and education. The aim of CCTs in these efforts is to reduce short-term poverty and to improve family members' prospects of overcoming poverty and participating more fully in the economy in the long term.

One CCT program is *Oportunidades*, the Mexican government's social safety net program for poor households, which was previously known as *Progresa*. *Oportunidades* provides CCTs to poor households in an attempt to break the cycle of poverty, poor nutritional status and poor health, and limited educational attainment by enabling families to engage in better health and education practices. Like many CCT programs, *Oportunidades* selects its participants by targeting geographic areas with high levels of poverty. The program then targets only those with incomes below a certain level.[37]

In 2005, *Oportunidades* provided a monthly cash transfer to participating families that averaged about $20, which constituted about 23 percent of the amount needed at that time to be above the poverty line in Mexico. The transfers included:[37]

- $13 per household
- $8–17 per child of primary school age
- $25–32 per child of secondary school age
- $12–22 per child as a one-time grant for school supplies

In exchange for the cash transfers, families had to meet certain conditions, or "co-responsibilities." These included:[37]

- Full immunization and participation in growth monitoring of children under 2 years of age
- Participation in growth monitoring of children 2 to 5 years of age three times a year
- Attendance at four prenatal visits by pregnant women
- Two postpartum care visits for breastfeeding women
- Once a year physical exams for adult family members
- Attendance at health education sessions by adult family members

Oportunidades also aims to promote gender equality by creating social and economic opportunities specifically for women. For example, *Oportunidades* delivers CCTs to women, which contrasts with traditional social programs that are often geared toward economic empowerment of the head of household, who is usually a male. Moreover, *Oportunidades* provides larger CCTs for girls enrolled in secondary school than boys, to counter social norms that drive gender discrimination and cause girls to drop out of school. Finally, the visibility of women in the community is enhanced though the election of women to serve as liaisons between program beneficiaries and *Oportunidades* officials.

Oportunidades was the first national, government-run CCT program. The program incorporates unique approaches to target poor households, empower women, engage beneficiaries, and evaluate program outcomes. By 2006, the program reached more than 5 million beneficiaries.

In 2009, when a major evaluation of the program was completed, *Oportunidades* had been associated with significant gains in a number of areas. These included a more than 10 percent increase in household expenditure, a substantial increase in the number of health visits, and a 44 percent reduction in stunting. The gains associated with the program also included a reduction in illness among its participants and a decrease in maternal mortality of between 2 percent and 11 percent. In addition, the enrollment in secondary schools increased by 20 percent for girls and 10 percent for boys.[37]

Partly based on the successes of *Oportunidades*, many other countries have developed similar programs in an effort to alleviate poverty and improve health, nutrition, and education. The first countries to engage in such efforts were in Latin America, with Brazil also having a large national program of importance. However, countries in Asia and Africa have also used CCTs to achieve greater demand for health and education, such as a girls' secondary school scholarship scheme in Bangladesh and CCTs for hospital-based delivery in India.

An important research agenda is being carried out on CCTs that focuses, among other things, on their effectiveness, especially compared to transfers that are not conditional; the cost-effectiveness of CCT programs, including compared to interventions meant to alter supply rather than demand; and the impact of CCT programs on health outcomes. Research is also needed to examine the quality of the ongoing CCT programs to ensure that participation leads to impact.[37]

Care Groups

The Problem: Preventable Child Deaths

Although many countries have achieved significant progress in reducing the mortality of under-5 children, some countries, especially in sub-Saharan Africa have not made sufficient progress.[38] Many of these preventable deaths are associated with undernutrition, which contributes to about one-third of under-5 child mortality globally.[39] One of the main priorities in child health, therefore, is how to reduce child deaths and malnutrition. Some of the most important ways to do this relate to the promotion of behavior change.[40]

What Needs to Be Done: Behavior Change

A number of behavioral interventions have been identified as effective in reducing childhood undernutrition in settings where 95 percent of the world's maternal and child deaths occur.[41] For example, exclusive breastfeeding for up to 6 months, appropriate complementary feeding, handwashing with soap and proper disposal of feces contribute to decreased risk of death; increased growth; improved nutritional status; and the prevention of pneumonia, diarrhea, and infection in very young children.[42,43] These practices are also among the 12 key family and community practices identified by UNICEF and the World Health Organization (WHO) to improve child survival, growth, and development.

Other practices that can reduce child death in evidence-based and cost-effective ways include scheduled immunizations, adequate micronutrient intake, use of bednets, enhancing psychosocial development, home care for illness, home treatment for infections, prompt care seeking, compliance with advice, and antenatal care.[44] Despite the fact that what needs to be done is known and needs to be taken to scale, there remain critical challenges around the uptake of these practices. Many efforts to promote uptake have focused on promoting these practices by reaching large numbers of mothers.[40]

A Possible Solution: The Care Group Model

World Relief, under the guidance of Dr. Peter Ernst, first developed the Care Group model as a way to reach large groups of mothers in Mozambique in 1995. Food for the Hungry then adopted the model in Mozambique in 1997. Since then, World Relief, Food for the Hungry, and more than 21 additional organizations have adopted the Care Group model in more than 20 countries.[45]

The Care Group model is a strategy for expanding coverage of key maternal and child health interventions through groups of "10–15 volunteer, community-health educators who regularly meet with project staff for training and supervision and . . . each volunteer is responsible for visiting 10–15 of her neighbors, sharing what she has learned and facilitating behavior change at the household level."[46]

This model aims to improve maternal and child health by promoting behavior change through peer-to-peer interaction at the community level. The model focuses on building teams of volunteer women who are trained by paid community health workers. Each paid community health worker trains 12 Care Group volunteers who then are responsible for approximately 10–12 families each.[40]

Care Group meetings occur every 2 weeks and include a reporting of events, teaching of the week's two or three health messages, group reflections, and other social activities. Between meetings, Care Group volunteers visit their assigned 10–12 households to share and teach the key health and nutrition weekly message. The paid promoters help supervise the process.[40]

Over the years, there have been various modifications to the Care Group model. However, central characteristics of the model include:[47]

- A strong peer-to-peer health promotion component
- Care group volunteers are chosen by the mothers who are being served or community leaders
- Care Group volunteers visit no more than 15 households
- Care Group meeting attendance is monitored
- Each beneficiary mother is contacted at least once every month
- Data on pregnancies, births, and death are collected by volunteers
- The majority of what is taught through Care Groups seeks to promote behavior change directed towards the reduction of mortality and malnutrition
- Care Group volunteers use some sort of visual teaching tool during household visits

Evidence of Success

The Care Group Model has been shown in many settings to improve multiple indicators of child health, including overall mortality reduction. Mozambique has one of the highest child mortality rates in the world and one of the longest and most studied Care Group programs is Food for the Hungry's Child Survival Program in Sofala province, Mozambique. Overall, a study of this program found that undernutrition declined by 31 percent from 2006 to 2010 in four districts that first received the Care Group intervention.

The study also showed that undernutrition declined by 42 percent from 2009 to 2009 in another group of three districts.[39] Demonstrated behavioral changes included an increase in exclusive breastfeeding from 17 to 77 percent, an increase in the percentage of children receiving one vitamin-A rich food per day from 29 to 88 percent, and an increase in the percentage of mothers who know at least three child danger signs from 29 to 93 percent.[40] Importantly, these results

were achieved in cost-effective ways, at an average cost of $2.78 per beneficiary per year.[39]

Using a modified version of the Care Group Model, World Relief's Tube Poka Child Survival Project in the Chitipa District of Malawi observed similar results. The percentage of children who were underweight decreased from 29.9 to 13.1 percent, while the percentage of children exclusively breastfed increased from 40 to 80 percent. In addition, the percentage of children with diarrhea who were treated with oral rehydration therapy increased from 8 to 64 percent.[48] Similar results in behavior change have been observed in Guatemala, Liberia, Rwanda, Cambodia, Zambia, Kenya, and Ethiopia, among other countries.[49]

Data collected by Care Group volunteers has also demonstrated reductions in child mortality. The magnitude of reduction varied by country. For example, in the Child Survival Program in Mozambique, a 42 percent decline in under-5 mortality was estimated. A 71.9 percent decline was estimated in the World Relief/Cambodia Light for Life Child Survival Program in Cambodia. Of the Care Group programs associated with USAID in some capacity, the rate of decline in under-5 mortality was 49 percent greater than that in similar USAID programs that do not implement Care Groups.[50] It is estimated that when Care Groups are implemented, the average cost per life saved is $2,204, and the average cost per disability-adjusted life year (DALY) averted is $67.25, which would be cost-effective in even the poorest country.

Lessons Learned

The Care Group model has been shown to be a cost-effective intervention in reducing preventable child deaths and overall child mortality, even in areas with the highest burden of child mortality. In particular, the Care Group model offers key lessons in promoting behavior change and reaching high impact with limited investment in cost-effective ways.

Although behavior change promotion can often be difficult to implement, the Care Group model has shown that it is possible to change behaviors quickly and sustainably by using peer-to-peer promotion programs.[51] This intervention demonstrates the value of engaging communities in behavior promotion and provides a mode to promote behavior change that builds on trusted and already established networks and relationships within a community.[51] In addition, for many women, becoming a Care Group volunteer is the first time they have held a recognized position of influence in their community, which has created a platform for them to promote behavior change.[39,52]

The Care Group focus on community-level health promotion also suggests that success does not depend on improvements in health facilities that are often difficult to achieve. The Care Group model has been implemented in countries and communities with some of the worst child health outcomes and some of the most limited access to healthcare services or health education. In fact, the encouraging results of this intervention suggest that health behaviors can be improved in low-resource communities with simple interventions that offer high impact at less than $2 a beneficiary a year.[39] Moreover, in areas with limited resources, Care Groups can help build the basis for long-term health system improvement. For example, the collection of data on key indicators can be used to help build a community health information system, a necessity for sustained improvement.[42] It is also possible that the Care Group model can be a foundation for behavior change in other key health areas, including, for example, HIV, TB, water, or sanitation.[49]

Ebola and Culture

Introduction

Culture affects how individuals think and feel, including about illness and disease. Cultural practices, beliefs, customs, and rituals can often increase or mitigate the risk of individuals being exposed to pathogens, which can then affect the transmission patterns of diseases. With this in mind, disease control efforts to be successful must take into account the unique beliefs and actions of different groups.

Sensitivity to cultural factors associated with the control of infectious and parasitic disease has increased in the past 20 years. However, relatively little attention has been given to cultural factors associated with emerging infectious diseases, especially diseases with high case fatality rates such as Ebola.[53] The challenges of the 2014 Ebola epidemic have brought to light the importance of paying much more attention to cultural issues when designing and implementing programs for the control of emerging and reemerging infectious diseases.

What Is Ebola?

Ebola virus disease (EVD) is an acute, serious illness that is transmitted to people from wild animals; it spreads in the human population through human-to-human transmission via direct contact with bodily fluids of infected people or surfaces contaminated with these fluids. People remain infectious as long as their blood and body fluids, including semen and breast milk, contain the virus. The average EVD case fatality rate is around 50 percent but case fatality rates have varied from 25 percent to 90 percent in past outbreaks.[54]

The first Ebola outbreak occurred in Yamuku, Democratic Republic of the Congo in 1976.[55] Major outbreaks have

also occurred in the Democratic Republic of the Congo in 1995, northern Uganda from 2000–2001, and the Democratic Republic of the Congo and Uganda around 2008. However, the most recent 2014 outbreak in West Africa is the most complex to date and has seen more cases and deaths than all previous other outbreaks combined.[54,56]

Impact of Culture on Ebola Transmission

Culture is related to Ebola outbreaks in several unique ways, including through burial practices, caregiving practices, and societal stigma. A greater understanding of the relationship between these cultural elements and Ebola virus disease has shed light on how Ebola is transmitted and allowed for more effective disease control interventions. The following illustrations are examples of how knowledge of local culture can help us understand the dynamics of disease transmission and disease control in certain settings.[57]

Burial practices are the most notable and discussed cultural practice related to Ebola. It is estimated that 60 percent of the cases in the 2014 outbreak in Guinea were associated with burial practices.[57] There is a risk of transmission of Ebola after a patient is deceased because the bodies and bodily fluids of the deceased patients remain contagious many days after death.[58] Nonetheless, many local customs call on a family member, often a paternal aunt, to wash and prepare the body for burial, potentially exposing this individual to a high viral load.[53]

Ebola infections can also occur during burials when family and community members perform religious rites that require directly touching the body.[59] Moreover, the potential exists for transmission to distant areas when visiting funeral attendants are exposed to the body itself and when family members distribute personal property of the loved one, which may have been infected with the virus.[59,60] In Liberia, for example, among Muslims, Christians, and followers of indigenous Liberian religious customs, it is common for family and friends of the deceased to hold a wake in the home before the burial, both to console each other and to celebrate the life of the deceased. At this occasion, family members usually handle the corpse themselves and funeral attendees pay their respects by touching or kissing the body of the deceased.[61] In November 2014, the World Health Organization released a safe burial protocol that acknowledges the necessity of religious washing before burial and other sacred rituals such as praying over the body and describes how these rituals can be maintained in a safe way. It also discussed safe alternatives to these practices.[59]

Interestingly, evidence exists that gender roles can explain why it has been observed that men are more likely to be infected early in an Ebola outbreak, whereas the number of female cases greatly exceeds the number of male cases over the course of the outbreak. Men are likely to be the ones hunting in many rural areas. This puts them at greater risk for coming into contact with forest animals, which often triggers the initial animal-to-human transmission of the virus.[62] However, as an outbreak continues, women are most affected by Ebola. This relates to the fact that women are usually the ones to feed and clean up after sick relatives, which heightens their exposure to the Ebola virus. In addition, women traditionally are also more likely to perform the funeral rituals.[61] Up to November 2014, in fact, Liberia reported that 75 percent of persons who died of Ebola were women.[63] Despite the evidence that women are often disproportionately affected, at the community level, men still seem to dominate meetings and remain the main participants in discussions of control strategies.[63] This imbalance suggests that women need to play a greater role in future campaigns.

Stigma on the local and international level can also complicate the Ebola response. In local areas, the stigma carried by Ebola survivors and family members of Ebola victims could exacerbate disease spread. In particular, misinformation can result in families hiding relatives and friends infected with Ebola to avoid being shunned by their own communities. Individuals remaining in their homes can undermine the need for treatment in hospitals. This can also pose threats to household members who are then put at risk for Ebola infection.[60,64]

On an international level, stigma can result from paranoia and fear of the disease, which can interfere with response efforts and humanitarian aid. Some countries have imposed harsh travel restrictions, travel bans, or compulsory quarantines for individuals upon return. These efforts to reduce risk limit the exchange of physical and human resources that disease-afflicted areas need.[64] In November 2014, the UN called on the global community to work to understand the roots of this stigma and to address these roots in order to promote solidarity,[65] or unity in action.[66] Many parallels have been drawn with the early HIV/AIDS epidemic, and, as a result, local education interventions for Ebola have been built off of the grassroots community-based stigma reduction initiatives developed to combat stigma associated with HIV/AIDS.[67]

In addition to the factors discussed here, there are many other important cultural factors related to Ebola transmission and control dynamics. For example, the use of bushmeat has been identified as the primary mechanism of spillover of the Ebola virus from wildlife reservoirs to humans. In Liberia, 75 percent of meat consumption is bushmeat.[57] In addition, traditional healers in the informal healthcare system in many areas also can influence disease parameters. Traditional healers often have significant power within local communities and sometimes will advocate for prevention or treatment efforts that differ from those suggested by the biomedical or foreign aid communities. However, traditional healers sometimes spread misinformation, such as in Northern Uganda when traditional healers shared that drinking bleach would cure Ebola. Yet they can also be used as important mechanisms to spread correct public health information. During the 2014 outbreak, traditional healers in one district of Sierra Leone, for example, have decided to stop treating patients until they have received appropriate training on the Ebola virus.[57]

Lessons Learned

Cultural practices are often referred to as barriers to controlling an epidemic. Overall, a limited number of studies have investigated the influence of cultural factors on disease transmission and control of emerging and reemerging diseases. The few studies that have been conducted, however, have identified that if cultural knowledge is embraced, it can be used as a tool to effectively craft a response that engages afflicted communities and resources in order to save lives as quickly as possible.

The first sociocultural study of Ebola, conducted in 2003, determined that although some cultural elements such as burial practices can amplify an outbreak at first, many in-place cultural belief systems or practices can be used to control outbreaks. This is because many of these belief systems have had to evolve to survive diseases with high fatality rates for many years.[53] For example, this first study conducted outside Gulu, Uganda, identified that residents, mostly of the Acholi ethnic group, came to identify Ebola as a *gemo*, a traditional explanation for the disease outside of a biomedical context. After this identification, the Acholi people modified their practices in a way that matched suggested WHO epidemic control measures, including isolation of patients and suspension of public events such as funerals. These adaptions were not achieved under a biomedical explanation for disease but rather one that reflects a more holistic understanding of illness, common in many parts of the world. Local and international health workers could then work with the Acholi people in an effective way to spread culturally relevant information to help combat the outbreak.[53]

Ebola outbreaks and outbreaks of other similar diseases are rare events. Nonetheless, the 2014 Ebola epidemic has heightened awareness of the relevance of cultural factors to understanding transmission. It also raised attention to the need for sensitivity to culture in designing control campaigns. However, these characteristics are relevant to particular groups of people in certain regions and also to a particular disease. Whether an Ebola outbreak occurs in a new region or an outbreak of a different disease arises, effective control campaigns must consider in sensitive ways the interplay of culture and disease transmission in order to help communities protect themselves and save lives.

MAIN MESSAGES

Culture is a set of beliefs and behaviors that are learned and shared. Culture operates, among other areas, in the domains of the family, social groups beyond the family, religion, art, music, and law. Culture is an important determinant of health in many ways. It relates to people's health behaviors, their perceptions of illness, the extent to which they use health services, and forms of medicine that they have practiced traditionally. This chapter examines the links between culture and health from the perspective of the extent to which a culture satisfies the physical and psychological needs of those who follow it.

Perceptions of illness vary considerably across cultures. What is seen as normal in some societies may be seen as illness in others. Different societies also have differing perceptions of the causes of illness and disease. In addition to perceptions related to the "Western medical paradigm," diseases may be viewed, for example, as a result of the body "being out of balance," supernatural causes, offending the gods, emotional stress, or witchcraft. Different cultures also take an array of steps, beyond the western medical paradigm, to prevent illness. Some of these include rituals, the wearing of charms, and the observance of certain food taboos.

When people believe themselves to be ill, they usually resort to trying home remedies first. Following that, people in traditional societies often visit some type of traditional healer. It may be some time before they consult a physician practicing "modern medicine," often only when they are certain that they are ill and when other forms of treatment have not brought relief.

Many forms of traditional behavior are conducive to good health. This might include, for example, traditional practices that allow the mother to spend some time with her baby before she returns to her normal work and household chores. Male circumcision, as practiced in many cultures, reduces the transmission of HIV. Other traditional practices, however, are not health promoting. Feeding sugar water to infants, for example, is not good for the health of the infants, who should be exclusively breastfed for 6 months. It is important to consider how healthy behaviors can be promoted.

There are a number of models of how behaviors can be changed, including the Health Belief model, the Diffusion of Innovations model, and the Stages of Change model. To encourage behavior change, of course, requires a good understanding of the behaviors that are taking place, how they relate to health, the underlying motivation for them, and the likely response to various approaches aimed at changing them.

When thinking about trying to change behavior on a large scale, such as promoting an immunization program, the use of seat belts, or the willingness to seek treatment for leprosy, several approaches are important. One way to engender change is to engage in community mobilization. Promoting messages about desirable and undesirable health behaviors can also be done effectively using mass media. Social marketing and health education efforts are also important. Conditional cash transfers are also being used increasingly to promote behavior change. An effective tool for setting the foundation for any efforts at investing in health or trying to change behaviors is to carry out a social assessment, which will identify the social basis of the health issues one is trying to influence, as well as the likely social impacts of the proposed activities.

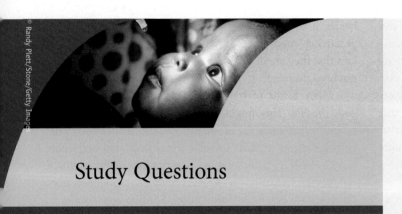

Study Questions

1. What is culture? Give some examples of aspects of culture that vary across different societies.

2. Why is it important to assess the relationship between culture and health in specific societies by the extent to which cultural practices promote or discourage good physical and mental health?

3. Name three cultural practices that are health promoting. Name three cultural practices that are harmful to health.

4. How does culture relate to people's perceptions of illness? Why would some cultures regard some illnesses as normal?

5. What would low-income people in traditional societies likely see as possible causes of illness?

6. What is the difference between illness and disease?

7. When an infant is ill in a traditional society in a low-income country, from whom and in what order are the parents likely to seek help?

8. Why would members of the community seek treatment for illness from traditional healers?

9. If you wanted to encourage the large-scale adoption of a healthy behavior, such as giving up cigarette smoking, what information would you want to know as you plan your effort?

10. Why are social assessments important? If they are done well, what gains would they produce that might not come if there were no such assessment?

REFERENCES

1. Scrimshaw, S. C. (2001). Culture, behavior, and health. In M. H. Merson, R. E. Black, & A. Mills (Eds.), *International public health: Diseases, programs, systems, and policies* (pp. 53–78). Gaithersburg, MD: Aspen Publishers.

2. Tylor, E. (1871). *Primitive culture.* London: J. Murray.

3. Haviland, W. A. (1990). The nature of culture. In *Cultural anthropology* (6th ed.). Fort Worth, TX: Holt, Rinehart & Winston, Inc.

4. Miller, B. (2004). *Culture and health.* Presentation given at George Washington University, Washington, DC.

5. Murphy, E. M. (2003). Being born female is dangerous for your health. *American Psychologist, 58*(3), 205–210.

6. Kleinman, A., Eisenberg, L., & Good, B. (1978). Culture, illness, and care: Clinical lessons from anthropologic and cross-cultural research. *Annals of Internal Medicine, 88*(2), 251–258.

7. Hopper, S. (1993). The influence of ethnicity on the health of older women. *Clinics in Geriatric Medicine, 9,* 231–259.

8. Letendre, A. D. (2002). Aboriginal traditional medicine: Where does it fit? *Crossing Boundaries, 1*(2), 78–87.

9. Jegede, A. S. (2002). The Yoruba cultural construction of health and illness. *Nordic Journal of African Studies, 11*(3), 322–335.

10. Pachter, L. M. (1994). Culture and clinical care. Folk illness beliefs and behaviors and their implications for health care delivery. *JAMA, 271*(9), 690–694.

11. Bolton, J. M. (1972). Food taboos among the Orang Asli in West Malaysia: A potential nutritional hazard. *American Journal of Clinical Nutrition, 25*(8), 788–799.

12. Chiwuzie, J., & Okolocha, C. (2001). Traditional belief systems and maternal mortality in a semi-urban community in Southern Nigeria. *African Journal of Reproductive Health, 5*(1), 75–82.

13. Trigo, M., Roncada, M. J., Stewien, G. T., & Pereira, I. M. (1989). [Food taboos in the northern region of Brazil]. *Revista de Saúde Pública, 23*(6), 455–464.

14. Sundararaj, R., & Pereira, S. M. (1975). Dietary intakes and food taboos of lactating women in a South Indian community. *Tropical and Geographical Medicine, 27*(2), 189–193.

15. Bhasin, V. (2003). Sickness and therapy among tribals of Rajasthan. *Studies of Tribes and Tribals, 1*(1), 77–83.

16. Fassin, D., & Badji, I. (1986). Ritual buffoonery: A social preventive measure against childhood mortality in Senegal. *Lancet, 18*(1), 142–143.

17. Institute of Health Metrics and Evaluation. (n.d.). *GBD 2010 heat map.* Retrieved September 24, 2014, from http://vizhub.healthdata.org /irank/heat.php.

18. Edberg, M. (2007). *Essentials of health behavior: An introduction to social and behavioral theory applied to public health.* Sudbury, MA: Jones & Bartlett.

19. Murphy, E. (2005). *Promoting healthy behavior. Health bulletin 2.* Washington, DC: Population Reference Bureau.

20. Rosenstock, I. M., Strecher, V. J., & Becker, M. H. (1988). Social learning theory and the Health Belief Model. *Health Education Quarterly, 15*(2), 175–183.

21. Rogers, E. (1983). *Diffusion of innovations* (3rd ed.). New York: Free Press.

22. Population Institute. (n.d.). *Soap operas: Making a difference in developing nations.* Retrieved February 28, 2014, from https://www.population institute.org/resources/populationonline/issue/1/7/.

23. Vanclay, F. (2003). *Social impact assessment: International principles.* Special Publication Series No. 2. Fargo, ND: International Association for Impact Assessment. Retrieved December 28, 2014, from http://www.iaia .org/publicdocuments/special-publications/SP2.pdf.

24. This policy and program brief is adapted with permission from a paper prepared in May 2010 by Josephine E.V. Francisco, titled *Barrier Analysis of Exclusive Breastfeeding Practices in Ruyigi and Cancuzo Provinces, Burundi.* This paper was part of a culminating experience to meet the requirements for the master of public health degree at The George Washington University.

25. UNICEF. (2014). *Infant and young child feeding.* Retrieved September 24, 2014, from http://data.unicef.org/nutrition/iycf.

26. Food for the Hungry. *Barrier analysis.* Retrieved April 23, 2011, from http://barrieranalysis.fhi.net.

27. Chan, M. (2014, February 11). *WHO director-general celebrates polio-free India.* Retrieved May 29, 2014, from http://www.who.int/dg /speeches/2014/india-polio-free/en/.

28. Centers for Disease Control and Prevention. (1998). *Progress toward poliomyelitis eradication—India, 1998. MMWR, 47*(37), 771–781.

29. The Communication Initiative Network. (2004). *Social mobilisation-communication polio eradication partnership—India.* Retrieved April 23, 2011, from http://www.comminit.com/en/node/127845/292.

30. UNICEF. India polio eradication. Retrieved April 23, 2011, from http://www.unicef.org/india/health_3729.htm.

31. Maps of India. Indian States and Union Territories. Retrieved June 5, 2015, from http://www.mapsofindia.com/states/.

32. Global Polio Eradication Initiative. (2011). *Monthly situation reports.* Retrieved April 23, 2011, from http://www.polioeradication.org/Mediaroom /Monthlysituationreports.aspx.

33. Chaturvedi, S., Dasgupta, R., Adhish, V., et al. (2009). Deconstructing social resistance to pulse polio campaign in two north Indian districts. *Indian Pediatrics, 46*(11), 963–974.

34. Obregón, R., Chitnis, K., Morry, C., et al. (2009, August). Achieving polio eradication: A review of health communication evidence and lessons learned in India and Pakistan. *Bulletin of the World Health Organization, 87*(8), 624–630.

35. Bhagat, P. (2005). *Vaccination campaign focuses on tackling social resistance to vaccine.* Retrieved April 23, 2011, from http:www.unicef.org /infobycountry/india_25290.html.

36. Gabrysch, S., Lema, C., Bedrinana, E., et al. Cultural adaptation of birthing services in rural Ayachucho, Peru. *Bulletin of the World Health Organization, 87*(9), 724–729.

37. Eichler, R., Levine, R., & Performance-Based Incentives Working Group. *Performance incentives for global health.* Washington, DC: Center for Global Development.

38. UNICEF. *Committed to child survival: A promise renewed.* Progress Report 2014. Retrieved November 25, 2014, from http://apr.norvenanino .website/wp-content/uploads/2015/02/APR-Progress-Report-2014.pdf.

39. Davis, T. P., et al. (2013). Reducing child global undernutrition at scale in Sofala Province, Mozambique, using Care Group volunteers to communicate health messages to mothers. *Global Health: Science and Practice, 1*(1): 35–51.

40. Davis, T. (2014, November). *Reducing malnutrition and child deaths using Care Groups.* Food for the Hungry presentation.

41. World Health Organization. (2012). *Countdown to 2015: Tracking progress in maternal, newborn and child survival. Accountability for maternal, newborn and child survival: an update on progress in priority countries.* Geneva: World Health Organization. Retrieved December 28, 2014, from http://www.countdown2015mnch.org/countdown-news/26-new-update -fosters-country-accountability.

42. Freeman, P., Perry, H. B., Gupta, S. K., & Rassekh, B. (2012). Accelerating progress in achieving the millennium development goal for children through community-based approaches. *Global Public Health, 7*(4), 400–419. doi:http://dx.doi.org/10.1080/17441690903330305

43. Center for High Impact Philanthropy, University of Pennsylvania. *Care Group programs case study.* Retrieved November 17, 2014, http://www.impact.upenn.edu/images/uploads/130412_Care_Groups.pdf.

44. World Health Organization. *Child health and development: Key family practices.* Retrieved November 20, 2014, from http://www.emro.who.int/child-health/community/family-practices#12.

45. CORE Group, Food for the Hungry, and World Relief. *Why critieria?* Retrieved November 18, 2014, http://www.caregroupinfo.org.

46. CORE Group. (2013). *Care Group definition.* Retrieved November 18, 2014, from http://www.caregroupinfo.org/.

47. *Care Group minimum criteria reviewer checklist.* Revised November 2012. Retrieved November 18, 2014, from http://www.caregroupinfo.org/.

48. Crespo, R., Kabaghe, V., Morrow, M., & Borger, S. (2009). *Tube Poka Child Survival Project. Final evaluation report.* USAID and World Relief.

49. CORE Group, Food for the Hungry, and World Relief. *Care Group journal articles.* Retrieved from http://caregroups.info/?page_id=48.

50. Perry, H., Morrow, M., Davis, T., Borger, S., Weiss, J., DeCoster, M., & Ernst, P. (2014). *Care Groups—An effective community-based delivery strategy for improving reproductive, maternal, neonatal and child health in high-mortality, resource-constrained settings: A guide for policy makers and donors.* Washington. DC: CORE Group.

51. Center for High Impact Philanthropy, University of Pennsylvania. Improving Child Health and Nutrition with Care Group Program: Q and A with Tom Davis of Food for the Hungry. Retrieved June 5, 2015, from http://www.impact.upenn.edu/2013/07/improving_child_health_nutrition_with_care_group_programs_qa_w_tom_davis_of/.

52. Casazza, L., et al. (2007). *Light for Life cost extension child survival project.* World Relief Cambodia and USAID. Retrieved from http://caregroups.info/docs/WRC_Cambodia_Final_Eval_2007.pdf.

53. Hewlett, B. S., & Amola, R. P. (2003, October). Cultural contexts of Ebola in Northern Uganda. *Emerging Infectious Diseases, 9*(10). Retrieved November 14, 2014, from http://wwwnc.cdc.gov/eid/article/9/10/02-0493.

54. World Health Organization. (2014, September). *Ebola fact sheet.* Retrieved November 14, 2014, from http://www.who.int/mediacentre/factsheets/fs103/en/.

55. Hewlett, B. S., & Hewlett, B. L. (2008). *Ebola, culture, and politics: The anthropology of an emerging disease.* Belmont, CA: Thomson Wadsworth.

56. Centers for Disease Control and Prevention. *Outbreaks chronology: Ebola virus disease.* Retrieved November 16, 2014, from http://www.cdc.gov/vhf/ebola/outbreaks/history/chronology.html.

57. Alexander, K. A., et al. (2014). What factors might have led to the emergence of Ebola in West Africa? *PLoS Neglected Tropical Diseases.* Retrieved from http://blogs.plos.org/speakingofmedicine/2014/11/11/factors-might-led-emergence-ebola-west-africa/

58. CDC and WHO. (1998). *Control for viral haemorrhagic fevers in the African health care setting.* Atlanta, GA: Centers for Disease Control and Prevention.

59. World Health Organization. (2014, November 7). *New WHO safe and dignified burial protocol—key to reducing Ebola transmission.* Retrieved from http://www.who.int/mediacentre/news/notes/2014/ebola-burial-protocol/en/.

60. Chowell, G., & Nishiura, H. (2014). Transmission dynamics and control of Ebola virus disease (EVD): A review. *BMC Medicine, 120.* Retrieved from http://www.biomedcentral.com/1741-7015/12/196.

61. Ravi, S., & Gauldin, E. (2014). Sociocultural dimensions of the Ebola virus disease outbreak in Liberia. *Biosecurity and Bioterrorism: Biodefense, Strategy, Practice, and Science, 12*(6). DOI:10.1089/bsp.2014.1002.

62. World Health Organization. (2007). *Addressing sex and gender in epidemic-prone infectious diseases.* Geneva: WHO. Retrieved from http://www.who.int/csr/resources/publications/SexGenderInfectDis.pdf?ua=1.

63. Wolfe, L. (2014, August 20). Why are so many women dying from Ebola? *Foreign Policy.* Retrieved November 16, 2014, from http://www.foreignpolicy.com/articles/2014/08/20/why_are_so_many_women_dying_from_ebola.

64. Hitchen, J. (2014, November 5). *Ebola in Sierra Leone: Stigmatization.* Africa Research Institute. Retrieved November 15, 2014, from http://www.africaresearchinstitute.org/blog/ebola-stigma/.

65. UN News Center. (2014, November 12). *Ebola: UN special envoy says combating stigma integral to overall crisis response.* Retrieved November 15, 2014, from http://www.un.org/apps/news/story.asp?NewsID=49320#.VGfA3PTF8_k.

66. Oxford Dictionaries. Solidarity. Retrieved November 19, 2014, from http://www.oxforddictionaries.com/us/definition/american_english/solidarity.

67. Davtyan, M., et al. (2014). Addressing Ebola-related stigma: Lessons learned from HIV/AIDS. *Global Health Action, 7,* 26058. Retrieved from http://dx.doi.org/10.3402/gha.v7.26058.

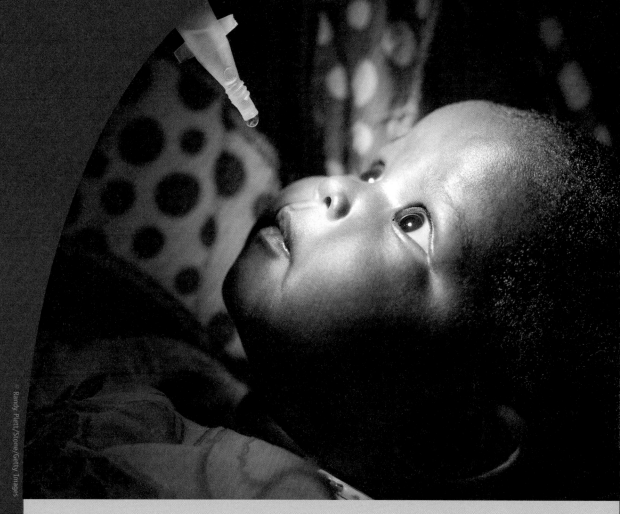

Randy Plett/Stone/Getty Images

PART III

The Burden of Disease

CHAPTER 7

The Environment and Health

LEARNING OBJECTIVES

By the end of this chapter the reader will be able to:

- Discuss the most important environmental threats to health in low- and middle-income countries
- Review the burden of disease from household and ambient air pollution and unsafe water and sanitation
- Examine the contribution of personal hygiene to reducing the burden of environmentally related health problems
- Comment on the costs and consequences of these environmental burdens
- Describe some of the most cost-effective ways of reducing the global burden of environmental health problems

VIGNETTES

Rashmi lived in the eastern part of Nepal in a modest home. She often had difficulty breathing. This was linked to the way Rashmi cooked, with an unvented household stove that was fueled by cow dung or wood. She cooked two meals a day on the stove, and she often held her new baby on her back as she did so. She heard about different stoves and about using kerosene or gas for fuel. However, she lacked the money to buy a new stove or to use kerosene or gas for cooking.

Sunisa was a young mother in a rural area in northern Laos. She had two children, a 1-year-old and a 3-year-old. Sunisa was not wealthy. Her house had no water supply. She collected water daily from the stream about half a mile from her house in containers she carried on her head. She stored the containers at the edge of her house, covered by cloth. Sunisa was not an educated woman and did nothing to purify the water. Her two daughters regularly had bouts of diarrhea, partly the result of drinking unsafe water.

Juan had lived in Mexico City his whole life and was now 70 years old. He remembered a time when the city was not so crowded, had few cars, and when the views from the city were magnificent. He lamented the fact that today the city was too crowded to enjoy, the traffic was overwhelming, and the air was often unbreathable. It was so polluted that on many days there was no view at all. Juan had a very hard time breathing because he suffered from chronic obstructive pulmonary disease (COPD). Juan suspected air pollution contributed to his illness.

Raj and his family lived in a slum at the edge of Patna, India. The slum was the size of a small city. Most of the houses were made of scrap wood with scrap metal roofing. The houses had no water connection and people had to walk to the edge of the slum to get their water from a standpipe or buy it from a tanker if the standpipe did not work. There were no private toilets either. There were a few toilets that were shared but they were always dirty. For this reason, many people in the slum, especially the women, waited until dark and then went to defecate in fields near the slum.

THE IMPORTANCE OF ENVIRONMENTAL HEALTH

Environmental health issues are major risk factors in the global burden of disease. One study, which took a broad view of environmental risk factors, concluded that between 25 and 33 percent of the global burden of disease can be attributed to environmental risk factors.[1] The World Health Organization (WHO) suggests that environmental risk factors affect more than 80 percent of the diseases on which it regularly reports. In addition, WHO has estimated that 24 percent of the global disease burden, 23 percent of all deaths, and 33 percent of the total disease burden in children are attributable to these environmental risk factors.[2] The *Global Burden of Disease Study 2010* and risk factors suggested that about 15 percent of the total deaths among all age groups globally are attributable to five environmental causes: unimproved water, poor sanitation, ambient air pollution, household air pollution, and lead.[3]

The importance of environmental risk factors to the global burden of disease should not be a surprise. The third-leading cause of death in low- and middle-income countries is chronic obstructive pulmonary disease, the fourth-leading cause of death is lower respiratory infections, and the fifth is diarrheal diseases.[4] Each of these is closely linked with environmental factors. In addition, environmental risk factors are even more important when considering the causes of death of children in low- and middle-income countries. Lower respiratory conditions are the leading cause of death for children 0–5 years of age in these countries, and diarrheal diseases are fourth. For children 5–9 years old, diarrheal diseases are the leading cause of death and lower respiratory conditions are third.[4]

Environmental health matters are also of special importance because addressing them effectively is central to the achievement of the Millennium Development Goals (MDGs), as shown in **Table 7-1**.

As shown in the table, reducing environmental risk factors is critical to meeting the poverty and hunger goal, given the large share of ill health and resulting economic losses from these risk factors. Improving access to water can be a major improvement in the lives of poor women in low- and middle-income countries, given the amount of time they have to spend getting water. Enhancing sanitation produces important social gains for women, as well, because in the absence of improved sanitation, they face major discomforts, inconveniences, and sometimes illness. Addressing environmental risk factors can clearly make a major contribution to reducing child mortality by reducing two of the leading causes of death in children. Reducing household air pollution can also lead to major improvements in the health of women and children. Environmental improvements can reduce the breeding grounds for malarial mosquitoes, and many measures that reduce the health risks of the environment will increase environmental sustainability.

This chapter aims to introduce some of the most important links between health and the environment. Environmental health is a very broad topic. Given the introductory nature of this text, this chapter focuses largely on only three

of the most important risk factors in terms of the burden of environmentally related diseases in low- and middle-income countries. These include unsafe water, sanitation, and hygiene; ambient air pollution; and household air pollution that comes from the use of solid fuels.[5]

The chapter begins by covering some of the most important terms and concepts that relate to environmental health. It then explores the burden of disease related to the three risk factors noted previously. After that, it briefly reviews the costs and consequences of the selected environmental risk factors.

The chapter concludes with policy and program briefs that discuss some of the most challenging environmental health issues and some of the most cost-effective ways to address them in low- and middle-income settings. Much has been written about environmental health. Readers who wish to explore environmental health in greater detail are encouraged to pursue those writings, possibly starting with an introductory text on environmental health.[6,7]

KEY CONCEPTS

It is important to understand how the word *environment* is used in this chapter. In some cases, the word *environment* in a health context is defined very broadly, meaning everything that is not genetic. In other cases, when considering health, the word *environment* includes only physical, chemical, or biological agents that directly affect health. For the purposes of this chapter, the environment is largely defined as "external physical, chemical, and microbiological exposures and processes that impinge upon individuals and groups and are beyond the immediate control of individuals."[8,p379] The chapter, however, also looks at some behavioral matters related to water and sanitation and household air pollution.

It is also valuable to understand the meaning of *environmental health*. This generally refers to a set of public health efforts that "is concerned with preventing disease, death, and disability by reducing exposure to adverse environmental conditions and promoting behavior change. It focuses on the direct and indirect causes of disease and injuries and taps resources inside and outside the healthcare system to help improve health outcomes."[9]

The World Health Organization takes a broad view of the environment and says:

> Environmental health comprises those aspects of human health, including quality of life, that are determined by physical, chemical, biological, social, and psychosocial factors in the environment. It also refers to the theory and practice of assessing, correcting, controlling,

TABLE 7-1 Key Links Between Environmental Health and the MDGs

Goal 1: Eradicate Poverty and Hunger

Link: Reducing environmental risk factors is central to eradicating poverty by reducing the burden, which falls largely on the poor, of environmentally related morbidity and mortality.

Goal 2: Achieve Universal Primary Education

Link: Children who do not have access to clean water and sanitation are more likely to suffer from undernutrition due to the effects of diarrheal disease. There is a correlation between nutritional status and learning. Children with poor nutritional status are not as likely to stay in school or learn as much as healthy children.

Goal 3: Promote Gender Equality and Empower Women

Link: Improving access to water can improve the lives of poor women in the low- and middle-income world by reducing the amount of time required to get water. Reducing household air pollution can also substantially improve the lives of women because they suffer a disproportionate burden when they are cooking.

Goal 4: Reduce Child Mortality

Link: Addressing environmental risk factors can reduce the two leading causes of death in children—diarrheal diseases and pneumonia. Diarrheal disease can be reduced through improved access to clean water and sanitation. Pneumonia can be reduced through improvements in household air quality.

Goal 5: Improve Maternal Health

Link: Diarrheal disease associated with poor sanitation and unsafe water can harm the nutritional status of the mother. Clean water and sanitary conditions are needed for safe births.

Goal 6: Combat HIV/AIDS, Malaria, and Other Diseases

Link: Environmental improvements can reduce the breeding grounds for malarial mosquitoes and vectors for other infectious diseases, such as schistosomiasis and dengue fever.

Goal 7: Ensure Environmental Sustainability

Link: Measures to improve water supply, sanitation, and personal hygiene promote sustainability, especially when they are carried out in community-based ways.

Modified from Millennium Development Goals., © 2015, United Nations, http://www.un.org/millenniumgoals/goals. Reprinted with the permission of the United Nations.

and preventing those factors in the environment that can potentially affect adversely the health of present and future generations.[10]

It is important to note that in discussing the burden of disease and other topics, this chapter will use terms from WHO. What one usually refers to as "ambient air pollution" is referred to in the burden of disease study as "ambient particulate matter pollution" and by WHO as "ambient air pollution." This chapter will use the term *ambient air pollution*. What one commonly refers to as "household air pollution" is referred to in the global burden of disease study as

TABLE 7-2 Typical Environmental Health Issues: Determinants and Health Consequences

Underlying Determinants	Selected Adverse Health Consequences
Household	
Unsafe water, inadequate sanitation and solid waste disposal, improper hygiene	Diarrhea and vector-related diseases, such as malaria, schistosomiasis, and dengue
Crowded housing and poor ventilation of smoke	Respiratory diseases and lung cancer
Exposure to naturally occurring toxic substances	Poisoning from arsenic, manganese, and fluorides
Community	
Improper water resource management, including poor drainage	Vector-related diseases, such as malaria and schistosomiasis
Exposure to vehicle emissions and industrial air pollution	Respiratory diseases, some cancers, and reduced IQ in children
Global	
Climate change Ozone depletion	Injury/death from extreme heat/cold, storms, floods, and fires Indirect effects: spread of vector-borne diseases Aggravation of respiratory diseases, population dislocation, water pollution from sea level rise, etc. Skin cancer, cataracts Indirect effects: compromised food production, etc.

Adapted with permission from The World Bank. Environmental health. Retrieved February 27, 2015, from http://siteresources.worldbank.org/INTPHAAG/Resources/AAGEHEng.pdf.

"household air pollution from solid fuels" and referred to by WHO as "household air pollution." This chapter will refer to "household air pollution."

Table 7-2 highlights some examples of environmental health issues, their determinants, and their consequences. It organizes these examples by their level of impact: the household, the community, or global.

KEY ENVIRONMENTAL HEALTH BURDENS

This section very briefly examines the most important health conditions that relate to the environmental issues that are discussed in this chapter. The section then examines the burden of disease from those conditions.

Household Air Pollution

WHO estimates that about 3 billion people in the world depend on solid fuel for their cooking and heating. The household air pollution that is discussed here is related to these uses. Such fuels include the fossil fuel coal and the biomass fuels of cow dung, wood, logging wastes, and crop waste.[11,12] In the cases that most concern us, cooking and heating are done on open stoves that are not vented to the outside. These are generally used by poorer segments of society, because people usually move to kerosene or gas for cooking and switch to improved stoves and better ventilation as their family income grows.

Biomass fuels and coal do not completely combust when they are burned. Instead, they leave behind breathable particles of a variety of gases and chemical products. The amount of these substances in a poorly ventilated home can exceed WHO norms by more than 20 times.[12] Smoke from burning biomass inside the home can produce conjunctivitis, upper respiratory irritation, and acute respiratory infection. The carbon monoxide produced can lead to acute poisoning.

Other gases and smoke are associated over the long term with cardiovascular disease, chronic obstructive pulmonary disease, adverse reproductive outcomes, and cancer.[12] Women and children are especially vulnerable to the effects of household air pollution.

Ambient Air Pollution

Many pollutants can be found in the ambient air. The most common effects of ambient air pollution are respiratory symptoms, including cough, irritation of the nose and throat, and shortness of breath.[13] Table 7-3 indicates some of the most common pollutants in the ambient air, examples of their sources, and the most important health effects. Certain preexisting health factors make some people susceptible to being harmed by air pollution. In addition, older and younger people are generally most susceptible to the health effects of ambient air pollution.

There have been a number of instances in which severe air pollution has been associated with considerable excess mortality in a very short time. Among the most famous cases was in London, England, in 1952. Because of what is called a temperature inversion, a dense fog, full of pollutants, hung over the city center for several days. The value of certain particulates in the air was 3 to 10 times the normal level. On December 13, 1952, the city administration reported a death rate per 100,000 people that was more than four times the normal daily death rate for that period.[13]

Water, Sanitation, and Hygiene

Only about 60 percent of the people in the world have access to improved sanitation. This ranges from about 80 percent in Latin America and the Caribbean to only about 30 percent in sub-Saharan Africa.[14] Many of the large cities in Africa have no modern sanitation system, and in Asia large shares of the populations in some areas also have no access to sanitary disposal of human waste. UNICEF and WHO estimated that about 2.4 billion people would be without improved sanitation in 2015.[15]

There is good evidence that improved disposal of human waste is associated with reductions in diarrheal disease,

TABLE 7-3 Common Air Pollutants and Their Health Effects

Name of Pollutant	Example of Source	Health Effects
Carbon monoxide	Combustion of gasoline and fossil fuels; cars	Reduction in oxygen-carrying capacity of the blood
Lead	Leaded gasoline, paint, batteries	Brain/central nervous system damage; digestive problems
Nitrogen dioxide, nitrogen oxides	Combustion of gasoline and fossil fuels; cars	Damage to lungs and respiratory system
Ozone	Variety of oxygen formed by chemical reaction of pollutants	Breathing impairment; eye irritation
Particulate matter	Burning of wood and diesel fuels	Respiratory irritation; lung damage
Smog	Mixture of pollutants, esp. ozone; originates from petroleum-based fuels	Irritation of respiratory system and eyes
Sulfur dioxide	Burning of coal and oil	Breathing problems; lung damage
Volatile organic compounds (VOCs)	Burning fuels; released from certain chemicals (e.g., solvents)	Acute effects similar to those of smog; possible carcinogen

Data from U.S. Environmental Protection Agency. *The plain English guide to the Clean Air Act: The common air pollutants*. Retrieved March 28, 2005, from http://www.epa.gov/airquality/peg_caa/cleanup.html; U.S. Environmental Protection Agency. Air & radiation: Six common air pollutants. Retrieved February 27, 2015, from http://www.epa.gov/air/urbanair/.

intestinal parasites, and trachoma. Failure to dispose properly of human waste contaminates water and food sources and leads to an increase in transmission of pathogens through the oral–fecal route. Failure to improve sanitation is also associated with the spread of parasitic worms, such as ascaris and hookworm.[16] Improved sanitation reduces the burden of trachoma, because the flies that are significantly involved in the spread of that disease breed, among other places, in human waste.[16]

UNICEF and WHO also estimated that about 90 percent of the world's population had access to an improved water source in 2012. However, this still left almost 750 million people without such access and almost 200 million people who depend on open water sources.[15] In parts of sub-Saharan Africa and Oceania, less than 50 percent of the population has access to an improved water source. In much of sub-Saharan Africa, Yemen, Pakistan, Afghanistan, Cambodia, and Laos, less than 75 percent of the population has access to an improved water source.[17] However, even the water that people do have access to and that is deemed safe in official statistics often contains dangerous pathogens.

In fact, waterborne diseases are among the most important in terms of the burden of disease, and they are numerous in low- and middle-income countries. **Table 7-4** indicates how

TABLE 7-5 Selected Waterborne Pathogens

Enteric protozoal parasites
- *Entamoeba histolytica*
- *Giardia intestinalis*
- *Cryptosporidium parvum*
- *Cryptosporidium cayetanensis*

Bacterial enteropathogens
- *Salmonella*
- *Shigella*
- *Escherichia coli*
- *Vibrio cholerae*
- *Campylobacter*

Viral pathogens
- Enteroviruses
- Adenoviruses
- Noroviruses

Modified from Friis, R. H. (2007). Water quality. In *Essentials of environmental health* (p. 211). Sudbury, MA: Jones and Bartlett.

TABLE 7-4 Classification of Water-Related Infections

Transmission	Water-Related Infections
Waterborne	The pathogen is in water that is ingested
Water-washed (or water-scarce)	Person-to-person transmission because of a lack of water for hygiene
Water-based	Transmission via an aquatic intermediate host
Water-related insect vector	Transmission by insects that breed in water or bite near water

Data from Cairncross, S., & Valdmanis, V. (2006). Water supply, sanitation, and hygiene promotion. In D. T. Jamison, J. G. Breman, A. R. Measham, et al. (Eds.), *Disease control priorities in developing countries* (2nd ed., p. 775). Washington, DC and New York: The World Bank and Oxford University Press.

water-related diseases may be classified. Some of the most important waterborne pathogens are shown in **Table 7-5**.

These pathogens are associated with diarrhea and a host of other gastrointestinal problems. They can be deadly when they lead to severe diarrhea and dehydration. Such diseases are especially risky for the very young, the very old, and people who have compromised immune systems, such as people living with HIV/AIDS.

THE BURDEN OF ENVIRONMENTALLY RELATED DISEASES

The *Global Burden of Disease Study 2010* estimated that:

- About 3.5 million deaths and 4.3 percent of global DALYs were attributable to household air pollution[18]
- 3.1 million deaths and 3.1 percent of global DALYs were attributable to ambient air pollution[18]
- 0.3 million deaths and 0.9 percent of global DALYs were attributable to unimproved water and sanitation[4,19]

The sections that follow explore further the burdens of household air pollution, ambient air pollution, and unimproved water and sanitation. One section also comments on hygiene.

Household Air Pollution

Many people believe that the most important environmental risk factor in low- and middle-income countries is ambient air pollution; however, this is not true. Rather, household air pollution is the fourth most important risk factor globally and in low- and middle-income countries.[4]

WHO estimated that about 4.3 million deaths in 2012 from stroke, ischemic heart disease, acute lower respiratory infections, lung cancer, and chronic obstructive pulmonary disease were attributable to household air pollution. The WHO regions of South-East Asia and the Western Pacific shared most of that burden, with 1.69 and 1.62 million attributable deaths, respectively. This largely relates to the large burdens in India and China.[20]

These figures include only those diseases for which there is solid evidence of a link to household air pollution from the use of solid fuels. However, this may be an underestimate of the real burden of disease from household air pollution because there is some evidence that household air pollution of this type is also associated with cataracts and tuberculosis. There is also tentative evidence of links with adverse pregnancy outcomes, especially low birthweight, and two types of cancer other than lung cancer.[11]

Almost all the burden of disease from household air pollution from the use of solid fuels is in low- and middle-income countries. It is estimated that 41 percent of all of the deaths attributable to household air pollution are among females.[20] Young children in low- and middle-income countries are often carried by their mothers on their backs as they attend to household and work chores, such as cooking. They also tend to spend long hours at home with their mothers. Therefore, they are also exposed more than others to household air pollution. It is estimated that 13 percent of all deaths attributable to household air pollution are among children younger than 5 years.[20]

Ambient Air Pollution

WHO estimates that ambient air pollution contributed to 6.7 percent of all deaths in 2012.[21] WHO estimates that about 16 percent of the lung cancer deaths, 11 percent of the deaths from COPD, and more than 20 percent of ischemic heart disease and stroke are attributable to ambient air pollution.[21] Fifty-three percent of the deaths attributable to ambient air pollution were among men, 44 percent women, and 3 percent children under five years of age.[22]

India and China have major burdens of disease that relate to ambient air pollution from particulate matter. In fact, about two-thirds of the global burden of disease from ambient air pollution is in the low- and middle-income countries of Asia. A number of countries in Eastern Europe also face a high burden of disease from this pollution.[22]

Water, Sanitation, and Hygiene

The *Global Burden of Disease Study 2010* estimated that unimproved water and sanitation contribute to 0.3 million deaths and 0.9 percent of DALYs in 2010.[18] WHO estimated that 842,000 deaths and 1.5 percent of the global burden of disease was attributable in 2012 to poor water, sanitation, and hygiene.[23] Earlier estimates suggested that within the African region, about 85 percent of the DALYs from these risk factors are related to the oral–fecal route of disease transmission and to diarrheal disease, primarily among young children.[5]

We should expect globally that the burden of disease related to these risk factors will fall disproportionately on children, who suffer such a large share of the burden of disease from diarrhea. In fact, the global burden of disease study estimated that unimproved water and sanitation account for 1 percent of child mortality.[18] The burden of these risk factors will also fall overwhelmingly on poor and less educated people in the poorer countries of South Asia and of sub-Saharan Africa. They have less access than others to improved water supply and sanitation and to the knowledge of good hygiene they need to avoid illness in the face of unsafe water and sanitation.

It is very complicated to try to assess individually the relative contribution of unsafe sanitation, unsafe water, and poor hygienic practices to the burden of diarrheal disease, partly because they are all so closely linked with each other. Nonetheless, both historical experiences in what are now the high-income countries and a number of studies in low- and middle-income countries suggest that improving water supply alone will not reduce diarrheal disease as needed. This seems to stem from the large amount of diarrhea that is associated with food that is unsafe and with poor personal hygiene. More will be said about these later.

Separate from any impact on the reduction of diarrheal disease, improvements in water supply are associated with important reductions in the burden of disease from dracunculiasis, schistosomiasis, and trachoma.[16]

THE COSTS AND CONSEQUENCES OF KEY ENVIRONMENTAL HEALTH PROBLEMS

For a number of reasons, the social and economic consequences of the key environmental health issues that have been discussed are enormous. First, the fact that about 25 percent of the total global burden of disease is due to environmental risk factors[24] suggests substantial social and economic costs related to these issues.

Second, as indicated earlier, the burden of these risk factors and their related causes of disease falls disproportionately on relatively poorer people. It is poorer people who cook with biomass fuels and coal, not better-off people. These burdens also fall on low- and middle-income countries more than on high-income countries. People in high-income countries do not customarily cook with biomass fuel or coal and they do not have to contend with the problems of unsafe water and sanitation that people in lower- and middle-income countries face. Their knowledge of good hygiene practices is also superior to the level of knowledge of most people in low- and middle-income countries.

Third, these environmental health burdens have very negative consequences on productivity. The consequences of household air pollution, for example, are very costly to women in terms of morbidity and disability and days of reduced productivity from both acute and chronic illnesses. In addition, the economic and social consequences of ill health for women in many low- and middle-income countries go considerably beyond just women's health. Rather, they spill over onto the health of the rest of her family, especially young children, whose own health and survival depend in important ways on the health of the mother.

Young children are especially at risk from all three environmental issues discussed in this chapter. They are especially vulnerable to unsafe water, and diarrheal disease can put them into a cycle of infection and malnutrition, ultimately retard their growth and development, or be deadly. Household air pollution can also lead to a cycle of illness and respiratory infection, death from pneumonia, or disability from asthma. To a lesser extent, ambient air pollution can do the same. The elderly face particular risks from ambient air pollution. This can exacerbate chronic health problems they already have, leading to additional disability and its attendant reduction in productivity.

REDUCING THE BURDEN OF DISEASE

Important progress has been made in some settings in addressing the environmental health issues discussed here. The next section examines some of the lessons learned to date and some of the most cost-effective measures that can be taken to enhance health in low- and middle-income countries by addressing selected environmental health issues.

Ambient Air Pollution

Ambient air pollution is a very broad topic and there is relatively little published data on the cost-effectiveness of approaches to addressing it in low- and middle-income countries. The studies that have been done on high-income countries, however, suggest that low- and middle-income countries could take a number of cost-effective steps to reduce the health burden of ambient air pollution.[25]

A number of cities, for example, including Jakarta, Manila, Kathmandu, and Mumbai, participated in a World Bank–assisted effort to assess their ambient air pollution and take measures to reduce it. They examined:[25]

- The amount and type of pollution
- How it was being dispersed
- The health impacts of reductions in particulate matter
- Time and cost to implement reductions
- Health benefits
- The value of those health benefits
- How the benefits compared to the costs of the intervention

Some of the first measures that these cities and some other large cities in low- and middle-income countries have taken to reduce ambient air pollution have included:[25]

- The introduction of unleaded gasoline
- Low-smoke lubricant for two-stroke engines
- The banning of two-stroke engines
- Shifting to natural gas to fuel public vehicles
- Tightening emissions inspections on vehicles
- Reducing the burning of garbage

It would also be reasonable to ensure that governments in low- and middle-income countries use their regulatory authority to incorporate information about ambient air pollution in their policies on transportation and industrial development.[25] In line with this, many of the low-income countries do not yet have a significant problem of ambient air pollution. It will be much more effective for those countries to put in place cost-effective approaches now to minimize ambient air pollution and its health effects than it will be to try later to mitigate those effects. In doing so, they should take account of vehicular and industrial pollution.

Household Air Pollution

There are a number of areas in which actions could be taken to reduce household air pollution from the burning of solid fuels for cooking and heating. In terms of the source of pollution, cooking devices can be improved, less polluting fuels can be used, and families can reduce their need for these fuels by using solar cooking and heating. Some changes can also be made to the living environment. Mechanisms for venting smoke can be built into the house, for example, or the kitchen can be moved away from the main part of the house. People can also change their behaviors to reduce pollution or exposure to it by using dried fuels, properly maintaining their stoves and chimneys, and keeping children away from the cooking area.[26]

Public policy can also play a helpful role in trying to reduce household air pollution. The public sector, for example, can promote information and education about such pollution and how to reduce it in schools, in the media, and in communities. The government can also use tax policy to reduce the cost of cooking appliances and fuels that will reduce this pollution. If necessary, it could subsidize the cost of improved fuels and appliances for those below a certain income level. Governments could also undertake surveillance of the problem and, if possible, set and enforce standards for household air pollution, although this will certainly be beyond the capacity of most low-income countries.[26]

Calculating the cost-effectiveness of different approaches to reducing the health effects of household air pollution is a very complicated matter and requires many assumptions. Nonetheless, the conclusions of the analyses that have been done are instructive. The main finding is that the most cost-effective approach to reducing household air pollution in sub-Saharan Africa and South Asia, where the needs are greatest, would be to promote the use of improved stoves. The most cost-effective approach in East Asia would be to promote the use of better fuels, such as kerosene and gas. Of course, this conclusion presumes that the stoves get maintained and the fuels are of good quality, which may not always be the case and the failure of which would detract from the effectiveness of these approaches.[26]

In addition, a number of lessons have been learned about how to encourage the uptake of better stoves and better fuels, some drawn from extensive experiences in China and India. These include:[26]

- Involve end users, especially women, in helping to assess needs and design approaches.
- Promote demand for better stoves and fuels to encourage the development of competitive suppliers and market choice.
- Consider subsidies and microcredit for selected interventions to help defray the cost of improvements for the poor.
- Establish national and local policies that encourage the needed changes in stoves and fuels.

Sanitation

There are a number of different levels of technology associated with excreta disposal, many different forms of toilets, and a wide array of costs associated with them. Sanitation could range from the simple technology of bucket latrines to modern urban sewage systems. **Table 7-6** lists the different

---

TABLE 7-6 Selected Sanitation Technologies

- Simple pit latrine
- Small bore sewer
- Ventilation-improved latrine
- Pour-flush
- Septic tank
- Sewer connection

Data from Cairncross, S., & Valdmanis, V. (2006). Water supply, sanitation, and hygiene promotion. In D. T. Jamison, J. G. Breman, A. R. Measham, et al. (Eds.), *Disease control priorities in developing countries* (2nd ed., p. 780). Washington, DC and New York: The World Bank and Oxford University Press.

---

approaches to excreta disposal. Although we usually think of toilets as owned by individuals, they can also be public and shared by many individuals and families.

The cost per person for methods of sanitary removal of human waste varies considerably. At the bottom levels of service, it appears that pour-flush latrines, ventilation-improved latrines, and simple pit latrines can be constructed in low- and middle-income settings for about $60. Assuming that these last approximately 5 years, the annual cost per capita would be about $12. The construction cost of conventional sewage systems in some countries is more than 10 times that amount. In addition, they need water to function properly and water is often in short supply.[16] Work is ongoing to develop more cost-effective toilets, and in Bangladesh a simple pour-flush pan has been developed that costs only about $0.27 per household to construct.[16]

Contrary to what we might believe, all of these systems can be operated in a hygienic manner that addresses health concerns. A very important review that was done in the early 1980s, for example, concluded that from the point of view of health, pit latrines would be just as hygienic as modern sewage systems, even if they were considerably less convenient.[27]

Given the relatively low cost of simple methods of sanitation and their relative effectiveness, it might be surprising that such a small share of households in low- and middle-income countries have a sanitary means of excreta disposal. Yet, besides the cultural constraints to their use, there are some other important constraints, as well:[16]

- *Lack of knowledge of options*: The poor in particular may not understand the options available to them and may believe that toilets cost more to install than they do.

- *Cost*: Even at relatively low prices, the poor may not have the money to pay for the up-front costs of a toilet.
- *Construction*: There may be a lack of skills to help install the toilets.
- *Local laws*: Particularly in urban areas, local laws may forbid low-cost sanitation, even if the area has no modern sewage system.

In some countries the public sector leads the effort to build low-cost sanitation systems. The public sector may also subsidize the cost of toilets for the poorest families, given that these sanitation improvements provide benefits to society as a whole. In addition, the public sector can try to enforce regulations to require the use of toilets. Although such regulatory authority is weak in most low-income and many middle-income countries, one of the main cities in Burkina Faso was able to promote toilet construction by taking away the title of homes if their owners did not install a toilet within a specific period of time.[16]

It is also possible, if the private sector believes that there is a market for low-cost sanitation, for such efforts to be handled in the private sector. In this case, the public sector may confine its role to areas needed to encourage private sector involvement and public demand for the toilets. This would include, for example, promoting the use of toilets, encouraging private sector involvement, setting technical standards, and helping to train people in installation and maintenance techniques.[16]

Promotion of improved sanitation can also be done with a public–private partnership and led by nongovernmental organizations (NGOs). Two of the most successful cases of improving low-cost sanitation were led by NGOs in Zimbabwe and Bangladesh. In Zimbabwe, an NGO was able to help communities construct 3,400 latrines for about $13 per unit, or only about $2.25 per person served.[28] In Bangladesh, an NGO has helped to make 100 villages free of open defecation for a cost of only about $1.50 per person served.[29] In both of these cases, the families in these communities paid for the latrines themselves.

The largest impact of improved sanitation is in the reduction of diarrhea. Some studies[30] suggest that improved sanitation facilities in low- and middle-income countries result in an average reduction in cases of diarrhea of 28 percent. It is very important to note that having a toilet seems to also increase the handwashing habits of families, which itself brings benefits, as discussed later.

Finally, the benefits of sanitary excreta removal go beyond reducing diarrhea. Improving sanitation should reduce the prevalence of several worms, including ascaris, trichuris, and hookworm.[16] Given the low cost of some forms of latrines, they would be cost-effective approaches to reducing the prevalence of these worms. As noted earlier, the same would be true in terms of the positive impact and low costs of reducing trachoma through improved sanitation.[31]

Water Supply

There are many analogies between water supply and sanitation. For water, as well as for sanitation, there are many different levels of technology and the costs vary considerably according to the level of technology employed. One could get water, for example, from the following types of improved water sources:

- House connection
- Standpost
- Borehole
- Dug well
- Rainwater collection

This section examines the relative cost-effectiveness of different approaches to achieving health benefits from improved water supply. In considering these costs and benefits, reasonable access to water was considered to be access to at least 20 liters per day from one of these sources from not more than 1-kilometer distance.[16]

Improving water supply can lead to a variety of health benefits. The most important studies that have been done have shown that providing a continuous supply of water with good bacteriological quality can reduce the morbidity of a number of diseases, as shown in **Table 7-7**. Studies showed a median reduction in trachoma, for example, of 27 percent, schistosomiasis of 77 percent, and dracunculiasis of 78 percent.[16]

Other studies have looked at the health benefits from different combinations of investments in water quantity, water quality, sanitation, and the promotion of hygiene. The results of these studies are somewhat surprising to those not involved in the environmental field. They suggest that the largest reductions in diarrhea morbidity—approximately 30 percent—come from investing in sanitation only, water and sanitation, or hygiene only. The lowest reductions, between 15 percent and 20 percent, came from investing in water quantity only, or a combination of water quality and quantity, all without complementary investments in hygiene or in sanitation.

As noted earlier, many of the pathogens that are waterborne are also carried on food. Thus, sanitation has a large potential impact on reducing those pathogens. However,

TABLE 7-7 Potential Morbidity Reduction from Excellent Water Supply

Condition	Percentage Reduction
Scabies	80
Typhoid fever	80
Trachoma	60
Most diarrheas and dysentery	50
Skin and subcutaneous infections	50
Paratyphoid, other *Salmonella*	40

Modified with permission from Cairncross, S., & Valdmanis, V. (2006). Water supply, sanitation, and hygiene promotion. In D. T. Jamison, J. G. Breman, A. R. Measham, et al. (Eds.), *Disease control priorities in developing countries* (2nd ed., p. 776). Washington, DC and New York: The World Bank and Oxford University Press.

water alone may not yield the results that sanitation would. For this, among other reasons, complementary investments for the promotion of hygiene are critical to realizing gains from water and sanitation.[16]

Another important lesson is that the greatest effect of investments in water is realized when people have water connections in their homes. Unfortunately, community standpipes, for example, do not produce the same level of health gains as individual household water connections.[16] A review in New Guinea, for example, showed that there was 56 percent less diarrhea in homes with an individual connection than in homes that got their water from standpipes.[16] This may partly be the case because people with individual connections use considerably more water than those without such connections and much of the additional water may be used to engage in better hygiene.

Hygiene

Unfortunately, there have been relatively few studies of the impact of hygiene promotion on actual health behaviors and on related reductions in the burden of disease. The studies that have been done showed that investing in hygiene promotion led to a 33 percent reduction in diarrhea. They also found that hygiene promotion efforts need to focus on simple

messages about handwashing and avoid trying to promote too many messages at once, if they are to be successful and sustainable. It appears that the messages that families acquire through hygiene promotion do stay with them and that retraining is necessary only once every 5 years.[16] Studies have also been done on the impact of handwashing on respiratory infections. Handwashing was associated in these studies with a significant reduction in acute respiratory infections.[16]

Integrating Investment Choices About Water, Sanitation, and Hygiene

When the information from the studies previously discussed is reviewed together, it appears that the promotion of hygiene, the promotion of sanitation, and the construction of standposts are all likely to be cost-effective in low- and middle-income countries. However, using public funds to provide individual household connections to water supply systems is likely to be above the cutoff for cost-effective investments. This is shown in **Table 7-8**.

The costs of hygiene and sanitation promotion compare favorably, for example, with the costs per DALY averted of oral rehydration. In addition, such investments might help to reduce the burden of diarrhea and decrease the need for oral rehydration.

TABLE 7-8 Cost per DALY Averted of Selected Investments in Water, Sanitation, and Hygiene

Investment	$/DALY Averted
Hygiene promotion	3.35
Sanitation promotion only	11.15
Water sector regulation and advocacy	47.00
Hand pump or standpost	94.00
House connection	223.00
Construction and promotion	270.00

Modified with permission from Cairncross, S., & Valdmanis, V. (2006). Water supply, sanitation, and hygiene promotion. In D. T. Jamison, J. G. Breman, A. R. Measham, et al. (Eds.), *Disease control priorities in developing countries* (2nd ed., p. 791) Washington, DC and New York: The World Bank and Oxford University Press.

On that basis, what would be a sensible approach to improving health through investments in water supply, sanitation, and hygiene in low- and middle-income countries? First would be to promote hygiene. This is necessary both for its own sake and to maximize the value that will accrue from investments in water supply and sanitation. Second, governments should promote low-cost sanitation schemes. In doing this, they should encourage the private sector to invest in this business, encourage demand from consumers, try to ensure that there are skills to install the latrines, and try to set and enforce standards to which they have to be built. Third, low-cost water supply schemes should also be developed. This can often be done best in conjunction with communities and with community-based approaches. Finally, the government should use its regulatory and other authority to be sure that it helps consumers meet the costs of these schemes and also encourages investment in water supply schemes with household connections that families pay for. Much has been written about approaches to water and sanitation. Those interested in how such schemes get designed, built, operated, and financed are encouraged to review some of the literature on those topics, which is beyond the scope of this text.

POLICY AND PROGRAM BRIEFS

Four policy and program briefs follow. The first brief discusses a program for handwashing with soap in Senegal. The second concerns a campaign for "total sanitation" in East Java, Indonesia. Both cases were largely successful in meeting their goals and have valuable lessons for other countries trying to improve hygiene and sanitation. The third brief is on water-related poisoning in Bangladesh due to arsenic. The last brief summarizes the findings of some of the most important studies done to date on possible links between climate change and health.

Handwashing with Soap in Senegal

Handwashing with soap is key to preventing the spread of disease because it kills various agents, such as harmful bacteria, that can cause infection. Nonetheless, the rate of handwashing with soap in Senegal is relatively low, as it is in many low- and middle-income countries. According to a study conducted in Senegal in 2004, for example, the rate of handwashing with soap was 18 percent after cleaning a child, 18 percent before handling food, and 23 percent after going to the toilet.[32] Distance between soap and a source of water, soap being controlled by people who do not want to share it, and the lack of a designated place for handwashing are all barriers to handwashing with soap in Senegal.

The Public-Private Partnership for Handwashing with Soap (PPPHW) was created in Senegal in 2003 with the mission to promote handwashing with soap. With technical assistance from an international partnership housed at the World Bank, the Water and Sanitation Program (WSP), PPPHW was originally sited within the Senegalese government unit that oversees sanitation within the Ministry of Health.

The PPPHW launched a communications campaign in 2004 with the goal of educating people about the importance of using soap when washing hands, in addition to the most critical times for handwashing. "Water rinses but soap cleans" was the main message of this first phase of communications efforts.

The campaign made use of a number of communications methods to send its message. Television and radio spots were aired nationally, especially during times when mothers were preparing meals. More than 87 percent of Senegalese own radios and 40.1 percent own televisions, explaining why mass media can be an effective tool for exposing the campaign's slogan and visual aspects. Billboards, which are prevalent in Senegal, were also used.

The campaign also hosted interactive local community events to extend its messages directly to the population. Local marketplaces and schools hosted live entertainment and demonstrations to educate women and children about the importance of handwashing with soap. In addition, small-group discussions were held at women's associations and waiting rooms of local health centers to facilitate communication among the people about the importance of using soap.

The PPPHW project introduced a second phase of activities to promote handwashing with soap in 2008 after being incorporated into the WSP's Global Scaling Up Handwashing Project, which seeks to "apply innovative promotional approaches to behavior change to generate widespread and sustained improvements in handwashing with soap."[32,p1] The project expanded in this phase to reach 8 of the 11 regions in Senegal with a more defined target of women of reproductive age and primary school–aged children ages 5 to 9. The goal was to improve handwashing with soap practices of over 500,000 mothers and children.

Studies in 2008 identified which behavioral determinants were correlated with handwashing with soap in an attempt to incorporate a wider spectrum of behavioral determinants into the second phase of the behavior change program. At this point, the majority of the 2,040 mothers who participated in the study understood the campaign message of the first phase, or the importance of using soap when handwashing.

Fifty-two percent disagreed with the statement that "water alone is enough." Mothers also understood the link between handwashing with soap and disease prevention, with close to 80 percent agreeing or strongly agreeing that removing dirt and invisible germs requires handwashing with soap. However, research suggested that access to and availability of soap and water in the household is a key determinant for handwashing with soap and had to be planned for.

Based on the assumption that most mothers now understood the importance of handwashing with soap, the second phase of the program aimed to "awaken, fortify, and support" intentions to wash hands with soap. The campaign encouraged mothers to act upon intentions by planning for handwashing, such as designating a certain place for handwashing with soap. The campaign message was delivered through the same communications channels used in the first phase. With technical assistance and guidance from WSP, local communications and consulting firms and NGOs designed, planned, and carried out different components of the project.

New billboards and radio and television spots were created with the intention of positively reinforcing mothers' and children's commitment to washing hands with soap. From June to December 2009, 92 television and 1,496 radio spots aired. At local soccer games and other community locations, respected community members gave handwashing demonstrations and testimonials of their pledge to wash hands with soap. The 161 events that were held through December 2009 reached an estimated 140,000 people.

Workers from local NGOs also visited homes to discuss with mothers tangible ways of turning into action the intention of washing hands with soap. The 150 trained workers helped mothers plan the necessary steps for setting up a designated handwashing station, including making sure that water and soap were available and accessible.

Of course, the program faced a number of challenges. Engaging local partners, while still ensuring that campaign messages were communicated effectively and consistently, presented some initial challenges. At first, local advertising agencies created negative messages that emphasized germs and disease, rather than positive messages of healthy outcomes from handwashing with soap, as instructed. As a result, WSP worked closely with local agencies to coordinate advertisements.

Another challenge was making sure that outreach workers who visit homes go beyond offering information, by discussing mothers' obstacles to handwashing with soap and devising practical solutions through careful planning and building of handwashing stations. Performance monitoring

and coaching of workers has helped to ensure they do their job effectively. A lesson learned for changing behavior is that the use or demonstration of a tangible product that facilitates behavior change, such as a sample handwashing station, can be a powerful tool for turning intention into action.

This project also exemplifies the importance of continually revising campaign strategy to account for a project's past successes or failures. In addition to reevaluating the entire campaign message to launch the second phase, throughout this phase certain program elements were further revised to reflect current evaluations. The 2008 campaign advertisements originally portrayed men merely as social supporters; however, later monitoring of the program suggested that a man's role in the family as provider, protector, and role model gives him tremendous influence in promoting handwashing with soap. In fact, half of women surveyed considered their husbands the decision makers in purchasing soap. Thus, program planners recognized the significant role that men play in overcoming barriers to accessibility and availability of soap, and they adjusted the campaign to engage men more in selling the importance of handwashing with soap. Modified communication materials portray men as committed to handwashing with soap, thus fortifying men's intentions to do so and increasing the visibility of their influential role.[33]

Total Sanitation and Sanitation Marketing: East Java, Indonesia[34]

The Water and Sanitation Program is an international partnership housed at the World Bank that supports poor people in acquiring affordable, safe, and sustainable access to water and sanitation services.[35] One part of this program has been Total Sanitation and Sanitation Marketing (TSSM) projects in a number of countries. These are based on a three-pronged approach to rapidly increasing the number of people who use sanitary means of disposing of human waste:

- The development of a strategy for changing behaviors, based on consumer research
- The development of an approach to increasing the market for latrines, based on market research
- A community-led campaign for total sanitation—an approach that seeks to make a community completely free of open defecation

TSSM projects also pay particular attention to the monitoring of progress, continuous evaluation of results, and learning as you go. Special emphasis is also placed on creating an enabling environment for the project to meet its goals, by working to enhance the policy, institutional, and financial frameworks within which a sanitation program has to be carried out.

In 2007, a TSSM project was launched in East Java, Indonesia. At the time the project was launched, sanitation coverage was just below 70 percent in urban areas and only about 55 percent in rural areas. The intended project outcome was to provide access to sustainable sanitation services for 1.4 million people, in one of the most densely populated places in the world.[34]

This project paid greater attention than many earlier projects to involving the community in the design and development of the project, having the community participate financially in the project, increasing the community's demand for toilets, and ensuring that there would be a sufficient supply of appropriate toilets to meet that demand.[36]

Demand Creation

Districts had to volunteer to participate in the program. One of the first steps in the implementation of the project in East Java, therefore, was to create community-based and household-level demand for improved sanitation.

In order to garner government support of the behavior change program, discussions were held with local and district officials about the economic impact of poor sanitation at the country and district levels and the social and economic returns from investing in sanitation improvements.[34]

To create demand for improved sanitation, the project used the Community-Led Total Sanitation (CLTS) methodology, which mobilizes communities to completely eliminate open defecation. This approach focuses on community-wide sustainable behavioral change, rather than toilet construction for individual households. CLTS efforts try to help communities understand that, regardless of the number of toilets constructed, there is still a risk of disease if even one person continues to defecate in the open. As part of the CLTS approach, communities develop their own solutions to obtain improved sanitation and become free of open defecation.[34] An initial step in this process is mapping village boundaries and indicating where people defecate in the open.[37]

In addition, the program used marketing techniques to improve the demand for sanitation-related products and services, which included advertisements for desirable hygienic behaviors.[37] The program created and marketed, for example, a communication campaign with a character, "Lik Telek," or "Uncle Shit" in the local language, which personifies the open defecation habit. With flies dancing around his head, and a smug smile, Lik Telek goes behind a tree to defecate in the open, while onlookers advise him to use improved sanitation facilities.[38] The districts funded the campaign, which included a series of posters, radio commercials, and an 8-minute video drama.

Improvements in the Supply of Sanitation

The project conducted market research for 18 months to better understand the sanitation market as well as the demand for sanitation services. Market research revealed that there was no common definition of the ideal sanitation facility among consumers, sanitation suppliers, and engineers. Standards varied greatly and generated an impression that a good sanitation facility was unaffordable. In addition, open defecation into water was considered socially acceptable, convenient, safe, and clean because the feces are considered invisible, carried away by water or eaten by fish.

In light of these findings, the project worked with designers and suppliers to ensure that there would be a common definition of improved sanitation and that various sanitation options would be available, at a range of prices. To popularize a common definition of an ideal sanitation facility, the program created a "WC-ku Sehat," or "my latrine is healthy/hygienic," thumbs-up sign to identify facilities that meet the improved sanitation criteria. The program also prepared an Informed Choice Catalogue of improved WC-ku Sehat sanitation options at varying prices, which displays all possible combinations of belowground, on the ground, and aboveground sections of latrines.[34]

To further strengthen the quantity, quality, and appropriateness of the supply of sanitation, a technological training institute in East Java held mason training and accreditation programs. These aimed to ensure that a qualified mason would be available in every district to work on improved sanitation facilities. As of June 2009, a total of 600 artisans in 10 districts were trained in this way, and an additional 1,110 artisans were to receive training after that.[36]

Achievement of Project Goals

Overall, the program appears to have produced larger benefits than more conventional approaches to sanitation, because of the high level of community involvement and use of research-based strategies for increasing both demand and supply. The community-led approach in East Java yielded a 49 percent increase in access to improved sanitation within an 18-month period. More conventional approaches generally yielded increases of only about 10–15 percent over such a period. Moreover, between November 2007 and May 2009, more than 325,000 persons gained access to improved sanitation facilities in 21 districts of East Java. As important, again in contrast to the conventional approach, the poorest households in East Java established 715 open defecation–free villages and gained access to improved sanitation at higher rates than nonpoor households.

It was also anticipated that the TSSM approach taken in East Java would be more sustainable than less community-based approaches, because it involved active participation and community investment and was not dependent on external funding. Community households financed their own projects or collaborated with credit groups. Local governments co-funded project interventions. TSSM approaches were integrated into local governments' budgeting, planning, implementation, and monitoring systems, which should also make them more sustainable.[34] One year of the subsidy-free approach taken in this project led to 10 to 15 times more toilets being constructed than in conventional subsidized schemes.

Nonetheless, the TSSM program in Indonesia still faced a number of challenges, as the phase of the project described above was being completed. New interventions such as sanitation marketing, although effective, require significant inputs from skilled staff that were in short supply. They are also resource intensive and may be beyond the financial means of local governments. In addition, because Indonesia did not have a national sanitation program at the time the East Java program was launched, the government needed sustained political commitment and help from TSSM to scale up total sanitation efforts to other Indonesian provinces.[36]

Arsenicosis in Bangladesh

Universal access to safe and clean drinking water has been a long-standing priority on the global health agenda. To help Bangladesh achieve this goal, a program started in the 1970s has helped to install thousands of tube wells throughout the country. Unfortunately, due to unknown groundwater contamination, 33 to 77 million people have been put at risk of arsenicosis from drinking the water from these wells.[39] This mass exposure and its emerging consequences is already the largest mass poisoning in history. How did this happen and what can we learn from this experience?

What Is Arsenic?

Arsenic is a toxic element that has no apparent beneficial health effects for humans. Natural arsenic salts are present in all waters but usually in only very small amounts. Most waters in the world have natural arsenic concentrations of less than 0.01 mg per liter, but arsenic is much more concentrated in the rocks and soil of some regions. Arsenicosis is arsenic poisoning, which occurs after exposure to arsenic for a long time, usually 5–20 years. Symptoms can include skin lesions, hardening of the skin, dark spots on hands and feet, swollen limbs, and loss of feeling from hands and legs.

Lesions are easily infected, pose a threat of gangrene, and can be very painful. Although there is typically a long latency period of more than 20 years from the first exposure to arsenic, lesions can appear more quickly if arsenic concentrations are high enough.[40]

Drinking arsenic-rich water over a long period can result in various health effects, including skin cancer; cancers of the bladder, kidney, and lung; diseases of the blood vessels of the legs and feet; and possibly also diabetes, high blood pressure, and reproductive disorders. Approximately 1 in 100 people who drink water containing 0.05 mg arsenic per liter or more for a long period may eventually die from arsenic-related cancers.[41] Fortunately, these symptoms are usually reversible if detected early and if the contaminated drinking source is replaced.[40]

The Problem

Previously, Bangladesh struggled with providing safe water sources to its population because most of its surface water sources were contaminated with microorganisms. This led to a high level of gastrointestinal disease in children. Since the 1970s, tube wells have been installed to reduce disease from ingestion of pathogens from surface waters.[42]

These wells consist of tubes that are 5 cm in diameter that are inserted into the ground, usually at depths of less than 200 m.[43] It is now known that groundwater from depths greater than 150 m usually contains less arsenic and can be a sustainable drinking water source.[42]

In Bangladesh, the first case of arsenicosis was reported in 1987 and arsenic contamination in groundwater was first confirmed in 1993. By 1998, the extent of arsenic poisoning was evident. By 2008, a total of 4.7 million tube wells in Bangladesh had been tested and 1.4 million of those had been found to contain arsenic above the government drinking water limit of 50 mg per liter.[40] In 2013, it was estimated that over 25 million people had been exposed to arsenic levels over the national limit of 50 mg per liter and 5.6 million people had been exposed to drinking water with over 200 mg per liter of arsenic. By 2013, at least 40,000 people had symptoms of arsenicosis.[41]

Long-Term Consequences

Although the number of reported arsenic-related diseases and deaths in Bangladesh is already substantial, it will only increase in the future because the latency period after exposure can last several decades. Moreover, another a concern is a generation of "arsenic orphans" when the current generation of caretakers start to face premature death from arsenicosis.[42]

The social and economic consequences of arsenicosis are also debilitating. People with arsenic poisoning suffer enormous social stigma in Bangladesh because of the widespread belief that arsenic poisoning is contagious or a curse.[40] Moreover, some estimates suggest that by about 2,030 arsenic-related mortality in Bangladesh could lead to a loss of $12.5 billion in economic productivity.[42]

Lessons Learned

This public health emergency that occurred in Bangladesh has demonstrated that all groundwater drinking sources should be tested for potential contamination.[43] The events in Bangladesh have led to greater global attention about the risk of environmental groundwater contamination. It is now known that arsenic contamination exists in more than 70 countries, and half of these discoveries have been made in the last 10–15 years.[41]

Although the long-term consequences of arsenic exposure can be mitigated by eliminating exposure, the public health response to the emergency was not as rapid as it should have been. Three years after the contamination was confirmed, interventions had reached only a few hundred villages and by the year 2000 millions of wells still needed to be tested. Much of the response was delayed while long-term solutions were investigated.[43]

Climate Change and Health

Background

Climate change refers to the increase in the earth's average temperature that has been observed and the consequences that might be associated with this rise in temperature.[44] It is estimated that the earth has warmed by 1.4°F (0.8°C) in the past 100 years.[44] Accompanying the rising temperature has been a change in rainfall levels; an increase in the frequency of extreme weather such as floods, droughts, or heat waves; and the melting of glaciers, warming of the oceans, and the rising of sea levels.[44] The United Nations Secretary-General has said that climate change is the major, overriding environmental issue of our time.[44] Climate change is also considered a significant threat to the fight to improve the health of poor people in the poorest countries.[45]

The Problem

According to WHO estimates, climate change will cause an additional 250,000 deaths per year between 2030 and 2050.[46] Specifically, WHO has estimated that climate change will lead to approximately 38,000 additional deaths due to heat exposure in elderly people, 48,000 deaths due to diarrhea,

60,000 deaths due to malaria, and 95,000 deaths due to childhood undernutrition.[47]

The United Nations Intergovernmental Panel on Climate Change, the leading international body for the assessment of climate change, reported 95 percent certainty in 2013 that human activities have caused most of the warming of the planet's surface that has occurred since the 1950s.[48] These findings place increased pressure on the global society to act to reverse the observed trends, especially because those predicted to be affected the most by the effects of climate change have contributed least to its causes.[48]

How Does Climate Change Affect Health?

There are many mechanisms through which climate change can affect health. For example, extreme weather patterns such as droughts, flooding, and heat waves can lead to direct increases in mortality as a result of their effect on infrastructure, disruption of daily activities, and severe conditions placed on the human body. Droughts are thought to have the greatest global disaster effects because they often affect large regions.[49] In addition, variable rainfall patterns can result in a lack of a safe water supply, which can compromise hygiene and can lead to increased risk of diarrheal disease.[47] Changes in rainfall can also indirectly affect the nutritional status of populations by altering agricultural production. Higher temperatures contribute to deaths associated with respiratory and cardiovascular disease as the body is subjected to harsher conditions. High temperatures can also exacerbate air pollution levels, which can lead to a greater incidence of asthma cases. Changing weather patterns can also influence the balance of ecosystems and biodiversity of a region. Even small changes in rainfall and temperature can alter the distribution of disease carriers, such as mosquitoes, which can then affect the prevalence of vector-borne diseases, such as dengue or malaria.[50]

Who Is Affected?

A *Lancet* Commission has indicated that all people are at risk to be negatively affected by climate change and the well-being of billions will be put at risk. Nonetheless, some groups of people are more vulnerable than others.[51] In particular, low-income countries, and in some cases middle-income countries as well, could be affected to a greater extent because areas with weak health infrastructure will be least prepared to respond and adapt to the changes in weather and corresponding changing health and disease patterns. In addition, it is anticipated that urban areas will be affected to a greater extent by any negative impacts of air pollution or rises in temperature, whereas rural areas will be more affected by changes in weather patterns that affect agricultural production.[47]

Within all countries, children and the elderly will be among the most vulnerable to the diseases climate change is likely to influence. Children will be affected by increased risk of diarrheal disease, malaria, and undernutrition, whereas the elderly will be most affected by increased risk of heat-related conditions and also extreme weather patterns, given their more fragile physical state.[47,52]

What Must Be Done?

Climate change is likely to have high human and economic costs. In fact, the World Health Organization estimates that by 2030, the damage to health will be between $2–4 billion per year.[47] The potential health and economic consequences can be mitigated with cost-effective interventions. The climate change response proposed by the United Nations Environment Program involves both adaptation strategies that build resilience to climate change in the short run and mitigation strategies that aim to reduce long-term carbon emissions.[53] All mitigation and adaptation strategies offer direct health benefits as a result of either preventing the effects of climate change on health or preparing the health community to better respond to these effects.

In the short term, the public health community can prepare for any negative climate change effects by enhancing public health education surrounding emergency preparedness, warnings of high pollution, and general public health education, including boil water notices during floods, public awareness on vector-borne diseases, and promotion of good hygiene.[54]

In the long term, mitigation efforts revolve around reducing emissions of greenhouse gases, particularly carbon and methane emissions.[55] Assuming a world population of 9 billion by 2050, reductions of more than two-thirds in emissions would be needed to avoid doubling preindustrial revolution levels.[50] Effective control efforts would avoid 0.6 to 4.4 million deaths related to particulate matter and 0.04 to 0.52 ozone-related deaths and can also increase annual crop yields by 30 to 135 million metric tons due to ozone reductions in 2030 and beyond.[56,57] Benefits of methane emissions reductions have been estimated at $700 to $5,000 per metric ton.[57]

The United Nations Environmental Program suggests many strategies to control carbon and methane emissions, but given that the largest contributor to greenhouse emissions is the burning of fossil fuels, reducing this activity should be a priority.[55] Fossil fuels can be controlled both directly and indirectly. For example, on a policy level, regulations can be put in place that directly limit the magnitude of emissions or that require manufacturing processes that are more environmentally friendly and less wasteful.[55]

In addition, research and support of energy sources other than fossil fuels must be sustained as a mitigation strategy in order to offer an alternative to the burning of fossil fuels. These commitments need to be made in low- and middle-income countries, as well as in high-income countries, and there have already been successful and cost-effective interventions in resource-poor settings. In Jaipur, India, for example, a 350-bed health facility cut its total energy bill in half between 2005 and 2008 through solar-powered water heaters and lighting. In Brazil, one efficiency initiative reduced the demand for electricity of a group of 101 hospitals by 1035 kilowatts at a cost savings of 25 percent.[52]

Another mitigation strategy is the halting of deforestation and forest degradation. Agricultural expansion, forest clearing, infrastructure development, destructive logging, fires, and other similar activities contribute almost 20 percent of the global greenhouse gas emissions, the second-leading contributor.[55] These activities can be discouraged through offering alternative economic means for organizations and individuals engaged with them, such as creating carbon markets in which governments or businesses are rewarded for their efforts made to reduce carbon emissions.[55]

Other mitigation strategies can include reducing agricultural waste and inefficiency through investing in new farming and storing technologies, reducing waste associated with the construction industry, investing in improved recycling infrastructure, or promoting sustainable tourism that engages local communities and protects natural ecosystems.[55] The *Lancet* Commission and other actors have stated that interventions must be implemented on the individual, local, national, and international levels in order to best mitigate the looming potential effects of climate change on health.[51]

FUTURE CHALLENGES

Many challenges will be associated with reducing the burden of disease that is related to hygiene, water supply, and sanitation; household air pollution; and ambient air pollution. One important challenge has to do with population growth. The population is continuing to grow in many low- and middle-income countries and will do so for some time. As the population grows, and as increasing numbers of people move to cities, for example, will low- and middle-income countries be able to provide the necessary infrastructure for improved water supply and sanitation?

At the same time, if the economies of low- and middle-income countries grow at a relatively rapid and sustained pace, how will they manage the pollution that is related, for example, to increased use of energy and greater use of automobiles by better-off people? In addition, will relatively poorly governed societies be able to manage and regulate industrial forms of pollution that could further harm air and water quality?

Many of the health impacts related to household air pollution and unsafe water and sanitation exact a larger toll on rural people than urban people, on the poor rather than the better-off, and on women and children. In this light, many countries will need to explore ways to reduce household air pollution and improve the safety of the water supply through community-based approaches. Such approaches will often have to link the public, private, and NGO sectors with communities and will have to explicitly focus on women and children.

Reducing the burden of environmentally related health problems will also require that people be better informed about that burden. At the societal level, people and communities will need to understand more about the links between their health and the environment. At national, regional, local, and family levels, people will also need to be more aware of the solutions to these problems that might be available to them. The need for better and more information about issues and options for addressing them will be especially important among the poor, the poorly educated, the rural, and women.

Another challenge of addressing environmental health issues is that efforts to address them generally require action outside the health sector. Urban water supply systems are usually under the control of public or private companies. Urban sanitation is usually managed by individual cities. In rural areas, water supply and sanitation are most likely to be controlled by communities and individuals. Household air pollution is an issue that can best be addressed by working with families and communities to change the way they cook and the fuel they use for cooking. Ambient air pollution comes, among other things, from industrial plants and vehicles, the control of which depends on an array of economic and policy matters beyond the scope of the health ministry.

MAIN MESSAGES

Environmental health issues have a large impact on the global burden of disease. These impacts occur at the individual, household, community, and global level. Broadly speaking, about one-third of the total global burden of disease is related to environmental factors.[58] About 8 percent of the global burden of disease is associated with the environmental factors discussed in this chapter, including ambient air pollution, household air pollution from the use of sold fuels, and water, sanitation, and hygiene.[5]

The risks of these environmental factors are greatest for poor women and their children due to their exposure to household air pollution from the burning of solid fuel and to poor-quality water. The risks of environmental impacts on health are greatest in the low-income countries of Africa and Asia. Environmental risk factors are especially important causes of illness and death from diarrhea and acute respiratory infections among young children. They also have a large impact on the burden of disease from certain parasitic infections, such as worms. Given the prominence of these risk factors, it is essential that improvements be made in water, sanitation, and hygiene.

The burden of household air pollution stems largely from cooking on unventilated stoves with solid biomass fuels or coal, as done by a large share of poor people in the world. The sources of ambient air pollution are many, and vehicle emission is among the most important in most cities. Poor sanitation allows pathogens in human waste to spread, but only about 60 percent of the people in the world have access to improved sanitation. Unsafe water carries pathogens. The lack of water prevents people from engaging in appropriate hygiene practices. Poor hygiene practices, including open defecation and the failure to engage in handwashing with soap, are common in low- and middle-income countries, especially among people who lack education.

Data are weak on cost-effective approaches to reducing ambient air pollution in low- and middle-income countries. However, it appears that a number of measures could be taken to reduce pollution and enhance health, including eliminating leaded gasoline, eliminating two-stroke engines, strengthening emissions standards, and shifting vehicle fuel to natural gas. In Africa and South Asia, the most cost-effective approach to reducing household air pollution will be to promote the use of improved stoves. In East Asia, the most cost-effective approach would be to encourage a shift from biomass fuels and coal to kerosene or gas.

The most cost-effective approach to reducing the burden of water-related diseases, especially diarrhea, is to invest in low-cost sanitation and standposts for water and to promote handwashing. Investments in water can have numerous benefits, including saving the time of women who are usually charged with getting water and often have to expend large amounts of energy to do so. The provision of water can also contribute to reduction in certain parasitic diseases. However, in the absence of improved hygiene, the provision of improved access to water alone still fails to address an important share of the burden of diarrheal disease.

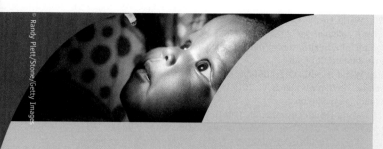

Study Questions

1. Why are environmental health issues important in global health? Which of them are the most important and why?

2. Why would the burden of disease from household air pollution in low- and middle-income countries be larger than that from ambient air pollution?

3. In what regions of the world would the burden from household air pollution be the greatest? Why?

4. What are the different ways in which unsafe water is related to the spread of disease? Give some examples of specific diseases that are spread in various water-related ways.

5. What are some of the health problems associated with ambient air pollution?

6. Why is it important to promote handwashing?

7. What approach would you take in a low-income African country to enhance the access of the poor to better water supplies? Why?

8. How would you try to expand access to low-cost sanitation in Nepal? Why?

9. What would constrain poor people in Nepal from investing their own resources in improved low-cost sanitation? How could those constraints be overcome?

REFERENCES

1. Smith, K. R., Corvalan, C. F., & Kjellstrom, T. (1999). How much global ill health is attributable to environmental factors? *Epidemiology, 10*(5), 573–584.

2. Prüss-Üstün, A., & Corvalán, C. (2006). *Quantifying environmental health impacts: Preventing disease through healthy environments: Towards an estimate of the environmental burden of disease.* Geneva: World Health Organization. Retrieved February 25, 2014, from http://www.who.int /quantifying_ehimpacts/publications/preventingdisease/en/.

3. Institute of Health Metrics and Evaluation. *GBD cause patterns.* Retrieved October 6, 2014, from http://vizhub.healthdata.org /gbd-cause-patterns/.

4. Institute of Health Metrics and Evaluation. *GBD 2010 heat map.* Retrieved October 6, 2014, from http://vizhub.healthdata.org/irank/heat .php.

5. Lopez, A. D., Mathers, C. D., Ezzati, M., Jamison, D. T., & Murray, C. J. L. (2006). Measuring the global burden of disease and risk factors 1990–2001. In A. D. Lopez, C. D. Mathers, M. Ezzati, D. T. Jamison, & C. J. L. Murray (Eds.), *Global burden of disease and risk factors.* New York: Oxford University Press.

6. Friis, R. H. (2007). *Essentials on environmental health.* Sudbury, MA: Jones and Bartlett.

7. Yassi, A., Kjellstrom, T., de Kok, T., & Guidotti, T. L. (2001). *Basic environmental health.* New York: Oxford University Press.

8. McMichael, A. J., Kjellstrom, T., & Smith, K. R. (2001). Environmental health. In M. H. Merson, R. E. Black, & A. Mills (Eds.), *International public health: Diseases, programs, systems, and policies.* Gaithersburg, MD: Aspen Publishers.

9. The World Bank. *Environmental health.* Retrieved February 27, 2015, from http://siteresources.worldbank.org/INTPHAAG/Resources /AAGEHEng.pdf.

10. World Health Organization. *Public health, environmental and social determinants of health.* Retrieved February 27, 2015, from http://www.who .int/phe/en.

11. World Health Organization. *Household air pollution and health.* Fact Sheet No. 292. Retrieved December 28, 2014, from http://www.who.int /mediacentre/factsheets/fs292/en/index.html.

12. Yassi, A., Kjellstrom, T., de Kok, T., & Guidotti, T. L. (2001). Health and energy use. In *Basic environmental health* (pp. 311–331). New York: Oxford University Press.

13. Yassi, A., Kjellstrom, T., de Kok, T., & Guidotti, T. L. (2001). Air. In *Basic environmental health* (pp. 180–208). New York: Oxford University Press.

14. World Bank. *Improved sanitation facilities (% of population with access).* Retrieved February 27, 2015, from http://data.worldbank.org /indicator/SH.STA.ACSN/countries?display=graph.

15. UNICEF. (2013). *2.4 million people will lack access to improved sanitation in 2015.* Retrieved October 14, 2014, from http://www.unicef.org /media/media_69091.html.

16. Cairncross, S., & Valdmanis, V. (2006). Water supply, sanitation, and hygiene promotion. In D. T. Jamison, J. G. Breman, A. R. Measham, et al. (Eds.), *Disease control priorities in developing countries* (2nd ed., pp. 771–792). New York: Oxford University Press.

17. UNICEF and WHO. (2014). *Progress on sanitation and water 2014 update.* Geneva: WHO.

18. Lim, S. S. et al. (2013). A comparative risk assessment of burden of disease and injury attributable to 67 risk factors and risk factor clusters in 21 regions, 1990–2010: A systematic analysis for the Global Burden of Disease Study 2010. *Lancet, 380*(9859), 2224–2260.

19. Institute of Health Metrics and Evaluation. (2014). *GBD Compare.* Retrieved October 15, 2014, from http://vizhub.healthdata.org /gbd-compare/.

20. World Health Organization. (2014). *Burden of disease from household air pollution for 2012.* Retrieved June 3, 2014, from http://www .who.int/phe/health_topics/outdoorair/databases/FINAL_HAP_AAP _BoD_24March2014.pdf.

21. World Health Organization. (n.d.). *Mortality from ambient air pollution.* Retrieved March 6, 2015, from http://www.who.int/gho/phe /outdoor_air_pollution/.

22. World Health Organization. (2014). *Burden of disease from ambient air pollution for 2012.* Geneva: World Health Organization.

23. World Health Organization. (2014). *Water sanitation health.* Retrieved June 22, 2015, from http://www.who.int/water_sanitation_health /en/.

24. World Health Organization. *Preventing disease through healthy environments: Towards an estimate of the environmental burden of disease.* Retrieved February 25, 2014, from http://www.who.int/quantifying_ehimpacts /publications/preventingdisease/en/.

25. Kjellstrom, T., Lodh, M., McMichael, A. J., Ranmuthugala, G., Shrestha, R., & Kingsland, S. (2006). Air and water pollution: Burden and strategies for control. In D. T. Jamison, J. G. Breman, A. R. Measham, et al. (Eds.), *Disease control priorities in developing countries* (2nd ed., pp. 817–832). New York: Oxford University Press.

26. Bruce, N., Rehfuess, E., Mehta, S., Hutton, G., & Smith, K. (2006). Household air pollution. In D. T. Jamison, J. G. Breman, A. R. Measham, et al. (Eds.), *Disease control priorities in developing countries* (2nd ed., pp. 793–816). New York: Oxford University Press.

27. Feachem, R., Bradley, D., Garelick, H., & Mara, D. (1983). *Sanitation and disease: Health aspects of excreta and wastewater management.* Chichester, U.K.: John Wiley & Sons.

28. Waterkeyn, J. (2003). *Cost-effective health promotion: Community health clubs.* Paper presented at the 29th WEDC Conference, Abuja, Nigeria.

29. Allan, S. (2003). *The WaterAid Bangladesh/VERC 100% sanitation approach; Cost, motivation and subsidy.* Unpublished master's thesis, London School of Hygiene.

30. Pruss-Ustun, A. et al. (2014). Burden of Disease from Inadequate Water, Sanitation and Hygiene in Low- and Middle-income Settings: A Retrospective Analysis of Data from 145 Countries. *Tropical Medicine and International Health, 19*(8), 894–905.

31. Emerson, P. M., Lindsay, S. W., Alexander, N., et al. (2004). Role of flies and provision of latrines in trachoma control: Cluster-randomised controlled trial. *Lancet, 363*(9415), 1093–1098.

32. This brief is based on Water and Sanitation Program. (2010). *Senegal: A handwashing behavior change journey.* Retrieved October 20, 2010, from http://www.wsp.org/wsp/sites/wsp.org/files/publications/WSP_SenegalBC Journey_HWWS.pdf.

33. Water and Sanitation Program. (2010). *Involving men in handwashing behavior change in Senegal.* Retrieved October 26, 2010, from http://www .wsp.org/wsp/sites/wsp.org/files/publications/WSP_InvolvingMen_HWWS .pdf.

34. This brief is based largely on Water and Sanitation Program. (2009). *Total Sanitation and Sanitation Marketing Project: Indonesia country update. Learning at scale.* Retrieved October 11, 2010, from http://www.wsp.org /wsp/sites/wsp.org/files/publications/learning_at_scale.pdf.

35. Water and Sanitation Program. Home. Retrieved October 12, 2010, from http://www.wsp.org/.

36. Water and Sanitation Program. (2009). *Annual report 2009.* Retrieved October 12, 2010, from http://www.wsp.org/wsp/global-initiatives /Global-Scaling-Up-Handwashing-Project/Annual-Progress-Report-2009.

37. Water and Sanitation Program. *Scaling up rural sanitation: Core components.* Retrieved October 12, 2010, from http://www .wsp.org/global-initiatives/global-scaling-sanitation-project/Sanitation -core-components#applying_total_sanitation.

38. Water and Sanitation Project. Global Scaling Up Sanitation Project Second Annual Progress Report. Retrieved February 27,2015, from http://www.wsp.org/sites/wsp.org/files/publications/gsp_annual_progress_report.pdf.

39. Smith, A. H., Lingas, E. O., & Rahman, M. (2000). Contamination of drinking-water by arsenic in Bangladesh: A public health emergency. *Bulletin of the World Health Organization, 78*, 1093–1103.

40. UNICEF. (2008). *Arsenic mitigation in Bangladesh*. Retrieved August 8, 2014, from http://www.unicef.org/bangladesh/Arsenic.pdf.

41. UNICEF. (2013). *Arsenic contamination in groundwater*. Position Paper No. 2. Retrieved August 8, 2014 from http://www.unicef.org/media/files/Position_Paper_Arsenic_contamination_in_groundwater_April_2013.pdf.

42. Flanagan, S. V., Johnston, R. B., & Zheng, Y. (2012). Arsenic in tube well water in Bangladesh: Health and economic impacts and implications for arsenic mitigation. *Bulletin of the World Health Organization, 90*, 839–846. doi: 10.2471/BLT.11.101253.

43. Smith, A, H., Lingas, E. O., & Rahman, M. (2000). Contamination of drinking-water by arsenic in Bangladesh: A public health emergency. *Bulletin of the World Health Organization, 78*, 1093–1103.

44. Environmental Protection Agency. (2014). *Climate change: Basic information*. Retrieved October 16, 2014, from http://www.epa.gov/climatechange/basics/.

45. World Bank. (2014). *Climate change overview*. Retrieved November 4, 2014, from http://www.worldbank.org/en/topic/climatechange/overview#1.

46. Hales, S., Kovats, S., Lloyd, S., & Campbell-Lendrum, D. (2014). *Quantitative risk assessment of the effects of climate change on selected causes of death, 2030s and 2050s*. Geneva: World Health Organization.

47. World Health Organization. (2014). *Climate change and health*. Fact Sheet No. 266. Retrieved from http://www.who.int/mediacentre/factsheets/fs266/en/.

48. Intergovernmental Panel on Climate Change. (2013). *Climate change 2013: The physical science basis*. Contribution of Working Group I to the fifth assessment report of the Intergovernmental Panel on Climate Change. Cambridge, UK and New York, NY: Cambridge University Press.

49. McMichael, A. J., Woodruff, R. E., & Hales, S. (2006). Climate change and human health: Present and future risks. *Lancet, 367*, 859–869.

50. Haines, A., Kovats, R. S., Campbell-Lendrum, D., & Corvalan, C. (2006). Climate change and human health: Impacts, vulnerability and public health. *Public Health, 120*, 585–596.

51. Costello, A., et al. (2009). Managing the health effects of climate change. Lancet and University College London Institute for Global Health Commission. *Lancet, 37*, 1693–1733. doi: 10.1016/S0140-6736(09)60935-1.

52. Neira, M. (2012). *Environmental health and sustainable development*. Geneva: World Health Organization. Retrieved November 4, 2014, from http://ec.europa.eu/environment/archives/soil/pdf/may2012/02%20-%20Maria%20Neira%20-%20final.pdf.

53. United Nations Environment Programs. *Climate change*. Retrieved October 15, 2014, from http://www.unep.org/climatechange/Introduction.aspx.

54. United Nations Environment Programs. *Climate change adaptation*. Retrieved November 4, 2014, from http://www.unep.org/climatechange/adaptation.

55. United Nations Environment Programs. *Climate change mitigation*. Retrieved November 4, 2014, from http://www.unep.org/climatechange/mitigation/Home/tabid/104335/Default.aspx.

56. Anenberg, S. C. (2012). Global air quality and health co-benefits of mitigating near-term climate change through methane and black carbon emission controls. *Environmental Health Perspectives, 120*, 831–839.

57. Shindell, D., et al. (2012). Simultaneously mitigating near-term climate change and improving human health and food security. *Science, 335*(6065), 183–189.

58. Smith, K. R., Corvalan, C. F., & Kjellstrom, T. (1999). How much global ill health is attributable to environmental factors? *Epidemiology, 10*(5), 573–584.

CHAPTER 8

Nutrition and Global Health

By the end of this chapter, the reader will be able to:

- Define key terms related to nutrition
- Describe the determinants of nutritional status
- Discuss nutrition needs at different stages of the life course
- Discuss the burden of nutrition problems globally
- Review the costs and consequences of those burdens
- Discuss measures that can be taken to address key nutrition concerns

VIGNETTES

Shireen was a 1 year old who lived in Dhaka, the capital of Bangladesh. Shireen was born with low birthweight. In addition, her family lacked the income needed to provide her with adequate food after she was no longer breastfeeding. Shireen had also repeatedly been ill with respiratory infections and diarrhea and she was hospitalized again with pneumonia. Despite the best efforts of the hospital, Shireen died after 2 days there.

Ruth lived in Liberia and was pregnant with her first child. Ruth had been anemic for all of her adult life, from not having enough iron-rich foods in her diet. She also had no access during pregnancy to iron and folic acid tablets or to foods that were fortified with vitamins and minerals. Ruth went into labor one evening and delivered the baby with the help of a traditional birth attendant. After the baby was born, however, Ruth began to bleed severely. Her family was not able to get her to a hospital and Ruth died.

Dorji was 15 years old and lived in the mountains of northern India. Dorji was very short and had severe intellectual disabilities. Dorji was not the only one in his village with these problems. Dorji lived in an area in which the soils had little iodine. Although the government of India was encouraging the fortification of salt with iodine, such salt was not sold in Dorji's region of the country.

Rachel and her mother lived in Mombassa, a port city in Kenya. Rachel had already received her first polio vaccine and she was soon to get another. When the children participated in "polio days" they got not only a polio vaccine; they also got a dose of vitamin A. Until recently, there were many young children in Kenya and elsewhere who were blind due to the lack of vitamin A. Since the polio campaign started and children got extra vitamin A as part of that campaign, however, almost no children had become blind.

Fai Ho was a 7-year-old boy who lived in South China. He was an only child. As his family had done increasingly well economically, they began to eat fewer and fewer traditional foods and more Western and processed foods, such as soft drinks and potato chips. The family also began to watch more television and get less exercise. In addition, whenever the family wanted to do something special with their son, they took him to a fast-food restaurant for a cheeseburger and French fries. Despite the low rates of obesity among children and adults in China traditionally, Fai Ho was already obese.

THE IMPORTANCE OF NUTRITION

Some things are more important than others, and the role of nutrition in health is one of the more important ones. As noted in **Table 8-1**, and elaborated on throughout this chapter, nutritional status has a profound relationship with health status.

Nutritional status is fundamental to the growth of young children, their proper mental and physical development, and their health as adults. In addition, because of the impact of nutrition on health, nutritional status is intimately linked with whether or not children enroll in school, perform effectively while there, and complete their schooling. Nutritional status, therefore, has a profound effect on labor productivity and people's prospects for earning income.

Despite the importance of nutrition to health, an exceptional number of people in the world are undernourished. This is especially the case for poor women and children in low-income countries, particularly in South Asia and

sub-Saharan Africa. In fact, childhood underweight is the leading risk factor for death of under-5 children globally and suboptimal breastfeeding is the second leading attributable risk factor for those deaths.[1] In addition, about 16 percent of children under 5 globally were underweight in 2011, with the overwhelming majority of such children living in low- and middle-income countries.[2] Moreover, about 26 percent of children globally are stunted, with especially high rates of stunting in South Asia and sub-Saharan Africa.[2] A recent review of maternal and child nutrition in low- and middle-income countries suggested that about 45 percent of all child deaths, or more than 3 million child deaths each year, are attributable to nutrition-related causes.[3] Remarkably, that would be the equivalent of more than 8,000 nutrition-related child deaths in the world every day.

These issues related to maternal and childhood undernutrition are even more difficult to accept because there are a number of low-cost, but highly effective, nutrition interventions that can dramatically improve nutrition status, which are not being implemented sufficiently. Many improvements in nutrition can be enabled largely by communication efforts, such as the promotion of breastfeeding, the introduction of appropriate complementary foods, and the eating of foods that are rich in certain micronutrients. Such communication efforts, however, are not put in place frequently enough or effectively enough. The fortification of salt with iodine has been carried out in high-income countries for more than 50 years but uniodized salt is still sold in many low-income countries. The importance of iron and folic acid to successful outcomes of pregnancy has also been well known for decades,[4] yet many women in low-income countries, like Ruth in the vignette, do not get supplements of iron and folic acid or eat food that is fortified with iron and folate.

Moreover, the nutritional picture of the world has changed dramatically in the last few decades. At the same time as so many people are undernourished, about 2.1 billion people—nearly 30 percent of the world's population—are overweight or obese. This includes close to 7 percent of the world's under-5 children who are overweight.[2] Obesity was once considered a problem unique to high-income countries. However, the vast majority of overweight and obese people in the world today live in low- and middle-income countries. In fact, many countries will have to deal simultaneously for some time to come with several different types of malnutrition, including underweight, micronutrient deficiencies, and overweight and obesity.[5]

Overweight and obesity are especially important for several reasons. First, the prevalence of these problems has been increasing in almost all countries. Second, they are closely linked with a number of noncommunicable diseases,

TABLE 8-1 Selected Links Between Nutrition and the Health of Mothers and Children

Good maternal nutrition and avoiding obesity is essential for good outcomes of pregnancy for the mother and the child.

Exclusive breastfeeding for 6 months promotes better health and better cognitive development for infants than mixing breastfeeding with other foods during that period.

Nutritional deficits in fetuses and in children under 2 years of age may produce growth and development deficits in infants and young children that can never be overcome.

About 45 percent of all deaths in children under 5 years worldwide are associated with nutritional deficits.

Underweight and micronutrient deficiencies in children make those children more susceptible to illness, cause illnesses to last longer, and can lead to deaths from diarrhea, measles, pneumonia, and malaria that might have been preventable.

Rapid weight gain in children who were underweight is associated later in life with obesity and noncommunicable diseases.

Obesity in women—and men—is associated with a range of noncommunicable diseases, such as heart disease, stroke, and diabetes.

Data from Black RE, Victora CG, Walker SP, et al. Maternal and child undernutrition and overweight in low-income and middle-income countries. *Lancet.* August 3, 2013;382(9890):427–451.

TABLE 8-2 Key Links Between Nutrition and the MDGs

Goal 1: Eradicate Poverty and Hunger

Link: Poor nutritional status is both a cause and a consequence of poverty. Improving income and nutritional status will improve health status.

Goal 2: Achieve Universal Primary Education

Link: Children who are properly nourished enroll in school at higher rates than undernourished children, attend school for more years, and perform better while they are there than undernourished children.

Goal 3: Promote Gender Equality and Empower Women

Link: Women suffer very high rates of some nutritional deficiencies, such as iron deficiency anemia, that constrain their health and their productivity. Overweight and obesity are also associated with diseases that can constrain the productivity of females. Improving the nutritional status of women will enhance their income earning potential and ability to be more productive in all of their work.

Goal 4: Reduce Child Mortality

Link: About 45 percent of all child deaths worldwide are associated with malnutrition. It will not be possible to make major strides in reducing child mortality without significant improvements in the nutritional status of young children.

Goal 5: Improve Maternal Health

Link: Maternal health and pregnancy outcomes for women and for children are intimately connected to the nutritional status of the pregnant women. Some problems arise from nutritional deficits. Others are linked to overweight and obesity.

Goal 6: Combat HIV/AIDS, Malaria, and Other Diseases

Link: Poor nutritional status makes people more susceptible to illness and to being sick for longer periods of time. Good nutrition is especially important for people suffering from some health conditions, such as tuberculosis and HIV/AIDS.

Data from United Nations. Millennium Development Goals. Available at: http://www.un.org/millenniumgoals/. Accessed June 6, 2015; and Black RE, Victora CG, Walker SP, et al. Maternal and child undernutrition and overweight in low-income and middle-income countries. *Lancet*. August 3, 2013;382(9890):427–451.

such as heart disease, stroke, and diabetes, that exact an enormous toll on people's health and productivity and on the costs of health care. Third, prevention of the problems associated with overweight and obesity is complex and involves strategies in a variety of sectors and across individual, local, national, and global spheres. Finally, treating these problems can be extremely costly.

Nutrition is central to the achievement of the Millennium Development Goals (MDGs). Directly or indirectly, nutrition is related to almost all of these goals, as noted in **Table 8-2**. In fact, this table makes clear that there are *no* prospects for meeting the MDGs without substantial improvements in nutrition. The hunger goal is completely linked with nutrition, and nutrition deficits are intimately connected to whether or not people are poor. The large number of children who are poorly nourished will challenge the realization of the education goal. In addition, if about 45 percent of all child deaths are related to nutrition, then how can the child mortality goal be met unless nutrition problems are tackled more effectively? The nutritional concerns that are particular to women will constrain their productivity, limit improvements in their economic and social status, preclude gains in the reduction of maternal mortality, and have a deleterious impact on the children to whom they give birth.

In light of the exceptional importance of nutrition to human health, this chapter provides an overview of the most critical matters concerning nutrition globally. First, it introduces you to the most important terms used in discussing nutrition. It then examines the determinants of nutritional status. After that, the chapter explores the most important nutritional needs of people at different stages in their life course. It will then review key issues concerning the nutritional state of the world and the costs and consequences of selected nutrition problems. This is followed by six policy and program briefs and two case studies that illustrate key themes covered in this chapter. The chapter concludes by examining some of the challenges of trying to further improve nutritional status worldwide.

This chapter deals with undernutrition and overweight and obesity. The comments on undernutrition focus largely on children under 5 and pregnant women.

DEFINITIONS AND KEY TERMS

A number of terms related to nutrition are used throughout this chapter. These terms are defined in **Table 8-3**.

The term *malnutrition* should be used to refer to those who do not get proper nutrition, whether too little, too much, or of the wrong kind. This is the way that this text uses that term. In addition, people who lack sufficient energy and nutrients are referred to as "undernourished," "stunted," or

TABLE 8-3 Key Terms and Definitions

Anemia—Low level of hemoglobin in the blood, as evidenced by a reduced quality or quantity of red blood cells.

Body mass index (BMI)—Body weight in kilograms divided by height in meters squared (kg/m^2).

Iodine deficiency disorders (IDDs)—The spectrum of IDDs includes goiter, hypothyroidism, impaired mental function, stillbirths, abortions, congenital anomalies, and neurological cretinism.

Low birthweight—Birthweight less than 2,500 grams.

Malnutrition—Various forms of poor nutrition. Underweight or stunting and overweight, as well as micronutrient deficiencies, are forms of malnutrition.

Obesity—Excessive body fat content; commonly measured by BMI. The international reference for classifying an individual as obese is a BMI greater than 30.

Overweight—Excess weight relative to height; commonly measured by BMI among adults. The international reference for adults is as follows:
- 25–29.99 for grade I (overweight)
- 30–39.99 for grade II (obese)
- > 40 for grade III

For children, overweight is measured as weight-for-height two z-scores above the international reference.

Stunting—Failure to reach linear growth potential because of inadequate nutrition or poor health. Stunting is measured as height-for-age two z-scores below the international reference.

Undernutrition—The three most commonly used indexes for child undernutrition are height-for-age, weight-for-age, and weight-for-height. For adults, underweight is measured by a BMI less than 18.5.

Underweight—Low weight-for-age; that is, two z-scores below the international reference for weight-for-age. It implies stunting or wasting and is an indicator of undernutrition.

Vitamin A deficiency—Tissue concentrations of vitamin A low enough to have adverse health consequences such as increased morbidity and mortality, poor reproductive health, and slowed growth and development, even if there is no clinical deficiency.

Wasting—Weight, measured in kilograms, divided by height in meters squared, that is two z-scores below the international reference.

Z-score—A statistical term, meaning the deviation of an individual's value from the median value of a reference population, divided by the standard deviation of the reference population.

Data from The World Bank. Repositioning Nutrition as Central to Development. Washington DC: The World Bank; 2006: xvii.

"wasted," as appropriate. People who have low weight for their age are called "underweight." People who are nourished to the point of being too heavy for their height are called "overweight" or "obese," depending on their body mass index.

DATA ON NUTRITION

There are many gaps in the data on nutrition. It is difficult, for example, to find a single consistent data set that treats issues from low birthweight to micronutrient deficiencies to overweight and obesity, organized by World Bank region. In addition, some critical data on nutrition are not broken down into consistent age groups. Moreover, existing data on nutrition are often shown using different regions. Some data is presented by World Health Organization (WHO) regions but other data may be available by UNICEF regions, World Bank regions, or the subregions of the *Global Burden of Disease Study 2010.*[6]

Given these data issues, this chapter has made as much use as possible of a data set on nutrition that was produced jointly by UNICEF, WHO, and the World Bank.[2] However, it also complements those data with data from other sources, as needed, including the *Global Burden of Disease Study 2010.*

THE DETERMINANTS OF NUTRITIONAL STATUS

Undernutrition

Nutritional status depends on a number of factors, as shown in **Figure 8-1**, which follows a framework developed by UNICEF.[7] This framework was originally designed to highlight the determinants of undernutrition. However, as we will see later, it is also sheds light on the determinants of overweight and obesity.

In line with this framework, we can consider first the immediate causes of undernutrition. The two most important are inadequate dietary intake and illness. People may get an insufficient amount of food or not enough of some of the nutrients they need. These factors weaken the body, open the person to illness and infection, and lead to longer and more frequent illness than would otherwise be the case. Inadequate dietary intake becomes part of a vicious cycle of illness and infection, which makes it harder for people to eat, more difficult for them to absorb what they do take in, and actually raises the need for some nutrients. The relationship between infection and nutritional status is very important to keep in mind, especially when considering how to improve the nutritional status of poor children in low- and middle-income countries.

The UNICEF framework also includes a set of underlying causes for inadequate dietary intake and infectious disease that include "inadequate access to food in a household; insufficient health services and an unhealthful environment; and inadequate care for children and women."[7] Whether people get enough food within a household depends on a number of factors, including access to land, the ability to produce food

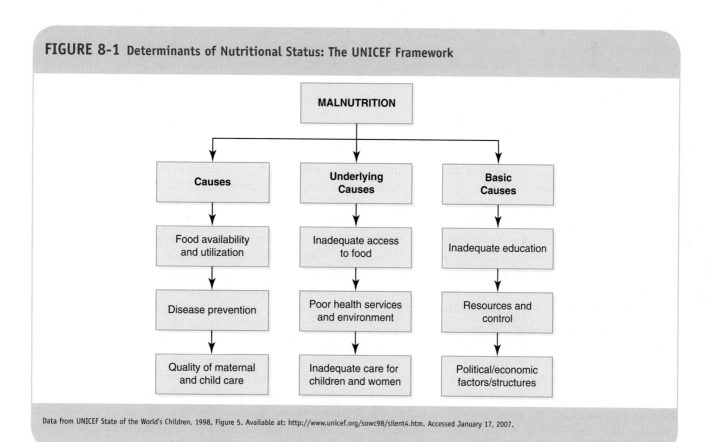

FIGURE 8-1 Determinants of Nutritional Status: The UNICEF Framework

Data from UNICEF State of the World's Children, 1998, Figure 5. Available at: http://www.unicef.org/sowc98/silent4.htm. Accessed January 17, 2007.

for those living in rural areas, and having access to food and the money to purchase it. In addition, the amount and type of food one gets depend in many families on social position, with women and girls sometimes getting less food or less nutritious food than men and boys get. It is also important to note that in rural areas in low-income countries, there may be a hungry season, in which families have exhausted the food from their last harvest, have not yet produced the food for the current year, and do not have the income to buy food, even if a market is accessible to them.

The lack of safe water and sanitation are extremely important causes of diarrheal disease and, therefore, greatly contribute to the cycle of infection and undernutrition. This is made worse when people live in generally unhygienic circumstances, in which food is often handled in unhygienic ways. These are also the circumstances under which people, especially children, are likely to get parasitic infections, such as worms, which sap the energy of children and make it harder for them to absorb what they do eat.

Child caring practices affect the nutritional status of children in similar ways to the manner in which they affect children's health status. If a child is exclusively breastfed for 6 months, if complementary foods that are of sufficient quality and quantity are introduced, and if food and water are handled in hygienic ways, then the nutritional status of young children will be enhanced. In addition, as discussed earlier, the nutrition and health status of the mother is an exceptionally important determinant of whether the child will be born with low birthweight and will thrive thereafter.

Access to appropriate health services is also very important to nutritional status, in a manner similar to its importance for health status. Receiving basic childhood immunizations is an important way to avoid illness and infection. The same is true for vitamin A supplements that are provided by many health services, zinc as an adjunct to oral rehydration therapy for diarrhea, and multiple micronutrient supplementation for pregnant women.[8] Medicines to rid children of worms can also be very important to their nutritional status. Unfortunately, there are still too many health systems that are not capable of effectively providing even these basic services.

Of course, at the root of nutritional status are the factors that UNICEF calls "basic causes." These relate to the social determinants of health. In a manner similar to the factors that determine health, the root causes of nutritional status also have to do with socioeconomic status, family income, the level of knowledge people have of appropriate health and nutritional practices, and the amount of control that people have over their lives. Governmental and global policies that affect agricultural production, marketing, and distribution as well as education, health, and nutrition programs can have a profound effect on the nutritional status of individuals, communities, and societies.

Overweight and Obesity

Obesity and overweight are caused by numerous factors that also relate to immediate causes, underlying causes, and basic causes. The most immediate cause is an increase in total energy intake coupled with a decrease in energy expenditure. This may be related to the genetic composition of some people. However, in broad terms, the rising global rate of obesity is being driven by global financial and trade liberalization, increased income and socioeconomic status, and urbanization, as discussed further later.

Genes play a role in the development of obesity, as they govern the body's response to changes in its environment. Genetic variations can influence behaviors, such as a drive to overeat or tendency to be sedentary. They also govern metabolism, causing some people to store body fat at higher rates than others.[9] These differences have been documented across racial and ethnic backgrounds and even within families.[9] There is also emerging evidence of gut microbes affecting metabolism and obesity, although this research is still in early stages.[10] Despite this biological role, it is crucial to understand that obesity is a result of the interaction between genetic susceptibility and the unhealthy environmental factors that are discussed further next; genetic variations just make people more or less susceptible to these environmental factors.[11]

There are a number of cultural and region-specific factors that contribute to the prevalence of overweight and obesity. In Egypt and Saudi Arabia, for example, women are discouraged from participating in physical activity.[12] In many cultures, boys do fewer household chores than girls, leading to less physical activity around the house.[13] Furthermore, in some Arab and African countries, as examples, being overweight is considered a sign of prosperity.[14]

Genetic and cultural factors associated with overweight are not new. Yet, both overweight and obesity have been increasing in almost all countries. The evidence suggests that these increases have been driven by three macro-level factors related to globalization: global financial and trade liberalization, increased per capita income and socioeconomic status, and increased urbanization.[15]

These factors have led to increased availability and consumption of sugar-sweetened beverages and energy-dense, nutrient-poor foods, along with changes in lifestyle and living environment. Together, these are helping to fuel the global obesity epidemic.[16]

Many countries, for example, implemented more market-oriented or liberal agricultural trade policies from the 1970s through the 1990s, which altered the price and availability of foods in their countries.[15] In addition, foreign direct investment in a range of countries also changed the types of foods available, their prices, and the way they are sold and marketed.[17]

Per capita income is rising globally and is expected to continue doing so for some time.[18] Rapid economic growth in low- and middle-income countries is associated with nutritional and lifestyle changes, including increased television viewing and consumption of highly processed foods. In high-income countries, body weight decreases with income, as better-off people can afford healthier food choices and more exercise.[19] At this stage of the development of many low- and middle-income countries, however, body weight tends to increase with increased socioeconomic status.[15]

There has also been an increase in urbanization in low- and middle-income countries, which in turn leads to overweight and obesity through a multitude of factors. Although in theory urbanization provides greater access to health services and education, which are both preventative measures for obesity, many low- and middle-income countries undergo urbanization at such a rapid pace that essential infrastructure lags behind.[16] Urbanization facilitates obesity through changes in diet, occupation, environment, and behavior, which all contribute directly to increased energy intake and decreased energy expenditure.

In the end, as noted previously, increased energy intake contributes to obesity and there are a number of factors leading directly to increased energy intake globally, stemming from changes in diet. Across all national income levels, it has been shown that countries that maintain their traditional food culture have less obesity.[20] However, globalization and urbanization have caused a nutrition transition away from traditional diets, opening access to cheap, energy-dense, and nutritionally poor food through fast food outlets, supermarkets, and an energy-dense, sugar-laden diet prominently featuring animal products. This has been accompanied by reduced access to fresh local produce, as urbanization has displaced farmers and farmland.[21]

Fast food has been linked to obesity and its related comorbidities, due to its high calorie content, large portion sizes, highly processed meat, highly refined carbohydrates, sugar-sweetened beverages, and high levels of salt, sugar, and fat.[22] Over the past 40 years, a large number of fast-food outlets have opened across the globe.[23] McDonald's, for example, the world's leading global food-service retailer, increased its international presence from 951 outlets in 1987 to over 35,000 outlets in over 100 countries today.[24,25]

The spread of multinational and regional supermarkets has also contributed to the obesity epidemic, as these markets increase access to sugar-sweetened beverages and high-energy, highly processed foods packed with sugar, salt, and fat.[26] Research has shown that supermarkets encourage consumers to eat more, regardless of the food.[27] Supermarkets are growing quickly, especially in Latin America but also in Asia, Eastern Europe, and Africa.[28,29]

In higher income countries such as the United States and Canada, proximity to supermarkets has been shown to reduce the prevalence of obesity and overweight in communities, as those markets provide access to a wider variety of fresh, healthier food than smaller stores that mainly sell highly processed, packaged foods.[30] However, although fruits and vegetables are an important component of supermarkets worldwide to attract consumers and generate profits, many consumers in low- and middle-income countries continue to rely on street fairs and small shops for their produce and use supermarkets as outlets for foods higher in sugar, salt, and fat.[28]

Accompanying the influx of fast food and supermarkets has been an exponential growth in food marketing and advertising, which creates major shifts in food demand, as marketing leads people to increase their consumption of advertised products.[31] The content of food ads aimed at children especially favors foods of poor nutritional quality.[32]

These factors have led to notable trends in diets in many settings. Intake of added sugars has dramatically increased across the globe over the past 4 decades, largely in the form of sugar-sweetened beverages (SSBs). As national income per capita and the proportion of the population residing in urban areas increases in low- and middle-income countries, sugar intake also increases.[33] Sugar-sweetened beverages are the largest sources of added sugars in the American diet,[34] and in Mexico, around 10 percent of total energy intake in all age groups comes from SSBs.[35]

Consumption of animal products is also increasing, and intake of red and processed meat is associated with weight gain, type II diabetes, heart disease, some cancers, and mortality.[36–40] Between 1989 and 2000, global consumption of foods from animal sources more than tripled in rural areas and almost quadrupled in urban areas.[41] There has been a subsequent decrease in global consumption of whole grains, fruits, and vegetables.[11,42]

At the same time as there has been an increase in energy intake in many settings, there has been a shift in those settings towards increased sedentary work, increased sedentary leisure time involving television or other electronic media, and increased use of motorized transport.[43]

Current guidelines recommend 30 or more minutes of moderate physical activity on most days of the week for the prevention of chronic diseases.[44] Yet, the lack of space for outdoor recreation in dense urban areas and people's fear of urban crime often limits opportunities for physical activity.[45] Additionally, in many low- and middle-income countries, there has been a movement away from jobs with high-energy expenditure such as farming, mining, and forestry, toward employment in less active jobs, including manufacturing and office-based work.[42]

Moreover, there is evidence that as cities expand from a population of 100,000 to 250,000 inhabitants to a population of over 5 million inhabitants, the proportion of travel by foot decreases from 37 percent to 28 percent and by bicycle from 26 percent to 9 percent.[46] Urban living is associated with a decrease in sleep duration, which is associated with weight gain in children and adults.[47] Stress, another risk factor for obesity, could be more common in rapidly urbanizing low- and middle-income countries, due to increased work hours and reduced societal support in comparison with traditional village settings.[43]

Technological advances have also encouraged indoor entertainment via television or computer, instead of outdoor recreation.[25] Time spent watching television has been linked to weight gain in children and adults, and a reduction in sedentary behavior has been shown to have beneficial effects on weight, independent of exercise.[48]

GAUGING NUTRITIONAL STATUS

The nutritional status of infants and children is largely gauged by measuring and weighing these children and then plotting their weight and height on growth charts, like the one shown in **Figure 8-2**. These growth charts have been standardized internationally. The place of the child on the growth curves indicates how the child is growing compared to the international reference standard.

Table 8-3 showed key terms that relate to measures of nutritional status. Among the most important such measures for infants and children are:

- birthweight—a child has a low birthweight if the child's weight at birth is below 2,500 grams
- height-for-age—a child is stunted if its height-for-age is two z-scores below the international reference height-for-age
- weight-for-age—a child is underweight if its weight is two z-scores below the international reference weight-for-age

- weight-for-height—a child is wasted if its weight, measured in kilograms, divided by height, in meters squared, is more than two z-scores below the international reference

We usually think of deficits in nutrition as being large and evident; however, it is extremely important to note that this is not necessarily the case. Rather, a large share of the nutritional deficits that exist globally are mild or moderate and may not be very obvious. Nonetheless, even mild and moderate malnutrition can have very negative consequences on the biological development of people, on their health, and on their productivity, and some of these negative effects may be irreversible.

The nutritional status of adults is generally determined on the basis of a body mass index (BMI). BMI is the body weight in kilograms, divided by height in meters squared. Although some countries have their own standards, generally, an adult is considered:

Underweight if his/her BMI is less than 18.5
Of normal weight if his/her BMI is 18.5 to 25
Overweight if his/her BMI is greater than 25
Obese if his/her BMI is greater than 30.[49]

KEY NUTRITIONAL NEEDS

The Needs of Young Children and Pregnant Women

Many nutrients are important. However, when thinking about the needs of pregnant women and young children, particularly in low- and middle-income countries, several are of paramount importance. These include protein, energy, and the five micronutrients: vitamin A, iron, iodine, zinc, and calcium. This section briefly examines each of these topics, and **Table 8-4** summarizes the sources of these nutrients and their key impacts.

In order to thrive, people have to take in enough energy and micronutrients to fulfill their physiological needs. When this does not happen, undernutrition results. According to UNICEF, undernutrition is defined as "the outcome of insufficient food intake (hunger) and repeated infectious diseases. Undernutrition includes being underweight for one's age, too short for one's age (stunted), dangerously thin for one's height (wasted), and deficient in vitamins and minerals (micronutrient malnutrition)."[50,para.1]

Stunting or chronic undernutrition is the result of cumulative deficiencies in dietary intake (inadequate amounts of energy and micronutrients) and recurrent bouts of infectious diseases.[50] This causes linear growth failure, resulting in low height-for-age.[51]

FIGURE 8-2 Model Growth Chart

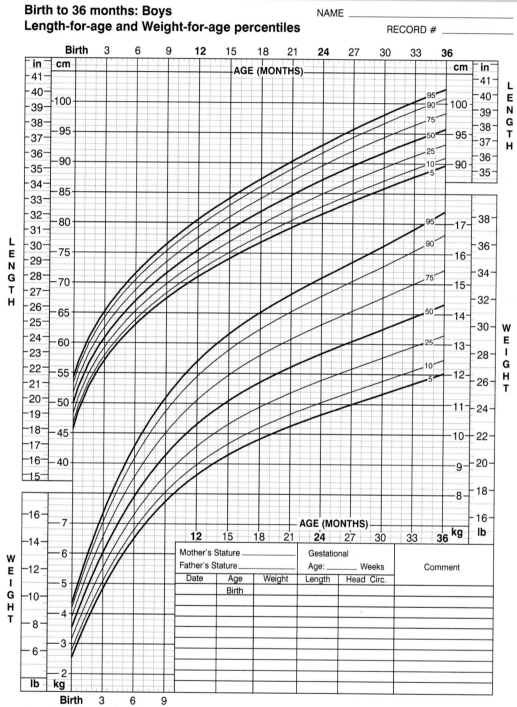

Birth to 36 months: Boys
Length-for-age and Weight-for-age percentiles

NAME _____

RECORD # _____

Published May 30, 2000 (modified 4/20/01).
SOURCE: Developed by the National Center for Health Statistics in collaboration with
the National Center for Chronic Disease Prevention and Health Promotion (2000).
http://www.cdc.gov/growthcharts

TABLE 8-4 Key Nutritional Needs, Sources, and Selected Functions

Key Nutritional Needs	Sources	Selected Functions
Protein	Milk, eggs, chicken, and beans	Proper growth of children and immune functions
Vitamin A	Liver, eggs, green leafy vegetables, orange and red fruits and vegetables	Proper immune function and prevention of xerophthalmia
Calcium	Milk and dairy products; some green leafy vegetables such as broccoli, kale, mustard greens, and bok choy or Chinese cabbage; almonds, Brazil nuts, and beans	Building strong bones and teeth; Clotting blood; Sending and receiving nerve signals; Reduces problems of hypertension in pregnant women
Folic acid	Leafy green vegetables; Fruits; Dried beans, peas, and nuts; Enriched breads, cereals and other grain products	Helps body make new cells and is essential for preventing children being born with neural tube defects
Iodine	Selected seafood and plants grown in iodine-containing soil	Growth and neurological development
Iron	Fish, meat, poultry, grains, vegetables, and legumes	Prevent iron deficiency anemia, prevent low birthweight and premature babies
Zinc	Red and white meat and shellfish	Promote growth, immune function, and cognitive development

Data from the *Journal of Nutrition*. Nutrient information. Retrieved February 8, 2007, from http://jn.nutrition.org/nutinfo/; Bhutta, Z. A., Das, J. K., Rizvi, A., et al. (2013, August 3). Evidence-based intervention for improvement of maternal and child nutrition: what can be done and at what cost? *Lancet, 382*(9890), 452–477; MedlinePlus. (n.d.). *Calcium in diet*. Retrieved May 14, 2015, fromhttp://www.nlm.nih.gov/medlineplus/ency/article/002412.htm; MedlinePlus. (n.d.). *Folic acid*. Retrieved May 14, 2015, from http://www.nlm.nih.gov/medlineplus/folicacid.html.

Underweight or low weight-for-age is a composite measure of being too thin (wasted) and too short (stunted). It is the indicator used in Millennium Development Goal 1 (eradicate extreme poverty and hunger) to measure progress in addressing undernutrition at the individual level.

Wasting is the outcome of weight loss that is often associated with acute shortages of food and infection. Sometimes wasting is related to shocks such as drought or famine. However, wasting can also be a result of substantial acute energy deficits related to other factors that help to determine nutritional status.

Severe acute malnutrition (SAM) is generally defined by a very low weight-for-height measurement of below minus 3 standard deviations of the median WHO growth standards. Severe acute malnutrition is an extreme form of undernutrition. Wasting, including that associated with severe acute malnutrition, needs to be treated as an emergency.[52]

Undernourishment greatly raises the risk of illness, especially for children. In addition, being malnourished in childhood is associated with decreased intellectual capacity. Somewhat ironically, young children who are malnourished but who rapidly gain weight later in childhood and adolescence are at high risk as adults of nutrition-related chronic diseases such as diabetes, high blood pressure, and high cholesterol.[53]

In addition, undernourished women of short stature have greatly increased risks of dying of pregnancy-related causes. Furthermore, undernourished women have a greatly increased risk of delivering premature or low-birthweight babies. Such babies are, in turn, at much greater risk than full-term babies or babies with a birthweight of over 2,500 grams (5.5 pounds) of growing poorly, not developing properly, or dying.[51] More will be said later about the consequences of undernutrition in children and in pregnant women.

Vitamin A

Vitamin A is found in a variety of plants but mostly in green leafy vegetables, yellow and orange fruits that are not citrus, and carrots. It is also found in some animal products, including liver, milk, and eggs.[51] The lack of vitamin A is associated with the development of a condition known as xeropthalmia. The person with this condition first gets "night blindness." Later, the eye dries out, which can lead to permanent blindness.[54]

What is less well known, however, is that vitamin A is extremely important to the proper functioning of the immune system and to a child's growth. Trials of vitamin A supplements on newborns reduced the risk of deaths from infections by 25 percent and from prematurity by about 66 percent.[55] Deficiency in vitamin A has a profound impact on the severity of certain illnesses and whether a child will survive a bout of pneumonia, malaria, measles, or diarrhea.[51]

Iodine

Iodine is generally found in some types of seafood and in plants that are grown in soil that naturally contains iodine.[56] People who live in mountainous areas often do not get enough iodine in their diets, because they do not consume much seafood and mountainous soils often lack iodine. This was the case, for example, for Dorji, in the vignette at the start of this chapter. The lack of iodine is most often associated with a growth on the thyroid, called a goiter, and the failure to develop full intellectual potential.[56] However, iodine deficiency disorders "can also include fetal loss, stillbirth, congenital anomalies, and hearing impairment."[51,p554] In fact, iodine deficiency most often manifests itself in mild intellectual disabilities,[51] and people with cretinism have an IQ that is on average 10 to 15 points below that of people who do not suffer this deficit.[57] In extreme forms, iodine deficiency may also lead to severe mental retardation and being both deaf and mute. In fact, iodine deficiency has been a preventable but, nonetheless, major cause of impaired cognitive development in children.[58]

Iron

The most easily absorbable form of iron is found in fish, meat, and poultry. Less absorbable forms can be found in fruits, grains, vegetables, nuts, and dried beans. The lack of iron is most often associated with iron deficiency anemia, which we usually associate with weakness and fatigue. This is especially a problem for adolescent women and pregnant women, because women who are iron deficient have an increased risk of giving birth to a premature or low birthweight baby or of hemorrhaging and dying in childbirth.[59]

Iron deficiency is also associated with poor mental development and reduced immune function.[51] In addition, iron is a critical requirement for children in the 6- to 24-month age group to ensure optimal development of their cognitive and motor skills.

Zinc

The best sources of zinc are red and white meat and shellfish.[60] Severe deficiency in zinc is associated with "growth retardation, impaired immune function, skin disorders, hypogonadism, and cognitive dysfuncion."[51,p554] Mild to moderate deficiency increases susceptibility to infecion.[51] Indeed, children who receive zinc supplementation when they have diarrhea recover more rapidly than those who do not,[60,61] and zinc deficiency is a major risk factor for morbidity and mortality from diarrhea, pneumonia, and malaria, as discussed later.[51,55]

Folic Acid and Calcium

Folic acid and calcium are especially important for pregnant women and for successful birth outcomes. Folic acid is a B vitamin that helps the body to make new cells. Folic acid is found in leafy green vegetables, some fruits, beans, peas, and nuts, and in enriched products, such as flour. Deficiencies of folic acid in pregnant women are associated with neural tube defects in their children, such as spina bifida.[62] Calcium is generally found in dairy products but can also be gotten from some green leafy vegetables, some fish with small bones, and from some nuts and seeds. Diseases in pregnancy that relate to high blood pressure are among the leading causes of maternal death. Supplementation with calcium has been shown to reduce the risk of hypertensive disorders of pregnancy.[8]

Overweight and Obesity

A balanced, healthy diet is crucial for the prevention of obesity and noncommunicable diseases. A systematic review of dietary recommendations defined by expert panels has identified a number of basic components to a healthy diet, namely vegetables, fruits, whole grains, legumes, and nuts, with limited amounts of red and processed meat.[63] Such a diet provides a high intake of dietary fiber and micronutrients and a low intake of saturated and trans fats, cholesterol, added sugars, and salt.[63] Various dietary components are playing a large role in the growth of global obesity and overweight. These components are elaborated upon next.

Fats

Monounsaturated and polyunsaturated fats, found in nuts, plant-based oils, and fish, are associated with a number of health benefits. They can help reduce levels of bad cholesterol in the blood, lowering risk of heart disease, while also providing essential fats that the body cannot manufacture itself, such as omega-6 and omega-3 fatty acids.[64] On the other hand, saturated and trans fats have been shown to be harmful to cardiovascular health by raising bad cholesterol levels.[65–67] Saturated and trans fats are found largely in red meat and dairy products; trans fats are also prominent in processed foods made with partially hydrogenated oils, used to extend shelf life.

Sodium

High sodium intake can lead to hypertension, which is a major risk factor for stroke and fatal coronary heart disease.[68] Sodium is found in high quantities in restaurant and processed foods.[68] Evidence suggests that limiting sodium intake to no more than 1.7 grams per day is beneficial in reducing blood pressure; this translates to an overall salt intake of less than 5 grams per day.[69]

Added Sugars

Overconsumption of added sugars (this excludes sugars from milk, fruits, and vegetables) threatens the nutritional quality of diets by providing large amounts of energy without supplying specific nutrients, and has been shown to lead to obesity and diabetes.[69] The consumption of sugar-sweetened beverages (SSBs) in particular has been scientifically shown to promote weight gain, type 2 diabetes, and coronary heart disease.[35,70–72] Adults who drink one SSB or more per day are 27 percent more likely to be overweight or obese than nondrinkers, regardless of income or ethnicity.[73] The World Health Organization has called for a reduced daily intake of added sugars to less than 10 percent of total energy intake, amounting to 12 teaspoons of added sugars for a diet of 2,000 calories a day.[74]

Dietary Fiber and Refined Carbohydrates

Dietary fiber, sources of which include whole grains, legumes, fruits, and vegetables, has many potential health benefits, including the prevention of obesity, diabetes, cardiovascular diseases, and various cancers.[69] However, whole grains are often processed to produce refined carbohydrates, which effectively removes the majority of fiber and other nutrients from the grain. Most of what remains is starch, giving a high glycemic index and load, rapidly increasing blood glucose, and increasing the risk of obesity and type II diabetes.[75] Examples of refined carbohydrates include white bread, white pasta, and white rice. Studies have shown that for each incremental serving of white rice per day, the type II diabetes

risk increases by 11 percent; the risk is more evident in overweight and obese individuals.[76,77]

NUTRITIONAL NEEDS THROUGHOUT THE LIFE COURSE

Nutritional needs vary with one's place in the life course. Having outlined some of the most important nutritional needs that concern global health issues, therefore, it will now be valuable to examine how those needs change from pregnancy, through infancy, childhood, adolescence, adulthood, and old age. This will assist us in getting a better understanding of the nature of the nutrition problems globally, the burden of disease related to nutrition, and how this burden might be addressed.

Pregnancy and Birthweight

The nutritional status of a pregnant woman is especially important to the outcome that she will have in pregnancy, both for herself and for her newborn. It is critical that a pregnant woman stay well nourished and healthy. During pregnancy, the woman will need to get a sufficient amount of protein and energy from the food she eats, and it is generally recommended that she consume 300 calories more per day than when she is not pregnant. In addition, iron, iodine, folate, zinc, and calcium will be very important to the health of the woman and her newborn.[78]

The birthweight of a baby is an extremely important determinant of the extent to which a child will thrive and become a healthy adult. Fetuses that do not get sufficient and appropriate nutrition from the mother may suffer a number of problems, including stillbirth, mental impairment, or a variety of severe birth defects. They could also undergo a general failure to grow properly, referred to as intrauterine growth retardation. Babies who are born at term but who are low birthweight have a much greater risk of getting diarrhea and pneumonia than babies born above 2,500 grams. Those born with a birthweight from 1,500 to 1,999 grams are 8 times more likely to die from birth asphyxia and infections than those born with a birthweight of 2,000 to 2,499 grams.[55]

Infancy and Young Childhood

An important share of a child's biological development takes place between conception and 2 years of age. This period is often called the "window of opportunity." It is essential to understand that nutritional gaps that arise during this period may produce problems in stature or mental development that may never be overcome. They may also lead to more frequent infection and infections that last longer than would be the case in a better-nourished child. Thus, it is extraordinarily important that infants and young children get a sufficient amount of protein, energy, and fat from their foods. They also need sufficient amounts of iodine, iron, vitamin A, and zinc.

There is very strong evidence worldwide that infants will grow best and stay healthiest if they are exclusively breastfed for the first 6 months of their lives. In fact, it has been estimated that in 2011 about 800,000 deaths a year, or almost 15 percent of all child deaths, were associated with suboptimal breastfeeding.[3] Children will also thrive best if foods other than breast milk or infant formula begin to be introduced in hygienic ways around 6 months of age, while breastfeeding continues.[79] Especially in low-income countries in which nutritional deficits are likely to be considerable, such foods will be especially valuable if they are fortified with key vitamins and minerals.

The nutrition needs of the infant continue into young childhood, but the nutritional status of many children faces risks as the child stops breastfeeding, as noted earlier. At this stage, the child's nutritional status depends on the ability of the family to provide an adequate diet and to help the child avoid illnesses and infections. Among the most critical issues concerning childhood nutrition is that stunted children have very little chance to catch up in their growth and that most of the damage done to their development, both physical and mental, cannot be changed.[80]

This fact has enormous implications for public policy aimed at enhancing nutrition status. It means that the focus of attention in addressing undernutrition and its consequences must be on children from conception to 2 years of age, and it must start by trying to ensure that pregnant women are well nourished and healthy enough to give birth to healthy babies of acceptable birthweight. As previously noted, there is a window of opportunity for ensuring that children grow properly and reach their biological potential. This window opens at conception and closes, at least most of the way, around the time the child is 2 years of age.[57]

Adolescence

Adolescent girls who are well nourished grow faster than adolescent girls who are not well nourished. Adolescent girls who are poorly nourished, but still growing, are much more likely than well-nourished girls to give birth to an underweight baby. This may stem from the fact that the fetus and the girl are competing for nutrients in the adolescent who is still growing.[79] Poorly nourished and very small adolescent girls also have more complications of pregnancy than do older girls who are taller. This relates partly to the difficulties of very small women giving birth, because of their

size. In addition, all adolescents go through a growth spurt, although children who are stunted are unable to make up in adolescence for their retarded growth. For adolescents to grow properly and become healthy adults, they need appropriate protein and energy. They also have particular needs for iodine, iron, and folic acid. Because of their growth during this period, calcium is also especially important for adolescents.[79]

Adulthood and Old Age

Adults need appropriate, well-balanced nutrition to stay healthy and productive. All people, including adults, also need to pay particular attention in their diets to foods that can be harmful to their health, such as foods that contain too much fat, cholesterol, sugar, or salt. Older adults have special nutritional needs that are very important but often forgotten. The ability of older people to live on their own and to function effectively depends in many ways on their nutritional status; however, many older people lack the income or the support needed to eat properly. Like other adults, they need to get enough protein, energy, and iron and avoid obesity. They also have to pay particular attention to getting enough calcium to reduce the risk of osteoporosis, which is a condition in which bones become fragile and can break.[81]

THE NUTRITIONAL STATE OF THE WORLD

Undernutrition

There has been important progress in reducing the burden of undernutrition over the last 2 decades. The most recent estimates suggest, for example, that the rate of underweight in children younger than 5 years of age in low- and middle-income countries fell from about 28 percent in 1990 to about 17 percent in 2011.[2] In addition, a number of countries, including Bangladesh, China, Indonesia, Mexico, and Vietnam, made especially rapid progress in reducing levels of undernutrition in their under-5 children over that period.[82] Important progress has been made in addressing micronutrient deficiencies as well. The number of households using iodized salt, for example, has increased from about 20 percent in 1990 to about 80 percent today.[5] There has also been a dramatic increase in the share of the world's children who receive vitamin A supplements, which now stands above 70 percent in almost all low- and middle-income countries.[5]

Despite this progress, a large number of pregnant women and children in the world are undernourished. About 100 million children globally suffer from moderate or severe underweight, about 165 million are stunted, and more than 50 million are wasted.[2] Many poor women in the world are also underweight. A large share of the poor women and children in the world also suffer from deficiencies in important micronutrients. Nutritional problems remain a fundamental cause of ill health and of premature death for infants, children, and pregnant women. The economic costs of undernutrition are great. The section that follows examines the burden of nutrition disorders that relate to undernutrition and reviews undernutrition as a risk factor for ill health and death.

Low Birthweight

Figure 8-3 presents data on low birthweight, which refers to babies born under 2,500 grams. Unfortunately, the data are incomplete. It is also for some, but not all, UNICEF regions. Given the extent of undernutrition in South Asia, it should not be a surprise that almost 30 percent of the babies born in South Asia are born with low birthweight. Sub-Saharan Africa has the next highest prevalence of low birthweight, at about 12 percent.[83]

More than 100 million children under 5 years of age, or about 16 percent of the children younger than 5 years of age globally, were moderately or severely underweight in 2011.[2] As shown in **Figure 8-4** the regional rates of underweight vary from 1.5 percent in the Americas to about 25 percent in Africa and about 47 percent in South-East Asia.

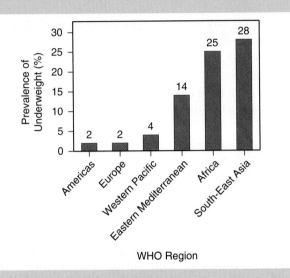

FIGURE 8-4 Prevalence of Underweight in Children Under 5 Years of Age, by WHO Region, 2011

Data from UNICEF, WHO, and The World Bank. Levels & Trends in Child Malnutrition: Joint Child Malnutrition Estimates. 2012. Accessed May 10, 2015. http://www.who.int/nutgrowthdb/jme_unicef_who_wb.pdf.

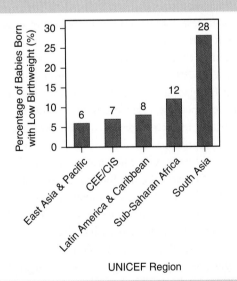

FIGURE 8-3 Prevalence of Low Birthweight, by UNICEF Region, 2007–2011

Note: CEE/CIS stands for Central and Eastern Europe and the Commonwealth of Independent States; No data available for the region Middle East & North Africa.
Data from UNICEF. Improving Child Nutrition: the achievable imperative for global progress. 2013. http://data.unicef.org/corecode/uploads/document6/uploaded_pdfs/corecode/NutritionReport_April2013_Final_29.pdf. Accessed May 6, 2015.

Wasting

In addition to the large number of children who are underweight, it is estimated that about 51 million children globally are moderately or severely wasted.[2] This would be equal to about 8 percent of all of the under-5 children globally. **Figure 8-5** shows the rates of wasting by WHO region. The South-East Asia region of WHO has the highest rates of wasting by a substantial margin but the Africa and Eastern Mediterranean regions also have very high rates of wasting among children under 5 years of age.

Stunting

Almost 165 million children were also estimated in 2011 to be stunted globally.[2] This was just over a quarter of all under-5 children. As shown in **Figure 8-6** About 40 percent of all children under 5 in the WHO Africa region suffered from moderate or severe stunting in 2011, as did about 35 percent of the under-5 children in the South-East Asia region. More than a quarter of the under-5 children in the Eastern Mediterranean region also suffered from stunting.[2]

Selected Micronutrient Deficiencies

Table 8-5 provides information on the prevalence of deficiencies in vitamin A, zinc, iodine, and iron. Some of the

FIGURE 8-5 Prevalence of Wasting in Children Under 5 Years of Age, by WHO Region, 2011

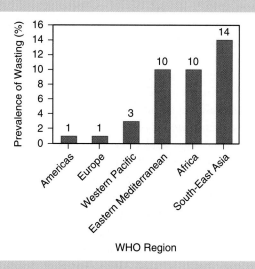

WHO Region

Data from UNICEF, WHO, and The World Bank. Levels & Trends in Child Malnutrition: Joint Child Malnutrition Estimates. 2012. Accessed May 10, 2015. http://www.who.int/nutgrowthdb/jme_unicef_who_wb.pdf.

FIGURE 8-6 Prevalence of Stunting in Children Under 5 Years of Age, by WHO Region, 2011

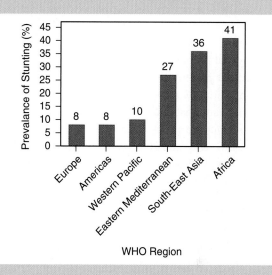

WHO Region

Data from UNICEF, WHO, and The World Bank. Levels & Trends in Child Malnutrition: Joint Child Malnutrition Estimates. 2012. Accessed May 10, 2015. http://www.who.int/nutgrowthdb/jme_unicef_who_wb.pdf.

TABLE 8-5 Selected Micronutrient Deficiencies, by UN Region

Region	Prevalence of Vitamin A Deficiency (%)		Prevalence of Zinc Deficiency (%)	Prevalence of Iodine Deficiency (%)	Prevalence of Iron Deficiency Anemia (%)	
	Children < 5	Pregnant Women	Overall	Overall	Children < 5	Pregnant Women
Africa	41.6	14.3	23.9	40.0	20.2	20.3
Americas & Caribbean	15.6	2.0	9.6	13.7	12.7	15.2
Asia	33.5	18.4	19.4	31.6	19.0	19.8
Europe	14.9	2.2	7.6	44.2	12.1	16.2
Oceania	12.6	1.4	5.7	17.3	15.4	17.2

Note: Vitamin A deficiency definition used is serum retinol < 0.70 μmol/L (1995–2005); zinc deficiency defined as inadequate zinc intake and is determined from a weighted average of country means (2005); iodine deficiency defined as urine iodine concentration < 100 μg/L (2013); iron deficiency anemia defined as hemoglobin < 110 g/L (2011).

Data from Black, R. E., et al. "Maternal and child undernutrition and overweight in low-income and middle-income countries." *The Lancet* 382(9890): 427–451.

information is on children under 5 years of age and pregnant women, some is only on under-5 children, and the zinc data are for all age groups. The data are arranged by UN region.

Africa and Asia have the highest rates of deficiency of vitamin A, zinc, and iron. Europe has the highest rate of iodine deficiency. Given the importance of vitamin A and zinc to overall immune functions, it is of great concern that more than 40 percent of the under-5 children in the Africa region and about 33 percent in the Asia region are deficient in vitamin A and that about 24 and 20 percent of the people in those regions are at risk of zinc deficiency. It is also striking that between 10 and 20 percent of under-5 children and between 15 and 20 percent of all pregnant women are iron deficient in all regions.

Deaths Associated with Undernutrition

Only a small share of the deaths of under-5 children globally are a direct result of undernutrition.[1] However, undernutrition, as discussed earlier, is an exceptionally important risk factor for illness, disability, and death from other causes, including diarrhea, pneumonia, measles, and other communicable diseases.[3] In addition, anemia is a risk factor for more than 25 percent of maternal deaths and calcium deficiencies contribute to maternal death from preeclampsia.[3]

As noted earlier, about 45 percent, or 3 million under-5 child deaths a year, can be attributed to nutrition-related causes. This is estimated to be the total number of deaths related to the joint effects of fetal growth restriction, suboptimal breastfeeding, stunting, underweight, wasting, and vitamin A and zinc deficiencies. About 1.3 million of these deaths are attributable to the joint effects of just fetal growth restriction and suboptimal breastfeeding. About 875,000 deaths are attributable to wasting and 1 million to stunting underweight. Zinc and Vitamin A deficiencies are thought to be associated with about 116,000 and 157,000 under-5 child deaths a year, respectively. Fetal growth restriction is related to low birthweight, as discussed earlier, for babies carried to term. Clearly, any efforts to reduce child deaths will have to focus on addressing these issues, which are so fundamental to whether children survive and thrive.[3]

Overweight and Obesity

Once considered a problem unique to high-income Western countries, obesity is now a major contributor to the global burden of disease, affecting people of all ages and incomes around the world.[25,84] Today, 2.1 billion people, nearly 30 percent of the world's population, are obese or overweight.[85] In fact, worldwide obesity has nearly doubled since 1980.[86] According to the World Health Organization, overweight

and obesity are also responsible for 44 percent of the diabetes burden, 23 percent of the ischemic heart disease burden, and between 7 percent and 41 percent of certain cancer burdens.[87] Low- and middle-income countries, including sub-Saharan Africa, India, parts of southeast Asia, China, and most of South America, now carry the majority of the obesity and chronic disease burden, and are predicted to continue to do so for some time.[88] See **Figure 8-7**.

Among the world's adult population, 37 percent is overweight or obese, representing a 27.5 percent increase since 1980.[85] Broken down by sex, the worldwide proportion of overweight and obese adults has increased from 28.8 percent to 36.9 percent in men and from 29.8 percent to 38.0 percent in women.[85] As seen in Figure   8, women have higher rates of obesity than men in all of the WHO regions. Of note, an obesity prevalence of over 50 percent is seen for both men and women in Tonga and for women in Kuwait, Kiribati, the Federated States of Micronesia, Libya, Qatar, and Samoa.[85] Of all countries in sub-Saharan Africa, women in South Africa have the highest obesity rates, at 42 percent.[85] See **Figure 8-8**.

Childhood obesity has emerged as one of the most serious public health challenges of the 21st century in part

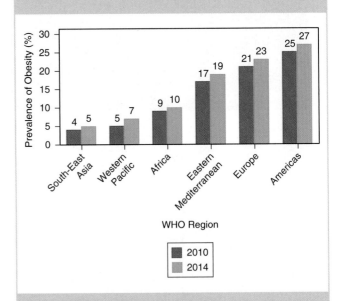

FIGURE 8-7 Prevalence of Obesity in Adults, 2010 and 2014, by WHO Region

Note: Obesity: BMI ≥ 30; Age-standardized estimates
Data from WHO. Global Health Observatory Data Repository: Obesity (bodymassindex>=30) (age-standardized estimate) Data by WHO Region. http://apps.who.int/gho/data/view .main.2480A?lang=en. Accessed May 6, 2015.

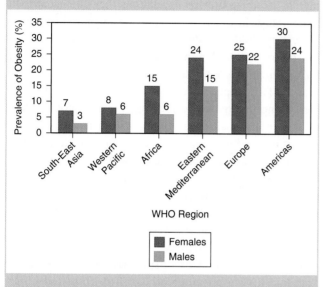

FIGURE 8-8 Prevalence of Obesity in Adults, by Sex and WHO Region, 2014

Note: Obesity: BMI ≥ 30; Age-standardized estimates
Data from WHO. Global Health Observatory Data Repository: Obesity (bodymassindex>=30) (age-standardized estimate) Data by WHO Region. http://apps.who.int/gho/data/view .main.2480A?lang=en. Accessed May 8, 2015.

because it tends to continue into adulthood, increasing the risk of chronic diseases later in life.[44,89] Among children and adolescents, worldwide obesity and overweight have increased by 47.1 percent since 1980.[85] According to the World Health Organization, an estimated 43 million children globally were overweight or obese in 2010, and 35 million of these children were living in low- and middle-income countries.[90] In high-income countries, 23.8 percent of boys and 22.6 percent of girls were overweight or obese in 2013.[85] Prevalence of childhood overweight and obesity in low- and middle-countries has also increased, from 8.1 percent in 1980 to 12.9 percent in 2013 for boys and from 8.4 percent to 13.4 percent in girls.[85] The increase in childhood obesity has occurred more rapidly than adult rates in several countries, including the United States, Brazil, and China.[11] Particularly high rates of child and adolescent obesity are seen in Middle Eastern and North African countries, especially among girls.[85] See **Figure 8-9** for data on under-5 overweight, including obesity.

In terms of individual countries, the United States has the highest proportion of the world's obese people (13 percent), whereas China and India together represent 15 percent of the world's obese population. Countries in the Middle East

FIGURE 8-9 Prevalence of Overweight, Including Obesity, in Children Under 5 Years of Age, by WHO Region, 1990 and 2011

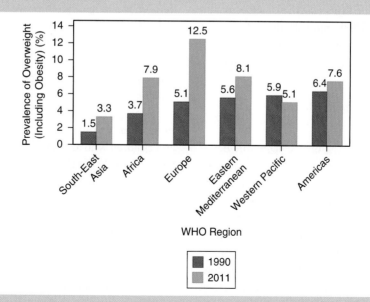

Data from UNICEF, WHO, and The World Bank. Levels & Trends in Child Malnutrition: Joint Child Malnutrition Estimates. 2012. Accessed May 10, 2015. http://www.who.int/nutgrowthdb/jme _unicef_who_wb.pdf

and North Africa, Central America, and island nations in the Pacific and Caribbean have extremely high rates of overweight and obesity, at 44 percent or higher. In terms of world regions, the highest rates of overweight and obesity overall in 2013 were seen in the Middle East and North Africa, where more than 58 percent of men and 65 percent of women were overweight or obese. In Central America, more than 57 percent of adult men and more than 65 percent of adult women were overweight or obese, with the highest prevalence (greater than 50 percent among both men and women) found in Colombia, Costa Rica, and Mexico. In the Pacific Islands, nearly 44 percent of men and more than 51 percent of women are overweight or obese, and in the Caribbean, 38 percent of men and more than 50 percent of women are overweight or obese.[85]

Although the overall prevalence of overweight and obesity has increased worldwide over the last 30 years, there have been large variations in rates. In high-income countries, increases in obesity began in the 1980s, accelerated from 1992 to 2002, and have slowed since 2006. Middle Eastern countries such as Saudi Arabia, Bahrain, Egypt, Kuwait, and Palestine are experiencing some of the largest worldwide increases in obesity.[85] Over the next 2 decades, the largest proportional increase in overweight and obesity will likely occur in low- and middle-income countries, with predicted increases of 62 to 205 percent for overweight and 71 to 263 percent for obesity.[88]

Obesity and overweight are among the leading risks for global deaths and are responsible for around 3.4 million adult deaths annually, 3.9 percent of years of life lost, and 3.8 percent of disability-adjusted life years (DALYs).[85] Obesity and overweight are now responsible for more deaths globally than underweight. They are also responsible for more deaths than underweight in all high-income and most middle-income countries.[87]

NUTRITION, HEALTH, AND ECONOMIC DEVELOPMENT

Nutrition has an important bearing on the economic development prospects of people, communities, and countries. In some of the early thinking about economic development, many economists saw nutrition as something that people consumed, but they did not see it as a productive investment. However, as we will see later, nutrition is an extremely important contributor to human health and the development of human intellectual and biological potential. It, therefore, has an extremely important link with what people learn, their strength and ability to use their own labor, and other factors relating to their potential productivity. The following comments follow the life course.

First, nutritional deficits can take an enormous toll on maternal health, with important economic consequences. Women are responsible for child care in most low- and middle-income countries. In addition, they often contribute to household income. The death of a woman in the prime of her life, in childbirth, due to undernutrition or deficiencies in iron or vitamin A, can leave poor families with reduced income and needs for child care they cannot meet. It is common, in fact, in poor families in low-income countries for very young children to die not long after their mothers die.

The nutritional status of a woman can also have a major impact on the birthweight of a child and the child's future nutritional status and can lead to neural tube defects.[91] A number of forms of malnutrition contribute to the failure of infants and children to grow or to achieve their full mental potential. Children who are undernourished and small in stature enroll in schools at lower rates or later in age than students who are perceived by their parents to be normal in size. Children who are undernourished have IQs that are lower than students who are properly nourished. These undernourished students are less attentive in class and less able to learn than other students. Children who are undernourished fall ill more than well-nourished children. Thus, they miss more school, learn less from school, and are much more likely than well-nourished children to drop out of school, with its attendant economic consequences.

Nutritional status also plays an important part in the productivity of adults. Numerous studies have shown that improvements in nutritional status, such as eliminating iron deficiency anemia, can improve worker productivity by 5–15 percent.[92] The contribution of nutrition to maintaining good health also has important economic returns. It helps people to avoid disease and the costs associated with treating disease. These points are well illustrated by the policy and program brief on Guatemala later in the chapter.

Moreover, through its impact on health, nutritional status also has an important bearing on life expectancy. Infants and children who are better nourished live longer than those who are poorly nourished, and they also can contribute to the economy for longer. Adults who are properly nourished get sick less and for shorter periods, live longer, and work more years than adults who are not well nourished. Thus, they, too, can make more contributions to the economy than people who are not well nourished.

A look at social and economic history also speaks to the importance of nutrition to economic development. Studies that have been done of the economic development of England showed that improvements in nutritional status of adults in England in the late 19th century were important to improving the stature and strength of workers, their health, and their economic outputs.[93] Other studies have shown that there is a correlation between height and wages. Rubber tappers in Indonesia significantly improved the amount of rubber they could tap when their anemia was treated with iron supplements, and road construction workers in Kenya were 4–12.5 percent more productive after getting calorie supplements.[94] Female mill workers in China increased their production efficiency by 17 percent after being given iron supplements for 12 weeks.[95] A major review of nutrition by the World Bank noted that reducing micronutrient deficiencies in China and India could increase their gross domestic product (GDP) by $2.5 billion per year.[57] Other studies have shown that losses from deficiencies in individual micronutrients can cost 1–2 percent of GDP and that losses from stunting can be as high as 8–10 percent of GDP.[91]

Obesity and overweight also take an immense toll on society. First, obesity and overweight are extremely detrimental to health, with economic consequences for individuals and society at large. Obesity and overweight are major risk factors for morbidity and mortality from many noncommunicable diseases, including cardiovascular disease, type II diabetes, hypertension, musculoskeletal disorders, and some forms of cancer, including endometrial, breast, and colon cancer.[96-98] Obesity and its associated comorbidities have high medical costs that can trap poor households in cycles of debt and illness, exacerbating poverty and perpetuating health and economic inequalities, especially in low- and middle-income countries.[99]

These costs can also be crippling on a national scale. In the United States, 5 to 10 percent of all medical spending is used for obesity-related health care, costing $190 billion annually, and over 25 percent of these costs are paid through public expenditures.[100,101] Expenditures in India and China are rapidly increasing.[102] From 2012 to 2030, diabetes and cardiovascular disease are projected to cost India $2.4 trillion and China $8.74 trillion.[103] It is possible that these costs will overwhelm the health system of China and slow China's economic growth.[11]

Overweight and obesity also affect worker productivity, further burdening society with a loss in economic production. Obese employees are more likely to have higher levels of absenteeism than their lean counterparts due to more health problems.[104] Higher staff turnover and lost earnings due to premature death from obesity-related diseases also result in a loss of worker productivity.[105] It is estimated that between 2006 and 2015, $84 billion in economic production will have been lost in low- and middle-income countries due to obesity and its related chronic diseases.[106] The cumulative cost of decreased productivity and increased health care due to noncommunicable diseases (NCDs), for which overweight and obesity are leading risk factors, was estimated to be about $1.4 trillion globally in 2010.[107] Over the next 2 decades, cardiovascular disease, chronic respiratory disease, cancer, diabetes, and mental health will be responsible for a cumulative output loss of $47 trillion. This loss represents 75 percent of global GDP in 2010.[108]

Finally, obesity can have significant effects on mental health, which can be especially harmful to children and their academic achievement.[109] Obesity and overweight have been shown to cause low self-esteem, anxiety, depression, poor body image, and suicidal thoughts and actions. Bias and bullying in schools, along with their emotional consequences, can seriously hinder academic achievement for overweight and obese children and adolescents. Obese adolescents are less likely to attend college or attain a degree, thus preventing them from earning as much money later in life and setting them up for a cycle of illness and debt as they age.[110]

POLICY AND PROGRAM BRIEFS

Six policy and program briefs follow. The first describes the impressive efforts that Nepal has undertaken to address micronutrient deficiencies, despite being a very poor country. The second discusses an effort in Kenya to launch a flour fortification effort in an exceptionally short period of time, despite many years of not having done so previously. The third brief illustrates the long-term impact of nutrition supplementation. It reviews the findings of a study on Guatemala that examined the long-term impact of improved nutrition on the stature, intellectual abilities, and wages of adults. The fourth discusses South Korea's efforts to encourage the maintenance of traditional diets. The fifth reviews a program in Brazil for encouraging physical activity. The last examines efforts by Finland to reduce salt consumption.

Nepal Addresses Micronutrient Deficiencies

Many Nepali families lack the income needed to consistently buy nutrient-rich foods. Many families also lack the knowledge of a healthy diet needed to ensure their children are well nourished. These issues have resulted in high rates of undernutrition and micronutrient deficiencies, particularly in women and children.[111]

In the 1990s, for example, more than half of the under-5 children in Nepal were stunted.[111,112] In addition, nearly 75 percent of pregnant women and over half of all children were anemic. The coverage of nutritional programs was low. Many pregnant women did not receive iron and folic acid supplements,[111] and there was little fortification of food.

More recently, however, Nepal has become a leader in addressing micronutrient deficiencies. To address anemia, the government initiated the National Anemia Control Strategy and Iron Intensification Program in 2003, with support from WHO, UNICEF, and the Micronutrient Initiative. This program provides iron supplements for pregnant women distributed by female community health volunteers, in addition to deworming services, maternal care, and fortified foods. A monitoring system was established to identify pregnant women as soon as possible and to ensure that women fully participate in the recommended services.

In addition, the United States Agency for International Development (USAID) and the Ministry of Health collaborated to integrate zinc into the national diarrhea management plan. In 2006, only 0.4 percent of caregivers provided zinc during any bout of diarrhea in the previous 2 weeks. To increase the use of both oral rehydration therapy (ORT) and zinc when treating diarrheal disease, USAID has supported training for private sector healthcare providers. In addition, efforts were undertaken to increase the availability of zinc in the private sector. Linked with these efforts, public and private sector programs to increase the use of zinc reached 65 percent of the population by 2009.[112] The Micronutrient Initiative has also helped the government to improve popular knowledge and awareness about zinc through local radio advertising, the delivery of zinc in the public and private sectors, and has helped to strengthen the monitoring and reporting system for zinc usage and the zinc supply chain.[113]

Vitamin A tablets are being distributed to children twice a year to help enhance children's immunity, prevent night blindness, and reduce morbidity and mortality from measles, pneumonia, and diarrhea. The Micronutrient Initiative has also helped the government to pilot a vitamin A supplementation program for newborns.[113]

Community health worker volunteers (CHWV), usually women who live in the community, play an important role in implementing these programs. They administer the needed supplements in their communities, recording the children or women who receive the supplements. Additionally, the CHWVs spend time educating parents, particularly women, on nutrition topics such as the importance of eating nutrient-rich foods and micronutrient supplements, good hygiene habits, and breastfeeding.[114] Nongovernmental organizations (NGOs) have played an important role in addressing issues related to micronutrient deficiencies by helping to train CHWVs to perform the tasks mentioned previously.[114]

The collaborative efforts of the government, NGOs, community volunteers, and Nepal's development partners have led to a number of successes. By 2009, over 80 percent of pregnant women were receiving iron and folic acid supplements, and anemia had dropped 35 percent among these women. The usage of zinc had increased from less than 1 percent in 2005 to nearly 16 percent in 2008, with 85 percent of users correctly taking zinc and oral rehydration salts together, and 67 percent correctly taking zinc for the recommended 10 full days.[114] By 2009, there was also 95 percent coverage of vitamin A supplementation among children.[111] Linked to these efforts on micronutrient supplementation, among other programs, Nepal saw a decrease in mortality of children under the age of 5 from 142 per 1,000 in 1990 to 51 per 1,000 in 2009.[113]

Nepal has demonstrated that it is possible for a country with limited finances to carry out cost-effective programs to address micronutrient deficiencies with substantial results. This has been achieved in Nepal largely through strong political support, the use of community health worker volunteers, effective spread of knowledge about the importance of micronutrients, and careful program supervision and monitoring. It has also been assisted by close collaboration with a number of Nepal's development partners.

Rapid Results Initiative for Food Fortification in Kenya

For many years, African countries have fortified salt with iodine and have even made salt fortification a requirement. However, progress on food fortification in the Africa region has been relatively slow and in 2011 there were no requirements in the region for the fortification of other foods. This is despite the substantial nutritional gaps in Africa that could be addressed at least partly through fortification.[115]

Until recently, Kenya was among the countries that had successfully fortified salt but had not fortified other staple foods. The failure to move on fortification stemmed at least partly from difficulty in getting the public and private sectors to work together on fortification. In order for fortification to succeed, these parties must collaborate, because both play an important role in food fortification. The public sector is responsible for food safety. The private sector is responsible for producing and selling the fortified foods.[116]

The Kenyan National Food Fortification Alliance (KNFFA) was established to mobilize food companies and government organizations to fortify foods.[116] Initially, the process proved to be slow and little progress was made. Food companies felt that the government would not create and monitor food standards and the government felt that food companies would not willingly fortify foods.

To help overcome these barriers, the KNFFA leadership decided to collaborate with the Micronutrient Initiative (MI) and the Rapid Results Institute (RRI) to produce a fortified food in 100 days or less. The MI is a nonprofit organization based in Canada that is the leading global agency focusing exclusively on addressing micronutrient deficiencies, particularly in poor women and children in low-income countries. The RRI is a nonprofit organization that focuses on helping countries achieve rapid and sustainable results in key areas of health, education, water supply, and related social investments.

In order to move ahead on a fortification program, the stakeholders were brought together to address concerns surrounding food fortification, such as quality standards and standard enforcement, and to invite participation in the project. Second, a training meeting was held for stakeholders, such as food companies and government organizations. During this time, goals were set: in 130 days, a fortified food certification process would be developed and three brands of edible oils would be fortified with vitamin A.[115,116]

Through this effort, Kenya was able to meet its goal and achieve in a very short amount of time what it had not been able to do at all previously. By the end of the 130 days, three brands of oil, or 15 percent of the edible oil market, met international standards for vitamin A fortification in edible oils. Additionally, fortification standards, a fortification certification process, and a fortification logo, which can be put on a product to show that it meets standards, were developed.[116] The Kenya Bureau of Standards monitors food fortification standards and the Ministry of Health now regulates the certification process.[116] As a result of the initiative, there has been increased collaboration and trust between the public and private sectors, laying the foundation for future fortification of additional staple foods.

Childhood Nutrition Supplementation and Adult Productivity in Guatemala

A number of countries have undertaken efforts to provide supplementary food to undernourished children. Some of those programs, such as the Tamil Nadu Nutrition Project, have been evaluated carefully. However, very rarely has anyone followed for more than 2 decades the children who participated in a supplementary feeding program in order to gauge long-term program impact in adulthood. One such study was done for a program in Guatemala, as described in this section.

In four Guatemalan villages between March 1, 1969, and February 28, 1977, the Institute of Nutrition of Central America and Panama (INCAP) initiated the first phase of a study on nutrition supplementation and child development among 2,392 children who were under the age of 7. Researchers randomly assigned one of two treatments to each of the children. In two villages, children were offered a dietary supplement called "atole" that provided protein and energy. This supplement consisted of dry skim milk, Incaparina (a protein mixture), and sugar. In the other two villages, children were offered a supplement called "fresco." Unlike atole, fresco did not provide fat or protein and offered only minimal energy. Both supplements were equally fortified with micronutrients before being distributed twice daily from a central location in each village.[117]

The study followed the cohort of children over time and compared the effects of the nutritional supplement on schooling, adult intellectual functioning, child birthweight, and individual productivity. As part of this effort, between 2002 and 2004—25 years after the nutrition supplementation ended—researchers, in collaboration with Emory University, surveyed 1,448 of those who participated in the original study as children.[117] In order to measure literacy and reading comprehension, the InterAmerican Series Test was used. The Raven Progressive Matrices Test was used to determine cognitive development.

Children who had received the supplement of protein and energy, atole, scored higher on both tests as adults than those who received fresco. Among men, there was no significant relationship between the type of supplement taken and the amount of school completed. However, women who received atole completed 1.2 more years of school than the other women.[53] Overall, after controlling for the number of years of school completed, it was found that receiving the atole supplement was positively related for both men and women to higher adult intellectual functioning.[117]

Researchers also examined the relationship between economic productivity of individuals, measured through their wages, and which of the supplements was given in the INCAP nutrition intervention. Boys who were under the age of 3 when they first received atole had 46 percent higher wages as adults, compared to the boys who received fresco in the original study. There was no significant increase in economic productivity in women who received one supplement, compared to the other group.[118]

However, a girl's involvement in the INCAP intervention positively affected her offspring. Compared to those who received fresco, women who had received atole as children were found to have babies, especially sons, with a higher birthweight, a larger head circumference, and a greater height at birth. Additionally, their offspring had greater height-for-age and weight-for-age.[119]

Overall, this study has helped to shed light on the value of nutritional supplementation among children. The protein- and energy-based atole nutritional supplement resulted in higher literacy rates and cognitive development among men and women, higher employment wages for men, and offspring with a higher birthweight. This study further supports the premise that some forms of food supplementation in the early years of life can affect the remaining years of life in substantial and positive ways.

South Korea's Promotion of and Adherence to a Traditional Diet

South Korea's economy grew rapidly after its recovery from the Korean War (1950–1953).[120] This growth was accompanied by changes in lifestyle, including the rapid introduction of a more Western diet; fast-food restaurants in particular were popular among the younger generation, especially after the country hosted the Olympics in 1988.[121] A transition in the cause of death from communicable to noncommunicable diseases is estimated to have occurred in South Korea around 1970, compared with 1940 for the United States and 1950 for Japan.[122]

Unlike other Asian countries, however, South Korea maintained many of the aspects of its low-fat, high-vegetable traditional diet through its economic and nutrition transition. Based on its level of economic development, a 1998 dietary evaluation found that South Korea had lower than expected levels of fat intake (by 16.7 percentage points) and obesity prevalence, found to be largely due to government programs encouraging the retention of the traditional South Korean diet.[120]

The Korea Dietetic Association (KDA), a private organization, provided nutrition education through seminars and obesity camps, aided nutrition services at local health centers, and offered nutrition information for citizens on its website.[120] The KDA also monitored food and nutrition advertising disseminated through mass media and organized national nutrition campaigns.[120] The association also provided a variety of traditional menus to elementary schools, along with letters about preserving traditional dietary culture to students' homes. It also held lectures for parents.[123]

The combination of these efforts led to a retention of the traditional Korean diet and subsequent positive health outcomes. Vegetable consumption in South Korea was among the highest in Asia in 1998, comprising around 20 percent of total food consumption (280 grams daily per capita).[120] Kimchi remained the most consumed food after rice, accounting for approximately 40 percent of the total vegetable intake.[124] In addition, the daily per capita intake of fruits in South Korea increased significantly during the economic transition period; the increase was especially rapid in the 1990s. In 1998, 197.5 grams of fruits were consumed daily per capita,

more than a tenfold increase from the 18.9 grams consumed in 1970.[120]

Daily per capita fat intake in South Korea more than doubled from 16.9 grams in 1969 to 41.5 grams in 1998, and animal fat increased from 30.6 percent of total fat consumed in 1970 to 48.2 percent in 1998.[120] However, the proportion of fat-derived energy was still significantly lower than in other Asian countries, in part due to a traditional cooking style involving small amounts of oil.[121] Furthermore, the majority of meat consumed was cooked in a Korean style, as opposed to a Western style, and was typically accompanied by vegetables.[120]

Obesity rates in South Korea in 1998 remained quite low, at 1.7 percent for men and 3.0 percent for women. These rates were much lower than Western and other Asian countries.[120] Obesity rates in Korea today remain among the lowest in the Organisation for Economic Co-operation and Development (OECD), at 4 percent of the adult population. However, 30 percent of the population is overweight, and OECD projections indicate that rates of overweight will increase by a further 5 percent within 10 years.[125]

Through this initiative, South Korea has demonstrated the potential for effective public/private collaboration in the pursuit of a healthy diet. Using a combination of information dissemination and provision of skills, the country was able to adapt its message to contemporary society and successfully retain its traditional diet, preventing the spread of obesity.

Brazil: The Agita São Paulo Program Uses Physical Activity to Promote Health

Starting in the 1970s, Brazil began experiencing rapid economic growth and major socioeconomic shifts, resulting in lifestyle changes promoting obesity and overweight. By 1990, 69.3 percent of the adult Brazilian population led a sedentary lifestyle.[126]

After 2 years of preparatory consultation with the Pan-American Health Organization and other international agencies, the Agita São Paulo Program was launched in 1996 to address São Paulo's growing problem of obesity and overweight. The objective was to increase the level of knowledge among the São Paulo population about the importance of physical activity by 50 percent and the level of actual physical activity by 20 percent over a period of 10 years.[127] School children, the workforce, and the elderly were the main targets. The program concentrated on feasible, low- or no-cost ways to achieve at least 30 minutes of moderate-intensity physical activity per day, most days of the week. The goal was to convince the population that this physical activity could come from routine, daily activities such as walking to and from work or household chores, as opposed to less convenient exercises more likely to cause injury, such as structured fitness programs in gyms or organized sports.[127]

The program was structured as a partnership between government, industry, nongovernment organizations, and academic communities. Coordinated by the Studies Center of the Physical Fitness Research Laboratory of São Caetano do Sul (CELAFISCS), it was largely funded by the São Paulo State Secretariat of Health.[127] It was an extremely cost-effective program. Its annual budget ranged from $150,000 to $400,000, representing an investment of less than $0.01 per state inhabitant per year. In contrast, the estimated costs of illness related to a sedentary lifestyle in the state were about $1.00 per person per year.[128]

The program was overseen by a scientific board and an executive board. The scientific board consisted of Brazilian and international academics and doctors and provided the program's scientific foundation, assessed its implementation, and allowed it to better integrate with the medical community.[127] The executive board included more than 300 governmental, nongovernmental, and private organizations representing a wide range of sectors. These organizations were directly responsible for planning, organizing, and carrying out the program's activities.[129]

The program used three main types of activities to reach its target groups of students, workers, and the elderly: mega-events, actions carried out with partner institutions, and partnerships.[127] Mega-events were intended to reach the majority of cities in São Paolo state and involved at least a million people. Often coinciding with major cultural or seasonal holidays, they raised awareness of the importance of an active lifestyle through their activities and broad media coverage. Different mega-events were tailored to promoting specific activities for students, workers, and the elderly, but the most popular was "Agita Galera" ("Move, Crowd" or "Active Community Day"). It was celebrated across the 6,800 public schools in the state, reaching 6 million students and 250,000 teachers. Schools received a handbook and poster, as well as flyers for students and their families communicating the program's message. Students were also encouraged to prepare their own materials on the subject of physical activity and spread the message of the program in their communities while getting exercise. Partner institutions were also crucial to the program's success. The diversity in focus and type of partners encouraged innovation and a greater exchange of ideas for new activities. Each partner used a variety of pamphlets, manuals, advertising tools, and scientific information to promote physical activity among their employees and the communities they served. Finally, the program partnered

with more than 50 municipalities to establish 50 municipal communities throughout the state, that each planned, implemented, and monitored physical activities in their area.[127]

Various evaluations of the program were conducted and found positive effects for both increasing physical activity awareness and physical activity itself. Over a 3-year period, recall of the main program objective rose from 9.5 percent to 24.0 percent across the states. Recall increased with socioeconomic status level, reaching 67 percent of the most educated.[127] Furthermore, people who were aware of the program were more likely to be physically active; 54.2 percent of those familiar with the program were physically active in 2002, versus a rate of 31.9 percent for those who were not familiar with the program.[13] An analysis supported by the World Bank, the Centers for Disease Control and Prevention, and CELAFISCS concluded that the program was a good public health investment, achieving a cost-effectiveness ratio of less than R$50,000/QALY (quality-adjusted life year).[128]

Agita São Paulo has been a role model for similar local and national programs across Brazil and in other Latin American countries.[128] The World Health Organization has praised it as a model for other low- and middle-income countries, and it has since spurred an international mega-event celebrated annually to promote worldwide physical activity.[127]

Finland Uses Labels to Reduce Salt Consumption

Finland has traditionally had a diet high in salt, as it was used for conservation of food before other methods were available.[130] In the 1970s, Finnish salt intake was estimated to be approximately 12 grams per day (4,800 mg/day sodium), more than twice the value recommended by the World Health Organization, putting the population at risk for hypertension, stroke, and coronary heart disease.[131] This high intake spurred Finland's National Nutrition Council to recommend in 1978 steps to reduce salt consumption nationally.[132,133] From 1979 to 1982, a community-based intervention to reduce population-wide sodium intake called the North Karelia project was conducted to reduce mortality associated with cardiovascular disease.

Multiple stakeholders were involved with the project, including health service organizations, schools, nongovernmental organizations, media outlets, and the food industry.[130] The project was expanded to span the entire country after 3 years. Finnish media aided the effort by releasing numerous reports on the harmful health effects of salt, which raised both public and government awareness of salt and lower-sodium alternatives.[134] Health education of consumers and training programs for healthcare professionals, teachers, and caterers on how to reduce salt were also important components of the project.[130]

Building on the momentum from this movement, a number of labeling systems were implemented to inform consumers and discourage them from consuming high amounts of sodium. In 1993, the Ministry of Trade and Industry and the Ministry of Social Affairs and Health implemented salt-labeling legislation for food categories that contribute high amounts of sodium to the diet, such as breads, sausages and other meat products, fish products, butter, soups and sauces, ready-made meals, and spice mixtures containing salt, requiring that such foods be labeled with percentage of salt by weight.[135] The legislation required a "high salt content" label on foods with high levels of sodium, while allowing low sodium foods to carry a "low salt" label.[132,134] In 2000, the Finnish Heart Association began putting a "Better Choice" label on low-sodium products, and the Pansalt logo was used on products with sodium-reduced, potassium- and magnesium-enriched mineral salts.[132,134] It is estimated that these labeling initiatives caused the industry to reduce the salt content of targeted foods by about 20–25 percent.[136]

Salt intake was monitored using urinary sodium excretion every 5 years. By 2002, mean sodium intake was 3,900 mg/day for men and 2,700 mg/day for women. Diastolic blood pressure also decreased substantially, by more than 10 mm Hg.[130] This was caused by a combination of consumers choosing lower-sodium products and food companies discontinuing or reformulating their products to avoid high-salt labels through the use of alternatives such as mineral salts.[132,136] There was an 80 percent reduction in death rates from stroke and heart disease among the middle-aged population, contributing to a reduction in overall mortality in Finland and an increase in life expectancy by several years for both men and women.[136]

CASE STUDIES

There are a number of investments in improving nutrition status on a large scale that have made a significant difference to the communities in which they took place. One of the best known is the Tamil Nadu Nutrition Project in India. China has also made considerable progress in the last 10 years in controlling iodine deficiency.

Tamil Nadu State, India[137]

Background

The Tamil Nadu Integrated Nutrition Project in India is one of the most important efforts ever undertaken to improve nutritional status on a large scale. This project began in 1980 in the South Indian state of Tamil Nadu. It aimed at improving the nutritional status of poor women and children in the rural areas of the state through a set of well-focused interventions.

These specific goals were set for several reasons. First, the levels of malnutrition in poor women and children in Tamil Nadu were very high at the time the project was conceived. Second, malnutrition persisted despite considerable investments that had already been undertaken to improve nutrition status. Third, studies that had been done on those investments showed that they were not working as planned and were not cost-effective. Rather, the children who needed assistance most were not getting it. In addition, food that was given to children at feeding centers that was meant to be supplementary to their regular diet often replaced their regular food or was taken home and consumed by family members other than the intended children. The form of the food supplement was also difficult for children to eat. Moreover, little attention had been paid to nutrition education for families or to health investments that could complement the investments made in nutrition.

The project design was based on the idea that much of the malnutrition present in Tamil Nadu was because of inappropriate childcare practices, rather than just a lack of money to buy food. Thus, the project focused considerable attention on nutrition education and efforts to improve care and feeding practices for young children. In addition, because deficits at an early age often produce irreversible damage to children's physical and mental development, project interventions focused on pregnant and lactating women and on children younger than 3 years of age.

The Intervention

In line with this approach, the project included a package of services that were delivered by health and nutrition workers that consisted of nutrition education, primary health care, supplementary on-site feeding for children who were not growing properly, vitamin A supplementation, periodic deworming, education of mothers for managing childhood diarrhea, and the supplementary feeding of a small number of women.

An important innovation of the project was that it used growth monitoring of the children as a device for mobilizing community action. Groups of mothers met regularly to weigh their young children. They then plotted their weight-for-age on a growth chart. Together with the community nutrition worker, they identified which children were not growing properly. A related innovation of great importance was that supplementary feeding was targeted only to the children identified as faltering. In addition, children received food supplements only while they were not growing well. This was done in conjunction with nutrition education for mothers. The intent of this approach was that short-term feeding, combined with better childcare practices, could return the child to normal growth. This was a major change compared with previous practice in which supplementary feeding was more universal and longer term.

Impact

The nutrition interventions of the project were largely implemented as planned, but the health efforts were not fully implemented. Nonetheless, through careful evaluation the project was shown to have significantly reduced the levels of malnutrition of the targeted children. These improvements also continued over a substantial time, suggesting that the gains of the project were sustainable. The project was also more cost-effective than other investments that had tried to achieve similar aims in India.

Lessons Learned

This project was pioneering and revealed some very important lessons, including:

- Growth monitoring, coupled with short-term supplementary feeding of children who are faltering, can be a cost-effective way of improving nutritional status.
- More universal and longer term feeding of children is not necessary to achieve improvements in nutrition.
- Women can be organized to participate actively in growth monitoring efforts.
- Nutrition education can have a permanent and sustainable impact on child care and child feeding practices, even in the absence of other interventions.

The Challenge of Iodine Deficiency Disease in China

Background

For many years China had the heaviest burden of iodine deficiency in the world. In 1995, 20 percent of children ages 8 to 10 showed signs of goiter. Overall, some 400 million people in China were estimated to be at risk of iodine deficiency disorders, constituting 40 percent of the global total. Fortunately, iodine deficiency can be simply remedied by adding iodine to salt, a cheap and universally consumed food. Implementing this in a relatively poor and vast country like China at that time, however, was far from simple.

The Intervention

Scientific evidence linking iodine deficiency to mental impairment was seen by the Chinese government as a threat to its one-child-per-family policy, and so the government strengthened its resolve to tackle this widespread health risk. In 1993, China launched the National Iodine Deficiency Disorders Elimination Program, with technical and financial assistance from the donor-funded Iodine Deficiency Disorders Control Project. The public needed to be made aware of the risk of iodine deficiency, especially in regions where goiter was so common that it was regarded as normal. A nationwide public education campaign was launched, using posters on buses, newspaper editorials, and television documentaries to inform consumers and persuade them to switch to iodized salt. Provincial governors ensured that government education efforts reached even the most remote villages. The supply of iodized salt was increased by building 112 new salt iodination factories and enhancing capacity at 55 existing ones. Bulk packaging systems were installed to complement 147 new retail packaging centers, with packaging designed to help consumers easily recognize iodized salt. The sale of noniodized salt was banned, and technological assistance was provided to salt producers to adopt iodination. Salt quality was monitored, both at production, where the amount of iodine added needs to be just right, and in distribution and sales, because iodine in salt dissipates easily, reducing the shelf life of iodized salt. China's nationally controlled network of production and distribution made licensing and enforcement of legislation easier.

The Impact

By 1999, iodized salt was reaching 94 percent of the country, compared to 80 percent in 1995. The quality of iodized salt also improved markedly. As a result, iodine deficiency was reduced dramatically, and goiter rates for children ages 8 to 10 fell from 20.4 percent in 1995 to 8.8 percent in 1999.[138]

Costs and Benefits

At the time of these efforts, fortifying salt with iodine cost about 2 to 7 cents per kilogram, or less than 5 percent of the retail price of salt in most countries. The Chinese government invested approximately $152 million in the program, recovering some of this cost by raising the price of iodized salt. The World Bank, one of several donors, deemed the project extremely cost-effective.

Lessons Learned

China's success in reducing iodine deficiency offers valuable lessons for future efforts to reduce other micronutrient deficiencies such as iron and vitamin A through fortification. The government made a firm and long-standing commitment to tackle the problem and brought about administrative, legal, technical, and sociocultural changes that were needed to do so. Donor coordination was strong and effective and was managed by the Chinese government and the donors themselves, and the major players offered mutual support across all activities. The financing strategy was clearly defined from the start. The salt industry seized the opportunity of the investment in eliminating iodine deficiency to restructure and modernize the industry, gaining a firmer commercial footing and positioning itself to compete in the international market, given its cost advantages.

China's iodination program continues, with special targeting of resources on areas where the consumption of iodized salt is particularly low, usually in poor and remote mountainous regions where residents see iodized salt as too costly, especially when salt can be obtained cheaply from local salt hills, dried lakes, or the sea. Research will be needed to determine the best way to ensure iodine intake in these areas—through price subsidies, iodination of well or irrigation water, or even iodine capsules or injections, in the case of nomadic peoples. Through a variety of approaches, China is fast approaching the day when iodine deficiency will be unknown throughout its population. A more detailed review of this case is available in *Case Studies in Global Health: Millions Saved.*[139]

ADDRESSING FUTURE NUTRITION CHALLENGES

As noted earlier, the world has made progress in the last several decades in addressing key nutrition problems. Nonetheless, the world's nutritional status still faces critical issues in undernutrition, overweight and obesity, and the dietary risks to good health. Problems of undernutrition are especially severe in South Asia and sub-Saharan Africa. Problems of overweight and obesity are growing in many low- and middle-income countries. The world will not meet the MDGs that relate to nutrition. What steps will have to be taken to speed the world's progress on nutrition?

If the world is to do better in nutrition, it will have to take a number of steps in a variety of domains. First, policymakers who work both globally and in individual countries need to understand the exceptional importance of nutrition to good health and human productivity and act accordingly. About 45 percent of the under-5 child deaths globally are associated with nutritional causes. In addition, low-cost, highly effective solutions are available to deal with a number of critical nutrition issues, but they are not being implemented sufficiently. Thus, much greater attention needs to be paid by all concerned parties to nutrition as an underlying health issue. Nutrition does not fit neatly into governmental bureaucracies because it touches many government units, such as agriculture, health, and education. Thus, governments will also need to think creatively about how to ensure that there are government units accountable and responsible for promoting enhanced approaches to nutrition.

Improving government policy and action on nutrition will also require a good understanding of the nature of the nutrition problem in different settings. Nutritional concerns vary considerably by income group, gender, and ethnicity, and solutions to these problems will need to be carefully tailored to local circumstances. Moreover, almost all low- and middle-income countries will have to deal simultaneously with undernutrition and overweight and obesity.

In addition, governments need to work more effectively with the food industry to improve the way in which foods are fortified and to be sure that processed foods are healthy. Legal and financial arrangements need to be made in many countries so that more fortification can take place and the demand for fortified foods will be increased, as noted in the policy brief on Kenya. Similar arrangements will need to be made to limit sugar, salt, and some fats in processed foods. We have also seen the power in Tamil Nadu, for example, of focusing efforts on community-based action, in which affected people are involved in the design, implementation, and oversight of nutrition activities.

Although there is much knowledge of what works in nutrition, there are also other areas in which additional knowledge could fill important gaps. The world needs to continue gathering scientific knowledge about how key nutrition issues can be addressed. It would be very valuable to the world's nutrition status and health if more easy-to-make, nutritious, and inexpensive food supplements were available; if better formulas were available for some of the vitamin and mineral supplements that could be given less frequently, very cheaply, and without side effects; and, if additional cost-effective ways were found for fortifying foods. It will also be essential that today's low- and middle-income countries get a better sense of what works and at what cost to reduce the nutritional risks to good health.

Lastly, it is important for all societies to make the health and nutritional well-being of their citizens a national priority. One way to do this would be to create partnerships of civil society, government, and the private sector that can work together to identify nutrition issues, plan on how they can best be addressed, and then collaborate with each other and with communities to implement solutions to these problems.

As we consider the measures that can be taken to address key nutritional issues, as rapidly as possible and in cost-effective ways, it is essential to consider interventions in three domains:

- Nutrition-specific interventions—those interventions that can have a direct impact on nutrition, such as promotion of exclusive breastfeeding, micronutrient supplementation, and food fortification
- Nutrition-sensitive interventions—those interventions that address the underlying determinants of malnutrition, such as vaccination programs or

nutrition programs to enable farmers to increase the yield of crops that they consume

- The enabling environment for nutrition—this concerns laws, policies, resources, and institutional issues that relate to the approach countries take to nutrition and how effective they are at formulating, implementing, and monitoring nutrition interventions.[5] This could include, for example, taxing sweetened beverages or foods high in fat.

Additional comments on other measures for addressing undernutrition and overweight and obesity follow.

Undernutrition

It has already been noted that knowledge and behaviors are important determinants of what foods people eat, how they cook them, and how they consume them. Studies have shown that people can improve what they eat, how they cook, and how they eat their food by improvements in knowledge, even in the absence of improvements in income.[140] Nutrition education needs to be spread much more widely and in more appropriate ways to promote appropriate breastfeeding and complementary feeding and to help people eat better and more nutritious foods.

Growth monitoring and promotion programs, like that in Tamil Nadu, as well as others that were carried out in Honduras, Indonesia, and Madagascar, can also be important to improving nutrition outcomes at low cost. It is especially important that these programs be community-based. In addition, mothers who participate in these programs need to understand the importance of child growth and how they can carry out improved feeding and caring practices, such as exclusive breastfeeding, appropriate introduction of complementary foods, and the management of diarrhea. To succeed, growth monitoring and promotion programs must be coupled with programs for behavior change communication.[141]

The two-way relationship between infection, disease, and nutrition status has been noted. Many infections and diseases reduce one's ability to eat or ability to absorb food. At the same time, poor nutritional status reduces immunity to disease. To set the foundation for improvements in the nutritional status of poor people in low- and middle-income countries, especially poor infants, children, and women, it is very important to improve the control of parasitic infections such as hookworm and to control diarrheal diseases, malaria, and measles. Of course, doing this will also demand renewed efforts at health education; more effective basic health services, such as immunization; and improvements in water supply and sanitation.

Some people will simply not eat enough food or enough of the right foods, largely because of income gaps. These problems are also the result of, or are compounded by, natural disaster and conflict. Under these circumstances, it may be necessary that people receive food supplements like a high-protein, high-calorie ready-to-use therapeutic food. Alternatively, some people may receive vouchers for food, such as food stamps, which are cash transfers that can be used only to buy certain health and nutrition services or the right to buy certain foods at reduced prices. Conditional cash transfer programs are also being used to promote better nutrition, and smart cards are increasingly taking the place of food stamps or transfers of cash.

Vitamin and mineral supplementation is widespread in the world, is not expensive, and is often used as a way of improving the micronutrient status of large numbers of people, especially infants, children, and pregnant and lactating mothers. These can be given in capsules or syrups. Vitamin A should be given twice per year and should be integrated with child survival and other health services to minimize the cost of distribution.[57] In the last decade or so, vitamin A has been given orally to infants and children during national polio immunization days in many countries. These efforts can be expanded. At the same time, additional and carefully monitored efforts can be made to provide iron and folate to pregnant women. Unfortunately, these efforts have not worked as well as planned and need to be carefully reviewed and refined to enhance both coverage of supplementation and the extent to which women take the pills they do get.

Food fortification is practiced in many countries for a number of micronutrients. In fact, fortification in the industrialized countries has contributed greatly to the disappearance of several deficiencies. The fortification of salt with iodine is a very widespread practice and is very inexpensive, as we have seen in the China case noted earlier. About two-thirds of the world now consumes iodized salt, and the impact of fortification of salt could be further expanded through its double fortification with iron, as well as iodine. In addition, many different food products can be fortified. The key to effective fortification is to find a food product that is very widely consumed, for which there are no technical impediments to fortification, and for which fortification is inexpensive.[142] Thus, increasingly one could fortify flour, cooking oil, margarine, soy sauce, and other products, as well as salt. Multiple vitamin and mineral supplements are also being manufactured, which can be sprinkled on children's food to fortify it. Fortification can cost as little as 3 to 5 cents per person reached per year.[57] Clearly, fortification is a good way to harness the resources of commercial marketing networks to enhance the health of the population. Given the difficulties of iron supplementation, it may be that the most effective way of reducing iron deficiency in women is to operate an effective program of fortification for iron and folic acid.

Efforts are also under way for biofortification. The aim of this work is to use technologies to improve the nutritional content of foods, such as rice, yams, or other vegetables.

The latest studies show that young child deaths could be reduced by about 15 percent if the appropriate countries could take to scale a package of nutritional interventions, including:[8]

- Folic acid supplementation or fortification for pregnant women
- Balanced energy protein supplementation for pregnant women
- Calcium supplementation for pregnant women
- Multiple micronutrient fortification for pregnant women
- Promotion of appropriate breastfeeding practices
- Appropriate complementary feeding
- Supplementation with vitamin A and zinc for children aged 6 to 59 months
- Appropriate management of severe acute malnutrition
- Appropriate management of moderate acute malnutrition

Moreover, the evidence suggests that this package would be highly cost-effective at a cost per DALY averted of about $179.[91] In fact, a range of these and related nutrition interventions are cost-effective or have a high ratio of benefits to costs. **Table 8-6** indicates the cost per DALY averted of a number of measures to address undernutrition, as well as the benefit-cost ratio of some nutrition interventions.

These interventions compare favorably in their cost-effectiveness with a range of other health interventions that are cost-effective. The cost-effectiveness of several vaccines and bednets for malaria control, for example, is around $10 per DALY averted. Condom promotion to prevent transmission of HIV has a cost per DALY averted of about $40. Even the most expensive nutrition interventions, such as food supplements for young children, have a cost-effectiveness that is similar to that of antiretroviral therapy for HIV/AIDS or the use of aspirin to prevent heart disease.[91]

Overweight and Obesity

The obesity epidemic poses a serious global problem, especially in low- and middle-income countries. Given its scope, it is important to use policy measures across multiple levels

TABLE 8-6 Cost-Effectiveness and Benefit: Cost Ratios of Selected Nutrition Interventions

Cost per DALY Averted:

$5–$15 for vitamin A and zinc supplements
$40 for community-based management of severe acute malnutrition
$50–$150 for behavior change interventions taken to scale
$66–$115 for iron fortification
$90 for folic acid fortification

Benefit: Cost Ratios

6:1 for deworming
8:1 for iron fortification of staples
30:1 for salt iodination
46:1 for folic acid fortification

Data from Horton S. Economics of nutritional interventions. In: Semba RD, Bloem M, eds. Nutrition and Health in a Developing World, third edition. Totowa, New Jersey: Humana Press; 2015. Forthcoming.

to prevent obesity and reverse its trend. Strategies should include efforts on the international, national, local, and individual levels. The involvement of the food industry, healthcare providers, schools, urban planners, the agricultural sector, and the media is also essential.

International organizations can have a large impact on obesity by setting global nutrition and physical activity standards. They can also encourage surveillance, monitoring, and evaluation systems, to insure nutrition standards are met and to identify countries where obesity policies are most needed. In September 2011, the United Nations General Assembly convened a summit on global noncommunicable diseases, identifying key targets for strengthening and shaping primary prevention to reduce risk factors for NCDs, including obesity.[143] The World Health Organization has also done a large amount of work on the subject, including developing best buy cost-effective interventions to address NCDs. For diet and physical activity, WHO recommends reduced salt intake in food, replacement of trans fat with polyunsaturated fat, and public awareness through mass media on diet and physical activity. To address cardiovascular disease and diabetes, WHO recommends counseling and multidrug therapy for people with a high risk of developing heart attacks and strokes, including those with established cardiovascular disease, and treatment of heart attacks with aspirin.[108]

On a national scale, there are many opportunities to address obesity. Many governments set dietary guidelines, as well as age-specific physical activity guidelines.[144,145] Additional government campaigns addressing health can be implemented, such as the Let's Move campaign in the United States, spearheaded by the first lady. A comprehensive initiative dedicated to reducing national childhood obesity, Let's Move also established a task force to review programs and policies related to childhood nutrition and physical activity and developed a national action plan with fixed benchmarks.[146] Effective national prevention strategies in low- and middle-income countries are especially important, as many of these countries are still in a nutrition transition, presenting the added challenge of developing policies and programs to address overweight and obesity and undernutrition, while not hindering progress on either issue. There must be coordination and resource allocation across multiple sectors of government to create successful large-scale campaigns.

Aligning national dietary goals with nutritional and agricultural policies can be an effective tool for reducing obesity and overweight within a country. Food price modification is an effective way to promote health. Taxation of unhealthy foods and sugar-sweetened beverages is one strategy, with the hopes of decreasing consumption and generating revenue to fund programs that promote health.[147] Over the past 5 years, sugar-sweetened beverage taxes have been enacted in Denmark, Hungary, France, Mexico, and Berkeley, California in the United States. Although their effectiveness has yet to be fully determined, preliminary results from Mexico have shown that their excise tax has decreased sales of sugar-sweetened beverages by about 10 percent and increased sales of plain water by about 13 percent.[147] Food prices can also be modified through the removal of subsidies on oils, sugar, and foods from animal sources, increasing product costs globally and leading to reduced consumption, especially among the low-income population.[148] Prices for healthier foods such as fruits and vegetables can simultaneously be decreased through agricultural subsidies, likely increasing consumption with the proper infrastructure in place allowing such products to be accessible.[149] This has been the case in China, where subsidies on fruits, vegetables, and soybeans have increased production and consumption of these products.[150]

As we saw in Finland, governments can require nutrition labeling on packages listing the caloric and nutrient content of foods to help consumers make healthier, more informed choices and incentivize companies to reformulate products and introduce healthier options.[151] As new research develops,

government can mandate labels to list nutrients of specific concern, such as in Canada, the United States, and Brazil, where trans fat content is required to be listed on food packages.[152–155] Front-of-package labeling systems can be used to convey essential nutritional information simply and prominently using a short label or basic symbols. These labels can help the consumer identify nutritionally beneficial and harmful foods and beverages using color-coding, just by glancing at the package. For example, the UK traffic light front-of-package labeling system shows whether the product has high (colored in red), medium (yellow), or low (green) levels of fat, saturated fat, sugar, and salt.[156] Nutrition-labeling initiatives are growing in popularity among low and middle-income countries, including India, China, Brazil, Mexico, and South Africa. Along similar lines, calorie labeling on menus in restaurants and fast food outlets is being utilized in some parts of the United States. Preliminary research has shown beneficial effects on food choices and health.[157] Educational campaigns must be implemented alongside any type of labeling campaign to raise awareness about the initiative and the reasons for it, so that consumers can understand why the labels are important, where to find them, and what they mean.

Another way to promote healthier eating through nutritional policy is for governments to incentivize production and use of healthier substitutes, such as the use of oil with omega-3 fatty acids instead of partially hydrogenated oils. This requires collaboration between the agricultural and food industry sectors. The food industry, including restaurants, supermarkets, food manufacturers, and caterers, can also take voluntary action to reduce sugar, salt, fat, and caloric content from their food over time. Although these initiatives are under way in some high-income countries, similar initiatives should be translated to low- and middle-income countries.[158,159]

Legislation can be used to restrict unhealthy food marketing aimed at children through television, Internet, other media, and their environment, thus decreasing their consumption of those products and subsequently decreasing childhood obesity.[160] Zoning laws can also be instituted to limit the number of fast-food restaurants in a given area.[40] Although the World Health Organization has recommended that governments and industry reduce the amount of advertising and marketing of unhealthy foods to children, few countries have taken steps towards this goal.[161]

A healthy food environment in schools can encourage healthier eating for children in general, especially in conjunction with nutritional education for both students and parents.[162] School meal programs can provide healthy, low-cost or free meals to children, simultaneously addressing undernutrition and overweight and obesity. Policies can also be implemented to remove vending machines selling sugar-sweetened beverages and less healthy snacks, increasing the healthy snacks sold, and banning bake sales on school premises. The amount of physical education required during the school day can also be extended, and food marketing within schools can be eliminated.

The World Health Organization's Global Action Plan for the Prevention and Control of Noncommunicable Diseases 2013–2020 calls for a voluntary global target of a 10 percent relative reduction in the prevalence of insufficient physical activity.[87] To work toward achieving this goal, countries can adopt national physical activity guidelines and education campaigns to encourage over 30 minutes of moderate physical activity on most days of the week, such as we saw in Brazil.[44] Steps can also be taken to reduce television viewing and Internet usage via mandatory or voluntary action. For instance, the television network Nickelodeon designates one day a year as a "Worldwide Day of Play," in which they suspend programming across all of their TV channels and websites for 3 hours, encouraging children to "get up, go outside and play."[163] This concept could be extended to other networks for more regular, longer periods of time.

Improving the safety of and access to recreational spaces and facilities through urban planning at the national or regional level is important to encourage an active, pedestrian-friendly community. Governments can promote the use of public transportation and bicycles to increase physical activity levels in cities by providing incentives, such as discounted transportation fares, bike sharing programs, cycling safety classes, and secure bicycle parking.[15] The creation of sidewalks, parks, safe bicycle lanes, and buildings with accessible staircases can also be beneficial.

The media have leveraging power to frame obesity as a common challenge and to promote specific policy changes via digital and printed media and social marketing campaigns.[164] Media advocacy in this realm can direct political attention to obesity, generate public debate about policy options, and ultimately persuade the public and lawmakers to support specific policies.[164] The media can also serve to educate the public about the importance of the food environment; this dissemination of nutrition education, in conjunction with environmental, diet, and physical activity changes, has been shown to have positive effects on weight loss and health.[165,166]

Doctors can play a large role in the prevention and treatment of obesity and overweight. As part of standard doctor visits, physicians and other healthcare providers should measure body weight and provide continual nutritional and weight-management advice to encourage a healthy lifestyle.[166] Healthcare providers need to be trained to implement behavioral change strategies and to recognize their own weight stigma.[167] Medical organizations and nongovernmental organizations can also advocate for and influence policy on issues related to health and the environment.[15] For example, the American Heart Association released a scientific statement detailing interventions to reduce cardiovascular risk factors that has been cited hundreds of times and can be used as a roadmap for doctors and healthcare institutions to address overweight and obesity.[168]

Although food availability and the physical and social environment have a strong influence over choice, it is ultimately the individual who must eat healthily and exercise. Individuals should limit their energy intake, especially from sugars, and avoid excess salt, saturated fat, and trans fats. Adults should also get 150 minutes of physical activity a week, and children should exercise for 60 minutes a day.[44]

MAIN MESSAGES

Undernutrition

Nutritional status is a major determinant of health status. It has an important bearing on the health of pregnant women and on pregnancy outcomes for both mothers and children. It is a major determinant of the birthweight of children, how children grow, and the extent to which their cognitive functions develop properly. Nutrition status is also closely linked with the strength of one's immune system and one's ability to stay healthy.

In addition, nutritional status has an important bearing on people's capacity to learn and on their productivity. Nutritional deficits can seriously hamper the ability of children to attend school, concentrate while they are there, and learn effectively. Numerous studies have shown that workers who are anemic produce less than workers who do not suffer from iron deficiency anemia.

From the global health perspective, the most important concerns related to undernutrition are breastfeeding practices, whether or not people get enough of the right foods to have sufficient energy and protein, and the extent to which people have a sufficient intake of vitamin A, iodine, iron, zinc, and calcium. The importance of these nutrients and micronutrients varies with the place of people in their life course, with needs differing for adolescents, pregnant and lactating women, infants, children, adults, and older adults.

More than 1 billion people in the world today suffer from energy and protein malnutrition and deficiencies in key micronutrients. These problems often stem from people's lack of income to purchase enough food or food of appropriate quality. However, these problems also relate to culture, customs, and eating behaviors. Malnutrition of all types disproportionately affects poor people, marginalized people, and females.

Energy and protein malnutrition is associated with low birthweight, being underweight, failing to grow properly, and a weakening of immunity. Vitamin A deficiency is well known for its impact on vision but is also closely associated with general immunity and child growth. The lack of iron is the primary cause of iron deficiency anemia, which leads to weakness and fatigue; however, it is also associated with maternal morbidity and mortality, poor and stunted growth in children, and poor mental development in children. The lack of iodine causes thyroid problems, goiter, and important deficits in mental abilities. Iodine is also essential for proper child growth. The lack of zinc is associated with general immunity, the growth of children, and the development of children's cognitive and motor abilities. About 45 percent of the deaths in the world today of children under 5 years of age are associated with undernutrition.

There are cost-effective solutions to the most important nutritional concerns. People can wash their hands more frequently with soap to reduce the rate of infections and diarrhea that take such terrible tolls on nutritional status. Efforts can be enhanced to promote exclusive breastfeeding for 6 months, followed by the appropriate introduction of hygienically prepared complementary feeding. Food supplements can be given to those people who are not getting enough protein and energy. Nutritional supplements can be provided for vitamin A and iron. Salt can be fortified with iodine. Pregnant women can receive multivitamins. Zinc can be given along with oral rehydration to reduce the severity of diarrheal disease. Families can also learn, even in the absence of income gains, to improve what they eat. These actions will be most successful if they are tied to approaches that are taken by communities.

It is also critical to remember that the window of opportunity for ensuring that children are well nourished and develop properly is a small one. It begins at conception and lasts until the children are about 2 years of age. Damage done to children's development in this period is largely irreversible.

The most critical interventions to deal with undernutrition, therefore, are to:

- Ensure that pregnant women are well nourished and have sufficient amounts of needed micronutrients
- Promote exclusive breastfeeding for all children until they are 6 months of age
- Encourage the provision of appropriate complementary foods for infants beginning at 6 months of age
- Support effective programs in supplementation and fortification, based on nutritional needs at the local level, and embed them in community-based approaches

- Fight infection and illness through better hygiene, improved water and sanitation, and appropriate food and health behaviors
- Focus on South Asia and sub-Saharan Africa

These can be achieved by taking some of the following steps, among others, in the short, medium, and longer run:[141]

Short run

- Initiate community-based growth monitoring and promotion
- Carry out supplementation with vitamin A and iron
- Provide zinc for the management of diarrhea
- Selectively provide therapeutic food

Medium run

- Consolidate community-based growth monitoring and promotion
- Implement food supplementation through programs such as vouchers, smart cards, and conditional cash transfers
- Fortify locally appropriate foods with needed micronutrients, including completing the agenda on the fortification of salt with iodine

Long run

- Improve the education of women and take other appropriate measures to enhance the social standing of women in society
- Use technologies to improve the nutritional content of foods

Overweight and Obesity

The worldwide increase in overweight, obesity, and related chronic diseases has largely been driven by globalization, through a combination of global trade liberalization, economic growth, and rapid urbanization. These factors are causing dramatic changes in diet, lifestyles, and living environments, in turn promoting positive energy balance. Nutritional transitions in low- and middle-income countries involve increases in the consumption of fast food, increased prevalence of supermarkets, and a diet heavy in added sugar and animal products. Coupled with reductions in physical activity, and linked behavioral, cultural, and biological factors, obesity and overweight rates are increasing at alarming rates, especially in low- and middle-income countries.

A balanced, healthy diet consisting of vegetables, fruits, whole grains, legumes, and nuts is crucial to the prevention of obesity. Such a diet must limit red and processed meats, saturated and trans fats, added sugars, salt, and refined carbohydrates.

Unfortunately, the vast majority of the world is not receiving a healthy diet, as reflected by the 2.1 billion people worldwide who are overweight or obese. In high-income countries, poorer men are most at risk for obesity and overweight, whereas in low- and middle-income countries wealthier women are at a higher risk. Childhood obesity is of particular concern, as 43 million children are currently obese or overweight, and will likely continue this trend into adulthood.

Obesity and its related diseases have high costs in terms of health expenditures and quality of life, so prevention strategies are paramount, particularly in low-income and middle-income countries that must manage a double burden of malnutrition. Due to the scope and complexity of the obesity epidemic, prevention strategies and policies across multiple levels are needed in order to have a measurable effect. Changes should include high-level global policies from the international community to identify nutritional goals and guidelines. In addition, coordinated efforts by governments, organizations, communities, and individuals will be required to positively influence behavioral and environmental change. Policies and prevention efforts must also involve the industry, media, doctors, farmers, and urban planners.

Some of the most important and cost-effective interventions for addressing overweight, obesity, and the dietary risks to good health include measures that can be taken by governments, by industry, and by individuals:

- Reduce salt intake in food through government-mandated labeling, sodium limits, or taxes; voluntary industry sodium reduction; and individual action to read labels and make informed decisions about food choices.
- Replace trans fat with polyunsaturated fat through government-mandated bans on trans fat, incentives for production and use of healthier fats, and individual action to read labels and make more informed decisions about food choices.
- Increase public awareness through mass media on diet and physical activity, linked with mass media campaigns organized by government, local health departments, private organizations, and schools.
- Provide counseling and multidrug therapy for people with a high risk of developing heart attacks and strokes, including those with established cardiovascular disease; this should be linked with doctor–patient consultation; and medical organizations should include obesity prevention/discussion as standard for routine medical visits.
- Treat heart attacks with aspirin, linked to doctor-patient consultation.

It is also essential to note that addressing nutrition problems of all types will require action in three domains: nutrition-specific, nutrition-sensitive, and areas related to the enabling environment for nutrition.

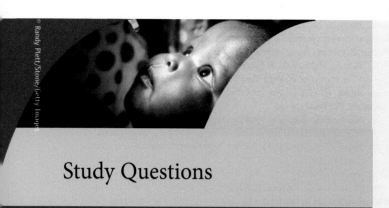

Study Questions

1. What is the importance of nutrition to the MDGs?

2. What are *stunting* and *wasting*?

3. What are some of the direct and indirect causes of undernutrition?

4. What are some of the direct and indirect causes of overweight and obesity?

5. What are the links between nutrition and health?

6. How are growth charts used to gauge nutrition status?

7. What are the most important micronutrient deficiencies and what health problems do they cause?

8. Why is anemia a special risk in pregnancy?

9. Why is exclusive breastfeeding for the first 6 months so important?

10. What parts of the world have the worst nutritional problems?

11. What are the links between nutrition and economic development?

12. What are some of the most important cost-effective interventions that could be made to address undernutrition in under-5 children?

13. What are some of the most important cost-effective interventions that could be made to address overweight and obesity?

REFERENCES

1. Institute of Health Metrics and Evaluation. (2015). *GBD 2010 heat map*. Retrieved May 12, 2015, from http://vizhub.healthdata.org/irank/heat.php.

2. United Nations Children's Fund, World Health Organization, The World Bank. (2012). *UNICEF-WHO-World Bank joint child malnutrition estimates*. New York: UNICEF; Geneva: WHO; Washington, DC: World Bank.

3. Black, R. E., Victora, C. G., Walker, S. P., et al. (2013, August 3). Maternal and child undernutrition and overweight in low-income and middle-income countries. *Lancet*, *382*(9890), 427–451.

4. UNICEF and The Micronutrient Initiative. (2004). *Vitamin and mineral deficiency: A global progress report*. Ottawa: The Micronutrient Initiative.

5. International Food Policy Research Institute. (2014). *Global nutrition report 2014: Actions and accountability to accelerate the world's progress on nutrition*. Washington, DC: International Food Policy Research Institute.

6. Lancet. (2010). *Global burden of disease study 2010*. Available at http://www.thelancet.com/global-burden-of-disease.

7. UNICEF. (1998). *State of the world's children: Focus on nutrition*. New York: Oxford University Press.

8. Bhutta, Z. A., Das, J. K., Rizvi, A., et al. (2013, August 3). Evidence-based intervention for improvement of maternal and child nutrition: What can be done and at what cost? *Lancet*, *382*(9890), 452–477.

9. Centers for Disease Control and Prevention. *Genomics and health*. Retrieved September 18, 2014, from http://www.cdc.gov/genomics/resources/diseases/obesity/index.htm.

10. Cox, A. J., West, N. P., & Cripps, A. W. (2014). Obesity, inflammation, and the gut microbiota. *The Lancet Diabetes & Endocrinology*, *3*(3), 207–215.

11. Popkin, B. M. (2006). Global nutrition dynamics: The world is shifting rapidly toward a diet linked with noncommunicable diseases. *American Journal of Clinical Nutrition*, *84*(2), 289–298.

12. Nakamura, Y. (2002). Beyond the hijab: Female Muslims and physical activity. *Women in Sport & Physical Activity Journal*, *11*(2), 21.

13. Matsudo, S. M., Matsudo, V. R., Araújo, T., Andrade, D., Andrade, E., Oliveira, L., et al. (2002). Nível de atividade física da população do estado de São Paulo: Análise de acordo com o gênero, idade, nível sócio-econômico, distribuição geográfica e de conhecimento. *Revista Brasileira de Ciência e Movimento*, *10*(4), 41–50.

14. Benjelloun, S. (2002). Nutrition transition in Morocco. *Public Health Nutrition*, *5*(1a), 135–140.

15. Malik, V. S., Willett, W. C., & Hu, F. B. (2012). Global obesity: Trends, risk factors and policy implications. *Nature Reviews, Endocrinology*, *9*(1), 13–27.

16. Fuster, V., & Kelly, B. B. (Eds.). (2010). *Promoting cardiovascular health in the developing world: A critical challenge to achieve global health*. Washington, DC: National Academies Press.

17. Hawkes, C., Chopra, M., & Friel, S. (2009). Globalization, trade, and the nutrition transition. In R. Labonté, T. Schrecker, C. Packer, & V. Runnels, *Globalization and health: Pathways, evidence and policy* (pp. 235–262). New York: Routledge.

18. Kearney, J. (2010). Food consumption trends and drivers. *Philosophical Transactions of the Royal Society B: Biological Sciences*, *365*(1554), 2793–2807.

19. Caballero, B. A. (2005). A nutrition paradox—underweight and obesity in developing countries. *New England Journal of Medicine*, *352*(15), 1514–1516.

20. Johns, T., & Eyzaguirre, P. B. (2006). Linking biodiversity, diet and health in policy and practice. *Proceedings of the Nutrition Society*, *65*(2), 182–189.

21. Wang, Y., Mi, J., Shan, X. Y., Wang, Q. J., & Ge, K. Y. (2007). Is China facing an obesity epidemic and the consequences? The trends in obesity and chronic disease in China. *International Journal of Obesity*, *31*(1), 177–188.

22. Pan, A., Malik, V. S., & Hu, F. B. (2012). Exporting diabetes mellitus to Asia: The impact of Western-style fast food. *Circulation*, *126*, 163–165.

23. Ritzer, G. (2002). An introduction to McDonaldization. *McDonaldization: The Reader*, 4–25.

24. McDonald's. *Company profile*. Retrieved September 1, 2014, from http://www.aboutmcdonalds.com/mcd/investors/company_profile.html.

25. Misra, A., & Khurana, L. (2008). Obesity and the metabolic syndrome in developing countries. *Journal of Clinical Endocrinology and Metabolism*, *93*(11, Suppl. 1), S9–S30.

26. Kimenju, S. C., Rischke, R., Klasen, S., & Qaim, M. (2015). Do supermarkets contribute to the obesity pandemic in developing countries? *Public health nutrition*, 1–10.

27. Hawkes, C. (2008). Dietary implications of supermarket development: A global perspective. *Development Policy Review*, *26*(6), 657–692.

28. Reardon, T., Timmer, C., Barrett, C., & Berdegue, J. (2003). The rise of supermarkets in Africa, Asia, and Latin America. *American Journal of Agricultural Economics*, *85*, 1140–1146.

29. Wagner, K. H., & Brath, H. (2012). A global view on the development of non communicable diseases. *Preventive Medicine*, *54*, S38–S41.

30. Cummins, S., & Macintyre, S. (2006). Food environments and obesity—Neighbourhood or nation? *International Journal of Epidemiology*, *35*(1), 100–104.

31. Popkin, B. M., Adair, L. S., & Ng, S. W. (2012). Global nutrition transition and the pandemic of obesity in developing countries. *Nutrition Reviews*, *70*(1), 3–21.

32. Horgen, K. B., Choate, M., & Brownell, K. D. (2001). Television and children's nutrition. In D. G. Singer & J. L. Singer (Eds.), *Handbook of children and the media* (pp. 447–461). Thousand Oaks, CA: Sage.

33. Popkin, B. M., & Nielsen, S. J. (2003). The sweetening of the world's diet. *Obesity Research*, *11*(11), 1325–1332.

34. Welsh, J. A., Sharma, A. J., Grellinger, L., & Vos, M. B. (2011). Consumption of added sugars is decreasing in the United States. *American Journal of Clinical Nutrition*, *94*(3), 726–734.

35. Malik, V. S., Popkin, B. M., Bray, G. A., Després, J. P., Willett, W. C., & Hu, F. B. (2010). Sugar-sweetened beverages and risk of metabolic syndrome and type 2 diabetes: A meta-analysis. *Diabetes Care*, *33*(11), 2477–2483.

36. Mozaffarian, D., Hao, T., Rimm, E. B., Willett, W. C., & Hu, F. B. (2011). Changes in diet and lifestyle and long-term weight gain in women and men. *New England Journal of Medicine*, *364*(25), 2392–2404.

37. Pan, A., Sun, Q., Bernstein, A. M., Schulze, M. B., Manson, J. E., Willett, W. C., et al. (2011). Red meat consumption and risk of type 2 diabetes: 3 cohorts of US adults and an updated meta-analysis. *American Journal of Clinical Nutrition*, *94*(4), 1088–1096.

38. Bernstein, A. M., Sun, Q., Hu, F. B., Stampfer, M. J., Manson, J. E., & Willett, W. C. (2010). Major dietary protein sources and risk of coronary heart disease in women. *Circulation*, *122*(9), 876–883.

39. Chan, D. S., Lau, R., Aune, D., Vieira, R., Greenwood, D. C., Kampman, E., et al. (2011). Red and processed meat and colorectal cancer incidence: Meta-analysis of prospective studies. *PLoS One*, *6*(6), e20456.

40. Pan, A., Sun, Q., Bernstein, A. M., et al. (2012). Red meat consumption and mortality: Results from 2 prospective cohort studies. *Archives of Internal Medicine*, *172*(7), 555–563.

41. Popkin, B. M. (2009). *The world is fat: The fads, trends, policies, and products that are fattening the human race*. New York: Penguin Group.

42. Popkin, B. M., & Gordon-Larsen, P. (2004). The nutrition transition: Worldwide obesity dynamics and their determinants. *International Journal of Obesity*, *28*(Suppl. 3), S2–S9.

43. Hu, F. B. (2008). *Obesity epidemiology*. New York: Oxford University Press.

44. World Health Organization. (2010). *Global recommendations on physical activity for health*. Geneva: WHO.

45. Sallis, J. F., Slymen, D. J., Conway, T. L., Frank, L. D., Saelens, B. E., Cain, K., et al. (2011). Income disparities in perceived neighborhood built and social environment attributes. *Health & Place, 17*(6), 1274–1283.

46. Singh, S. K. (2005). Review of urban transportation in India. *Journal of Public Transportation, 8*(1), 79–97.

47. Patel, S. R., & Hu, F. B. (2008). Short sleep duration and weight gain: A systematic review. *Obesity, 16*(3), 643–653.

48. Muntner, P., Gu, D., Wildman, R. P., Chen, J., Qan, W., Whelton, P. K., et al. (2005). Prevalence of physical activity among Chinese adults: Results from the International Collaborative Study of Cardiovascular Disease in Asia. *American Journal of Public Health, 95*(9), 1631–1636.

49. World Health Organization. (n.d.). *BMI classification*. Retrieved May 14, 2015, from http://apps.who.int/bmi/index.jsp?introPage=intro_3.html.

50. UNICEF. (2006). *Progress for children. A report card on nutrition, No. 4*. Retrieved May 8, 2011, from http://www.unicef.org/progressforchildren/2006n4/index_undernutrition.html.

51. Caulfield, L. E., Richard, S. A., Rivera, J. A., Musgrove, P., & Black, R. E. (2006). Stunting, wasting, and micronutrient disorders. In D. T. Jamison, J. G. Breman, A. R. Measham, et al. (Eds.), *Disease control priorities in developing countries* (2nd ed., pp. 551–567). New York: Oxford University Press and The World Bank.

52. World Health Organization. (2006). *Severe acute malnutrition*. Retrieved June 15, 2015 from http://www.who.int/nutrition/topics/malnutrition/en/.

53. Victora, C. G., Adair, L., Fall, C., et al. (2008). Maternal and child undernutrition: Consequences for adult health and human capital. *Lancet, 371*(9609), 340–357.

54. GP Notebook: *Xerophthalmia*. Retrieved May 30, 2015, from http://www.gpnotebook.co.uk/simplepage.cfm?ID=664403984.

55. Black, R. E., Allen, L. H., Bhutta, Z. A., et al. (2008). Maternal and child undernutrition: Global and regional exposures and health consequences. *Lancet, 371*(9608), 243–260.

56. Government of Australia. *Iodine explained*. Retrieved June 27, 2006, from http://www.betterhealth.vic.gov.au/BHCV2/bhcarticles.nsf/pages/Iodine_explained?open.

57. World Bank. (2006). *Repositioning nutrition as central to development*. Washington, DC: World Bank.

58. World Health Organization. (2015). Micronutrient deficiencies. Iodine deficiency. Retrieved June 15, 2015, from http://www.who.int/nutrition/topics/idd/en/.

59. US National Library of Medicine. Medline Plus. Iron. Retrieved July 7, 2015, from http://www.nlm.nih.gov/medlineplus/iron.html.

60. World Health Organization. (2015). Zinc supplementation in the management of diarrhea. Retrieved June 15, 2015, from http://www.who.int/elena/titles/bbc/zinc_diarrhoea/en/.

61. Brown, K. H., & Wuehler, S. E. (2000). *The micronutrient initiative*. Ottawa: The Micronutrient Initiative.

62. MedlinePlus. *Folic acid*. Retrieved May 14, 2015, from http://www.nlm.nih.gov/medlineplus/folicacid.html.

63. World Cancer Research Fund. (2007). *Food, nutrition, physical activity and the prevention of cancer: A global perspective*. Washington, DC: World Cancer Research Fund.

64. American Heart Association. (2015). *Polyunsaturated fats*. Retrieved September 21, 2014, from http://www.heart.org/HEARTORG/GettingHealthy/NutritionCenter/HealthyEating/Polyunsaturated-Fats_UCM_301461_Article.jsp.

65. Appel, L. J., Sacks, F. M., Carey, V. J., et al. (2005). Effects of protein, monounsaturated fat, and carbohydrate intake on blood pressure and serum lipids: Results of the OmniHeart randomized trial. *JAMA, 294*(19), 2455–2464.

66. Mozaffarian, D., Micha, R., & Wallace, S. (2010). Effects on coronary heart disease of increasing polyunsaturated fat in place of saturated fat: A systematic review and meta-analysis of randomized controlled trials. *PLoS Medicine, 7*(3), e1000252.

67. Mente, A., de Koning, L., Shannon, H. S., & Anand, S. S. (2009). A systematic review of the evidence supporting a causal link between dietary factors and coronary heart disease. *Archives of Internal Medicine, 169*(7), 659–669.

68. World Health Organization. (2014). *Guideline: Sodium intake for adults and children*. Retrieved September 18, 2014, from http://apps.who.int/iris/bitstream/10665/77985/1/9789241504836_eng.pdf.

69. Nishida, C., Uauy, R., Kumanyika, S., & Shetty, P. (2004). The joint WHO/FAO expert consultation on diet, nutrition and the prevention of chronic diseases: Process, product and policy implications. *Public Health Nutrition, 7*(1a), 245–250.

70. Malik, V. S., Willett, W. C., & Hu, F. B. (2009). Sugar-sweetened beverages and BMI in children and adolescents: Reanalyses of a meta-analysis. *American Journal of Clinical Nutrition, 89*, 438–439.

71. Fung, T. T., Malik, V., Rexrode, K. M., Manson, J. E., Willett, W. C., & Hu, F. B. (2009). Sweetened beverage consumption and risk of coronary heart disease in women. *American Journal of Clinical Nutrition, 89*(4), 1037–1042.

72. De Koning, L., Malik, V. S., Kellogg, M. D., Rimm, E. B., Willett, W. C., & Hu, F. B. (2012). Sweetened beverage consumption, incident coronary heart disease and biomarkers of risk in men. *Circulation, 125*(14), 1735–1741.

73. Babey, S. H. et al. (2009) *Bubbling over: Soda consumption and its link to obesity in California* (Healthy Policy Brief). Los Angeles: UCLA Center for Health Policy Research.

74. World Health Organization. (2015). *Guideline: Sugars intake for adults and children*. Geneva: WHO. Retrieved March 22, 2015, from http://apps.who.int/iris/bitstream/10665/149782/1/9789241549028_eng.pdf?ua=1.

75. Gross, L. S., Li, L., Ford, E. S., & Liu, S. (2004). Increased consumption of refined carbohydrates and the epidemic of type 2 diabetes in the United States: An ecologic assessment. *American Journal of Clinical Nutrition, 79*(5), 774–779.

76. Sun, Q., Spiegelman, D., van Dam, R. M., Holmes, M. D., Malik, V. S., Willett, W. C., et al. (2010). White rice, brown rice, and risk of type 2 diabetes in US men and women. *Archives of Internal Medicine, 170*(11), 961–969.

77. Villegas, R., Liu, S., Gao, Y. T., Yang, G., Li, H., Zheng, W., et al. (2007). Prospective study of dietary carbohydrates, glycemic index, glycemic load, and incidence of type 2 diabetes mellitus in middle-aged Chinese women. *Archives of Internal Medicine, 167*(21), 2310–2316.

78. Ohio State University. (2009). *Nutritional needs of pregnancy and breastfeeding* (Fact Sheet). Retrieved May 30, 2015, from http://ohioline.osu.edu/hyg-fact/5000/pdf/5573.pdf.

79. Black, R. E., Morris, S. S., & Bryce, J. (2003). Where and why are 10 million children dying every year? *Lancet, 361*(9376), 2226–2234.

80. Gillespie, S., & Flores, R. (n.d.). *The life cycle of malnutrition*. Washington, DC: International Food Policy Research Institute. Retrieved July 7, 2015, from http://ebrary.ifpri.org/cdm/ref/collection/p15738coll2/id/125440.

81. National Osteoporosis Foundation. *What is osteoporosis?* Retrieved May 30, 2015, from http://nof.org/articles/7.

82. UNICEF. *Nutrition: What are the challenges?* Retrieved June 28, 2006, from http://www.unicef.org/nutrition/index_challenges.html.

83. UNICEF and World Health Organization. (2004). *Low birth weight: Country, regional, and global estimates*. New York: UNICEF.

84. Finucane, M. M., Stevens, G. A., Cowan, M. J., et al. (2011). National, regional, and global trends in body-mass index since 1980: Systematic analysis of health examination surveys and epidemiological studies with 960 country-years and 9.1 million participants. *Lancet, 377*(9765), 557–567.

85. Ng, M., Fleming, T., Robinson, M., et al. (2014). Global, regional, and national prevalence of overweight and obesity in children and adults during 1980–2013: A systematic analysis for the Global Burden of Disease Study 2013. *Lancet, 384*(9945), 766–781.

86. Flegal, K. M., Carroll, M. D., Kit, B. K., & Ogden, C. L. (2012). Prevalence of obesity and trends in the distribution of body mass index among US adults, 1999–2010. *JAMA, 307*(5), 491–497.

87. World Health Organization. (2013). *Global action plan for the prevention and control of noncommunicable diseases 2013–2020*. Retrieved September 4, 2014, from http://apps.who.int/iris/bitstream/10665/94384/1/9789241506236_eng.pdf.

88. Kelly, T., Yang, W., Chen, C. S., Reynolds, K., & He, J. (2008). Global burden of obesity in 2005 and projections to 2030. *International Journal of Obesity, 32*(9), 1431–1437.

89. Singh, A. S., Mulder, C., Twisk, J. W., van Mechelen, W., & Chinapaw, M. J. Tracking of childhood overweight into adulthood: A systematic review of the literature. *Obesity Reviews, 9*(5), 474–488.

90. De Onis, M., Blossner, M., & Borghi, E. (2010). Global prevalence and trends of overweight and obesity among preschool children. *American Journal of Clinical Nutrition, 92*(5), 1257–1264.

91. Horton, S. (in press). Economics of nutritional interventions. In R. D. Semba & M. Bloem (Eds.), *Nutrition and health in a developing world* (3rd ed.). Totowa, NJ: Humana Press.

92. Hunt, J. M. (2002). Reversing productivity losses from iron deficiency: The economic case. *Journal of Nutrition, 132*(Suppl. 4), 794S–801S.

93. Fogel, R. (1991). *New sources and new techniques for the study of secular trends in nutritional status, health, mortality, and the process of aging*. Cambridge, MA: National Bureau of Economic Research.

94. Wolgemuth, J. C., Latham, M. C., Hall, A., Chesher, A., & Crompton, D. W. (1982). Worker productivity and the nutritional status of Kenyan road construction laborers. *American Journal of Clinical Nutrition, 36*(1), 68–78.

95. Li, R., Chen, X., Yan, H., Deurenberg, P., Garby, L., & Hautvast, J. G. (1994). Functional consequences of iron supplementation in iron-deficient female cotton mill workers in Beijing, China. *American Journal of Clinical Nutrition, 59*(4), 908–913.

96. World Health Organization. (2009). *Global health risks: Mortality and burden of disease attributable to selected major risks, 2009*. Geneva: WHO. Retrieved September 4, 2014, from http://www.who.int/healthinfo/global_burden_disease/GlobalHealthRisks_report_full.pdf.

97. Danaei, G., Ding, E. L., Mozaffarian, D., Taylor, B., Rehm, J., Murray, C. J., et al. (2009). The preventable causes of death in the United States: Comparative risk assessment of dietary, lifestyle, and metabolic risk factors. *PLoS Medicine, 6*(4), e1000058.

98. Prospective Studies Collaboration, et al. (2009). Body-mass index and cause-specific mortality in 900,000 adults: Collaborative analyses of 57 prospective studies. *Lancet, 373*, 1083–1096.

99. Beaglehole, R., Bonita, R., Horton, R., et al. (2011). Priority actions for the non-communicable disease crisis. *Lancet, 377*(9775), 1438–1447.

100. Centers for Medicare & Medicaid Services. (2013). *National health expenditures 2013 highlights*. Retrieved September 4, 2014, from http://www.cms.gov/Research-Statistics-Data-and-Systems/Statistics-Trends-and-Reports/NationalHealthExpendData/downloads/highlights.pdf.

101. Cawley, J., & Meyerhoefer, C. (2012). The medical care costs of obesity: An instrumental variables approach. *Journal of Health Economics, 31*(1), 219–230.

102. Popkin, B., Horton, S., & Kim, S. (2001). The nutrition transition and prevention of diet-related chronic diseases in Asia and the Pacific. *Food and Nutrition Bulletin, 22*(4), 1–58.

103. Bloom, D. E., Cafiero, E. T., McGovern, M. E., Prettner, K., Stanciole, A., Weiss, J., et al. (2013). *The economic impact of non-communicable disease in China and India: Estimates, projections, and comparisons* (NBER Working Paper No. 19335). Cambridge, MA: National Bureau of Economic Research.

104. Thompson, D., Edelsberg, J., Kinsey, K. L., & Oster, G. (1998). Estimated economic costs of obesity to U.S. business. *American Journal of Health Promotion, 13*(2), 120–127.

105. World Health Organization. (2000). *Obesity: Preventing and managing the global epidemic* (No. 894). Geneva: World Health Organization.

106. Abegunde, D. O., Mathers, C. D., Adam, T., Ortegon, M., & Strong, K. (2007). The burden and costs of chronic diseases in low-income and middle-income countries. *Lancet, 370*(9603), 1929–1938.

107. Food and Agriculture Organization of the United Nations. (2013). *The state of food and agriculture, 2013*. Rome, Italy: Author. Retrieved September 4, 2014, from http://www.fao.org/docrep/018/i3300e/i3300e.pdf.

108. Bloom, D. E., Cafiero, E., Jané-Llopis, E., Abrahams-Gessel, S., Bloom, L. R., Fathima, S., et al. (2011). *The global economic burden of noncommunicable diseases*. Geneva: World Economic Forum.

109. Kolotkin, R. L., Meter, K., & Williams, G. R. (2001). Quality of life and obesity. *Obesity Reviews, 2*(4), 219–229.

110. Friedman, R. R., & Puhl, R. M. (2012). *Weight bias: A social justice issue*. New Haven, CT: Yale University, Rudd Center for Food Policy and Obesity.

111. Basnet, A. S., & Mathema, P. (2010). *Micronutrient supplementation brings new hope for children in Nepal*. Retrieved January 10, 2011, http://www.unicef.org/infobycountry/nepal_56023.html.

112. Micronutrient Initiative. (2009). *Investing in the future: A united call to action on vitamin and mineral deficiencies. Global report 2009*. Ottawa, Ontario, Canada: Author. Retrieved January 10, 2011, http://www.united calltoaction.org/documents/Investing_in_the_future.pdf.

113. Micronutrient Initiative. *Nepal*. Retrieved January 10, 2011, from http://www.micronutrient.org/english/view.asp?x=605.

114. UNICEF. (2003). *Getting to the roots: Mobilizing community volunteers to combat vitamin A deficiency disorders in Nepal*. Kathmandu, Nepal: UNICEF Regional Office for South Asia. Retrieved May 31, 2015, from http://www.unicef.org/rosa/Getting.pdf.

115. Micronutrient Initiative. (2007). *Accelerating food fortification: A Rapid Results Initiative in Kenya*. Retrieved May 31, 2015, from http://rapidresultsinstitute.info/wp-content/uploads/2012/02/Kenya-Micro-Nutrients.pdf.

116. Micronutrient Initiative. *Accelerating food fortification in Kenya: A results based approach to forming public-private partnerships*. Retrieved June 15, 2015, from http://www.rapidresults.org/wp-content/uploads/2015/06/Accelerating-Food-Fortification-in-Kenya.pdf.

117. Stein, A. H., Wang, M., DiGirolamo, A., et al. Nutritional supplementation in early childhood, schooling, and intellectual functioning in adulthood: A prospective study in Guatemala. *Archives of Pediatrics and Adolescent Medicine, 162*(7), 612–618.

118. Hoddinott, J., Maluccio, J. A., Behrman, J. R., Flores, R., & Martorell, R. (2008). Effect of a nutrition intervention during early childhood on economic productivity in Guatemalan adults. *Lancet, 371*(9610), 411–416.

119. Behrman, J. R., Calderon, M. C., Preston, S. H., Hoddinott, J., Martorell, R., & Stein, A. D. (2009). Nutritional supplementation in girls influences the growth of their children: Prospective study in Guatemala. *American Journal of Clinical Nutrition, 90*, 1372–1379.

120. Lee, M. J., Popkin, B. M., & Kim, S. (2002). The unique aspects of the nutrition transition in South Korea: The retention of healthful elements in their traditional diet. *Public Health Nutrition, 5*(1a), 197–203.

121. Kim, S., Moon, S., & Popkin, B. M. (2000). The nutrition transition in South Korea. *American Journal of Clinical Nutrition, 71*(1), 44–53.

122. Drewnowski, A., & Popkin, B. M. (1997). The nutrition transition: New trends in the global diet. *Nutrition Reviews, 55*(2), 31–43.

123. Korean Dietetic Association. Retrieved September 20, 2014, from http://www.dietitian.or.kr.

124. South Korean Ministry of Health and Welfare. (1969–1999). *Reports on 1969–95 National Nutrition Survey; Report on 1998 National Health and Nutrition Survey.* Seoul, South Korea: Ministry of Health and Welfare.

125. Organisation for Economic Co-operation and Development. *Obesity and the economics of prevention: Fit not fat. Korea key facts.* Retrieved September 24, 2014, from http://www.oecd.org/els/health-systems /obesityandtheeconomicsofpreventionfitnotfat-koreakeyfacts.htm.

126. Rego, A., Berardo, F., & Rodrigues, S. (1990). Fatores de risco para doenças crônico não-transmissíveis: Inquérito domiciliar no município de São Paulo, SP (Brasil). Metodologia e resultados preliminares. *Revista de Saúde Pública, 24,* 277–285.

127. Matsudo, S. M., Matsudo, V. R., Araujo, T. L., Andrade, D. R., Andrade, E. L., et al. (2003). The Agita São Paulo Program as a model for using physical activity to promote health. *Revista Panamericana de Salud Pública, 14*(4), 265–272.

128. National Social Marketing Centre. (2012). *ShowCase: Agita São Paulo.* Retrieved October 17, 2014, from http://www.consumerfocus.org.uk /files/2012/09/Agita-Sao-Paulo-FULL-case-study.pdf.

129. Organización Panamericana de la Salud. (2002). *A multisectoral coalition in health: Agita São Paulo, una coalición multisectorial en salud.* São Paulo, Brasil: Midiograf.

130. European Commission. (2008). *Collated information on salt reduction in the EU, 2008.* Retrieved September 23, 2014 from http:// ec.europa.eu/health/ph_determinants/life_style/nutrition/documents /compilation_salt_en.pdf.

131. World Health Organization & Food and Agriculture Organization. (2003). *Diet, nutrition and the prevention of chronic diseases* (Technical report series 916). Geneva: World Health Organization; Rome: Food and Agriculture Organization.

132. He, F. J., & MacGregor, G. A. (2009). A comprehensive review on salt and health and current experience of worldwide salt reduction programmes. *Journal of Human Hypertension, 23*(6), 363–384.

133. Laatikainen, T., Pietinen, P., Valsta, L., Sundvall, J., Reinivuo, H., & Tuomilehto, J. (2006). Sodium in the Finnish diet: 20-year trends in urinary sodium excretion among the adult population. *European Journal of Clinical Nutrition, 60*(8), 965–970.

134. Karppanen, H., & Mervaala, E. (2006). Sodium intake and hypertension. *Progress in Cardiovascular Diseases, 49*(2), 59–75.

135. Pietinen, P., Valsta, L. M., Hirvonen, T., & Sinkko, H. (2007). Labelling the salt content in foods: A useful tool in reducing sodium intake in Finland. *Public Health Nutrition, 11*(4), 335–340.

136. World Action on Salt & Health. (2009). *Finland: Salt action summary.* Retrieved September 24, 2014, from http://www.worldactiononsalt.com /worldaction/europe/53774.html.

137. The World Bank. (1994). *Impact evaluation report: Tamil Nadu Integrated Nutrition Project.* Washington, DC: World Bank.

138. Goh, C. C. (2002). Combating iodine deficiency: Lessons from China, Indonesia, and Madagascar. *Food and Nutrition Bulletin, 23*(3), 280–291.

139. Levine, R., & What Works Working Group. (2007). *Case studies in global health: Millions saved.* Sudbury, MA: Jones and Bartlett.

140. Griffiths, M., Dicken, K., & Favin, M. (1996). *Promoting the growth of children: What works: Rationale and guidance for programs.* Washington, DC: World Bank.

141. Levinson, F. J., & Bassett, L. (2008). *Malnutrition is still a major contributor to child deaths.* Washington, DC: Population Reference Bureau.

142. Lofti, M., Merx, R., Naber, P., & Van der Heuvel, P. (1996). *Micronutrient fortification of foods: Current prospectus, research and opportunities.* Ottawa: International Agriculture Centre.

143. United Nations General Assembly. (2011). *Draft political declaration of the high-level meeting on the prevention and control of non-communicable diseases.* Retrieved September 20, 2014, from http://www.un.org/en/ga /ncdmeeting2011/pdf/NCD_draft_political_declaration.pdf.

144. U.S. Department of Health and Human Services. (2008). *Physical activity guidelines for Americans.* Retrieved September 1, 2014, from http:// www.health.gov/paguidelines/.

145. U.S. Department of Agriculture. *Dietary guidelines from around the world.* Retrieved September 2, 2014, from http://fnic.nal.usda.gov /professional-and-career-resources/ethnic-and-cultural-resources/dietary -guidelines-around-world.

146. Let's Move Campaign. *Let's move: America's Move to raise a healthier generation of kids.* Retrieved September 2, 2014, from http://www.letsmove .gov/.

147. Knight, H. S. F. (2014, October 11). *Soda tax backers sweet on Mexico's sugar-fighting success.* Retrieved March 21, 2015, from http:// www.sfgate.com/bayarea/article/S-F-soda-tax-proponents-salute-Mexico -as-model-5815356.php.

148. Guo, X., Popkin, B. M., Mroz, T. A., & Zhai, F. (1999). Food price policy can favorably alter macronutrient intake in China. *Journal of Nutrition, 129*(5), 994–1001.

149. Cash, S. B., Sunding, D. L., & Zilberman, D. (2005). Fat taxes and thin subsidies: Prices, diet, and health outcomes. *Acta Agriculturae Scandinavica Section C, 2*(3–4), 167–174.

150. Zhai, F., Fu, D., Du, S., Ge, K., Chen, C., Popkin, B. M. (2002). What is China doing in policy-making to push back the negative aspects of the nutrition transition? *Public Health Nutrition, 5*(1a), 269–273.

151. Kramer, L. (1995). Nutrition labels help build deli, bakery sales. *Supermarket News, 20,* 21–24.

152. Benincá, C., Zanoelo, E. F., de Lima Luz, L. F. Jr., Spricigo, C. B. (2009). Trans fatty acids in margarines marketed in Brazil: Content, labeling regulations and consumer information. *European Journal of Lipid Science and Technology, 111*(5), 451–458.

153. Skeaf, C. M. (2009). Feasibility of recommending certain replacement or alternative fats. *European Journal of Clinical Nutrition, 63,* S34–S49.

154. Coombes, R. (2011). Trans fats: Chasing a global ban. *BMJ, 343,* d5567.

155. Ratnayake, W. M., L'Abbe, M. R., Farnworth, S., et al. (2009). Trans fatty acids: Current contents in Canadian foods and estimated intake levels for the Canadian population. *Journal of AOAC International, 92*(5), 1258–1276.

156. Kmietowicz, Z. (2012). EU law forces UK ministers to rethink food labelling. *BMJ, 344,* e3422.

157. Roberto, C. A., Larsen, P. D., Agnew, H., Baik, J., & Brownell, K. D. (2010). Evaluating the impact of menu labeling on food choices and intake. *American Journal of Public Health, 100*(2), 312–318.

158. Department of Health. *Calories to be capped and cut.* Retrieved September 17, 2014, from http://mediacentre.dh.gov.uk/2012/03/24/calories -to-be-capped-and-cut/.

159. The Healthy Weight Commitment Foundation. Retrieved September 3, 2014, from http://www.healthyweightcommit.org/.

160. Hawkes, C. (2007). Regulating and litigating in the public interest. Regulating food marketing to young people worldwide: Trends and policy drivers. *American Journal of Public Health, 97*(11), 1962–1973.

161. World Health Organization. (2004). *Global strategy on diet, physical activity and health.* Retrieved September 4, 2014, from http://apps.who.int /iris/bitstream/10665/43035/1/9241592222_eng.pdf?ua=1.

162. Hawkes, C., Smith, T. G., Jewell, J., Wardle, J., Hammond, R. A., Friel, S., et al. (2015, February 18). Smart food policies for obesity prevention. *Lancet, 385*(9985), 2410–2421.

163. Nickelodeon. Worldwide day of play. Retrieved September 3, 2014, from http://www.nick.com/road-to-wwdop/.

164. Huang, T. T. K., Cawley, J. H., Ashe, M., Costa, S. A., Frerichs, L. M., Zwicker, L., et al. (2015, February 18). Mobilisation of public support for policy actions to prevent obesity. *Lancet, 385*(9985), 2422–2431.

165. Pekka, P., Pirjo, P., & Ulla, U. (2002). Influencing public nutrition for non-communicable disease prevention: From community intervention to national programme—Experiences from Finland. *Public Health Nutrition, 5*(1a), 245–251.

166. Gortmaker, S. L., Peterson, K., Wiecha, J., Sobol, A., Dixit, S., Fox, M. K., et al. (1999). Reducing obesity via a school-based interdisciplinary intervention among youth: Planet Health. *Archives of Pediatrics and Adolescent Medicine, 153*(4), 409–418.

167. Dietz, W. H., Baur, L. A., Hall, K., Puhl, R. M., Taveras, E. M., Uauy, R., et al. (2015, February 18). Management of obesity: Improvement of health-care training and systems for prevention and care. *Lancet.*

168. Artinian, N. T., Fletcher, G. F., Mozaffarian, D., Kris-Etherton, P., Van Horn, L., Lichtenstein, A. H., et al. (2010). Interventions to promote physical activity and dietary lifestyle changes for cardiovascular risk factor reduction in adults: A scientific statement from the American Heart Association. *Circulation, 122*(4), 406–441.

CHAPTER **9**

Women's Health

VIGNETTES

Suneeta was pregnant with her first child. She lived in northern India where many families prefer to have sons rather than daughters, especially for their firstborn child. Eager to have a son, Suneeta's husband took her to get a sonogram to determine the sex of the baby. When they learned the baby would be a girl, they decided that Suneeta should abort the fetus and try to get pregnant again in hopes of having a boy.

Sarah lived in rural Pakistan and was pregnant with her second child. When she went into labor, Sarah called for the traditional birth attendant, as most women did in her town. As Sarah's labor continued, she and the birth attendant realized that the labor was complicated. Sarah needed to go to a hospital to deliver the baby. In this part of Pakistan, however, women could not be taken to hospitals without their husband's permission. Sarah's husband was working in another city and was not available to give such permission. Several hours later, Sarah and the baby died at Sarah's home.

Carmen lived in a slum in Guatemala City, Guatemala. She was not married but became pregnant after relations with a man she had met several months before. In her culture, pregnancy without being married was a source of great shame for a woman's family. Fearing the reaction of her family to her pregnancy, Carmen decided to get an abortion. Although abortions are illegal in Guatemala, except to save the life of the mother,[1] they are performed there by both licensed physicians and unlicensed medical practitioners. Carmen could not afford the fee charged by a physician and went instead to an unlicensed abortionist. Carmen's abortion was not performed properly. She bled profusely as a result of the procedure, and she died before she could be taken to a hospital.

Elizabeth was a 15-year-old girl in Cape Town, South Africa. She was a good student but came from a poor family and was always short of the money she needed to pay for school supplies, uniforms, and books. John had been eyeing Elizabeth for some time. He was 25 years old, had a good job, and was always interested in spending time with the young ladies at Elizabeth's school. At the start of the second semester, when Elizabeth was trying to get together the money for school, John convinced her to sleep with him in exchange for a small amount of money. Elizabeth knew about HIV, but John convinced her that he was healthy and there was no need to use a condom. About a year later, Elizabeth fell ill, was given an HIV test, and turned out to be HIV-positive.

THE IMPORTANCE OF WOMEN'S HEALTH

These vignettes suggest several reasons why women's health issues must be given a prominent place in the global health agenda:

- Being born female can be dangerous to your health, especially in low- and middle-income countries.
- In many societies women are subjected to discrimination and very prescribed roles, both of which can be harmful to their health.
- Women face a number of unique health problems by virtue of their sex and their place in society.
- There are often important and unjustifiable differentials in the health of men and women.
- Morbidity, disability, and premature death of women can have enormous social and economic consequences on the affected women, on their families, and on society more broadly.
- Many relatively low-cost investments in the health of women would result in substantial numbers of deaths and disability-adjusted life years (DALYs) averted.
- Improving the education and health of women and their place in society is one of the most powerful and cost-effective approaches that can be taken to promote social and economic development.

In addition, the health of women is intimately linked with the Millennium Development Goals (MDGs).[2] **Table 9-1** indicates how six of the eight goals have a powerful relationship to women's health.

This chapter aims to give the reader a sense of the following:

- The key challenges facing women in low- and middle-income countries that relate to reproductive health and violence against women
- Which women are most affected by these challenges
- The key risk factors for these challenges
- The social and economic consequences of health problems for women
- What can be done to address these problems in as cost-effective a manner as possible

The chapter also includes comments on some of the key differentials in the health of men and women worldwide. In addition, it contains a number of policy and program briefs and case studies that illustrate some of its main points. Other aspects of health that relate in particular ways to women are covered elsewhere in the book, specifically in the chapters on

TABLE 9-1 Key Links Between Women's Health and the MDGs

Goal 1: Eradicate Poverty and Hunger

Link: Poor health and nutritional status of women is both a cause and an effect of poverty. Enhancing the nutritional status of women will improve their health and the health of their babies, with many associated beneficial consequences for both.

Goal 2: Achieve Universal Primary Education

Link: Improving the health of females will enhance their enrollment in, attendance at, and performance in schools. Improving the educational attainments of females will lead to improvements in their health and the health of their children.

Goal 3: Promote Gender Equality and Empower Women

Link: Improvements in equity and empowerment will lead to better education for females, more income-earning opportunities for them, and less violence against them, all of which will improve their health status.

Goal 4: Reduce Child Mortality

Link: An important share of child mortality is linked with poor health and nutritional status of the mother. Improving the health and nutritional status of the mother is the starting point for reducing the share of children born with low birthweight, a major contributor to child morbidity and mortality.

Goal 5: Improve Maternal Health

Link: This is directly connected to the health of women.

Goal 6: Combat HIV/AIDS, Malaria, and Other Diseases

Link: Women are disproportionately affected by HIV/AIDS, which is a major cause of illness, disability, and death for women. Combating HIV/AIDS would have a major impact on the health of females and on their families as well.

Data from United Nations. *Millennium Development Goals.* Available at: http://www.unece.org/fileadmin/DAM/commission/2006/MDG_Report_final.pdf. Accessed February 10, 2015.

nutrition, communicable diseases, and noncommunicable diseases.

KEY DEFINITIONS

As one reviews the most important health issues that affect women worldwide, a number of terms will be used repeatedly. The most important of these are shown in **Table 9-2**.

THE DETERMINANTS OF WOMEN'S HEALTH

The determinants of a woman's health relate to both sex and gender. "Sex is biological."[3,p205] It has to do with being born a female. "Gender is cultural."[3,p205] Gender has to do with societal norms about the roles of women and their social position relative to men.[4] Some health issues are primarily determined by biology, such as the fact that women alone get ovarian

---

TABLE 9-2 Selected Definitions in Women's Health

Abortion—The premature expulsion or loss of embryo, which may be induced or spontaneous.

Caesarean delivery (section)—The surgical delivery of a fetus through abdominal incision.

Eclampsia—A serious, life-threatening condition in late pregnancy in which very high blood pressure can cause a woman to have seizures.

Family planning—The conscious effort of couples to regulate the number and spacing of births through artificial and natural methods of contraception.

Female genital mutilation—Traditional practices that are all related to the cutting of the female genital organs.

Gestational diabetes—Diabetes that develops during pregnancy because of improper regulation of blood sugar.

Hemorrhage (related to pregnancy)—Significant and uncontrolled loss of blood, either internally or externally from the body. Antepartum (prenatal) hemorrhage occurs after the 20th week of gestation but before delivery of the baby. Postpartum hemorrhage is the loss of 500 mL or more of blood from the genital tract after delivery of the baby. Primary postpartum hemorrhage occurs in the first 24 hours after delivery.

Maternal death—The death of a woman while pregnant, during delivery, or within 42 days of delivery.

Obstetric fistula—An injury in the birth canal that allows leakage from the bladder or rectum into the vagina, leaving a woman permanently incontinent.

Preeclampsia (previously called toxemia)—A condition characterized by pregnancy-induced high blood pressure, protein in the urine, and swelling (edema) due to fluid retention.

Sepsis—A serious medical condition caused by a severe infection, leading to a systemic inflammatory response.

Sex-selective abortion—The practice of aborting a fetus after a determination that the fetus is an undesired sex, typically female.

Data from Planned Parenthood. Glossary. http://www.plannedparenthood.org/learn/glossary. Retrieved April 14, 2015.
American Diabetes Association. Gestational diabetes. http://www.diabetes.org/diabetes-basics/gestational/. Retrieved April 14, 2015.
Medscape. Postpartum hemorrhage. http://emedicine.medscape.com/article/275038-overview. Retrieved April 14, 2015.
World Bank. Maternal mortality ratio (modeled estimate, per 100,000 live births). http://data.worldbank.org/indicator/SH.STA.MMRT. Retrieved April 14, 2015.
Medline Plus. Sepsis. http://www.nlm.nih.gov/medlineplus/ency/article/000666.htm. Retrieved April 14, 2015 .

cancer. Other women's health issues are determined mostly by social factors, such as sex-selective abortion of female fetuses. Most women's health issues, however, are determined by a combination of biological and social determinants, such as the case of Sarah in the opening vignettes, who died in childbirth for a number of biological and social reasons that interacted. Further comments are given now on the biological and social determinants of women's health.

Biological Determinants

Women face a number of unique biological risks. One is iron deficiency anemia related to menstruation. Other risks are associated with pregnancy, including complications of pregnancy itself, diseases that may be aggravated by pregnancy, and the effects of some unhealthy lifestyle choices, such as smoking, on pregnancy.[5] During pregnancy, there are a number of conditions, for example, that can cause women to become ill or to die, including hypertensive disorders of pregnancy. In addition, a woman can be left with a number of permanent disabilities related to pregnancy, including uterine prolapse and obstetric fistula. Women can also die of preeclampsia or eclampsia. It is hemorrhage, however, that is the leading cause of maternal mortality. The conditions that can exacerbate pregnancy-related health risks include malaria, hepatitis, tuberculosis, malnutrition, and obesity, as well as certain mental health issues, such as depression. Unsafe abortions lead to significant morbidity and mortality for women. In terms of the effects of lifestyles on pregnancy, it is clear that certain occupations and the use of alcohol, tobacco, and drugs are especially important to avoid during pregnancy.[5]

Women are also biologically more susceptible to some sexually transmitted infections than men are, including to the HIV virus.[6] This relates to the fact that women have a greater mucosal area that is exposed during sexual relations than men have. There are also certain health conditions specific to women for biological reasons, such as uterine cancer or ovarian cancer, as mentioned previously. There are other health conditions that affect men, but for which women have a disproportionate share of the burden of disease, such as breast cancer. As women age, they also have a higher rate of heart disease than men have, although it is diagnosed far less frequently.[4]

Social Determinants

The social determinants of women's health are also very important, especially in societies that favor males. These social determinants relate predominantly to gender norms, which assign different roles and values to males and females, usually to the disadvantage of females. In many societies,

women's inferior status leads to social, health, and economic problems that men do not face.

The social determinants of health begin even before women are born. In some societies where male preference is very strong, such as in India and in China, some families determine the sex of their unborn children with the use of sonograms and then abort females, especially for the birth of their first child.[7,8] This was the case for Suneeta in one of the opening vignettes.[9]

Female infants are often breastfed less than boys of the same age and then fed less complementary food when they become toddlers.[10] In addition, young girls in many societies are also fed less than their male siblings. Older women in some cultures feed men first and then eat only the portions that are remaining. Others eat less nutritious food than the men in their family eat. Poor nutrition, often stemming partly from social causes, makes women more susceptible to illness. It also contributes to stunting and small pelvic size, which are hazards to the health of pregnant women and to their offspring.

There are a number of critical social issues that relate to women's sexual experiences. The low social status of women in many societies is linked to the physical and sexual abuse of women. Furthermore, male dominance means that women often have a limited choice about when and how to have sexual relations, with whom, and whether or not to use protection. As a result, women are frequently forced to have sex, often at young ages, and many times without a condom or other contraceptives. For these social reasons, women face heightened risks of becoming pregnant, having repeated pregnancies at close intervals, and getting sexually transmitted infections, including HIV/AIDS. In addition, rape is common in many settings, especially in areas of conflict.

A dowry is the gift that a bride's family gives to the family of a groom, and another form of violence against women is "dowry death." The data on mortality for young women in India suggest that there is a disproportionate number of young married women who accidentally die of burns, which are often alleged to occur when women are cooking. It appears, however, that some of these deaths are not accidental. Rather, the husband's family sometimes perpetrates the burning of the young woman when they are not satisfied with the dowry that she has brought to her marriage.[11]

High levels of depression also appear to be related to the low status of women in different societies and the expectations that those societies have of them. There is also widespread reporting in many societies of general gynecologic discomfort without physical explanation, which may be related to the life stressors many women face.[3]

Especially in low-income populations, there are numerous households that are headed by females who are divorced, separated, or widowed, or by women whose husbands are working elsewhere. The poorest people in a community tend to live in these households. These women also tend to be among the least well-educated people in a community. Low income and limited education negatively impact the health of such women. In addition, divorced or widowed women face severe discrimination in a number of cultures.

The roles that women play in different cultures can also pose important hazards to their health. In many societies, for example, women cook indoors on open fires without adequate ventilation. This is strongly associated with respiratory problems for these women and for their children.

Poverty, lack of or low levels of education, and low social status of women in many societies seriously constrain the access of women to health services. In addition, girls and women who need health services often do not take advantage of such services in a timely way. There are numerous instances, for example, in which women cannot use health services without the permission of a husband or male relative or without having a male relative take them to health services. In some settings, even when women need emergency care, such as during complications of pregnancy, social constraints prevent them from seeking such care and inhibit their husbands from taking them for treatment, as reflected in the vignette about Sarah.

THE BURDEN OF HEALTH CONDITIONS FOR FEMALES

Having looked at the biological and social determinants of health for women, we can now look at some of the key health issues that females face, their prevalence, and the critical risk factors for those health conditions. This part of the chapter focuses on sex-selective abortion, female genital mutilation, sexually transmitted infections, violence against women, and complications of pregnancy, with brief mention of nutrition.

Sex-Selective Abortion

How common is sex-selective abortion worldwide? How many unborn children are affected? Sex-selective abortion appears to be more prevalent in India and China than in any other country.[12] A number of studies have been done of this phenomenon and one study suggested that close to 10 million female fetuses were aborted in India in the last 20 years.[13] A more recent study concluded that India now has between 300,000 and 600,000 abortions of female fetuses each year, about 2 to 4 percent of all pregnancies with a female fetus. The study further concluded that from 2001–2010, 3 to 6 million female fetuses were aborted.[9]

An important consequence of sex-selective abortion is the skewed ratios of males to females in a number of countries. Naturally, one would expect that there would be about 105 females born for every 100 males. However, in India today, about 112 males are born for every 100 females, and in China there are about 111 males born for every 100 females. This phenomenon used to be the case in a number of other countries, including Singapore and South Korea, but the sex ratios at birth in those countries are now closer to what one would naturally expect.[14]

There is considerable evidence worldwide that both family size and preferences for males decrease as income and education rise. In the case of the countries cited previously, however, this has not been the case. Rather, as incomes and education have risen, and as technology has become more available, some families have used their income, knowledge, and access to technology—ultrasound in this case—to express their preference for males by engaging in sex-selective abortion. In India, this takes place especially after the first-born child is a female.[9] The one-child policy in China has almost certainly exacerbated male preference.

Female Genital Mutilation

Female genital mutilation (FGM) is sometimes called female genital cutting (FGC) or is referred to as female genital mutilation/cutting. The World Health Organization (WHO) has grouped female genital mutilation into four types, generally varying from excision of the prepuce, the fold of skin surrounding the clitoris, to excision of part or all of the external genitalia and the stitching and narrowing of the vaginal opening. There are also a variety of related practices, including pricking of the genitalia or using chemicals to narrow the vaginal opening.[15]

It is estimated that half of the girls who undergo FGM will be cut before they are 5 years of age and the remainder will be cut before they are 15 years of age. The cutting is generally done with razor blades, knives, or glass. It is estimated that about 125 million women worldwide have had genital cutting performed on them. Estimates also suggest that as many as 3 million girls in sub-Saharan Africa and in Egypt have this cutting performed on them each year. In some countries, such as Egypt, Guinea, and Somalia, female genital mutilation is practically universal among women who are 15 to 49 years old. However, there are other countries in Africa, such as Cameroon, Niger, and Uganda, in which only a small share of the women have had FGM. The practice appears to be diminishing almost everywhere, with fewer younger girls being cut than their mothers. Female genital mutilation is very closely related to ethnicity. In addition, the higher the level of education of the mother, the less likely the daughter is to be cut.[16]

When FGM is performed initially, it can result in terrible pain or shock. It is also associated with infection, because the instruments used for cutting are not always clean, as well as with acute hemorrhage. Over the longer term, it can lead to the retention of urine, infertility, and obstructed labor. Studies have shown that those more severely cut are more likely than others to have postpartum hemorrhage, caesarean section, and long stays in hospital. In addition, the babies of such women are more likely than babies born to mothers who have not undergone FGM to need resuscitation immediately after birth, to be stillborn, or to die a neonatal death.[17] If infection and hemorrhage linked to the act of FGM are not addressed in a timely and appropriate manner, FGM can also lead to death.[15]

Sexually Transmitted Infections

This section addresses sexually transmitted infections (STIs) other than HIV. It is important as one reviews this section to note that women are more biologically susceptible to sexually transmitted infections because of more exposed mucosal surfaces, because they often show no symptoms of those diseases, and because their roles in society make them less likely to get treated for sexually transmitted infections than men.

Sexually transmitted infections, other than HIV, that are not treated in a timely and appropriate manner can have a number of long-lasting effects on the health of women. These include pelvic inflammatory disease, chronic pain, ovarian abscesses, ectopic pregnancies, and infertility.[18] When pregnant women cannot get STIs treated in appropriate and timely ways, it can lead to fetal wastage, stillbirths, low-birthweight babies, eye and lung damage in babies, and congenital abnormalities.[18] In fact, recent estimates suggest that syphilis in pregnancy results in 305,000 fetal and neonatal deaths annually.[19] In addition, the complications of syphilis can lead to the death of the infected person.[18] Human papilloma virus (HPV) is associated with cervical cancer[18] and is estimated to cause about 530,000 cases of HPV a year and 275,000 cervical cancer deaths a year.[19] Chlamydia bears special mention because it is nine times more prevalent in women than in men.[4] Chlamydia is very prevalent in low-income countries and is associated with chronic conjunctivitis, reproductive tract infections, genital ulcer disease, and infertility.[4]

The *Global Burden of Disease Study 2010* includes estimates of the burden of disease from STIs, other than HIV. That study suggests that about 0.5 percent of the burden of disease among men and women in low- and middle-income countries can be attributed to syphilis, gonorrhea, sexually

transmitted chlamydial diseases, gonococcal infection, and other sexually transmitted infections (besides HIV/AIDS). Women in those countries face a slightly disproportionate burden of STIs, compared to men. Sub-Saharan Africa faces a disproportionately high share of morbidity and mortality from STIs compared to other regions. The STIs noted here are associated with about 1.0 percent of the total burden of disease in sub-Saharan Africa and about 1.2 percent of the burden in women in that region.[20]

From the limited studies available, the prevalence of chlamydia, gonorrhea, and syphilis appears to vary widely. Earlier studies done in China showed that rates of chlamydia in different parts of China ranged from 1 to 24 percent.[18] Studies done in other parts of Asia indicated that the prevalence of syphilis ranged from almost negligible to about 15 percent.[18] Studies done in sub-Saharan Africa have shown ranges for chlamydia from 2 to 30 percent, for gonorrhea from 2 to 32 percent, and for syphilis from almost negligible to 23 percent.[18]

Young people are at special risk of STIs, because they are often forced to have sex, their sexual relations are often unplanned, and they may not have the power or skills to use a condom.[17]

The risk factors for a woman getting an STI are well known and include young age when engaging in sexual relations, often because of child marriage, especially in Asia and sub-Saharan Africa; multiple sexual partners; sex with high-risk partners, including partners considerably older than the woman; and inability to use a condom. The use of alcohol and drugs is also associated with unprotected sex, as is unequal power between the woman and the man who are engaging in sexual relations.

Violence and Sexual Abuse Against Women

Violence and sexual abuse against women occur with remarkable frequency throughout the world. Violence is usually episodic, it is often not reported, and it is often associated with sexual abuse.[10] Sexual abuse can include rape, sexual assault, sexual molestation, sexual harassment, and incest.[21] It is very hard to get reliable data on violence and sexual abuse against women. However, a 2006 UNAIDS study suggested that 10–50 percent of women worldwide have been abused physically by an intimate partner at least once in their lives. The UNAIDS study also noted that "between 20–48% of adolescent girls aged 10–25 report their first sexual encounter was forced."[22] Another study on intimate partner violence indicated that "one-third of women have been beaten, coerced into sex, or subjected to extreme emotional abuse."[23,p159] The most recent WHO estimates of intimate partner violence suggest that:[24]

- About 35 percent of all women have been subject to sexual violence and or physical violence from an intimate partner or nonpartner.
- Worldwide about 30 percent of all women have been subject to intimate partner violence, although in some regions this is close to 40 percent.
- Thirty-eight percent of all women who are murdered are murdered by intimate partners.
- Seven percent of all women have been subjected to sexual violence by someone who was not an intimate partner.

In addition, there have been a number of conflicts in which rape has been used systematically, as a "tool of war."[25]

Violence and abuse against women have a number of negative consequences for the health of women. These include injuries, unwanted pregnancies, STIs, depression, and sometimes permanent disability or death.[5] The risk factors for whether or not a woman will suffer violence can be complicated, are often a result of many factors, and are not well-documented. However, it appears that such violence is associated with factors such as young age of the male partner, a history of violence of the male partner, low socioeconomic status of the male and female involved, proximity to drugs or alcohol, social isolation, and gender inequality. The likelihood of violence is heightened in conflict and postconflict situations.[26]

Maternal Morbidity and Mortality

WHO estimates that 289,000 maternal deaths occurred in 2013, meaning deaths that occur during pregnancy, during childbirth, or until 42 days after the baby is born.[27,28] From 1990 to 2013, it is estimated that the number of maternal deaths that occur annually declined by about 45 percent, which represented a decline of about 2.6 percent annually over that period. Although this is important progress, it was less than the 5 percent rate of annual decline that is needed to achieve the MDG concerning maternal mortality.[27]

About 99 percent of these maternal deaths occur in low- and middle-income countries. Sub-Saharan Africa accounts for about 62 percent of these deaths and South Asia for 24 percent. One-third of the maternal deaths occur in India and Nigeria. Ten countries account for almost 60 percent of all maternal deaths: India, Nigeria, Democratic Republic of the Congo, Ethiopia, Indonesia, Pakistan, Tanzania, Kenya, China, and Uganda.[29]

The low estimate of the global maternal mortality ratio was 160 per 100,000 live births. It was also estimated that the maternal mortality ratio in low- and middle-income countries was 230, or 14 times higher than the rate of 16 in high-income countries. The lifetime risk of dying a maternal death was estimated at 1 in 190 for the world as a whole, 1 in 3,700 for high-income countries, but 1 in 160 in low- and middle-income countries. The highest maternal mortality ratio was in Sierra Leone, where it was 1,100. The highest lifetime risk of dying a maternal death was in Chad at 1 in 15 and Somalia at 1 in 18.[29] **Table 9-3** shows the maternal mortality ratio by World Bank region and the lifetime chance of maternal death in those regions.

Birth is the time of greatest risk for the mother and the baby. Studies suggest that 42 percent of maternal deaths happen during birth or the first day after birth[30] and that between 50 and 71 percent of maternal deaths occur in the postpartum period, with most of those occurring in the first week after birth.[5]

There are both indirect and direct causes of maternal death. About 28 percent of maternal deaths are from obstructed labor and indirect causes, meaning diseases that complicate pregnancy or that are complicated by pregnancy. These include malaria, anemia, HIV/AIDS, and cardiovascular disease.[5] The importance of these problems depends on the presence of these diseases in different communities and how effective the health system is in responding to them. About 80 percent of maternal deaths stem from direct causes, including hemorrhage, infection, and hypertensive disorders, Unsafe abortion is also an important contributor to maternal death.[27,31] **Figure 9-1** indicates the major causes of maternal death and the share of maternal deaths worldwide that are associated with them.

The risk of maternal death is a stark reflection of the disparities in the health status between different countries and within those countries. A woman in the high-income countries has only a 1 in 3,400 chance of dying a maternal death. In sub-Saharan Africa, however, a woman has a 1 in 38 lifetime chance of dying a maternal death. This means that a woman in some countries in sub-Saharan Africa faces almost 100 times the risk of dying a maternal death than a woman in high-income countries.[29]

There are a number of risk factors for maternal death. Among the first are the nutritional status and general health status of the mother. Similarly, being of short stature is an important risk factor for maternal death. There is also a very strong correlation between maternal death and the level of education and income of the mother. Clearly, well-educated

TABLE 9-3 Maternal Mortality Ratio and Lifetime Risk of Dying a Maternal Death, by Region, 2013

Region	Maternal Mortality Ratio	Lifetime Risk of Dying a Maternal Death (1 in X)
Europe and Central Asia	28	1,700
East Asia and Pacific	75	700
Latin America and the Caribbean	87	500
Middle East and North Africa	78	430
South Asia	190	190
Sub-Saharan Africa	510	38
High-income countries	7	3,400

Data from WHO, UNICEF, UNFPA, The World Bank, and the United Nations Population Division. (2014). *Trends in maternal mortality: 1990 to 2013*. Geneva, World Health Organization.

FIGURE 9-1 Maternal Death by Cause, Low- and Middle-Income Countries, Percentage Distribution

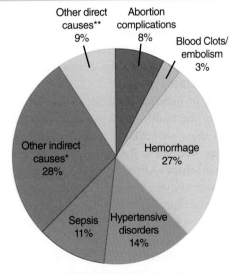

* Other direct causes includes complications of delivery, obstructed labor, and "other direct causes"
** Other indirect causes include HIV-related causes, preexisting medical condition that are exacerbated during pregnancy, and "other indirect causes"

Data from Say, L., et al. (2014). Global causes of maternal death: A WHO systematic analysis. *The Lancet Global Health* 2(6): e323-e333; WHO. Maternal mortality fact sheet. December 20, 2014 http://www.who.int/mediacentre/factsheets/fs348/en/.

women with comfortable incomes do not suffer many maternal deaths while uneducated and poor women do. Maternal death also varies with ethnicity and location, with rural women being at greater risk than urban dwellers. The risk of maternal death is also associated, among other things, with childbirth by adolescents,[10] women having their first child,[32] women having more than five children,[32] and childbirth at ages older than 35 years.[32] Short intervals between the births of subsequent children are also a risk factor for maternal death. Having a birth attended by a skilled healthcare provider and having access to emergency obstetric care are important to successful outcomes of pregnancy. In addition, consumption of alcohol, tobacco, and drugs during pregnancy can be harmful to both mother and child. Malaria and HIV/AIDS also pose substantial risks to pregnancy outcomes.

Maternal deaths are also more likely when women face what has been called "the three delays," which can occur at the level of the community and the health services:

"The delay in deciding to seek care;
"The delay in identifying and reaching a medical facility;
"The delay in receiving appropriate care at health facilities."[33]

This framework is discussed again later in the chapter.

Unsafe Abortion

A critical issue concerning abortions is whether they are safe or unsafe. WHO defines safe abortion as those abortions that are performed "by trained healthcare providers, with proper equipment, correct technique, and sanitary standards."[5] Unsafe abortions are essentially the opposite of that definition—performed by an untrained provider, with inappropriate equipment, poor technique, and unhygienic conditions.[5] It is thought that only about 60 percent of the abortions that are carried out every year worldwide are safe.[5]

Fewer than 1 woman per 100,000 who have a safe abortion will die as a result of the abortion. The mortality rate for unsafe abortions, however, is at least 100 times greater, although it varies by country, from about 100 per 100,000 such abortions to about 600 per 100,000. It is estimated that about 13 percent of the total maternal deaths that occur annually worldwide are due to unsafe abortions.[5,34]

WHO estimates that there are almost 22 million unsafe abortions in the world every year, of which almost 19 million take place in low- and middle-income countries. **Figure 9-2** shows the extent to which unsafe abortions take place in different regions of the world. The age of those having an unsafe abortion also varies by region. About 60 percent of the unsafe abortions in Africa take place among women younger than 25 years of age, compared to about 30 percent for women this age in Asia. In Latin America and the Caribbean, about half of the unsafe abortions are carried out on women 20 to 29 years of age.[5]

Obstetric Fistula

An obstetric fistula is a condition in which a hole opens up in a woman between the bladder and the vagina or between the rectum and the vagina. It is usually the result of prolonged or failed childbirth. As a consequence, urine or feces leak through the vagina. Obstetric fistula can have severe social and economic consequences, because women with fistula are often terribly stigmatized or abandoned.[35]

It is difficult to get good estimates of the number of women who suffer from obstetric fistula every year. Studies suggest that for every 100,000 births, between 50 and 80 women in sub-Saharan Africa, North Africa, and West and South Asia, and about 30 women in Latin America and China suffer a fistula.[36] At these rates, about 50,000 to 100,000 women each year will suffer a fistula.[37] It is thought that about 2 million women worldwide are living with fistula.[37]

The risk factors for fistula are those that are linked with an obstructed delivery, which is the precipitating factor for a fistula. These include undernutrition, young age at first birth, and having had multiple births. In addition, female genital mutilation and some traditional practices that damage the

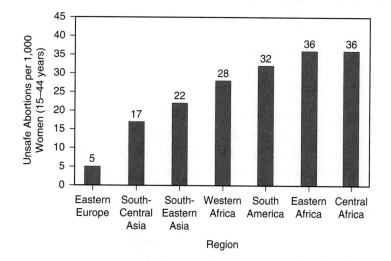

FIGURE 9-2 Unsafe Abortions by Region, 2008

Data from UNDP/UNFPA/WHO/World Bank Special Programme of Research, Development and Research Training in Human Reproduction (HRP). (2012). Unsafe abortion incidence and mortality-global regional levels in 2008 and trends, information sheet: WHO.

birth canal can also cause prolonged labor and lead to fistula. Fistula can also result from trauma, such as rape or sexual violence. The lack of access to emergency obstetric care and the failure to make use of such care, if available, also contribute to the prevalence of fistula.[37]

SOME KEY DIFFERENCES BETWEEN THE HEALTH OF MEN AND WOMEN

Much of the attention paid to the health of women in low- and middle-income countries over the last several decades has focused on reproductive health. More recently, however, greater focus has been put on females in all of their roles and on the extent to which gender discrimination has a negative impact on their overall health. Increasing amounts of information are available on the health of females compared to the health of males.[4] Overall, women have a higher life expectancy at birth than men. On average, women in low-income countries live 1 year longer than men and women in high-income countries live, on average, 7 years longer than men.[4]

However, an analysis of the extent to which females suffer a burden of disease greater than males identified 19 conditions that disproportionately affect females. Some of these relate to conditions that are specific to women, such as maternal conditions and cancers that overwhelmingly affect females. Some of these conditions are associated with the fact that females live longer than males, such as Alzheimer's disease, osteoarthritis, cerebrovascular and cardiovascular disease, and age-related vision disorders. In fact, it has been estimated that females lose 80 percent more DALYs from Alzheimer's disease, more than 60 percent more DALYs from osteoarthritis and age-related vision disorders, and more than 40 percent more DALYs from cerebrovascular and cardiovascular disease than men. Females also lose more than 50 percent more DALYs than males from depression and almost three times more DALYs than men from migraine headaches. As noted earlier, a condition affecting females that appears to be driven solely by discrimination is the excess burden of disease that women in South Asia suffer from fires and burns. In South Asia, females suffer more than 250 percent more DALYs from fire and burns than men do.[4] In fact, South Asia is the region of the world in which females are the least healthy compared to males.

THE COSTS AND CONSEQUENCES OF WOMEN'S HEALTH PROBLEMS

Women's health issues have enormous social costs. Violence against girls and women tends to isolate them socially. When a woman dies in childbirth, the social impacts are enormous. In most societies, women are the primary caregivers for children; therefore, when a mother dies, the death usually has a profound impact on the health of her children, with young children often dying soon thereafter. The social costs of some problems are particularly high. For example, women who have obstetric fistula are often socially isolated from their community.

Women are stigmatized for a variety of communicable diseases as well, such as TB, HIV/AIDS, and some of the neglected tropical diseases. There are also exceptional economic costs related to women's nutritional and health conditions but these are not often given the attention they deserve. The costs of violence against women, especially in low-income countries, have not been studied carefully but they are substantial. A study in Chile, for example, suggested that the costs of domestic violence were equal to 2 percent of Chile's gross domestic product (GDP). A similar study in Nicaragua indicated that such violence cost 1.6 percent of GDP. A review of intimate partner violence in the United States indicated that it led, in a single year, to 2 million injuries and costs of about $6 billion.[26]

The economic costs of maternal health conditions are also high but not well-documented. They also often fail to take account of morbidity associated with maternal health and not just mortality. These morbidities can seriously constrain women's productivity both in the home and outside the home. They can also significantly reduce the income that women can earn. When a woman dies a premature maternal death, the economic losses are substantial given the many years that the woman could have engaged in care of her family, work inside and outside the home, and the damage that will likely be done to the future prospects for economic well-being and economic contributions of any children who survive her. Illness associated with maternal conditions seriously constrains women's productivity and reduces the income they can contribute to their family. Similarly, depression in women also has high economic costs.

POLICY AND PROGRAM BRIEFS

Two policy and program briefs follow. The first examines the efforts of a nonprofit organization, Tostan, that works in community-based development in a number of countries in Africa and that has had some important successes in helping communities abandon FGM. The work of Tostan is especially interesting because it is embedded in the notion of educating and empowering communities to make decisions as communities in order to enhance their rights and improve their well-being. The second brief reviews the progress of Tamil Nadu state in India in reducing maternal mortality. This brief is significant, like the case study that follows it on Sri Lanka, because many countries have made only modest progress over the last 20 years in reducing maternal mortality and have not been able to put into place what has been learned elsewhere.

Addressing Female Genital Mutilation in Senegal[38]

Tostan is a U.S.-based nongovernmental organization (NGO) dedicated to community-led development in Africa. For more than 2 decades, Tostan has offered participatory, non-formal education about human rights and responsibilities to adults and adolescents in its Africa programs. In doing so, Tostan has sought to empower individuals and communities to initiate community dialogue and work to establish social change within their communities. Participatory education is intended to allow participants to have an active voice in the educational process, as they engage in group discussions that aim to foster collective learning.

As a central part of its work, Tostan developed and uses the Community Empowerment Program (CEP), a 30-month education program that consists of two parts: the *Kobi* and the *Aawde*. The Kobi, meaning "to prepare the field for planting," begins with sessions on democracy, human rights, and problem solving, and later covers health topics including hygiene, vaccinations, mental and physical development, the reproductive process, HIV/AIDS, STIs, and the risks involved in practices such as female genital cutting (FGC) and child/forced marriage. The Aawde, meaning "to plant the seed," is devoted to economic empowerment: helping participants draw on financial resources to have greater access to the local economy and choice in occupation, a freedom not traditionally given to individuals. Economic empowerment is achieved through literacy lessons and training in managing small projects. In addition, participants learn to use short message service (SMS) text messaging on mobile phones to practice their literacy skills.

A keystone of the Tostan program is "organized diffusion," whereby participants directly involved in the CEP share their knowledge with others. Participants "adopt" others with whom they share their newfound knowledge, while participating in the education program. Participants often choose spouses, friends, relatives, or neighbors as their adoptees. This process empowers participants to be both learners and teachers, as they discuss and reflect together on significant community issues.

Tostan conducts classes in local languages and draws on local traditions, including songs and oral stories. By engaging new themes in customary ways, it is hoped that participants will become confident, energized learners, who will begin to identify practices that affirm human rights, as well as other practices they wish to reinforce and harmful practices they want to abandon.

Tostan works with all members of the community in its education program: men, women, children, and religious and local leaders. By educating women and girls, the Tostan program facilitates their involvement in community planning and dialogue. In addition, Tostan believes that it would be impossible to create effective, sustainable change in a community without working with all community members and stakeholders.

Tostan and Female Genital Mutilation

Tostan has never been an anti-FGM organization, *per se*. Rather, Tostan is a community education organization that works with communities to encourage learning about both human rights and the corresponding responsibilities that result from those rights. For example, communities discuss how having the right to be free from all forms of violence relates to the corresponding responsibility to protect others from violence. This has contributed to the cessation of spousal abuse in many households and communities.

Through participation in the CEP, communities independently decided to abandon FGM. Because this was not part of its founding mission, Tostan was reluctant initially to become involved in it. However, the educational programs inspired participants to create a community-wide dialogue about FGM.

After the first village declared its abandonment of FGM, a local religious leader and participant in the Tostan program, Demba Diawara, approached Tostan and explained that to truly abandon FGM, a single village's declaration was insufficient. He explained that FGM was considered a prerequisite for marriage and that girls who had not undergone the practice could not get married, which would lead to a life of economic uncertainty and social exclusion. Moreover, because communities frequently marry outside their own community, it was clear that individual communities could not exclusively abandon FGM. Rather, the decision to abandon FGM in a significant number of communities within a social network would be necessary for abandonment to be both successful and sustainable. As a result, Tostan strategically chooses communities with which to work on FGM, focusing on interlinking social networks and connections to facilitate the spread of education and social change.

FGM is a social norm: an expected behavior that binds people together culturally. Many actors within a social group perpetuate it, and as such, it is impossible to hold any one person or one group responsible for its continuation. Tostan's educational approach encourages dialogue and deliberation about the assumptions and beliefs that hold social norms in place within communities. Such public deliberation has led to a shift in social norms and group expectations as thousands of communities have organized to abandon FGM.

Tostan's mission has not been to eradicate FGM or even ask that villages do so. Rather, its mission is concerned with educating participants about human rights and responsibilities so that they may become empowered to be leaders within their communities. Moreover, Tostan believes that in order to achieve lasting changes, communities must decide for themselves what is best for community members. Therefore, Tostan uses a holistic educational approach—one that addresses many different topics and issues faced within communities. This approach emphasizes within each community the practices that promote improved rights and well-being and provides the tools and forums to discuss what changes the community itself would like to see.

Program Impact

Tostan has worked at the grassroots level with thousands of communities in many African countries, including Senegal, Guinea, The Gambia, Mauritania, Somalia, Djibouti, Guinea Bissau, Burkina Faso, and Mali, learning from participants about their priorities, values, and hopes for the future. This deep knowledge of local conditions is a prerequisite for developing innovative strategies that are context-sensitive and responsive to villagers' lives and experiences. Because Tostan's pedagogical methods encourage lively participation and reflection, the organization receives constant participant feedback and is able to adapt quickly to changing circumstances. Tostan tries to foster a relationship of mutual empowerment between staff and participating communities, aiming to ensure that each gains confidence and strength through discussion, with each responsive to and learning from the other.

Tostan conducts internal reviews to assess its impact in the many areas the CEP addresses. This is typically done with reference to three types of communities: those with which it works directly, those that participate in CEP awareness-raising or declaration activities, and those that receive no intervention from Tostan. This approach allows for Tostan to better understand the interaction of social networks and their role in reshaping social norms through intercommunity discussion and debate. Tostan has found that villages with which it is either directly or indirectly involved have experienced a significant reduction in the rate of FGM following the completion of the CEP.

In addition to internal evaluations, organizations such as UNICEF and Macro International assessed the impact of

Tostan's CEP in 2008.[39] As of June 2010, and since the first Tostan-supported public declaration for the abandonment of FGC in 1997, 4,203 communities in Senegal, 364 in Guinea, 23 in Burkina Faso, 44 in The Gambia, and 36 in Somalia abandoned the practice. The long-term impact evaluation done by UNICEF and Macro International confirmed that the practice of FGM was reduced by 77 percent in the zones where Tostan had been active.

Tostan seeks to continuously evaluate its performance through internal and external assessments, as well as considering the invaluable feedback of CEP participants.[40] By maintaining a focus on human rights and responsibilities education, Tostan hopes to continue to support sustainable social change in a number of African countries.

Reducing Maternal Mortality in Tamil Nadu, India

The south Indian state of Tamil Nadu has made major improvements for more than 30 years in reducing maternal mortality. The experience in addressing maternal mortality in Tamil Nadu provides valuable lessons for other Indian states and for countries other than India about how to improve maternal health.

Although total fertility and maternal mortality have been lower in Tamil Nadu than in most Indian states for some time, the state government in the early 1980s still found them unacceptable. In 1980, for example, the maternal mortality ratio was 450 per 100,000 live births,[41] about where Zimbabwe is today.[29]

Despite an extensive family planning and reproductive health program in Tamil Nadu (the Family Welfare Program), an estimated 13 percent of families in the state still lacked access to family planning services as late as 1998–1999. In addition, as you read about earlier, there is considerable sex-selective abortion in India. Some of this is unsafe, and this, too, contributed to maternal mortality.[1] Moreover, in Tamil Nadu, as elsewhere, poor, rural, and young women suffer the greatest burden of maternal mortality. In addition, the state in the early 1980s was very rural, had high levels of poverty, and there was still substantial marriage and childbearing at a young age.[42]

The three delays noted earlier have also been major contributors to maternal mortality in Tamil Nadu, despite its progress in improving maternal health services. The delay in seeking appropriate obstetric care, which leads to late or no diagnosis, accounted for 40 percent of maternal deaths, even as late as 2004. The delay in transport to an appropriate facility in case of emergency was associated with 37 percent of maternal deaths in 2004. The delay in receiving emergency obstetric care at a referral facility accounted for 23 percent of maternal deaths in 2004.[42]

The government of Tamil Nadu responded to high rates of maternal and infant mortality by revamping its healthcare system in the 1980s to pay more attention to maternal and newborn health. With the object of making pregnancies safer and ensuring newborn survival, the initiatives have improved maternal health in a relatively short amount of time.

The strategy of the Tamil Nadu state government has included three components and seeks to combat the three delays. First, the policies aim to prevent and terminate unwanted pregnancies. A second objective is to provide greater access to obstetric care at the primary level, which would improve access to high-quality antenatal care, routine obstetric care, facility deliveries, and stabilization of emergencies before referral. Third, the policies seek to provide access to emergency obstetric care at the first referral level.[42]

To prevent unwanted pregnancies, the government increased accessibility and demand for family planning. In addition, the government increased the availability of safe abortion facilities in government-sponsored clinics. In conjunction with increased education, more economic development, and changing social norms, the total fertility rate in Tamil Nadu decreased to 1.7 in 2011.[42,43]

The state government addressed the delay in seeking appropriate care by improving the quality and accessibility of obstetric care at the primary level. Three staff nurses, who are also trained birth attendants, each work one 8-hour shift a day to ensure that care is available 24 hours a day. The nurses conduct antenatal checkups, attend deliveries, care for sick newborns, and arrange timely referrals if further care is necessary. Over 96 percent of mothers completed at least three antenatal visits during their last pregnancies in 2005–2006. Accessible obstetric care led to greater early registration of pregnancies and follow-up visits, causing earlier detection of pregnancy complications and the arrangement of life-saving referrals.[42]

The delay in transport to receive care has been significantly reduced through the introduction of an ambulance service. The government provides vehicles, and the service is managed by a local NGO. Poor pregnant women ride the ambulance free of charge, and wealthier patients are required to pay. Ninety-eight percent of deliveries took place in institutions in 2007–2008, compared to 67 percent in 1993–1994.[42]

Availability and access to emergency obstetric care were improved through the creation by 2008 of 62 Comprehensive Emergency Obstetric (CEmOC) and Newborn Care Centres. With an obstetrician and pediatrician on staff at all times and an anesthetist on call, these facilities provide all essential emergency obstetric and newborn care services 24 hours a day. There is an operating theater, laboratory, and blood bank. The CEmOC and Newborn Care Centres are located within one hour of any point in the state, and 86 percent of women reported they could reach one within half an hour or less in 2004–2005. Additionally, 83 percent of women said they received services within half an hour, showing that the delay of receiving treatment has been reduced. Access to emergency facilities is reducing maternal and newborn mortality, reflected by, among other things, the fact that 19 percent of deliveries were caesarean sections.[42]

As it has taken these steps to improve health services, the government has continued to promote education. Women are getting pregnant less frequently and later in life due to greater use of family planning.[42] In addition, there are fewer early marriages, greater awareness of family planning and nutrition as a whole, and improved literacy.[42] As these changes have occurred, Tamil Nadu was able to reduce the maternal mortality ratio from 450 per 100,000 live births in 1980 to 97 in 2011.[44]

The government of Tamil Nadu has pursued policies to improve maternal health, despite changes in the political party that has governed the state. The state has also tried to carefully monitor the investments it has made in strengthening primary and emergency health services, ensuring a more dedicated workforce, promoting the availability of essential drugs, and improving community engagement with health centers through outreach programs.[42]

Challenges remain, however, to sustaining the improvements Tamil Nadu has made in maternal health. These include reducing the high incidence of stillborn babies, closing regional disparities in maternal and neonatal mortality, further expanding access to emergency care facilities, and targeting urban health issues.[42]

CASE STUDIES

There has been some progress in a number of countries in dealing with the critical health issues discussed previously. The next section of this chapter examines two cases about efforts to address health conditions among women and promote family planning. The first deals with the reduction of maternal deaths in Sri Lanka, the second concerns efforts to encourage family planning in Bangladesh. The Sri Lanka and Bangladesh cases are well-documented success stories.

Maternal Mortality in Sri Lanka[45]

Background

Sri Lanka has had an impressive history of public-sector commitment to education and health, even when its income per capita was low. The female literacy rate in Sri Lanka has been more than double the South Asian average, and free health services have been available in rural areas since the 1930s.[45] Another unusual strength of Sri Lanka is that it has a good civil registration system that has recorded maternal deaths since about 1900.[46]

Interventions

Sri Lanka has taken a number of steps to reduce maternal deaths. First, Sri Lanka improved access to health services. Starting in the 1930s, Sri Lanka established health facilities throughout the country that were staffed by medical officers. In addition, Sri Lanka expanded secondary and tertiary facilities in the 1950s and around the same time established a working ambulance service.

Second, as early as the 1940s, Sri Lanka introduced policies to expand the number of midwives, who were the frontline workers dealing with pregnant women and child-birth. The focus on midwifery and on promoting easy access to higher-level health services in Sri Lanka has contributed to a wide acceptance by women and their families of giving birth with the assistance of a trained midwife at home or in the hospital. Midwives in Sri Lanka today serve a population of 3,000 to 5,000 people, and they provide an invaluable link between the local community and the health system.

Another step that Sri Lanka took to reduce maternal deaths was to make use of its civil registration data to identify what areas of the country had the most significant problems with maternal mortality. On this basis, the government was able to target its efforts to especially vulnerable groups, including women who were isolated both physically and socially, such as on distant tea estates. The government coupled these efforts with continuous activities, starting in the 1960s, to ensure that the quality of maternal health services was always appropriate. The lessons learned from individual maternal deaths, for example, were disseminated throughout the health system so that the quality of services could be improved and errors in dealing with obstetric problems could be reduced.

At the same time, the government made considerable progress in other health areas. This included efforts to improve health by improving sanitation and by measures to combat malaria and hookworm. These actions also contributed to improved health and lowered maternal mortality rates.

Impact

As a result of these efforts, Sri Lanka prior to 2008 had halved maternal deaths every 6 to 12 years since 1935. This has meant a decline in the maternal mortality ratio from between 500 and 600 maternal deaths per 100,000 live births in 1950 to 29 per 100,000 more recently.[47,48] Skilled medical practitioners now attend 97 percent of the births in Sri Lanka, compared with 30 percent in 1940.

One very important point to note about Sri Lanka is that it has achieved better maternal health outcomes than many countries that have higher per capita incomes or spend more on health than Sri Lanka. Low-cost, but dedicated and well-trained health personnel, including midwives, helped make the expansion of access to health care in Sri Lanka affordable.

Lessons

Sri Lanka's success in reducing maternal deaths can be attributed to widespread access to maternal health care, including emergency obstetric care, built upon a strong health system that provides free services to the entire population. The professionalism and broad use of midwives, the systematic use of health information to identify problems and guide decision-making, and targeted quality improvements for vulnerable groups were also ingredients for success. Sri Lanka's tradition of public-sector commitment to human development created conditions where gains were reinforced by good education, an emphasis on gender equity, the promotion of family planning, and a coordinated network of health services. Although factors such as the introduction of antibiotics and national efforts against malaria helped lower maternal mortality ratios, it was the step-by-step actions of the government rather than better living conditions alone that led to most of the improvements in maternal health. Sri Lanka's success offers important lessons for other low- and middle-income countries that have unacceptably high levels of maternal deaths. Detailed information on this case is available in *Case Studies in Global Health: Millions Saved.*[49]

Reducing Fertility in Bangladesh

Background

Despite the existence of several family planning methods, more than 150 million women in low- and middle-income countries who wish to limit or space childbearing do not use contraception. In Bangladesh, where more than half the women are illiterate and cultural traditions favor large families, each woman had, on average, almost seven children in the mid-1970s, thereby jeopardizing her health and that of her children. For a country with the world's highest population density where almost 80 percent of the people lived in poverty, it became clear that lowering population growth would be very important.

The Intervention

In 1975, the government of Bangladesh launched a program to reduce the national birth rate. The program had four components. First, young, married women were trained as outreach workers to visit women at home and offer information and contraceptive services. The number of these family welfare assistants (FWAs) eventually exceeded 40,000. Their outreach surpassed all expectations, with virtually all Bangladeshi women having been contacted at least once by an FWA, including many women isolated by cultural practices, geographical location, or poor transportation. The second element of the program was the provision of a wide range of family planning methods through a well-managed distribution system. The third component was the establishment of thousands of family planning clinics in rural areas to which outreach workers could refer clients for long-term family planning methods such as sterilization. The fourth element was the information, education, and communication (IEC) campaign. The IEC program successfully tailored its message to achieve different aims, such as persuading men to talk to their wives about contraception and winning social acceptance for FWAs by creating a story about a compelling soap opera heroine who eventually becomes an FWA. In fact, the IEC campaign's remarkable success has inspired similar mass media initiatives in other countries such as Kenya, Tanzania, and Brazil.[50]

The government's program evolved substantially over time, benefiting greatly from the existence of the Matlab Health Research Center that has operated for more than 40 years as a site for large-scale research on the operation of health, nutrition, and family planning programs. Within villages in the Matlab area, researchers have tested various approaches to the delivery of health services. Matlab evaluations have shaped maternal and child health programs in Bangladesh and in many other countries.

The Impact

The program resulted in virtually all women in Bangladesh becoming aware of family planning options. Contraceptive use increased from 8 percent in the mid-1970s to about 50 percent by 2007, and fertility declined from 6.3 births per woman in the early 1970s to about 3.3 in the mid-1990s.[51] Although other factors such as increased education and employment opportunities for women also increased demand for contraception, the family planning program has been shown to have had an independent effect on attitudes and behaviors.[52]

Costs and Benefits

The program is estimated to have cost about $100 million to $150 million per year, with more than half the funding coming from the United States Agency for International Development (USAID), the United Nations Development Program (UNDP), the World Bank, and other agencies.

Efforts are under way to increase program efficiency. The most expensive program component is that of FWAs, who were once critical to program success but are now valued by clients more as a convenience than as an essential source of information.[53] Research suggests that the most cost-effective strategy for the continued promotion of family planning is a fixed site approach that provides health and family planning services from clinics, complemented with targeted outreach to hard-to-reach clients.[54] However, some of those involved in women's health believe that "doorstep delivery" by FWAs would continue to be cost-effective if the FWAs delivered not only family planning but also other messages on sexual and reproductive health, such as safe motherhood, STIs, and HIV/AIDS. They also note the benefits of the FWAs as role models for women's status in rural areas.[21]

Lessons Learned

The success of the program can be attributed to four factors. The first was political commitment on the part of Bangladesh and the international agencies involved. The second was the broad use of FWAs, who carried the program's message into almost every home, however isolated. The third was the excellent use of mass media strategies to target audiences and change behavior. The fourth was the research and data provided by the Matlab Center that helped to constantly identify problems and improve the program. Although the program still faces a number of challenges, Bangladesh is one of the few low-income countries to have reduced fertility rapidly without resorting to coercive measures. More detailed information on this case is available in *Case Studies in Global Health: Millions Saved.*[49]

ADDRESSING FUTURE CHALLENGES

The health of females in low-income countries is a powerful reflection of biological susceptibility and gender norms that assign certain roles, restrictions, and values to females, compared to males. It also reflects the fact that the health systems in many countries have profound gender gaps and cannot or do not serve effectively the health needs of females. In this light, making major improvements in the future in the health of females in low- and middle-income countries will require attention to an array of social and public health measures.

One future challenge will be to improve the nutritional status of females, because it is poor nutrition *in utero* and from infancy that can later lead to women becoming stunted, not reaching their full biological potential, and experiencing a variety of health conditions.

Another challenge that is central to the long-term improvement in the health of females is access to education.

The empowerment of females socially is strongly associated with their level of education. Empowerment will improve the status of females and reduce the extent to which discrimination against them hurts their health. In addition, education improves access to important health information that can make a difference in women's and children's health. The education of females is among the most powerful contributors to overall development, as well.

Major changes must also be made in the perception that communities have of female roles and the health of females. This will require significant efforts at the level of communities and populations as a whole to put greater value on women's health. This will help to reduce the abortion of female fetuses and ensure that women in obstructed labor do not die because they lack appropriate and timely medical attention.

A continuing challenge will also be to put greater emphasis on the health of females as people, rather than as just women who give birth. This would encourage policymakers to take a number of steps that are essential to improving the health of females globally, including gaining a better understanding of the health conditions affecting females and what can be done about them, and making the health of females central to all health efforts. In addition, in many cultures, females are constrained in dealing with male medical workers, so it is also very important to train more female health workers and to deploy them appropriately to the places where they are most needed.

The next section comments on further measures that can be taken to deal with some of the particular health problems discussed previously, such as female genital mutilation, sexually transmitted infections, violence against women, and other reproductive health issues, including maternal mortality, unsafe abortion, and fistula.

Female Genital Mutilation

The policy and program brief on Tostan reflects the importance of ensuring that efforts that promote change need to be specifically tailored to local practices and to local beliefs. Linking these efforts with other measures that promote female empowerment, female education, and female control over economic resources will also be needed. FGM is intimately linked with deep-seated local beliefs and traditions that vary with ethnicity, education, income, and location. Only by taking account of these underlying issues will one be able to address FGM.[15]

Violence Against Women

We have already discussed the extent to which violence against women is usually a result of a complex set of factors and the interactions among them. Although there is increasing evidence on the factors linked to violence against women, there is little evidence about what works to reduce such violence and what are the most cost-effective approaches to doing so, especially in low- and middle-income countries.

Some studies have shown that protecting women against violence through legislation, as has been done in the United States and some other high-income countries, can have important positive effects in some settings. Shelters for abused women can also be used to reduce violence against them. Ensuring that the police, judges, and healthcare personnel are trained to deal with violence against women in more sensitive and more effective ways has also been useful. It also appears that many nongovernmental organizations can deal with violence against women as effectively and at a lower cost than some government services can do.[26]

Other studies have shown that a combination of measures adapted to local circumstances best addresses the constellation of factors that put women at risk of violence. Some of the most important of these measures are noted in **Table 9-4**. The Tostan experience also speaks to community-based efforts to reduce violence against women.

A recent study based on a review of literature about violence against women in low- and middle-income countries

TABLE 9-4 Selected Measures to Reduce Intimate Partner Violence

Prevention and education campaigns to increase awareness of intimate partner violence and change cultural norms about violence against women
Treatment for those who engage in intimate partner violence
Programs to strengthen ties to family and jobs
Couples counseling
Shelters and crisis centers for battered women
Mandatory arrest for offenders

Modified with permission from Rosenberg, M. L., Butchart, A., Mercy, J., Narasimhan, V., Waters, H., & Marshall, M. S. (2006). Interpersonal violence. In D. T. Jamison, J. G. Breman, A. R. Measham, et al. (Eds.), *Disease control priorities in developing countries.* (2nd ed., pp. 755–770). Washington, DC and New York: The World Bank and Oxford University.

suggests that the most successful programs of the small number that have been evaluated appear to be "participatory, engage multiple stakeholders, support critical discussion about gender relationships and the acceptability of violence, and support greater communication and shared decision making among family members, as well as non-violent behaviour."[55,p1555]

Sexually Transmitted Infections

Sexually transmitted infections are important not only because of the morbidity and mortality associated with them, particularly among women in sub-Saharan Africa, but also because they increase the chance of getting HIV/AIDS. It is critical, therefore, that the burden of these diseases be addressed. Some comments follow about addressing three of the most common STIs other than HIV among women: syphilis, gonorrhea, and chlamydia.

The goals of any program for reducing these sexually transmitted infections must be to reduce infection, reduce the complications of infections, and reduce the spread of STIs to infants when they are born.[18] It is much more cost-effective to prevent these diseases and to treat them before they lead to complications than it is to treat them later. Achieving these goals requires that young women initiate their first sexual relations at later ages; be able to refuse unwanted sex, even from their husbands; have relations with fewer partners; use condoms; and have any STIs diagnosed early and treated properly.

Meeting these aims will also require that young people get "the information and skills for making good decisions"; have access to "a range of health services that help them to act on those decisions"; and "live within a social, legal, and regulatory framework that supports health behaviors and protects young people from harm."[41,p153]

The successes in reducing STIs, other than HIV, to date have focused on a common set of health system interventions and capacities. First, the health system must have an ability to carry out surveillance of STIs. Second, there needs to be a health education program, targeted to those people most at risk of infection. Third, appropriately trained health workers need to be able to provide proper treatment of infection. Fourth, a system of partner notification must be in place so that the partners of the infected individuals can also be tested and treated, if necessary. Finally, there must be an effective program for access to health services, including condom use, generally referred to as "condom promotion."[18]

For example, Sweden made important strides in reducing chlamydia. Sweden offered free diagnosis coupled with a major health education campaign in schools, partner notification, and condom promotion. Linked to this, Sweden was able to reduce the prevalence of gonorrhea 15-fold and cut the prevalence of chlamydia by one-half over a 15-year period. Zambia also made good progress in reducing the burden of sexually transmitted infections by expanding the number of STI clinics, improving the training of health educators and clinicians, and expanding health education.[18] South Africa's "Love Life" initiative focuses on improving the sexual health of adolescents ages 12 to 17 years. Some reviews of this program suggest that it is associated with "better understanding of health risks, delayed debut of sexual relations, fewer partners, more assertive behavior regarding condom use, and better communication with parents about sex."[41,p154]

Maternal Mortality

We have already seen that about 300,000 women die each year of maternal causes, and that almost 40,000 die as a result of unsafe abortion. There is also considerable morbidity related to pregnancy. The fact that childbirth itself is such a risk in some settings is usually a result of the three delays: a delay in deciding to seek care, a delay in identifying problems and transporting the woman to a hospital, and a delay in providing appropriate emergency obstetric care in the hospital. There is also considerable disability, illness, and death related to unsafe abortion.

Unsafe Abortion

Most of the disability, morbidity, and mortality associated with abortion are the result of unsafe abortion, mostly in low- and middle-income countries in which abortion is legally restricted. To address the effects of unsafe abortion, it is essential that the health system in these settings be able to provide hygienic and appropriate post-abortion care at the lowest level of the health system possible. This means that they must be able to deal effectively with sepsis, hemorrhage, and shock. This may require a hospital stay, antibiotics, the ability to perform anesthesia, and the ability to transfuse blood.[10] Vacuum aspiration is a more cost-effective way to deal with incomplete abortion than to depend on the more surgical dilation and curettage approach. The drug misoprostol may also be a cost-effective means for dealing with an incomplete abortion in low-resource settings or could be used as a complement to vacuum aspiration. However, the use of the drug, which can be used to induce abortion raises political issues in a number of settings.[56] Prevention of unsafe abortion is also important, including universal access to family planning and services, including after abortion.[10]

In countries in which abortion laws are more liberal, it is essential that services be widely available so that women do not turn to unsafe abortion providers. Women also need to know that legal abortion is available. In addition, it is critical that legal abortions are safe and hygienic and that services be available to deal with any post-abortion complications. In these cases, including countries in Eastern Europe and Japan in which abortion is a common method of family planning, it is important that counseling be available about choices of family planning methods.[10]

Family Planning

"Family Planning Saves Lives" is the name of a long-standing publication and a phrase of considerable importance.[57] Indeed, because pregnancy and abortion are such important risks for disability, illness, and death, one way to avoid these problems is to reduce unwanted pregnancy through the promotion and widespread availability of family planning. In fact, it has been suggested that in countries with high maternal mortality ratios, as many as one-third of the maternal deaths could be avoided through an effective family planning program.[10] The importance of family planning is highlighted by the fact that many women in the world today would like to delay or avoid pregnancy or space their births, but they do not have the access to family planning needed to do this. Studies done in sub-Saharan Africa, for example, suggest that 20 percent of the women in the region who would like to avoid pregnancy do not have access to family planning.

There are permanent methods of family planning that include sterilization of either males or females, although only about 8 percent of the total number of sterilizations worldwide are among men.[58] There are also long-term methods of family planning, including intrauterine devices and implants. Short-term methods include contraceptive pills, injectables, and barrier methods, such as condoms or diaphragms. In addition, exclusive breastfeeding for at least 6 months—before the mother's menstrual period returns—acts as a natural contraceptive. There are also methods for natural family planning that focus on periodic abstinence.

A number of countries, including Bangladesh, Brazil, Colombia, Korea, and Vietnam, have made important progress in promoting the use of family planning. The experience from these countries suggests that an effective family planning program has to include information, education, and communication to promote informed choices by families about family planning; the need for a good selection of family planning technologies; the use of many points of service in both the public and private sector; services that are free or inexpensive enough for the poor to afford them; and health workers who are trained to work on family planning with knowledge and sensitivity, especially female health

workers for women who are reluctant to see male health workers.[59] There is considerable evidence that *social marketing* is an effective tool for promoting family planning, as well. Social marketing refers to the use of commercial marketing techniques to sell health-related measures, such as family planning.

Family planning is a cost-effective investment in reducing maternal death, but it is not clear which approach to family planning programs is most cost-effective compared to other approaches. The high rate of maternal death in sub-Saharan Africa and South Asia suggest that these are the two regions in which family planning would be most cost-effective to reduce maternal morbidity, disability, and mortality.[60] In addition, total fertility remains very high in many parts of sub-Saharan Africa and some parts of South Asia. It continues to be accompanied, as well, by young age of marriage and first birth and closely spaced births.

Complications of Pregnancy

The risks of complications of pregnancy increase when the general health of the mother is not good. Thus, the nutritional status of the mother is very important. In addition, malaria is very dangerous for pregnant women, especially in sub-Saharan Africa, and HIV/AIDS also complicates pregnancy outcomes for both women and their children.

Some of the conditions that affect pregnancy outcomes can be identified during prenatal care. However, although it is important for pregnant women to get regular medical exams during their pregnancy—and WHO recommends four such visits—some complications of pregnancy cannot be foreseen during those checkups. Thus, it is also critical to ensure that a skilled healthcare provider attends births in order to handle the complications of pregnancy and refer the pregnant woman to a facility where the complications can be addressed appropriately. In addition, it is important that communities have transportation to urgently get women to emergency obstetric care when there are complications of pregnancy and that health services be able to address the complications with high-quality care.

Studies show that there are several cost-effective packages of services that can reduce maternal death due to complications of pregnancy. The basic package of essential obstetric services that all countries should have is shown in **Table 9-5**. Countries that have more financial resources may wish to also provide some additional services that can address food, multivitamin supplements, malaria prophylaxis, the ability to deal with complicated deliveries of an HIV-positive mother, and arrangements for caring for a high-risk infant,[59] which are also shown on Table 9-5. As countries carry out these

TABLE 9-5 Basic Care Packages for Pregnancy at the Primary Level

Routine Prenatal Care
Clinical examination
Obstetric and gynecological examination
Urine test
Laboratory tests: hemoglobin, blood type and rhesus status, syphilis and other symptomatic testing for sexually transmitted diseases
Advice on emergencies, delivery, lactation, and contraception
Education
Iron and folic acid supplementation
Tetanus toxoid immunization
Screening and treatment for syphilis
Delivery Care
Clean delivery technique, clean cord cutting, clean delivery of baby and placenta
Active management of the third stage of labor
Episiotomy in appropriate cases
Recognition and first-line management of delivery complications
Intravenous fluid
Intravenous uterotonics, if bleeding occurs
Partograph
Essential newborn care
Intravenous antibiotics

Modified with permission from Graham, W. J., Cairns, J., Bhattacharya, S., Bullough, C. H. W., Quayyum, Z., & Rogo, K. (2006). Maternal and perinatal conditions. In D. T. Jamison, J. G. Breman, A. R. Measham, et al. (Eds.), *Disease control priorities in developing countries* (2nd ed., p. 515). Washington, DC and New York: The World Bank and Oxford University Press.

services, they are increasingly encouraged to make them part of a continuum of care that addresses maternal, newborn, and child health as a coherent package.

Of course, it is critical that appropriate services of good quality be available. However, it is also essential that there be a demand for such services from the people who need them. This is especially important in places where there are substantial barriers to overcoming the first and second delays of identifying a problem with the delivery and transporting the woman to a place where she can get emergency obstetric care. A number of countries have initiated conditional cash transfer schemes to encourage all women to have births in hospitals. These schemes are meant to overcome the social and economic constraints to hospital deliveries. Parts of India, for example, are implementing conditional cash transfer programs that offer a payment to the person attending the birth for bringing the woman to the hospital for delivery and offer the family a payment for coming for a hospital-based delivery. In many settings, there is a risk that increased demand for hospital-based delivery will not improve maternal outcomes unless there is an improvement in the quality of care. It will be important in such settings to couple incentives to increase the demand for services with other incentive programs to improve the amount and quality of emergency obstetric services.

MAIN MESSAGES

As discussed by a well-known scholar and practitioner of women's health, "being born female is dangerous for your health."[3,p205] Some of the health conditions that women face are biologically determined. Others are socially determined. Some result from the interplay between biological and social determinants of health. The inferior social status of women in many cultures, however, is reflected in certain health conditions that women face and in some of the differentials that favor men between the health of men and the health of women.

As one looks globally at the health of women, especially poor women in low- and middle-income countries, one notes the importance of several key health issues. One is nutrition. Another is sex-selective abortion. A third is discriminatory healthcare practices toward young girls that cause these girls to suffer higher rates of mortality before age 5 than boys. Sexually transmitted infections are an important cause of DALYs for women in the reproductive age group, especially in sub-Saharan Africa. Female genital mutilation is a practice that is widespread, especially in parts of Africa, and it is associated with important morbidity and disability for women. Violence against women is also a central cause of ill health for women.

Illness, disability, and death from maternal causes are also unnecessarily high. About 300,000 women die each year of maternal causes; about 40,000 of these deaths are due to unsafe abortions. Complicated labor that is not properly attended can also lead to problems, such as fistula, from which an estimated 2 million women suffer worldwide. The risk of maternal morbidity, disability, and mortality is increased by having a stunted mother, young age at marriage, young age at first birth, having more than five children, and having closely spaced pregnancies. The lack of access to family planning and the demand for it is at the foundation of some of these problems. This is particularly the case in some places in South Asia and much of sub-Saharan Africa, where total fertility remains high and the coverage of family planning remains low. Increasing the uptake of family planning to delay the age at first birth, increase birth intervals, and reduce the number of births per woman would save lives, especially in low- and middle-income countries with weak emergency obstetric care.

The costs of women's health problems are very substantial. In many societies, women are the primary caregivers to children, and when the health of the mother suffers, there is often a negative effect on the health of the children, as well. In addition, women play important economic roles in many families and the morbidity, disability, and mortality associated with particular problems of women's health have substantial economic implications.

Some countries, such as Sri Lanka, have been able to improve the health of women at relatively low levels of expenditure by making wise choices about investments in health and education. These included increasing female education, providing widespread access to midwives, and ensuring adequate backup for the midwives at hospitals.

Improving the health of women in the future will require that health systems provide a cost-effective package of services, including nutrition, family planning, prenatal care, deliveries attended by skilled healthcare providers, emergency transportation of women who are having complicated labors, and emergency obstetric services of appropriate quality at a hospital. A number of countries are now undertaking a variety of efforts, including incentive programs, to try to increase the demand for such services and the supply of these services at an appropriate level of quality. In the long run, it will be important to change the gender roles that favor males, promote the education and empowerment of females, promote their prospects for earning income, and educate communities to better understand the health conditions that females face and the measures that can be taken to address them. These measures could help, among other things, to reduce sex-selective abortion, female infanticide, and violence against women, and avoid the three delays that are associated with maternal morbidity, disability, and mortality.

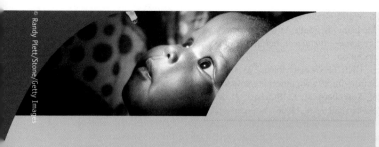

Study Questions

1. Why can it be said that "being born female is dangerous to your health"?

2. Why should we pay particular attention to the health of females?

3. In what ways do gender issues affect the health of females?

4. What are some of the key differences in the burden of disease between males and females?

5. What are the sources of those differences?

6. What are the three delays and why are they important?

7. What steps do countries need to take to deal with the complications of unsafe abortions?

8. What measures might be taken to reduce intimate partner violence?

9. How could one reduce the risk to women of sexually transmitted infections?

10. What are some of the most cost-effective investments that should be made to improve the health of women in low-income countries?

REFERENCES

1. Prada, E., Restler, E., Sten, C., Dauphinee, L., & Ramirez, L. (2005). *Abortion and postabortion care in Guatemala: A report from health care professionals and health facilities* (Occasional Report No. 18). New York: Guttmacher Institute. Retrieved January 17, 2015, from http://www.guttmacher.org/pubs/2005/12/30/or18.pdf.

2. United Nations. Millennium Development Goals. Retrieved March 15, 2006, from http://www.un.org/millenniumgoals.

3. Murphy, E. M. (2003). Being born female is dangerous for your health. *American Psychologist, 58*(3), 205–210.

4. Buvinic, M., Medici, A., Fernandez, E., & Torres, A. C. (2006). Gender differentials in health. In D. T. Jamison, J. G. Breman, A. R. Measham, et al. (Eds.), *Disease control priorities in developing countries* (2nd ed., pp. 195–210). New York: Oxford University Press.

5. World Health Organization. (2005). *The world health report 2005: Make every mother and child count.* Geneva: World Health Organization.

6. Quinn, T. C., & Overbaugh, J. (2005). HIV/AIDS in women: An expanding epidemic. *Science, 308*(5728), 1582–1583.

7. Abeykoon, A. T. P. L. (1995). Sex preference in South Asia: Sri Lanka an outlier. *Asia-Pacific Population Journal, 10*(3), 5–16.

8. Gu, B., & Roy, K. (1995). Sex ratio at birth in China, with reference to other areas in East Asia: What we know. *Asia-Pacific Population Journal, 10*(3), 17–42.

9. Jha, P., Kesler, M. A., Kumar, R., et al. (2011, May 24). Trends in selective abortions of girls in India: Analysis of nationally representative birth histories from 1990 to 2005 and census data from 1991 to 2011. *Lancet, 377,* 1921–1928.

10. Tinker, A. (1994). *A new agenda for women's health and nutrition.* Washington, DC: The World Bank.

11. Rov, K. (1999). *Encyclopaedia against women & dowry death in India.* New Delhi: Anmol Publications.

12. Gendercide Watch. *Case study: Female infanticide.* Retrieved June 10, 2006, from http://www.gendercide.org/case_infanticide.html.

13. Jha, P., Kumar, R., Vasa, P., Dhingra, N., Thiruchelvam, D., & Moineddin, R. (2006). Low female-to-male sex ratio of children born in India: National survey of 1.1 million households. *Lancet, 367*(9506), 211–218.

14. Central Intelligence Agency. The world factbook field listing: Sex ratio. Retrieved January 3, 2015, from https://www.cia.gov/library/publications/the-world-factbook/fields/2018.html.

15. UNICEF. (2005). *Female genital mutilation/cutting: A statistical exploration 2005.* New York: UNICEF.

16. UNICEF. (2014). *Female genital mutilation/cutting: A statistical overview and exploration of the dynamics of change.* New York: UNICEF.

17. Glasier, A., Gulmezoglu, A. M., Schmid, G. P., Moreno, C. G., & Look, P. F. V. (2006). Sexual and reproductive health: A matter of life and death. *Lancet, 368,* 1595–1607.

18. Rowley, J., & Berkley, S. (1998). Sexually transmitted diseases. In C. J. L. Murray, & A. D. Lopez (Eds.), *Health dimensions of sex and reproduction* (pp. 19–110). Geneva: World Health Organization.

19. World Health Organization. (2013). *Sexually transmitted infections (STIs).* Retrieved January 3, 2015, from http://apps.who.int/iris/bitstream/10665/82207/1/WHO_RHR_13.02_eng.pdf.

20. Institute of Health Metrics and Evaluation. (2013). *GBD compare.* Retrieved January 3, 2015, from http://vizhub.healthdata.org/gbd-compare/.

21. World Health Organization. (2015). Violence against women. Retrieved June 4, 2015, from http://www.who.int/mediacentre/factsheets/fs239/en/.

22. UNAIDS. *Violence against women and AIDS.* Retrieved February 28, 2006, from http://data.unaids.org/GCWA/GCWA_BG_Violence_en.pdf.

23. Williams, J. (2004). Women's Mental Health: Taking Inequality into Account. In J. Tew (Ed.), *Social Perspectives in Mental Health: Developing Social Models to Understand and Work with Mental Distress.* London: Jessica Kingsley.

24. World Health Organization, London School of Hygiene and Tropical Medicine, & South African Medical Research Council. (2013). *Global and regional estimates of violence against women.* Geneva: World Health Organization.

25. UNICEF. Sexual violence as a weapon of war. Retrieved April 14, 2015, from http://www.unicef.org/sowc96pk/sexviol.htm.

26. Rosenberg, M. L., Butchart, A., Mercy, J., Narasimhan, V., Waters, H., & Marshall, M. S. (2006). Interpersonal violence. In D. T. Jamison, J. G. Breman, A. R. Measham, et al. (Eds.), *Disease control priorities in developing countries* (2nd ed., pp. 755–770). New York: Oxford University Pres.

27. World Health Organization. (2014). *Maternal mortality* (Fact sheet no. 348). Retrieved January 3, 2015, from http://www.who.int/mediacentre/factsheets/fs348/en/.

28. Last, J. M. (2001). *A dictionary of epidemiology* (4th ed.). New York: Oxford University Press.

29. World Health Organization, UNICEF, UNFPA, The World Bank, & United Nations Population Division. (2013). *Trends in maternal mortality: 1990 to 2013.* Geneva: World Health Organization.

30. Lawn, J. E., Lee, A. C., Kinney, M., et al. (2009). Two million intrapartum-related stillbirths and neonatal deaths: Where, why, and what can be done? *International Journal of Gynaecology and Obstetrics, 107,* S5–S19.

31. Say, L., et al. (2014). Global causes of maternal death: A WHO systematic analysis. *The Lancet Global Health, 2*(6), e323–e333.

32. AbouZahr, C. (1998). Antepartum and postpartum hemorrhage. In C. J. L. Murray, & A. D. Lopez (Eds.), *Health dimensions of sex and reproduction: The global burden of sexually transmitted diseases, HIV, maternal conditions, perinatal disorders, and congenital anomalies* (pp. 165–190). Cambridge, MA: Harvard School of Public Health.

33. Measure Evaluation Population and Reproductive Health (PRH). (2014). *Safe motherhood.* Retrieved January 7, 2015, from http://www.cpc.unc.edu/measure/prh/rh_indicators/specific/sm.

34. World Health Organization. *Preventing unsafe abortion.* Retrieved January 4, 2015, from http://www.who.int/reproductivehealth/topics/unsafe_abortion/magnitude/en/.

35. Royal College of Midwives. (2010). *Obstetric fistula: A silent tragedy.* London: The Royal College of Midwives Trust.

36. AbouZahr, C. (1998). Prolonged and obstructed labor. In C. J. L. Murray, & A. D. Lopez (Eds.), *Health dimensions of sex and reproduction: The global burden of sexually transmitted diseases, HIV, maternal conditions, perinatal disorders, and congenital anomalies* (pp. 243–266). Cambridge, MA: Harvard School of Public Health.

37. Health & Development International. (2005). *Obstetric fistula as a catalyst: Exploring approaches for safe motherhood.* Meeting report, Atlanta, GA, October 3–5, 2005.

38. This case study is based on a draft case study that was provided by Tostan. More information about Tostan can be found at their website, http://www.tostan.org.

39. UNICEF. (2008). *Long-term evaluation of the Tostan Programme in Senegal: Kolda, Thies and Fatick regions.* New York: UNICEF.

40. Diop, N., Moreau, A., & Benga, H. (2008). *Evaluation of the long-term impact of the Tostan Programme on the abandonment of FGM-C and early marriage: Results from a qualitative study in Senegal.* New York: Population Council.

41. Providing interventions. (2006). In D. T. Jamison, J. G. Breman, A. R. Measham, et al. (Eds.), *Priorities in health* (pp. 129–154). New York: Oxford University Press.

42. World Health Organization. (2009). *Safer pregnancy in Tamil Nadu: From vision to reality.* Retrieved August 22, 2010, from http://whqlibdoc.who.int/searo/2009/9789290223566.pdf.

43. Jansankhya Sthirata Kosh (National Population Stabilisation Fund). (2011). *Why population matters.* Retrieved January 7, 2015, from http://www.jsk.gov.in/total_fertility_rate.asp.

44. Office of Registrar General India. (2011). *Maternal and child mortality and total fertility rates: Sample Registration System (SRS)*. Retrieved January 7 2015, http://censusindia.gov.in/vital_statistics/SRS_Bulletins/MMR_release_070711.pdf.

45. This case study is largely based on Pathmathan, I., Lijestrand, J., Martins, J. M., et al. (2003). *Investing in maternal health: Learning from Malaysia and Sri Lanka*. Washington, DC: The World Bank.

46. Wickramasuriya, G. A. W. (1939). Maternal mortality and morbidity in Ceylon. *Journal of the Ceylon Branch of the British Medical Association*, *36*(2), 79–106.

47. United Nations. (2003). *Human development report*. New York, NY: United Nations.

48. World Bank. (2014). *Maternal mortality ratio (modeled estimate per 100,000 live births*. Retrieved January 7, 2015, from http://data.worldbank.org/indicator/SH.STA.MMRT.

49. Levine, R., & What Works Working Group. (2007). *Case studies in global health: Millions saved*. Sudbury, MA: Jones and Bartlett.

50. Manoff, R. (1997). Getting your message out with social marketing. *American Journal of Tropical Medicine and Hygiene*, *57*(3), 260–265.

51. Mitra, S. N., Al-Sabir, A., Cross, A. R., & Jamil, K. (1997). *Bangladesh demographic and health survey 1996–1997*. Dhaka: National Institute for Population Research and Training.

52. Barkat-e-Khuda, Roy, N. C., & Rahman, D. M. (2000). Family planning and fertility in Bangladesh. *Asia-Pacific Population Journal*, *15*(1), 41–54.

53. Janowitz, B., Holtman, M., Johnson, L., & Trottier, D. (1999). The importance of field workers in Bangladesh's family planning programme. *Asia-Pacific Population Journal*, *14*(2), 23–36.

54. Routh, S., & Barkat-e-Khuda. (2000). An economic appraisal of alternative strategies for the delivery of MCH-FP services in urban Dhaka, Bangladesh. *International Journal of Health Planning and Management*, *15*(2), 115–132.

55. Ellsberg, M., Arango, D. J., & Morton, M., et al. (2014, November 20). Prevention of violence against women and girls: What does the evidence say? *Lancet*, 1703–1707.

56. Guttmacher Institute. Implementing Postabortion Care Programs in the Developing World: Ongoing challenges. Retrieved April 14, 2015, from https://www.guttmacher.org/pubs/gpr/17/1/gpr170122.html.

57. Smith, R., Ashford, L., Gribble, J., & Clifton, D. (2009). *Family planning saves lives* (4th ed.). Washington, DC: PRB.

58. Jamison, D. T. (2006). Maternal and perinatal conditions. In D. T. Jamison, J. G. Breman, A. R. Measham, et al. (Eds.), *Disease control priorities in developing countries* (2nd ed., pp. 499–529) New York: Oxford University Press.

59. Graham, W. J., Cairns, J., Bhattacharya, S., Bullough, C. H. W., Quayyum, Z., & Rogo, K. (2006). Maternal and perinatal conditions. In D. T. Jamison, J. G. Breman, A. R. Measham, et al. (Eds.), *Disease control priorities in developing dountries* (2nd ed., pp. 499–530). Washington, DC: Oxford University Press and The World Bank.

60. Jamison, D. T., Breman, J. G., Measham, A. R., et al. (Eds.), *Priorities in health*. New York: Oxford University Press.

CHAPTER **10**

The Health of Young Children

LEARNING OBJECTIVES

By the end of this chapter the reader will be able to:

- Understand the most important causes of illness and death among young children globally
- Discuss the importance of neonatal death
- Describe why some children survive and others die
- Describe the most cost-effective child health interventions
- Describe some examples of successful child health initiatives
- Discuss the importance of immunization and the progress made in expanding immunization in low- and middle-income countries
- Discuss some of the challenges of further enhancing the health of young children in these countries

VIGNETTES

Nassiba was born in a remote part of Tajikistan. At 3 years of age, she became very ill with measles. She died before her parents could get her to a health center. Nassiba's birth was never registered because the registration center was far from her home and her parents could not afford the registration fee. When Nassiba died, her death was not recorded either. According to the national records, she never existed.

Esther was born in Cape Town, South Africa, to an HIV-positive mother. At the time of Esther's birth, the health system did not offer drugs to prevent the transmission of HIV from mother to child. A few months later, Esther showed signs of HIV infection.

Tirtha was born in far western Nepal 7 months ago. She was the fourth child in her family. She was eating some baby foods as well as breastfeeding. One day Tirtha developed persistent diarrhea and became feverish. Her mother wanted to take Tirtha to the health center, but it was 2 hours away so she decided to see how Tirtha was feeling the next day. The next morning Tirtha was dead from dehydration.

Juan was born in the highlands of Bolivia to an indigenous family. The family did what they could to keep the new baby warm, but it was very cold in the mountains. Several days after birth, Juan began to breathe heavily. The family called the community health worker for assistance. The health worker treated Juan for pneumonia with an antibiotic that she had just learned to use through a program for saving newborn lives. She also gave the family advice about taking care of the baby. The last child born to the family died of pneumonia but Juan survived.

THE IMPORTANCE OF CHILD HEALTH

There are a number of reasons why the health of young children deserves its own chapter. First, it has recently been estimated that about 6.3 million children under 5 years of age die in the world each year.[1] This is equal to more than 17,000 children under 5 who die *each day*. The second reason to pay special attention to child health is that so many of these deaths are preventable. Young children, for example, almost never die in high-income countries[2] and it has been estimated that more than half of child deaths each year could be avoided through known, simple, and low-cost interventions.[3] Third, children have a special place in the global health agenda because they are so vulnerable. The measures needed to ensure that they are born healthier, breastfed properly, immunized on schedule, and raised in safe and hygienic conditions, for example, can be taken only by others who care for them. Their vulnerability also raises important ethical issues about the responsibility of adults to ensure the health and survival of children.

Child health is also closely linked with poverty. If children had access to safer water and better sanitation, then many of them would not succumb to diarrhea. If their families had more education, especially their mothers, then families would be better equipped to ensure that their children were better cared for. If families had more income, then they would have greater access to health, education, and other social services that would also serve children well.

There has been substantial progress in reducing the number of children who die each year globally. The number of young children dying each year has been sufficiently reduced between 1990 and 2013 so that about 90 million children survived who would otherwise have died.[4] **Figure 10-1** shows that progress and the rate of decline for each World Bank region and for the high-income countries.

However, despite this progress, the health of young children is also of particular concern because some parts of the world have not made sufficient progress in enhancing child health. This has been especially true in parts of sub-Saharan Africa and South Asia, as can also be seen in the figure.[4]

For all these reasons, children are featured prominently in the Millennium Development Goals (MDGs), as noted in **Table 10-1**.

This chapter highlights the most important issues concerning the health of young children in low- and middle-income countries. It will review the burden of disease for these children, with important comments on their first month of life. It will assess the risk factors for illness and death that occur in children under 5 years of age. It then examines measures that can be taken to reduce the burden

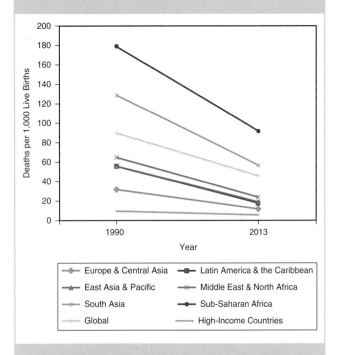

FIGURE 10-1 Decline in Under-5 Child Mortality by World Bank Region and for High-Income Countries, 1990–2013

Data from World Bank. World development indicators: Mortality. Retrieved February 24, 2015, from http://data.worldbank.org/indicator/SH.DYN.MORT/countries/1W-Z4-ZQ-Z7?display=graph.

TABLE 10-1 Key Links Between Child Health and the MDGs

Goal 1: Eradicate Extreme Hunger and Poverty
Link: More than 50 percent of child deaths worldwide are associated with malnutrition.

Goal 2: Achieve Universal Primary Education
Link: Enrollment, attendance, and performance of children in schools is closely linked with their health.

Goal 3: Promote Gender Equality and Empower Women
Link: Empowering women will enhance their health, their education, and their ability to raise healthier children.

Goal 4: Reduce Child Mortality
Link: This is directly related to child health.

Goal 5: Improve Maternal Health
Link: Maternal health is a major predictor of the birthweight of a child and the child's subsequent health and survival prospects.

Goal 6: Combat HIV/AIDS, Malaria, and Other Diseases
Link: HIV/AIDS and malaria are major killers of young children.

Goal 7: Ensure Environmental Sustainability
Link: An important share of childhood illnesses and deaths are related to unsafe water and poor sanitation. Indoor air pollution is also very detrimental to the health of children.

Data from United Nations. Millennium Development Goals. Available at: http://www.un.org/millenniumgoals.

of disease in young children. The chapter concludes with a review of some of the key challenges to further improving the health of young children in low- and middle-income countries. The chapter illustrates key concepts in a number of program and policy briefs and case studies.

This chapter focuses on the most important causes of illness and death in children: causes related to the deaths of neonates, plus pneumonia, diarrhea, malaria, the neglected tropical diseases, and vaccine-preventable diseases. This chapter is about children under 5 years of age, largely in low- and middle-income countries. The chapter generally refers to them as "young children" or "children."

It is also important to note that the chapter does not discuss stillbirths. The World Health Organization (WHO) defines a stillbirth as: "a baby born with no signs of life at or after 28 weeks' gestation."[5] Stillbirths are a very important issue, one that WHO has called an "invisible public health priority."[5] It is estimated that 2.6 million babies are stillborn each year, almost all of them in low- and middle-income countries.[5] Students who are interested can review this issue in greater detail, starting with materials from WHO and a *Lancet* series that extensively covered the latest findings on stillbirths.[6]

KEY TERMS

Some of the key indicators used in measuring and analyzing global health issues, which will be used extensively in this chapter, include the neonatal mortality rate, infant mortality rate, and under-5 child mortality rate.

In this chapter, we also speak of three different phases of the lives of young children:

Neonatal—referring to the first month of life
Infant—referring to the first year of life
Under-5—referring to children 0 to 4 years old

In addition, you will read about some of the most important causes of disease, disability, and death in children under 5 years, as shown in **Table 10-2.**

TABLE 10-2 Selected Terms Relating to Causes of Child Illness and Death

Asphyxia—A condition of severely deficient oxygen supply.

Diarrhea—A condition characterized by frequent and watery bowel movements.

Hookworm—A parasite that lives in the intestines of its host, which may be a mammal such as a dog, cat, or human. Two species of hookworm commonly infect humans, *Ancylostoma duodenale* and *Necator americanus*.

Malaria—A disease of humans caused by blood parasites of the species *Plasmodium falciparum, vivax, ovale, knowlesi,* or *malariae* and transmitted by *Anopheles* mosquitoes.

Pertussis—A highly contagious bacterial disease that is one of the leading causes of vaccine-preventable death. Pertussis is also known as whooping cough.

Pneumonia—An inflammation, usually caused by infection, involving the alveoli of the lungs. Pneumonia is one of several lower respiratory tract infections.

Polio—An infectious disease caused by poliovirus that can lead to paralysis.

Sepsis—A serious medical condition caused by a severe infection, leading to a systematic inflammatory response.

Tetanus—A bacterial infection usually contracted through a puncture wound with an unclean object. Neonates acquire tetanus when their umbilical cord is contaminated, often when cut with an unsterile object.

Data from Birley, M. H. *PEEM Guidelines 2—Guidelines for forecasting the vector-borne disease implications of water resources development*. Retrieved March 22, 2015, from http://www.who.int/water_sanitation_health/resources/peem2/en/. Doctors Without Borders. *Glossary*. Retrieved April 14, 2007, from http://www.doctors withoutborders.org/education/bol/Glossary.htm. World Health Organization. Soil transmitted helminth infections. Retrieved April 10, 2015, from http://www.who .int/mediacentre/factsheets/fs366/en/. World Health Organization. Pneumonia. Retrieved April 10, 2015, from http://www.who.int/mediacentre/factsheets /fs331/en/. Medline Plus. Sepsis. Retrieved April 10, 2015, from http://www.nlm.nih.gov/medlineplus/ency/article/000666.htm.

NOTE ON DATA

This chapter takes its data from a number of sources. Much of the basic data is taken from publications of the UN Inter-agency Group for Child Mortality Estimation. Other data come from WHO, UNICEF, the World Bank, and the *Global Burden of Disease Study 2010*. The chapter also takes data and considerable information from a *Lancet* series on newborns.

MORTALITY AND THE BURDEN OF DISEASE

Children Under 5 Years

As noted earlier, about 6.3 million children under 5 years of age died worldwide in 2013. About 99 percent of these deaths took place in low- and middle-income countries. Almost half of these deaths occurred in only five large countries: India, Nigeria, the Democratic Republic of the Congo, Pakistan, and China.[4] About 44 percent of the under-5 child deaths occurred among neonates, or children less than 28 days old.[1] Moreover, more than one-third of the children who died in the first 28 days died in the first day of life.[4]

Figure 10-2 depicts the neonatal mortality rate by World Bank region in 2013 and for high-income countries. The figure clearly shows the substantial differences in rates by region. As expected, the highest rates are in sub-Saharan

Africa and South Asia, with rates more than seven times the rate in of high-income countries.

Figure 10-3 shows the infant mortality rate by World Bank region and for high-income countries.

The pattern for infant mortality is similar to that for neonatal mortality, with sub-Saharan Africa having the highest rate and South Asia having the second-highest rate. In this case, however, sub-Saharan Africa has a rate over 12 times higher than that of high-income countries and South Asia nine times higher.

Figure 10-4 shows the rates of under-5 child mortality by World Bank region and for high-income countries.

The under-5 child mortality rate for sub-Saharan Africa is substantially higher than for any other region, including South Asia, and is more than 15 times the rate in high-income countries. South Asia again has the second-highest rate, in this case more than eight times the rate in high-income countries.

Figure 10-5 is a combination of the first three figures in this chapter and shows neonatal, infant, and under-5 child mortality by World Bank region and for high-income countries.

This figure makes a number of very important points:

- Sub-Saharan Africa has the highest rates for all indicators.

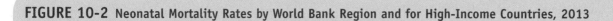

FIGURE 10-2 Neonatal Mortality Rates by World Bank Region and for High-Income Countries, 2013

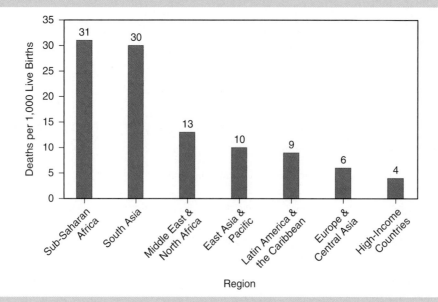

Data from the World Bank. World Development Indicators: Mortality. http://data.worldbank.org/indicator/SH.DYN.MORT/countries/1W-Z4-ZQ-Z7?display=graph. Accessed February 22, 2015.

FIGURE 10-3 Infant Mortality Rates by World Bank Region and for High-Income Countries, 2013

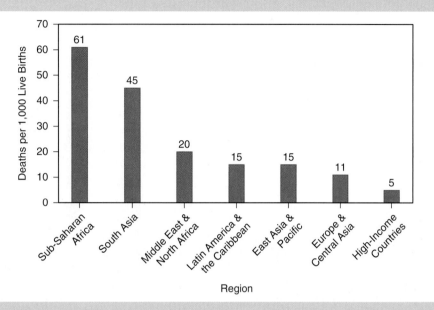

Data from the World Bank. World Development Indicators: Mortality. http://data.worldbank.org/indicator/SH.DYN.MORT/countries/1W-Z4-ZQ-Z7?display=graph. Accessed February 22, 2015.

FIGURE 10-4 Under-5 Child Mortality by World Bank Region and for High-Income Countries, 2013

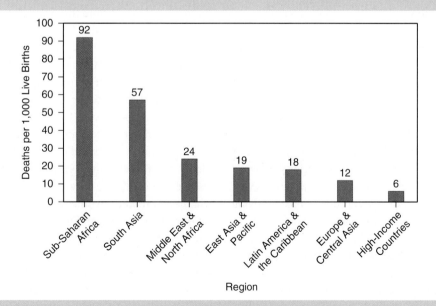

Data from the World Bank. World Development Indicators: Mortality. http://data.worldbank.org/indicator/SH.DYN.MORT/countries/1W-Z4-ZQ-Z7?display=graph. Accessed February 22, 2015.

FIGURE 10-5 Neonatal, Infant, and Under-5 Child Mortality Rates by World Bank Region and for High-Income Countries, 2013

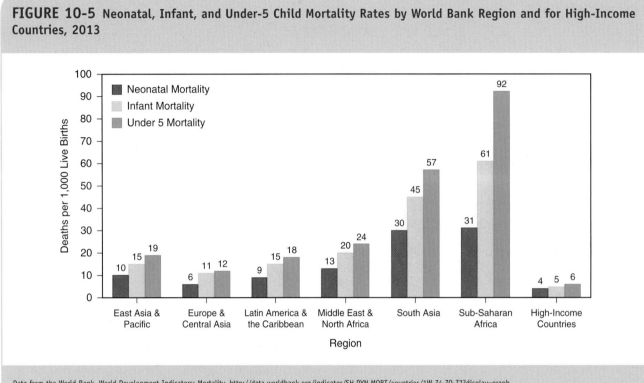

Data from the World Bank. World Development Indicators: Mortality. http://data.worldbank.org/indicator/SH.DYN.MORT/countries/1W-Z4-ZQ-Z7?display=graph.

- South Asia has the second-highest rates for all indicators.
- The rates tend to vary directly with the income group of the region.
- The higher the income group of the region, the more likely it is that children who die will die as neonates.
- In most low- and middle-income regions, the largest share of the children who die will die as neonates, but in some regions, there is still a significant risk of dying from the 1st month of life to the 12th month of life.
- In sub-Saharan Africa, uniquely, there are almost equal risks of dying in each of the periods shown—those living past the first month and those living past the first year still face substantial risks of dying between their first and fifth years.

As you would expect, the rates of infant and child mortality vary with income, education, and location. A study conducted by UNICEF several years ago showed that in sub-Saharan Africa, children from the lowest income quintile had almost twice the risk of dying before they were 5 years of age as children in the highest income quintile. The East Asia and Pacific, South Asia, and Middle East and North Africa regions, the poorest quintile children were almost three times more likely to die before they were 5 years old as those in the highest income quintile.

The differences by rural or urban location were less severe but still important. Rural populations in Latin America and the Caribbean were about 1.7 times more likely to die before their fifth birthday than urban populations, whereas those in South Asia were 1.5 times more likely, and those in sub-Saharan Africa were about 1.4 times more likely to die.[7]

For all low- and middle-income countries, under-5 children of mothers with no primary education were about twice as likely to die before they were 5 years of age, compared to children of mothers with a secondary education or higher. In most regions, other than South Asia, boys were more likely to die before they were 5 than girls. In the East Asia and Pacific region, however, boys and girls were equally likely to die before they were 5. These data suggest that in India and China, girls are still more likely to die under age 5 than boys are.[7]

Globally, the leading causes of death for children under 5 years of age are shown in **Table 10-3** by World Bank region and for high-income countries.

TABLE 10-3 Ten Leading Causes of Under-5 Deaths by World Bank Region, for High-Income Countries, and Globally, 2010

East Asia & Pacific	Europe & Central Asia	Latin America & the Carribean	Middle East & North Africa
1. Preterm birth complications	1. Lower respiratory infections	1. Preterm birth complications	1. Preterm birth complications
2. Lower respiratory infections	2. Congenital anomalies	2. Congenital anomalies	2. Congenital anomalies
3. Neonatal enceophalopathy	3. Preterm birth complications	3. Lower respiratory infections	3. Lower respiratory infections
4. Congential anomalies	4. Neonatal encephalopathy	4. Neonatal encephalopathy	4. Diarrheal diseases
5. Diarrheal diseases	5. Diarrheal diseases	5. Neonatal sepsis	5. Neonatal sepsis
6. Neonatal sepsis	6. Neonatal sepsis	6. Diarrheal diseases	6. Neonatal encephalopathy
7. Drowning	7. Meningitis	7. Forces of nature	7. Protein-energy malnutrition
8. Meningitis	8. Drowning	8. Protein-energy malnutrition	8. Road injury
9. Road injury	9. Stroke	9. Meningitis	9. Meningitis
10. Measles	10. SIDS	10. Road injury	10. Other cardiovascular and circulatory causes

South Asia	Sub-Saharan Africa	High-Income Countries	Global
1. Preterm birth complications	1. Malaria	1. Preterm birth complications	1. Preterm birth complications
2. Lower respiratory infections	2. Lower respiratory infections	2. Congenital anomalies	2. Lower respiratory infections
3. Diarrheal diseases	3. Diarrheal diseases	3. Neonatal encephalopathy	3. Malaria
4. Neonatal sepsis	4. Preterm birth complications	4. SIDS	4. Diarrheal diseases
5. Neonatal encephalopathy	5. Neonatal sepsis	5. Neonatal sepsis	5. Neonatal sepsis
6. Congenital anomalies	6. Protein-energy malnutrition	6. Lower respiratory infections	6. Neonatal encephalopathy
7. Meningitis	7. Neonatal encephalopathy	7. Road injury	7. Congenital anomalies
8. Protein-energy malnutrition	8. Meningitis	8. Drowning	8. Protein-energy malnutrition
9. Measles	9. HIV/AIDS	9. Interpersonal violence	9. Meningitis
10. Encephalitis	10. Congenital anomalies	10. Meningitis	10. HIV/AIDS

Institute for Health Metrics and Evaluation (IHME). GBD Heatmap. Seattle, WA: IHME, University of Washington, 2013. Available from http://vizhub.healthdata.org/irank/heat.php. Accessed February 27, 2015.

This table highlights several points:

- The lower the income group of the region, the more likely under-5 children are to die of infectious causes.
- The higher the income group of the region, the more likely under-5 children are to die of conditions related to birth, such as congenital anomalies.
- In sub-Saharan Africa uniquely, malaria and HIV/AIDS are also significant killers of young children.

Figure 10-6 shows the percentage share of different causes of death of under-5 children globally.

Almost all of these deaths are in low- and middle-income countries. As these countries have made progress in reducing under-5 child deaths, the leading causes of death globally have shifted toward prematurity and other issues around the period of the birth, such as birth asphyxia. Nonetheless, pneumonia is the second-leading cause of death of under-5 children globally, diarrheal diseases fourth, malaria eighth, and HIV, twelfth.

It is especially important for the formulation of policies to address the deaths of under-5 children to understand the causes of death at different times between birth and the end of the child's fourth year. Thus, **Figure 10-7** examines the causes of death among neonates globally. Preterm birth complications make up almost 35 percent of the total, birth asphyxia about 24 percent, sepsis and other infections 15 percent, congenital anomalies about 10 percent, and pneumonia about 5 percent.

As shown in **Figure 10-8**, pneumonia, diarrhea, malaria, and other communicable, perinatal, and nutritional conditions make up more than 60 percent of the total deaths of children in the post-neonatal period.

Additional Comments on Selected Causes of Morbidity and Mortality of Young Children

Pneumonia

Acute respiratory infections are very common causes of sickness and death in children younger than 5 years of age in

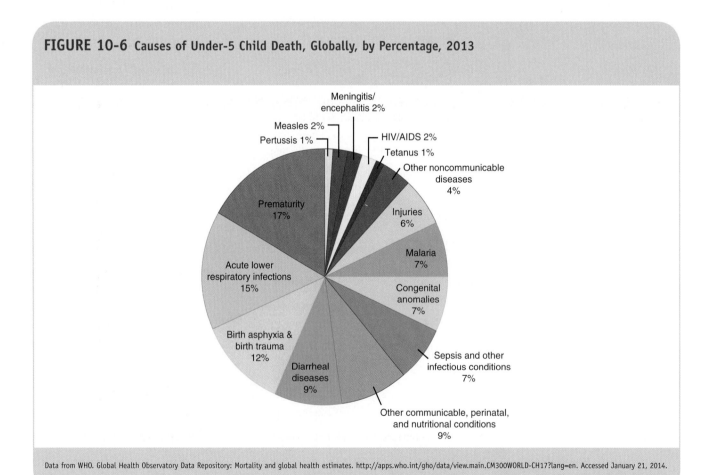

FIGURE 10-6 Causes of Under-5 Child Death, Globally, by Percentage, 2013

Data from WHO. Global Health Observatory Data Repository: Mortality and global health estimates. http://apps.who.int/gho/data/view.main.CM300WORLD-CH17?lang=en. Accessed January 21, 2014.

FIGURE 10-7 Causes of Neonatal Deaths, Globally, by Percentage, 2013

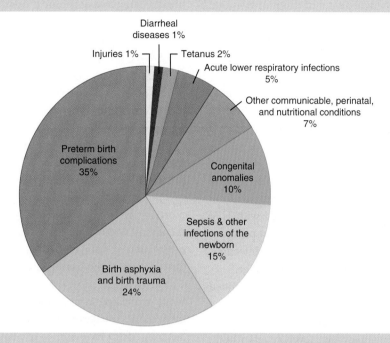

Data from World Health Organization. Global Health Observatory Data Repository. http://apps.who.int/gho/data/view.main.CM300WORLD-CH17?lang=en. Accessed February 6, 2015.

FIGURE 10-8 Causes of Post-Neonatal Under-5 Deaths (1–59 Months), Globally, by Percentage, 2013

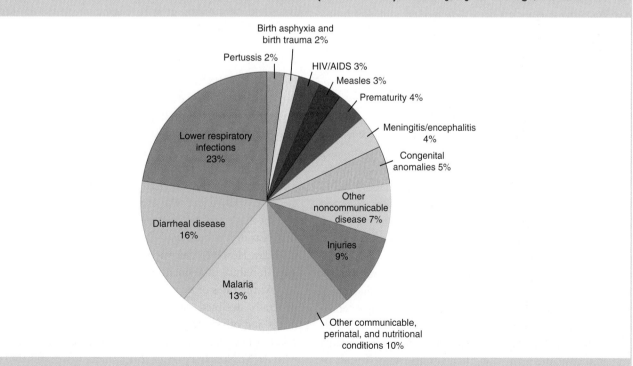

Data from WHO. Global Health Observatory Data Repository: Mortality and global health estimates. http://apps.who.int/gho/data/view.main.CM300WORLD-CH11?lang=en. Accessed February 28, 2015.

low- and middle-income countries where children average three to six acute respiratory infections per year. These cases are more severe and cause higher rates of death in low- and middle-income countries than in high-income countries. The most common acute respiratory infections are upper respiratory tract infections, such as the common cold and ear infections.[8]

The common lower respiratory infections are pneumonia and bronchiolitis. Pneumonia is caused by bacteria, viruses, and fungi. The most common forms of bacterial pneumonia are caused by *Streptococcus pneumoniae* (pneumococcus) and *Haemophilus influenzae,* type b (Hib).[8] The most common form of viral pneumonia is caused by respiratory syncytial virus. *Pneumocystis jirovecii* is a common form of pneumonia among children who are infected with HIV and the most significant cause of their death from pneumonia.[9] As noted earlier, pneumonia is the leading infectious cause of death globally of children under 5 years of age.

The most common way for pneumonia to be transmitted is via airborne droplets. However, it can also be transmitted through blood, especially around the time of birth.[9] Children who are sick with pneumonia may have fever, cough, wheezing, and difficulty breathing. Pneumonia can be diagnosed at the community level in resource-poor settings by the detection of rapid breathing of the sick child or the drawing in of the chest wall of the child during breathing, rather than its expansion, as is the case in a healthy person. Children who have bacterial pneumonia need to be treated with antibiotics, but only about one-third of the children who should receive such antibiotics actually get them. Most children with pneumonia can be treated in the community but very sick and very young children need to be treated in the hospital.[9]

Diarrhea

Diarrhea is the second-leading infectious cause of young child deaths, as noted earlier, and is caused by a number of different infectious agents, including bacteria, viruses, protozoa, and helminths.[10] Diarrhea is transmitted by what is known as the "fecal–oral" route of transmission, from the stool of one individual, eventually to the mouth of another. This is generally the result of unsafe water, poor sanitation, and poor hygiene.[10]

Dehydration, loss of nutrition and wasting, and damage to the intestines are all consequences of severe diarrhea.[10] Rapid dehydration due to diarrhea can be quickly fatal. In one study, infants with persistent diarrhea and severe malnutrition were at 17 times greater risk of dying than infants with mild malnutrition.[10] Children younger than 5 years of age in low- and middle-income countries have around three to four cases of diarrhea per year, with infants 6 to 11 months

of age having almost twice as many cases. As noted earlier, this is the age during which children usually stop exclusive breastfeeding and are at most risk of being exposed to unsafe water and foods.[10]

Malaria

Malaria is transmitted by the bite of one of several varieties of mosquito. It is an acute illness that arises in susceptible individuals 10 to 15 days after being bitten. Malaria should be diagnosed with either a blood smear or a rapid diagnostic test. It should be treated with artemisinin-based combination therapy (ACT) only upon a confirmed diagnosis but there are still significant gaps in following this approach.[11]

Malaria has an enormous impact on the morbidity and mortality of young children. The overwhelming majority of the almost 600,000 deaths a year that are caused by malaria occur among young children in sub-Saharan Africa.[11] In fact, malaria is the leading cause of death of children under 5 years of age in sub-Saharan Africa.[12] In addition, the morbidity associated with malaria in these children is staggering. One estimate suggested that people in endemic areas of sub-Saharan Africa have almost five episodes of malaria a year.[13] Moreover, the most severe form of malaria, cerebral malaria, has a case fatality rate of close to 20 percent, meaning that 20 percent of the children who get the disease die from it. Beyond the direct consequences of malaria on children are the indirect consequences. Malaria is associated with premature birth and intrauterine growth retardation, which are linked with low birthweight and reduced chances of survival.[13]

HIV/AIDS

One route of HIV transmission is from mother to child. This can take place either during birth or through breastfeeding. A newborn has a 15 to 45 percent chance of being infected with HIV from an HIV-positive woman who is not receiving antiretroviral therapy. This rate, however, can be reduced to 5 percent or lower by following proven protocols for the reduction of mother-to-child transmission.[14] Children who are HIV-positive and who are not treated with antiretroviral therapy have about a one-third risk of dying during their first year of life and a one-half risk of dying by their second birthday. However, starting treatment by their 12th week of life can reduce their chances of death by 75 percent.[15]

As the rates of new HIV infections among women have generally declined globally, and the use of antiretroviral drugs and other methods to prevent mother-to-child transmission has increased, fewer newborns have been infected with HIV. Nonetheless, in 2013, there were still 200,000 newborns infected with HIV and more than 90 percent of them were in sub-Saharan Africa.[15] As noted earlier, about

2 percent of the deaths of children under 5 globally are a result of HIV infection.

Measles

Measles is discussed further both in the section on immunization and in a policy brief on global efforts to reduce the burden of measles. For now, it is important to understand that measles is an acute respiratory infection that is spread through droplets in the air or contact with the nasal or throat secretions of an infected person. The initial symptoms are a runny nose, watery eyes, and white spots inside the cheeks. Later, a rash will break out, eventually spreading to the hands and feet.[16]

Measles can lead to complications including pneumonia, diarrhea, encephalitis, and blindness. Children who are younger than 5 years of age and either vitamin A deficient or HIV-infected are more vulnerable to measles complications and are more at risk of death than other children their age. Studies in sub-Saharan Africa suggest that between 0.5 and 10 percent of children who get measles will die from it.[17]

There has been an enormous amount of progress in increasing vaccination against measles in low- and middle-income countries and in reducing measles infections and deaths. In fact, such deaths decreased by 75 percent globally between 2000 and 2013.[16] Nonetheless, as noted earlier, measles is still among the leading killers of under-5 children globally, accounting for about 2 percent of their deaths. The role of vaccination in preventing measles and other diseases is discussed later in the chapter. However, it is essential to note here that, in the absence of vaccination, almost 100 percent of a population will get measles.[17]

Soil-Transmitted Helminths

Soil transmitted helminths are generally thought of as "worms" that infect humans. The most common such infections come from roundworm, hookworm, and whipworm. About 880 million children were at risk of infection from soil-transmitted helminths in 2012, but only about 30 percent of these children received appropriate treatment.[18] These infections can lead to severe morbidity, such as iron deficiency anemia, and are also associated with impaired physical and mental development in childhood.[19] Moreover, the burden of several species of worms is highest in children around 6 or 7 years of age.[20]

Additional Comments on Neonatal Mortality

There has been some progress in reducing the deaths of children younger than 5 years, as discussed earlier. However, there has been much less progress in reducing the neonatal death rate, except from neonatal tetanus.[21] Of the 6.3 million children under 5 years of age who died in 2013, about 44 percent of them, or about 2.8 million, died in the first month of life, and almost all of them lived in low- and middle-income countries.[1]

If the world is to further reduce child death rates, then it will have to reduce neonatal death rates. If the world is to do that, it will have to focus more precisely on when child deaths take place, where they take place, and why they occur. More than one-third of the children who die in their first month of life will actually die on their first day of life.[22] About 73 percent of the deaths that take place in the first month of life actually take place in the first week of life. Clearly, every day that a child lives increases the likelihood that he or she will stay alive. This may help to explain why children in a number of cultures are not named until after their first month of life. It may also help to explain why so many births are not registered with civil authorities, as was the case for Nassiba in the vignette that opened this chapter.

In thinking about neonatal deaths, just as in thinking about the deaths of all infants and children under 5 years, we must remember the relationship between the health of the mother and the health of the baby. Between 60 and 80 percent of neonatal deaths occur in low-birthweight babies. This generally reflects the poor health and nutritional status of the mother, including her being undernourished or having malaria, for example.[23] We also need to remember that an enormous number of child lives could be saved if the gap in child deaths between the richest and poorest segments of society were narrowed, even within most low- and middle-income countries.

RISK FACTORS FOR NEONATAL, INFANT, AND CHILD DEATHS

Why do so many children get sick and die of preventable causes? As mentioned earlier, an important part of the risks has to do with the social determinants of health. Poverty, for example, contributes to poor health and is a major underlying cause of morbidity and mortality among children. Where there is poverty, there is often inadequate nutrition. Where there is poverty, there is less access to safe water and sanitation, health services, and education. All of these are important determinants of child health. As noted earlier, there is a very strong correlation between family income and the likelihood that a neonate, an infant, or a child will survive. There is a similar correlation between the health and the educational status of the mother and the prospects that a child will survive birth and the first 5 years of life.

In fact, *The Millennium Development Goals Report 2006*, in commenting on progress toward the Millennium Development Goal of reducing child morbidity and mortality, revealed that higher household income and education for mothers doubled child survival rates. In families where the mother had no education or only primary education, child mortality averaged 157 deaths per 1,000 live births, whereas in families where the mother had secondary education or higher, mortality rates were close to 50 percent lower, at 82 per 1,000 live births.[24]

The health of the mother is also a critical determinant of the health of the newborn. The risk to the mother and child increases if the mother is a teenager or an older women, if the woman has had only a short birth interval between her last child and the next one, if the woman is of short stature, or if the woman is herself poorly nourished or suffering from malaria. These factors contribute to prematurity and low birthweight, both of which are important predictors of the well-being and survival of the child.[25]

The survival of a newborn is also closely linked with whether the birth took place in an appropriate healthcare setting and is attended by a trained healthcare provider.[26] A baby's chances of survival increase greatly when the baby is born in a setting that can deal with obstetric emergencies. The chances of survival also increase if the delivery is attended by a skilled birth attendant who can resuscitate babies who need it and can help counsel families about keeping babies warm and initiating breastfeeding early.

The environmental circumstances under which the child lives are also fundamental to child well-being. Indoor air pollution is an important risk factor for respiratory diseases. The lack of access to clean water and sanitation is linked with diarrheal disease and soil-transmitted helminths, among other problems. Living in zones that are endemic for malaria and other diseases poses a risk to young children. Moreover, the risk of unsafe hygiene increases greatly as the child begins to eat complementary foods and is no longer exclusively breastfed. We have also seen that better-educated families have more awareness about health risks, as well as safe behaviors that can improve their children's health and chances of survival.

Nutritional status has a profound impact, indirectly through the mother, and directly on the health and survival prospects of neonates, infants, and children younger than 5 years of age:[27,p2227]

- "Infants aged 0–5 months who are not breastfed have seven-fold increased risks of death from diarrhea and pneumonia, respectively, compared to infants who are exclusively breastfed."
- "35% of all child deaths are due to the effect of underweight status on diarrhea, pneumonia, measles, and malaria and relative risks of maternal body mass index for fetal growth retardation and its risks for selected neonatal causes of death."

- "In children with vitamin A deficiency, the risk of dying from diarrhea, measles, and malaria is increased by 20 to 24%. Likewise, zinc deficiency increases the risk of mortality from diarrhea, pneumonia, and malaria by 13 to 21%."

Wars and conflicts take a significant toll on children and are regrettable risk factors for child morbidity and mortality, particularly in sub-Saharan Africa and the Middle East. UNICEF estimated that in a typical 5-year war, under-5 mortality increases 13 percent.[28] In addition, the highest rates of neonatal death occur in conflict-ridden countries or countries just emerging from conflict, such as Liberia and Sierra Leone.[23]

Of course, family knowledge about health-seeking behaviors, the ability of families to actually seek appropriate health services, and their ability to get services of appropriate quality in a timely manner are also critical to whether children survive and thrive. As discussed further later, there are a number of low-cost and highly effective interventions that can reduce the burden of childhood deaths and disability-adjusted life years (DALYs). There are, for example, vaccines that can prevent some pneumonia and diarrhea and that can greatly reduce the burden of other vaccine-preventable diseases, such as measles. Families can be taught to diagnose pneumonia and community health workers can be taught to treat it with antibiotics. Oral rehydration can prevent deaths from diarrhea. Sleeping under a bednet can reduce the burden of malaria. Antiretroviral therapy can reduce mother-to-child transmission of HIV. Additionally, there are a range of nutrition interventions that are also low-cost and highly effective and that can enhance maternal and child health.

THE COSTS AND CONSEQUENCES OF CHILD MORBIDITY AND MORTALITY

One cannot measure direct losses in productivity that relate immediately to the morbidity and mortality of young children from the causes discussed in this chapter. There are, however, enormous costs and consequences to these illnesses. Some of them are short-term and relate to the family. Others are medium- or longer-term and relate to the child directly.

First, the direct and indirect costs of caring for a sick child can be very high. As noted earlier in this chapter, the average child in Africa is infected with malaria every 40 days. In addition, the average child in low- and middle-income countries will get three to six cases per year of acute respiratory infection and two to three cases of diarrhea. In this light, it is not surprising that families spend considerable parts of their limited financial resources on buying medical care for a sick child.[10] Moreover, caregivers devote special attention to the child who is ill, which prevents them from engaging in their normal income-earning activities.

Second, the medium- and long-term consequences of some childhood illnesses can be very high. Problems associated with prematurity, low birthweight, intrauterine growth retardation, and congenital abnormalities can lead to permanent disability and the associated costs to families and to society. A study on diarrheal disease in Brazil concluded that intelligence test scores were "25 to 65 percent lower in children with an earlier history of persistent diarrhea."[10,p375] The complications of measles can lead to encephalitis and blindness, as indicated earlier. By causing anemia, growth retardation, and the retardation of mental development, helminthic infections reduce children's enrollment, attendance, and performance in school and have consequences for later productivity.[20]

Finally, there is a range of social costs and consequences associated with childhood illness and death. Many poor families in low-income countries, knowing the odds are high that their newborn will die, have very high fertility to compensate for these deaths. In other words, in the hope of ensuring that the number of children they want will survive, they have more children than they would have otherwise.

IMMUNIZATION: A BEST BUY IN GLOBAL HEALTH

The Unique Importance of Immunization in Child Health

In a discussion of child health, immunization merits special attention because it is one of the most successful and cost-effective child health interventions that is available. Effective national immunization programs are essential to reduce under-5 morbidity and mortality globally. In fact, each year, routine immunization prevents between 2 and 3 million deaths and protects up to 100 million people against illness and disability.[29,30]

In 2013, 84 percent of the world's infants received vaccines to protect them from deadly diseases, which makes immunization closer to universal coverage than most other public health interventions.[31] The health benefits of immunization programs extend beyond the immunized individuals. For example, even unimmunized members of society may benefit from herd immunity where large portions of the population have been immunized against vaccine-preventable diseases. In addition, because immunization prevents illnesses that are typically treated with antibiotics, the risk of the development of antibiotic-resistant strains, which are more difficult and expensive to treat, is also diminished.

By maintaining population health, immunization also promotes economic growth and poverty reduction.[32] Recognized as a "best buy in global health," national immunization programs are investments in the individuals, families, communities, and countries in which they operate. Immunization makes economic sense. Studies suggest that scaling up existing vaccines in 72 of the poorest countries could save 6.4 million lives and avert $6.2 billion in treatment costs and $145 billion in productivity losses between 2011 and 2020.[33] Routine immunization generates economic benefits that derive from both productive human capital and medical costs averted by preventing disease.[34] These benefits increase family income and promote economic development at a societal level.

Immunization also allows children to become productive adults unburdened by the disability often associated with vaccine-preventable diseases. Immunization also improves life expectancy, and research suggests that a 5-year improvement in life expectancy results in 0.3 to 0.5 percent more annual growth in income per capita.[35,36] In addition, immunization prevents families of sick children from incurring the direct costs of treatment and hospitalization and the indirect costs associated with caregiving, such as inability to participate in the labor market while caring for a sick child. Moreover, in areas where the under-5 mortality rate is high, fertility rates also tend to be high as parents seek to ensure that some of their children will survive to adulthood. When population health improves and fertility rates drop, the age distribution becomes more favorable to economic growth, through "the demographic dividend."

Global Immunization Efforts

The international community has developed a variety of programs and initiatives to promote child health through immunization. The most significant of these programs is the Expanded Programme on Immunization (EPI). In 1974, the World Health Assembly launched EPI with the objective of vaccinating children throughout the world.[37] In its first phase, EPI focused on six diseases: tuberculosis (TB), poliomyelitis (polio), diphtheria, tetanus, pertussis (whooping cough), and measles. At the time EPI was created, only about 5 percent of the world's children were vaccinated against these six diseases, which were targeted by four vaccines.[38] EPI recommended vaccinating all eligible children from birth to 12 months against these diseases and giving pregnant women tetanus toxoid vaccinations.

Under EPI, individual countries were to create and implement their own national immunization programs, following guidelines set by WHO. Specifically, each state had to create and maintain a reliable cold supply chain, and transportation system to deliver doses of vaccine to health facilities, and vaccine stockpiles. In addition, states had to hire, train, and supervise healthcare workers, develop outreach programs to educate the public about vaccines and why they are important, and create a system for documenting which child has received which vaccine and when.[39]

States were also required to monitor their immunization programs using two methods: an administrative method and a community-based survey method. The former consists of gathering immunization data from clinics about the children who have been immunized during a specified period of time. Such data might include age, gender, doses, dates of vaccinations, and related information about each child. The survey method involves a two-stage cluster sampling approach developed by WHO.[39] Cluster sampling is a technique used when a researcher cannot get a complete list of members of the population he wishes to study but can get a list of groups within the population. In two-stage cluster sampling, first the entire population is divided into clusters and a random sample of clusters is selected, then a random sample of individuals who are members of those clusters are selected to, in this case, complete a survey. The surveys are conducted every 3 to 5 years, and the survey data are then used either as a primary source where official records are lacking or as a means by which to validate administrative reports. In addition, the Demographic and Health Surveys (DHS) Program and UNICEF's Multiple Indictor Cluster Surveys (MICS) are used routinely to collect data on children's vaccination coverage.[40]

Countries throughout the world progressively adopted EPI until the 1980s when the program became universal. When EPI was created in 1974, WHO established a standardized vaccine schedule that included four vaccines: Bacillus Calmette-Guérin (BCG), diphtheria-tetanus-pertussis (DTP), oral polio (OPV), and measles. For the first 20 to 30 years after EPI was created, global immunization efforts consistently included these four vaccines. Starting around the year 2000, however, scientific advances in the vaccines themselves and in logistics and storage, combined with a renewed global commitment to immunization, began to increase the number of introductions of new and underused vaccines (NUVIs), even in low- and middle-income countries.[41] Thus, EPI added hepatitis B (HepB), yellow fever in countries endemic for the disease, and *Haemophilus influenzae* b (Hib) vaccine to its recommended list of vaccines.

From the beginning of EPI, it was clear that the costs associated with national immunization programs would be prohibitive for some countries.[37,42] In 1977, therefore, the Pan American Health Organization (PAHO) created the PAHO Revolving Fund for Vaccine Procurement. This fund, which pooled the resources of 41 countries, allowed those countries to bargain as a group to buy large quantities of high-quality vaccines, syringes, and related supplies at the lowest possible price and then distribute them among the individual countries. This purchasing system helped enable the vaccination

of tens of millions of children in the Americas and avert millions of deaths from vaccine-preventable disease. In addition, it made it possible for the Region of the Americas to become the first of the six WHO regions to eliminate polio and the only region to eliminate indigenous transmission of measles and rubella.[43] The fund promotes self-sufficiency by using economies of scale to bring prices down to affordable levels. Today PAHO member states cover 95 percent of vaccination costs from their own national budgets.[43]

Low- and middle-income countries that were not members of PAHO were committed to EPI but consistently struggled to finance their national immunization programs. Then, in 1999, the Global Alliance for Vaccines and Immunization (GAVI; now referred to as Gavi) was created to improve child health by extending the reach of EPI to ensure that more children were vaccinated and that those vaccinations were complete. Gavi is a public-private partnership that works to promote and strengthen immunization programs in low- and middle-income countries. Through the International Finance Facility for Immunization and the Vaccine Fund, which is the funding arm of Gavi, eligible countries are provided with the financial resources to purchase vaccines and to fund the operational costs of national immunization programs and campaigns. In addition to cash grants, Gavi requires that countries co-finance immunization programs with the goal of graduating from Gavi eligibility and independently financing their programs. Gavi funding first became available to support national immunization programs in 2001, and there are currently 53 countries eligible to receive Gavi support.[44] Countries are eligible to receive Gavi support if their gross national income (GNI) per capita is equal to or below $1,570.[44] In order to qualify for support to introduce new or underused vaccines, Gavi-sponsored countries must also meet coverage levels of EPI vaccines.

Since 2000, Gavi-supported immunization programs have vaccinated 440 million children in some of the world's poorest countries.[45] Gavi supports the introduction of both new vaccines and new vaccine formulations in low- and middle-income countries. For example, with adequate funding, by 2015 Gavi plans to support the immunization of 90 million children with pneumococcal vaccines, 53 million with rotavirus vaccines, and 230 million with pentavalent vaccines.[46]

If Gavi is able to obtain $7.5 billion in additional investments for the 2016–2020 period, Gavi-supported countries will be able to immunize an additional 300 million children, resulting in 5 to 6 million lives saved.[47] This would increase the proportion of children who are fully protected with the 11 vaccines recommended by WHO from less than 5 percent to 50 percent.[47] The pentavalent vaccine, which will be discussed in more detail later, is key to this strategy because it combines five vaccines in one. This combination means that fewer shots are needed to fully vaccinate infants against five of the most deadly diseases. The pentavalent vaccine thus reduces the cost of stocking and administering additional vaccines and the number of healthcare visits. In addition, it is safer than administering the vaccines separately, decreases the risk of missed doses, and increases the number of fully vaccinated infants.

In 2002, EPI introduced the Reaching Every District strategy (RED), which sought to achieve 80 percent coverage of DTP3—the last of the DTP doses—in 80 percent of districts and to use contact with the healthcare system occasioned by routine immunization to deliver other child health interventions.[17] The RED initiative was implemented in 26 African countries between 2003 and 2005.[48] This measure succeeded in increasing the number of DTP3 vaccinations delivered.[49]

In 2005, WHO and UNICEF launched the Global Immunization Vision and Strategy (GIVS), 2006 to 2015. GIVS was the first 10-year framework aimed at decreasing morbidity and mortality associated with vaccine-preventable diseases by providing all people with equal access to immunization. GIVS had four key objectives: to immunize more people against more diseases, to introduce newly available vaccines and technologies, to integrate other critical health interventions with immunization, and to manage vaccination programs in the context of global interdependence.[46] Specifically, GIVS sought at least 90 percent national vaccination in all countries and at least 80 percent vaccination coverage in every district by 2010.[46]

In 2012 the Global Vaccine Action Plan (GVAP) was endorsed by the 194 WHO member states at the World Health Assembly. GVAP was designed to build upon the success of GIVS and sought to achieve key milestones in discovery, development, and delivery of lifesaving vaccines to the world's most vulnerable populations.[50] GVAP seeks to prevent millions of deaths by ensuring more equitable access to existing vaccines during the Decade of Vaccines, 2011–2020.[51] The Decade of Vaccines Global Action Plan is an effort to broaden the scope and reach of immunization globally. The plan seeks to ensure that all people, regardless of where they are born, who they are, or where they live, have the opportunity to lead lives free from vaccine-preventable diseases. Unlike efforts that came before it, GVAP is accompanied by a monitoring and accountability framework and a mechanism for independent review of progress, with the first review conducted in 2013.[50] Today WHO has expanded EPI recommendations to include vaccination against 11 diseases: diphtheria, pertussis, tetanus, poliomyelitis, TB, measles, HepB, Hib, pneumococcal disease, rotavirus, and human papillomavirus (HPV).[52]

Progress in Coverage of the Six Basic Vaccines and the Decline in Vaccine-Preventable Diseases

As noted, there are six core target diseases included in the national immunization programs of low- and middle-income countries: diphtheria, pertussis (whooping cough), tetanus, polio, tuberculosis, and measles. Much of the improvement that has occurred in the last 2 decades in child health is attributable to the increase in immunization coverage.[53] In fact, the number of deaths caused by the vaccine-preventable diseases originally targeted by EPI decreased from an estimated 900,000 in 2000 to 400,000 in 2010.[51] The dramatic effect of immunization coverage on disease prevalence is demonstrated in **Figure 10-9**, which illustrates the decline in the prevalence of measles. This graphic clearly portrays the increasing coverage of measles vaccine on the one hand, and the decline in the number of new measles cases on the other.

Next is an overview of the four core vaccines and the diseases they protect against.

Diphtheria-tetanus-pertussis (DTP) vaccine. Diphtheria, tetanus, and pertussis are potentially fatal bacterial diseases that primarily affect children. Vaccination against diphtheria, tetanus, and pertussis is accomplished together in a combined vaccine commonly referred to as DTP. In 2012, an estimated 83 percent (111 million) of infants worldwide were vaccinated with all three doses of DTP vaccine, compared with 76 percent in 1990.[54] In order to meet the MDG4 goal of achieving 90 percent vaccination for all three doses of DTP worldwide by 2015, an additional 13 million children will need to be vaccinated.[55] One dose of DTP, on average, costs $0.20.[56]

Polio vaccine. Poliomyelitis, commonly known as polio, is a highly infectious disease that mainly affects children under 5. One in 200 cases of polio leads to irreversible paralysis, and among those who become paralyzed, 5 to 10 percent die.[57] There is no cure for polio. The world has had a global eradication campaign against polio since 1988. Today there are just three polio-endemic countries, as compared with 125 polio-endemic countries in 1988.[57] In March 2014, the WHO South-East Asia Region was certified polio-free, which means that 80 percent of the world population now lives in polio-free areas. In just over 20 years, from 1990 to 2012, global coverage of infants with three doses of polio vaccine rose from 76 percent to 84 percent.[54] This coincided with a drop in the number of reported cases from 350,000 in 1988 to just 293 confirmed cases in 2012.[54] Current plans call for the progressive phase-out of oral polio vaccine and its replacement by inactivated polio vaccine (IPV) in the present decade,[58] to avoid the vaccine-derived polio that can occur, even if rarely, from the oral polio vaccine. The price per dose of OPV in 2015 was between $0.12 and $0.21, and the price

FIGURE 10-9 Reported Cases of Measles Globally and Coverage With the Measles Vaccine, 1980–2009

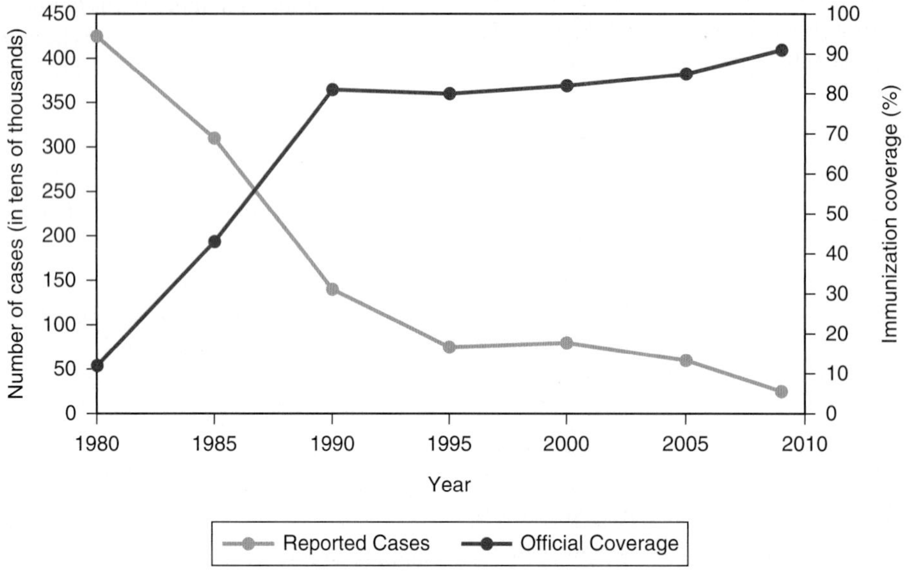

Modified from World Health Organization. WHO Vaccine-Preventable Diseases: Monitoring System, 2010 Summary. Retrieved March 3, 2015. http://whqlibdoc.who.int/hq/2010/WHO_IVB_2010_eng.pdf.

per dose of IPV was between $0.92 and $2.95.[56] A policy and program brief on the Global Polio Eradication Program is included in the next section. The chapter also includes a case study on the elimination of polio from the Americas.

Bacille Calmette-Guérin (BCG) vaccine. Tuberculosis (TB) is caused by a bacterium that most often affects the lungs. It is both preventable and curable but also highly contagious. Without proper treatment, up to two-thirds of people with TB will die.[59] Ninety-five percent of cases and deaths from TB occur in low- and middle-income countries in Asia and Africa. In 2012, half a million children became ill and 74,000 children died from TB.[59] The BCG vaccine, also known as the tuberculosis vaccine, has been available since 1921 and is administered to more than 80 percent of the world's infants as part of routine immunization programs.[60] Although BCG vaccine protects against meningitis and disseminated TB in children, it does not prevent reactivation of latent pulmonary infection.[60] The price per dose of BCG in 2015 was between $0.07 and $0.16.[56]

Measles vaccine. As discussed further in a policy and program brief later in this chapter, measles, which is a highly contagious viral disease, is one of the leading causes of death among children under 5 even though there is a safe

and cost-effective vaccine to protect against it. Since 2000, more than 1 billion children have been vaccinated against measles. In 2012, 84 percent of children worldwide received one dose of measles vaccine by their first birthday.[16] Sadly, even though measles vaccination reduced the number of measles deaths worldwide by 78 percent between 2000 and 2012, over 120,000 children died of measles in 2012.[16] The price per dose of measles vaccine in 2015 was between $0.23 and $0.48.[56]

Progress in Coverage of the Newer Vaccines

In the past 10 years, important advances have been made in the development and dissemination of new vaccines and in expanding the geographical reach of immunization programs. In recent years, additional vaccines have been developed to combat diseases beyond the six included in the original EPI. These newer and underused vaccines include HepB, Hib, pneumococcal conjugate vaccine, rotavirus, yellow fever, and HPV. Next is an overview of these vaccines and the diseases they protect against.

Hepatitis B vaccine. Hepatitis B is a viral infection that attacks the liver. The HepB vaccine, which is also included in the pentavalent vaccine discussed later, prevents hundreds of thousands of deaths every year, including those from liver cancer and cirrhosis.[61] The HepB vaccine is 95 percent effective and is the first vaccine to protect against a major cause of cancer.[61] As of 2012, the HepB vaccine had become part of national immunization schedules in 179 countries and had been introduced nationwide in 181 countries.[51] Today, global coverage of infants with three doses of HepB vaccine is estimated at 79 percent, compared to just 1 percent in 1990, though it varies by region.[56] One dose of HepB vaccine in 2015 cost between $0.16 and $0.38.

Haemophilus influenzae b (Hib) vaccine. Hib is a bacteria that causes meningitis and severe pneumonia in children under 5. In 2000, Hib was estimated to have caused 2 to 3 million cases of serious illness and 386,000 deaths in young children.[62] By the end of 2012, the Hib vaccine had become part of national immunization schedules in 173 countries and had been introduced in 184 countries, up from 177 countries in 2011.[33] Global coverage with three doses of Hib vaccine was estimated at 45 percent in 2012, reaching 91 percent in the Americas, but only 11 percent and 14 percent in the South-East Asia and Western Pacific Regions of WHO, respectively. The Hib vaccine may be administered alone or combined with DTP or other combinations including HepB and IPV. In 2015, one dose of the pentavalent vaccine, discussed further next, that includes Hib, cost between $1.34 and $2.80.[56]

Pentavalent vaccine. The pentavalent (five-in-one) vaccine, first introduced in 2001, is one of the most important scientific advances in immunization. This single vaccine, delivered in three doses, protects against diphtheria, pertussis, tetanus, HepB, and Hib. By permitting healthcare workers to immunize children against several diseases at once, this vaccine saves money and ensures broader coverage by minimizing the number of visits needed to administer the vaccine. In 2000, just one low-income country had introduced both Hib and HepB vaccines into its routine immunization program, but by the end of 2013 all low-income countries but one had introduced the pentavalent vaccine.[61] In 2014, South Sudan became the 73rd and last Gavi-supported country to introduce the pentavalent vaccine.[63] Global coverage of the pentavalent vaccine is expected to go from 50 percent in 2011 to more than 90 percent in 2020.[51,64]

Pneumococcal conjugate vaccine. Infection with pneumococcus, the bacterium that causes pneumonia, is responsible for half a million deaths of children under 5 each year.[61] Pneumonia is associated with 18 percent of all deaths of children under 5 globally, with the highest number of deaths occurring in low-income countries.[65] Current vaccines for pneumococcus are effective against the most common types

of pneumococcal bacteria. In the countries where they have been tested, pneumococcal conjugate vaccines have had positive effects on morbidity and mortality. Pneumococcal vaccine coverage is projected to rise from approximately 6 percent in 2011 to approximately 89 percent by 2020 across 94 low- and middle-income countries.[51,64] By the end of 2013, pneumococcal vaccine had been introduced in 102 countries, including 35 low-income countries.[61,66] By the end of 2013, 11 million children had been immunized against pneumococcal disease.[61] One dose of pneumococcal conjugate vaccine in 2015 cost between $3.30 and $7.00.[56]

Rotavirus vaccine. Rotaviruses are the most common cause of severe diarrheal disease among children under 5 worldwide. Although nearly every child in the world will contract rotavirus before the age of 5, nearly 95 percent of the related deaths occur in low-income countries where treatment is limited.[67] Although two rotavirus vaccines are available, they are not yet widely used in low-income countries. If rotavirus vaccines were used in all Gavi-eligible countries, it would be possible to avert an estimated 180,000 deaths and 6 million clinic and hospital visits each year, which would save $68 million per year in treatment costs. Based on significant reductions in morbidity and mortality resulting from the introduction of these vaccines, WHO recommends that all infants be vaccinated against rotavirus.[68] By the end of 2012, more than 20 Gavi-eligible countries had been approved for support for the rotavirus vaccine,[66] and by the end of 2013 six Gavi-supported countries had introduced it.[61] Rotavirus vaccine coverage is projected to rise from 2 percent in 2011 to 77 percent by 2020 across 94 low- and low-middle income countries.[64] A single dose of rotavirus vaccine in 2015 cost between $2.30 and $5.00.[56]

Yellow fever vaccine. Yellow fever is an acute viral hemorrhagic disease transmitted by mosquitoes. There are an estimated 200,000 cases causing 30,000 deaths per year worldwide, with 90 percent of cases occurring in Africa.[69] There is no cure for yellow fever, but one dose of the vaccine confers lifelong protection. WHO currently recommends vaccinating all infants over 9 months who live in yellow fever endemic areas. One dose of yellow fever vaccine in 2015 cost between $0.77 and $1.17.[56] WHO no longer recommends revaccination at 10-year intervals, as used to be the case.

Human papillomavirus (HPV) vaccine. Cervical cancer, 70 percent of which is caused by HPV, kills more than 270,000 women each year.[70] Of these deaths, roughly 85 percent occur in low- and middle-income countries.[70] Unlike the other vaccines discussed in this section, the HPV vaccine is not given to infants, but rather to children aged 9 to 13 (prior to initiation of sexual activity). Although previously WHO recommended three doses, current evidence supports the efficacy of two doses administered at least 6 months apart for girls less than 15 years of age. This reduction in the number of doses has both financial and health consequences, as the same number of doses can be administered to a larger number of girls and fewer girls are likely to be undervaccinated due to missed appointments or lack of vaccines.[55] A three-dose schedule, administered at 0, 1–2 months, and 6 months, is still recommended for girls over 15 years of age and for girls who are immunocompromised.[55] As of 2014, the HPV vaccine had been introduced in more than 45 countries.[33] In addition, pilot projects were begun in six Gavi-supported countries in 2013.[61] In 2015, one dose of HPV vaccine cost an average of $4.55.[56]

MenAfriVac. Up to 450 million people in Africa are at risk for meningococcal A meningitis, with major epidemics occurring every 7 to 14 years.[71] The Meningitis Vaccine Project (MVP), a partnership between PATH and WHO, worked with a consortium of international partners to develop a vaccine for use in sub-Saharan Africa that protects people 1 to 29 years of age against this type of meningitis. MenAfri-Vac is expected to reduce endemic meningitis by 50 percent and costs under $0.50 per dose.[71] Since its introduction in December 2010, more than 150 million people have received the vaccine.[72]

Next-Generation Vaccines and Vaccine Delivery

With the cooperation and support of organizations like Gavi, PATH, WHO, individual country donors, and the pharmaceutical industry, new vaccines and new vaccine delivery systems are currently being developed and tested. WHO anticipates that new vaccines against cholera, dengue, malaria, polio, and typhoid will be introduced during the Decade of Vaccines, which began in 2010.[51,64] In addition, research is under way to develop new vaccine formulations that are safer, easier to store and transport due to thermo-stability, and packaged in smaller vials to decrease waste.[73] An international cholera vaccine stockpile has been created, and discussions are under way to determine how best to distribute the vaccines.[55] Although there is currently no commercially available vaccine that protects against dengue, researchers predict that such a vaccine will reach the market in the next several years and that coverage of the new vaccine will rise to 49 percent by 2020.[64]

One of the most important recent developments in vaccine-preventable diseases relates to typhoid. Typhoid fever is caused by the salmonella typhi bacterium, and exposure usually occurs through ingestion of contaminated food or water. There are an estimated 21 million typhoid cases and between 216,000 and 600,000 typhoid-related deaths each year.[74] Existing vaccines do not provide long-term protection and are not safe for use among children under 2 years of age, when the disease is most lethal.[75] In fact, earlier vaccines were not approved for use among children under 5 years.[76] In 2013, Bharat Biotech, an Indian company, launched the first typhoid conjugate vaccine that has been clinically proven to provide long-term protection to adults and infants over 6 months of age.[77] Prices for the new vaccine are not yet available.

In July of 2014, a malaria vaccine that could be administered to children entered the final stages of review. When coupled with other interventions such as bednets, the new malaria vaccine has been shown to provide 46 percent protection against malaria when given to children 5 to 17 months old.[78] However, the vaccine has not yet been licensed in any country.

Progress Toward Universal Immunization of Children

Today, notwithstanding tremendous progress, vaccine-preventable diseases remain a major cause of morbidity and mortality around the world. In 2013, 111 million infants, or 84 percent of the world's children, were vaccinated against deadly diseases.[79] Unfortunately, millions of children each year are unvaccinated or undervaccinated. In 2012, nearly one in five infants (22.6 million children) did not receive the three doses of DTP vaccine they needed.[33,80] In 2013, 21.8 million infants were not vaccinated at all.[79] As a consequence, in 2012 1.5 million children died from vaccine-preventable diseases.[33]

Sadly, this burden is borne primarily by the most vulnerable populations: the poorest children living in the poorest parts of the world. Vaccination is consistent with the "inverse care law," which observes that the availability of good medical care tends to vary inversely with the need of the population.[81] Lower vaccine coverage rates are associated with socioeconomic determinants of health such as the educational status of the mother, geographical distance from health centers, and family income levels.[51] Race, ethnicity, whether a child lives in a rural or urban area, and the economic status of the country they live in are also important determinants of vaccine coverage, such that poor children living in rural areas or urban slums in parts of WHO's Africa and South-East Asia regions are among the least likely to be fully vaccinated. As noted earlier, WHO's Africa Region, consisting of 47 countries, has consistently lagged behind in immunization. Although three of WHO's regions report immunization coverage at or above

90 percent, the South-East Asia Region, which includes India, and the African Region lag far behind at just 77 percent and 75 percent, respectively.[79] Poor immunization coverage in the Africa Region may be explained in part by civil unrest, lack of human resources for health care, and limited funding for routine immunization services.[49]

Even within WHO regions, vaccination rates vary among countries, with high-income countries performing far better than low-income countries. DTP vaccination is widely considered a reliable marker of routine immunization.[49] The average coverage gap for all three doses of DTP between low-income countries and high-income countries has decreased from 30 percent in 2000 to 16 percent in 2010.[51] Nevertheless, of the 22.6 million children under 1 year of age worldwide who did not receive the DTP vaccine in 2012, more than 70 percent lived in 10 countries: the Democratic Republic of the Congo, Ethiopia, India, Indonesia, Iraq, Nigeria, Pakistan, Philippines, Uganda, and South Africa.[33] Similarly, of the estimated 20 million children worldwide who did not receive the first dose of measles vaccine in 2011, more than half lived in just five countries: the Democratic Republic of the Congo, Ethiopia, India, Nigeria, and Pakistan.[82] In 2011 large measles outbreaks were reported in all of these countries and several others.[82]

Vaccination rates vary within countries due to the relative wealth of a region, the healthcare facilities available, and the ease of travel to and from those facilities. Thus, children who live in isolated rural areas are among the least likely to be fully immunized. Coverage of the measles vaccine is a useful example. The measles vaccine coverage rate in some countries is up to 58 percent higher among the richest fifth of the population than among the poorest fifth.[51] Similarly, in some countries coverage of measles vaccine is 30 percent lower in rural areas as compared to urban areas.[51] Vaccination coverage also tends to be lower among the urban poor, especially in cities with transitory migrant populations, and among indigenous groups.[51] India provides an example of interregional differences in vaccination rates. Bihar has a three-dose DTP vaccine coverage rate of 40 percent, as compared to rates that are at least 30 percent higher in other Indian states such as Tamil Nadu and Kerala.[73]

Gaps in vaccination coverage are explained by a number of variables. Low-income countries lack the health infrastructure, human resources, and financing to maintain a predictable and sustainable national immunization program. The success of national immunization programs may also be inhibited by armed conflict, natural disasters, gaps in vaccine-preventable disease surveillance, and inadequate safety measures.[37] Critical challenges to universal coverage are discussed in the next section.

Critical Challenges to Universal Vaccine Coverage and What Is Being Done to Address Them

Today, there remain a number of critical challenges to universal childhood immunization. These challenges center on healthcare infrastructure and human resources, demand, supply, and financing. Low- and middle-income countries often do not have the healthcare infrastructure or human resources necessary to run a successful national immunization program on their own. In addition, lack of demand for immunization due to lack of information or traditional antivaccine beliefs is a significant impediment to universal immunization. Once demand has been stimulated, national immunization programs must be able to procure the necessary number of doses at an affordable price and on a predictable basis to ensure that children can be fully vaccinated according to recommended schedules. This requires an adequate supply provided at an affordable cost to the purchasing country. There are also challenges associated with financing these programs. A number of low-income countries will not have the resources needed in the short to medium run to finance effective immunization programs solely from their own funds. For these countries, universal immunization will require a combination of country-level action and support from public and private organizations, domestically and internationally.

Lack of infrastructure and human resources. Low-income countries often lack the most basic healthcare facilities and infrastructure. Delivering routine immunization services where the healthcare infrastructure is fragile or nonexistent is a major hurdle for many low-income countries. Although brick-and-mortar medical facilities may not be necessary to implement an immunization program, there must be a means by which to safely stockpile doses and transport them to the target population, as well as a reliable and accurate method for recording who has received vaccines and when. As new vaccines are introduced and scaled up, surveillance is needed to monitor outcomes and watch for changes in the epidemiology and disease characteristics.[66]

In addition to healthcare infrastructure, a successful national immunization program requires trained and adequately compensated healthcare personnel to administer the vaccines and to keep records of vaccinations. These workers must be managed and supervised to most efficiently deliver vaccines as part of a larger healthcare system. Of the 19.3 million underimmunized children in 2010, 6.6 million lived in Africa, and 60 percent of those children lived in just five countries where vaccines are available but the lack of delivery systems and a trained healthcare workforce to deliver the vaccines made implementation exceedingly difficult.[37] In recent years, Gavi has devoted considerable resources to health system strengthening in order to assist the poorest countries in developing an adequate and sustainable healthcare infrastructure.

Lack of demand. Demand creation is essential to the success of national immunization programs. A lack of demand may be the result of a lack of education or traditional beliefs that are at odds with vaccination. Political leaders and civil society must understand the risks and benefits of immunization and view routine immunization of all children as a government responsibility. Even after the original EPI vaccines are introduced, it is necessary to create demand for new and underused vaccines that are typically adopted later in low- and middle-income countries than in higher-income countries. For example, in 2010, just 13 percent of the birth cohort eligible for pneumococcal conjugate vaccine in high-income countries lived in places where it was not part of the national vaccine schedule.[51] In contrast, 98 percent of the birth cohort eligible for pneumococcal conjugate vaccine in low-income countries lived in places where the vaccine was not part of the national schedule.[51]

Stimulating demand by increasing awareness and understanding of the benefits of immunization is crucial in the effort to expand immunization programs. In places such as India where mobile phones are nearly ubiquitous, mobile phones and social networks can be used to educate the public about the benefits and risks of immunization, thereby stimulating demand.[51] Finally, ethical, cultural, ideological, or religious beliefs that are inconsistent with vaccination may need to be addressed before an immunization campaign will succeed.

Lack of supply. Once demand has been stimulated and a national program has been established, it is necessary to ensure that an adequate and reliable supply of vaccine will be available. Even if countries are willing to introduce new vaccines, it is often very difficult to obtain the necessary number of doses at an affordable price. An optimally effective immunization program requires that all eligible children receive vaccines and boosters on schedule. Gaps in supply may result in children who are unimmunized or underimmunized. The supply of vaccines may be jeopardized by the high cost of vaccines or by production or distribution problems as programs are scaled up.

As new vaccines become available and underused vaccines are administered more broadly, the supply and logistics systems will be further burdened. In some low-income countries, limited supply and lack of country preparedness are jeopardizing targets for pentavalent, pneumococcal, and rotavirus vaccine coverage rates.[61] To address gaps in supply, Gavi has developed an immunization supply chain strategy and has identified supply chain design and optimization as a priority for country-level funding.[83] In addition, WHO and UNICEF have developed an initiative to create supply chain hubs.[83] Supply-related challenges are also being addressed through advances such as the development of the pentavalent vaccine, which minimizes the number of vaccines and vaccine doses necessary to fully immunize a child.

New suppliers must also be encouraged to enter the vaccine market in order to ensure that an adequate and affordable supply is available at all times. Vaccines are expensive to produce due to increasingly complex manufacturing and regulatory schemes and the growing costs associated with research and development. In the short term, a limited initial supply of new vaccine typically leads to higher prices and an uncertain demand often leads to low-capacity investment in the manufacturing cycle, which eventually leads to delays in distribution of the vaccine. Thus, after a vaccine has been proven safe and effective, it has generally taken 15 to 20 years for it to be widely distributed among poor populations in low- and middle-income countries. To break this cycle in the case of pneumococcal vaccine, Gavi has funded the Pneumococcal Accelerated Development and Introduction Plan (pneumoADIP). Due to this program, the pneumococcal vaccine was introduced in low-income countries just 1 year after it was first introduced in high-income countries.[51]

In the long term, the availability of new vaccines creates greater market competition, which lowers the price of existing vaccines and increases the likelihood that they will reach children in low-income countries. Organizations like PATH are working to encourage the development of new vaccines and the entry of new companies into the vaccine market. With these goals in mind, PATH has developed a shared technology platform that provides information on methodologies, technology, material, and training for new manufacturers. In recent years, investment in vaccines has changed the global vaccine market, attracting new suppliers of high-quality vaccines at reduced prices.[61] These new suppliers are located throughout the world, including places like India, China, and Indonesia. In fact, emerging manufacturers now supply 86 percent of the core EPI vaccines to UNICEF.[84] The availability of long-term predictable funding for immunization programs and the increased demand for vaccines from low- and middle-income countries also encourage suppliers to provide vaccines at lower prices.[61]

Lack of financial resources. Costs associated with immunization are high and continue to rise. For example, the total cost for purchasing the original EPI vaccines rose from $1.37 per child in 2001 to more than $38.80 per child in 2011.[73] Experts predict that with the pneumococcal and rotavirus vaccines added to the original EPI vaccines, the cost of fully immunizing each child could reach $64.00.[37] WHO estimates that the costs to scale up immunization programs, introduce new and underused vaccines, and provide supplemental immunization sufficient to reach elimination and eradication goals in the world's 94 poorest countries will rise from between $3.5 billion and $4.5 billion in 2011 to between $6 billion and $8 billion in 2020.[51] That is, the cumulative cost of the Decade of Vaccines is expected to be between $50 billion and $60 billion.[51] Of these costs, 46 percent is for vaccines and injection supplies and 54 percent is for delivery costs and health systems.[64] Just three countries, Nigeria, India, and Pakistan, are expected to account for 37 percent ($21.1 billion) of these costs due to large birth cohorts and ambitious plans to scale up existing programs and introduce the pneumococcal and rotavirus vaccines.[64]

In addition, vaccines against cholera, dengue, malaria, polio (IPV), and typhoid are in various stages of development and are expected to comprise a growing proportion of immunization costs once they become available.[64] On the positive side, the costs of emergency response efforts will likely decrease as routine immunization programs expand and make progress toward the goals of controlling, eliminating, or eradicating vaccine-preventable disease.[64]

It is clear that without the market-shaping pressure, direct financial support, and encouragement of research and development by international organizations, even the core EPI vaccines would remain out of reach for many of the world's poorest populations. Innovations in financing have been pivotal in the effort to reach the goal of universal immunization. Efforts to stimulate funding and decrease prices have been successful. For example, by the end of 2013, the International Finance Facility for Immunisation (IFFIm) had raised $4.5 billion on the capital markets to help finance immunization programs worldwide. Since 2000, 440 million additional children have been immunized in Gavi-supported countries.[45,61] By 2015 Gavi planned to support the immunization of 90 million children with pneumococcal vaccines, 53 million with rotavirus vaccines, and 230 million with pentavalent vaccines.[46] Finally, through increased competition, improved technology, and international cooperation, the cost per dose for basic vaccines has dropped. For example, the weighted average price of pentavalent vaccine dropped 39 percent from $3.56 per dose in 2003 to $2.17 per dose in 2012, with a lowest price of $1.19 per dose from one supplier in 2013.[45]

The relative cost of vaccine and nonvaccine components in national immunization programs has changed over time. In the early years of EPI, the six basic antigens were relatively inexpensive, and the vaccines themselves accounted for just 20 percent of total program costs, with the remainder going to healthcare infrastructure, human resources, and supply chain and logistics infrastructure.[85] From 2000 to 2010, countries began to scale up the use of the pentavalent vaccine, and the total cost of immunization programs doubled or tripled, as the cost of the vaccines comprised an average of 50 percent of total program budgets.[85] This change was due in part to the fact that although the pentavalent vaccine itself was more expensive, the health system costs of introducing it were minimal. The pentavalent vaccine required no more office visits than the DTP vaccine it replaced, and the vaccine required little additional storage space in the vaccine cold chain. Today, as highly effective new vaccines are introduced into national programs, experts predict that the overall cost of these programs will increase significantly. The new vaccines are expensive, and upfront investments in nonvaccine components of national immunization programs, including training of healthcare human resources and maintaining in-country vaccination supply chains, will be necessary to ensure the success of these programs in the future.[85] A recent needs-based costing exercise conducted by WHO and UNICEF predicted that the average health system cost per child will rise from $24.90 during the period 2011 to 2015 to $32.60 from 2016 to 2020.[85]

Ultimately the goal for all countries is to be able to independently administer their national immunization programs with little or no outside support. One important step in this direction is the inclusion of immunization programs in national budgets. As of 2010, 154 of the 193 WHO member states reported having a specific budget line item for immunization, and 147 had multiyear national plans to sustain the gains achieved, enhance performance, and introduce appropriate new vaccines.[51] Although there remain serious challenges in the effort to achieve universal immunization, millions of lives have already been saved thanks to national political will in developing countries and the commitment and support of the international community.

POLICY AND PROGRAM BRIEFS

Given the importance of immunization, two policy and program briefs follow. The first reviews the progress of the Global Polio Eradication Initiative. The second examines progress against measles.

The Global Polio Eradication Initiative

In 1988, the World Health Assembly (WHA), the yearly meeting of the ministers of health of all member states of WHO, launched the Global Polio Eradication Initiative (GPEI).[86] At the time, polio was endemic in 125 countries on five continents and paralyzed 350,000 children a year, or 1,000 children per day.[87] In 2014, there were only 372 cases of polio in the world, and today polio is endemic in only three countries Afghanistan, Nigeria, and Pakistan.[88]

The GPEI is a public-private partnership led by national governments and directed by its founding partners, WHO, Rotary International, the U.S. Centers for Disease Control and Prevention (CDC), and UNICEF. It is the largest international public health effort to date, and the scale of its efforts is truly exceptional. Many international and national partners are now involved in both financing the program and carrying out its work.

The GPEI was built partly on earlier successes in eliminating polio. In the 1950s and 1960s, two effective polio vaccines were developed separately by Jonas Salk and Albert Sabin. In many high-income countries, initiatives promoting the use of the vaccines led to the elimination of polio.[89] The Salk inactivated polio vaccine, for example, reduced polio transmission in the United States from 20,000 cases per year in the 1950s to around 1,000 cases by the 1960s. The United States started to use Albert Sabin's oral polio vaccine in mass polio campaigns in 1963, and by 1979 transmission was stopped.

In addition, in 1979, Rotary International started its first polio vaccination project in the Philippines and succeeded in vaccinating 6 million children. Rotary then considered how it could provide the polio vaccine to all children in the world by 2005, the organization's 100th anniversary. In the next several years, therefore, Rotary collaborated with Sabin, raised $240 million, and then partnered with WHO, UNICEF, and the CDC to create the "PolioPlus" project in 1988.[90] That same year, UNICEF and WHO launched the Universal Childhood Immunization Initiative with the goal of reducing child mortality through immunization. PAHO also launched an initiative to eradicate polio in the Americas by 1990.[87]

The original goal of GPEI was to eradicate polio by 2000.[87] Although this goal was not met, by 2000, the number of polio cases globally had dropped to 1,000, a 99 percent reduction from the start of GPEI.[91] At that time, over 575 million children were being vaccinated annually with the oral polio vaccine through the efforts of 20 million volunteers in low- and middle-income countries.[86]

This success was achieved through the implementation of several key strategies: routine immunization of infants with oral poliovirus vaccine; mass immunization campaigns through National Immunization Days or supplementary national or regional activities; active surveillance for acute flaccid paralysis, a symptom of polio; enhancement of lab capacity to detect new cases; and "mop-up campaigns," which are targeted to a specific area and have a rapid response to disease outbreaks.[89,91]

These strategies have since been supplemented by health worker training, awareness campaigns, commitment of community and religious leaders, technological and scientific innovations such as geographic information system (GIS) mapping for surveillance and the introduction of new vaccine formulations, vaccine production and distribution, and the sharing of best practices.[89,92]

One of the great successes of the initiative has been the elimination of polio in India in 2014. In fact, many people thought this could never be accomplished, given challenges in India such as technical difficulties with the effectiveness of the vaccines among some children, very poor sanitation in much of India, active distrust of the polio program in a number of communities, especially in north India, and weak public health infrastructure.[93]

In recent years, however, the initiative has faced a number of difficult challenges as it seeks to take the final steps in eradicating polio. Some of these challenges are especially important in the three remaining endemic countries, in which not all children who should be vaccinated are being covered. Some factors contributing to the lack of coverage and the failure to stop transmission in these countries have been conflict, very weak public health infrastructure, poor sanitation, and religious or other social barriers that have reduced the ability of health workers to reach all children.[89] In 2012, the WHA stated that eradicating polio was a "programmatic emergency for global public health."[89]

GPEI also faces a range of other financial, political, and technical challenges. It has taken much longer than planned to eradicate polio, and the initiative has therefore cost dramatically more than its original estimates and led to some donor fatigue. In addition, no one foresaw the level of political antagonism to the program, such as the killing of polio workers in Pakistan by the Taliban, and overcoming these threats will not be easy. Moreover, the oral vaccine that is being used to promote the fastest reduction in new cases in low- and middle-income countries can itself cause vaccine-derived polio. Thus, the world must prepare to shift to the injectable form of the vaccine, which will be much more challenging to use than the oral form. Finally, vaccination will continue even after eradication, to avoid reintroduction of polio or of vaccine-derived polio.[94]

GPEI's strategic plan for 2013–2018 calls for the elimination of all wild poliovirus by 2014, which has not been achieved, and for a polio-free world by 2018. The plan focuses on four efforts:

- Routine immunization
- Supplementary immunization
- Surveillance
- Targeted mop-up campaigns

Central to the plan is the aim of strengthening national immunization systems by leveraging GPEI best practices and infrastructure and working closely with the Gavi Alliance.[94]

Measles—Progress and Challenges

Progress Against Measles—But Large Challenges Remain

There has been substantial progress against measles in the last decade, with measles deaths falling globally from 548,000 in 2000 to 158,000 in 2011.[95] Nonetheless, measles remains the 12th largest killer of children under 5 years of age globally.[96] In addition, measles is still a top 10 cause of death for children under 5 in South Asia and Southeast Asia.[96] Moreover, in 2012, 15 countries had large measles outbreaks, including countries in Europe, Africa, South Asia, and Southeast Asia.[95] This brief discusses what measles is, the vaccine against it, trends in the burden of disease, global goals, and the barriers the world faces in trying to address measles.

The Measles Virus

Measles is a highly contagious viral disease. In the absence of being vaccinated, almost anyone exposed to the virus will contract measles. The measles virus typically grows in the cells that line the back of the throat and lungs.[16] The virus that causes measles is transmitted by coughing and sneezing, as well as by close contact with infected nasal or throat secretions.[16] The virus continues to be active and contagious in the air or on infected surfaces for up to 2 hours.[16] It can be transmitted by an infected person from 4 days before symptoms start to occur to 4 days after the onset of symptoms.

The first sign of measles is usually high fever, which begins about 10 to 12 days after exposure to the virus.[16] In the initial stage of the virus, the symptoms include a runny nose, a cough, red and watery eyes, and small white spots inside the cheeks.[16] A rash will appear about 14 days after exposure to the virus and will last about 5 to 6 days.[16] The greatest risk of a severe reaction to measles is among poorly nourished young children, children with insufficient vitamin A, or those whose immune systems have been weakened by HIV/AIDS or other diseases.[16]

The Measles Vaccine

The measles vaccine is safe, effective, and inexpensive—it costs less than $1.00 to purchase and deliver[95] in low-income countries. The measles vaccine is often combined with a rubella vaccine, with the result known as "MR" vaccine. WHO recommends that each child receive two doses of the vaccine to ensure immunity and to prevent further outbreaks.[16] In countries where there is ongoing transmission of measles, WHO recommends the first dose be given to children when they are 9 months of age.[97] The second dose can be given through routine immunization programs or supplementary immunization.[98] Even with only one dose of the vaccine, however, there is an 85 percent chance that the child will develop immunity to the measles virus.[16]

Trends in the Burden of Disease

Despite the availability of a safe and cost-effective vaccine, about 20 million children who should receive the first dose each year do not do so. In addition, the African, Eastern Mediterranean, and European Regions of WHO are not on track to achieve their regional measles elimination goals.[99] In the Africa Region, large outbreaks continue in countries with weak immunization systems such as Angola, the Democratic Republic of Congo, and Ethiopia.[99] In the Eastern Mediterranean Region, there was a measles resurgence in Afghanistan, Pakistan, Somalia, and Yemen due to weak routine immunization systems and delayed follow-up campaigns.[99] Europe faces difficulties eliminating measles due to insufficient political commitment in Western Europe and health system weaknesses in Eastern Europe.[99] In the South-East Asia Region of WHO, there are many pockets in India and Indonesia that have not been vaccinated against measles due to children living in hard-to-reach areas.[99]

Any person who is not immune to measles can become infected. The most notable complications from measles include blindness, encephalitis, severe diarrhea and related dehydration, ear infections, and severe respiratory infections such as pneumonia.[16] Unvaccinated pregnant women are also at high risk of measles complications.[16] People who survive the measles virus remain immune for the rest of their lives.[16]

More than 95 percent of measles-related deaths occur in low-income countries, and death rates from measles can reach 10 percent in settings with high rates of undernutrition and poor health systems.[16] People who live in areas experiencing or recovering from a natural disaster or conflict are also at greater risk of contracting measles. This is largely because damage to health infrastructure and health services constrains routine immunizations and results in overcrowding in residential camps—both of which greatly increase the risk of infection.[16]

Global Goals

Millennium Development Goal 4 is to reduce the under-5 mortality rate by two-thirds between 1990 and 2015.[16] Routine measles vaccination coverage is an indicator of progress toward achieving this goal.[95] The Measles & Rubella Initiative that began in 2000 represents a collaborative effort of WHO, UNICEF, the American Red Cross, the Centers for Disease Control and Prevention, and the United Nations Foundation to achieve measles and rubella control goals.[16] Since 2000, the Measles & Rubella Initiative has reached over 1 billion children through mass vaccination campaigns.[16]

PAHO member countries have eliminated endemic measles and rubella from the Western Hemisphere.[100] Successful measles elimination strategies were implemented in PAHO member countries in 2000, and endemic measles transmission was successfully halted in the Americas in 2002.[100]

Addressing the Outstanding Challenges

There are several critical challenges in eliminating measles globally. First is the highly infectious nature of measles. Second, there are also technical challenges to measles elimination in high-density populations, such as parts of north India.[101] Third, some countries have not fully embraced measles control and reduction strategies.[101]

In 2012, the Measles & Rubella Initiative launched a new Global Measles and Rubella Strategic Plan, which covers the period 2012 to 2020.[95] The plans aims at measles and rubella elimination in at least five WHO regions by 2020.[16] The plan focuses on five concepts: to maintain high vaccination coverage with two doses of vaccines, monitor the disease using effective surveillance, develop and maintain outbreak preparedness, build public confidence and demand for immunization, and perform the necessary research and development to improve vaccination.[95]

Gavi has been an active partner in work against measles and has supported the financing of measles vaccine, syringes, and operational costs.[98] Gavi has also pledged $55 million to the Measles & Rubella Initiative until 2017 in Gavi-eligible regions.[98] Countries can apply and receive support from Gavi to provide children with the second dose of the vaccine if they received only the first dose. Gavi will also be providing support for supplementary immunization to six countries that are at high risk of outbreaks: Afghanistan, Chad, Ethiopia, the Democratic Republic of the Congo, Nigeria, and Pakistan.[98]

CASE STUDIES

Much of the important progress made so far in reducing the burden of disease in children has been associated with the spread of immunization programs and supplementing children with vitamin A. The following two cases look at successful examples in each of these areas that were affordable, effective, and had a substantial impact on reducing morbidity and mortality in young children. You can read about each of these cases in greater detail in *Case Studies in Global Health: Millions Saved.*[102]

Eliminating Polio in Latin America and the Caribbean

Background

In 1952, Jonas Salk discovered the inactivated polio vaccine. Mass immunizations between 1955 and 1961 led to a 90 percent drop in infections in the Western Hemisphere.[103] Ten years later, in 1962, Albert Sabin developed an oral polio vaccine that cost less, was easier to administer, and reduced the multiplication of the virus in the intestine.

The new oral polio vaccine became part of a package of six childhood vaccines included in the EPI launched by WHO in 1977. Latin America adopted the EPI in 1977, and the coverage of oral polio vaccine reached 80 percent within just 7 years. Between 1975 and 1981, the incidence of polio was nearly halved and the number of countries reporting polio cases dropped from 19 to 11.[104]

Intervention

Encouraged by the remarkable progress against polio, the PAHO launched a program to eradicate polio from Latin America and the Caribbean. Many international organizations joined together in the program, and regional and country-level Inter-Agency Coordinating Committees were established to oversee the program. Thousands of health workers, managers, and technicians were trained to implement the strategy for the eradication of polio, which included reaching every child with oral polio vaccination, identification of new polio cases, and aggressive control of any outbreaks. If polio was to be eradicated, then the campaign against it would build on the lessons learned from the smallpox eradication campaign.[105]

Impact

The last case of polio in the Latin America and the Caribbean region was reported in Peru in 1991. Polio reemerged briefly in the year 2000 when 20 vaccine-associated cases were reported in Haiti and the Dominican Republic, but no cases have been reported since 2000.

Costs and Benefits

The polio campaign in the Latin American and Caribbean region cost $120 million in its first 5 years—$74 million from national sources and $46 million from international donors—and $10 million annually from donor sources there-after. Taking into account the costs of treating polio and its disabling consequences, the investment paid for itself in only 15 years.[106] The program also generated vast improvements in the region's health infrastructure, and it advanced overall goals for immunization.

Lessons Learned

The success of eliminating polio from Latin America and the Caribbean in only 6 years was a result of exemplary political commitment, interagency and regional coordination, and tremendous social and community mobilization. The re-emergence of polio in 2000 alerted the region to the need for continued vaccination and surveillance. The success in Latin America and the Caribbean prompted the global effort to eradicate polio that was launched in 1988.[107] The importance of building trust with local leaders and working closely with communities is one of many lessons from the polio campaign in the Americas that is being put to good use in the Global Polio Eradication Initiative.

Reducing Child Mortality in Nepal Through Vitamin A

Background

Vitamin A deficiency is a leading determinant of child mortality in low- and middle-income countries. Until the last decade or so, vitamin A deficiency compromised the immune systems of nearly 40 percent of the children in low- and middle-income countries and led to almost 1 million deaths each year. Additionally, it contributed significantly to the burden of disease caused by malaria, diarrheal disease, acute respiratory infections, and measles.[108]

Vitamin A deficiency was especially important in Nepal, with 2–13 percent of preschool-aged children experiencing xerophthalmia, a form of blindness. Economic and geographic barriers helped to explain this high prevalence rate. First, difficult terrain made it hard to grow or access the types of food that supply vitamin A. Second, 38 percent of the Nepali population lived in absolute poverty, many of whom were socially excluded lower-caste families who frequently lacked the means to pay for nutritious foods.

Intervention

Prior to the late 1980s, it was widely held that micronutrient deficiencies were a result of diarrhea and other infant ill-nesses, rather than a cause of them. Yet, as early as the 1970s, Alfred Sommer noticed in conjunction with studies in Indonesia that vitamin A deficiency appeared to be linked with child death. A later randomized controlled trial conducted in Nepal by Keith West and Sommer indicated that periodic vitamin A delivery could reduce mortality in children ages 6 to 60 months by as much as 30 percent.[109]

In light of these research findings and Nepal's excessive infant mortality rate, the Nepalese Ministry of Health initiated a plan of action on vitamin A in 1992. The ministry worked closely with other government agencies and NGOs to develop a pilot program to deliver vitamin A capsules throughout Nepal. A technical assistance group was created to assist the health ministry in running the program. His Majesty, the King of Nepal, also demonstrated long-term commitment to this effort by incorporating Nepal's National Vitamin A Program into the Ten Year National Program of Action.

This program aimed to reduce child morbidity and mortality by prophylactic supplementation of high-dose vitamin A capsules to children 6 to 60 months of age, twice each year; the treatment of xerophthalmia, severe malnutrition, and prolonged diarrhea; and the promotion of behavior change to increase dietary intake of vitamin A and promote exclusive breastfeeding for the first 6 months of a baby's life.

The action plan on vitamin A focused on expanding the intervention in phases as Nepal's administrative capacity for the program was strengthened. The program was expanded to 32 priority districts at a rate of eight districts per year over 4 years. From 1993 to 2001, the program was brought to Nepal's remaining 43 districts. Children and new mothers in districts where the National Vitamin A Program was not yet established received one dose of vitamin A as part of national immunization campaigns. Once the National Vitamin A Program was operating in their district, the children received vitamin A supplementation twice a year.

Nepal's public health system faced severe problems at the time the vitamin A program was developed, from low utilization rates by people who had no confidence in the system to absenteeism by health workers. Consequently, the vitamin A intervention was revised to build upon and improve the existing networks of female community health volunteers (FCHVs) who helped deliver primary health care and family planning services to the villages of Nepal. Before the intervention, there were 24,000 FCHVs throughout 58 districts. However, many were not respected in their communities and had little incentive to remain committed to volunteering. The leader of the program's technical assistance group, Ram Shrestha, changed the way FCHVs were viewed by communities and themselves by focusing on notions of respect, recognition, and opportunity. Shrestha challenged deeply rooted gender biases by giving women responsibilities valued by their families and communities and the opportunity to make a difference.

A few years later, the number of FCHVs had more than doubled to 49,000 strong, and they were able to reach 3.7 million children twice a year with vitamin A capsules. By directly administering the capsules, the FCHVs served as a critical bridge between the public health sector and the community. Families were urged to bring their children to the distribution site, and many government sectors began to integrate messages about the importance of vitamin A into their programs.

Impact

An evaluation of the program indicated that under-5 mortality decreased by almost 48 deaths per 1,000 births, on average. Higher literacy rates among women, improved weight and nutritional status of children, and better vaccination rates were also associated with success. About 134,000 deaths were averted between mid-1995 and mid-2000 as a result of Nepal's Vitamin A Program.[110] Although it took nearly 8 years to achieve nationwide distribution, program coverage never dropped below 90 percent in districts, once they were covered.

Costs and Benefits

Compared to other micronutrient supplement programs, which can cost up to about $5 per child,[111] the vitamin A supplement program in Nepal was a relatively inexpensive approach to ease the burden of a national problem. The cost of the program per child covered was approximately $0.81 to $1.09 for a child receiving one capsule and $0.68 to $1.65 for a child receiving two capsules of vitamin A.[112] Additionally, given the 7,500 lives saved annually, the expanded program in 2000 was estimated to cost $345 per death averted or $11 to $12 per DALY averted.[113]

Lessons Learned

The success of Nepal's vitamin A supplementation program demonstrates how a technical innovation, when paired with an equally innovative operational plan, can result in a major population impact. Rather than trying to restructure the health system to accommodate the vitamin A program, Shrestha adapted the vitamin A program to the preexisting network of FCHVs and then refined it in a way that it could be successful. This approach also reinforced a multisectoral effort by involving the government, NGOs, and communities. Other key factors associated with this successful effort were partnership building, regular monitoring of quality, straightforward and effective public messages, and clarity of objectives and operational strategy. These lessons are all the more important given that this successful effort took place in a very poor country with extremely weak governance and poor administrative capacity.

ADDRESSING KEY CHALLENGES IN CHILD HEALTH

As noted earlier, there has been important progress in the last 25 years in reducing morbidity and mortality of children younger than 5 years of age. In fact, seven countries—Bangladesh, Malawi, Nepal, Liberia, Tanzania, Timor-Leste, and Ethiopia—reduced the rate of under-5 child mortality by more than two-thirds between 1990 and 2012. Eighteen other countries decreased the rate of under-5 child mortality by more than 50 percent but less than 66 percent over the same period.[4]

Despite this progress, the challenges to improving the health of children in low- and middle-income countries remain substantial. First, the progress that has been made has largely been in reducing the mortality rate of children between 1 and 5 years. Much less progress has been made in reducing the mortality rate of neonates.[1] Second, progress in reducing child deaths has remained insufficient in the two regions with the highest rate of such deaths—sub-Saharan Africa and South Asia. The only region with more under-5 children than in 1990 is sub-Saharan Africa, and this is the region where progress in reducing the under-5 mortality rate has been the lowest.[4]

In addition, many interventions that are known to be low-cost and effective at reducing morbidity and mortality in young children are not being implemented where they are needed most. Many mothers-to-be and mothers are not well-nourished and are not receiving appropriate prenatal care. A large number of births in low-income countries take place without the help of a skilled birth attendant who can assist the mother and, for example, resuscitate the baby if needed. Many families still do not use oral rehydration therapy (ORT) when their child gets diarrhea. Too often, the pneumonia that kills young children is not diagnosed or treated appropriately and in a timely way. Insecticide-treated bednets, which are known to reduce the transmission of malaria, are still not as widely used as they should be. There are also major gaps in the early diagnosis and appropriate treatment of malaria in children.

A large proportion of neonatal deaths in the low- and middle-income countries could be avoided with simple technologies that can be effectively implemented in low-income settings.[26] In fact, almost two-thirds of the child deaths that occur every year could be prevented by the effective implementation of measures such as these, that are both low-cost and effective.[27]

What can be done to increase the uptake of these approaches, especially in South Asia and sub-Saharan Africa? What can be done to decrease as quickly as possible the rate of neonatal deaths, again, largely in these two regions? Can measures be taken that will help children from low-income families with little education die as rarely as children from better-off and better-educated families?[114] The following section examines some of what has been learned about cost-effective interventions to prevent child deaths and how these efforts can be scaled up more rapidly. Some of the comments will be organized around the life cycle. Others will be organized by type of intervention.

Critical Child Health Interventions

An Overview of Key Interventions

There are several ways to think coherently about the interventions needed to reduce preventable deaths among children under five years of age. One is to take a life-course approach. In this case, we can think of the timing for different interventions:[115,116]

- Prepregnancy
- During pregnancy
- During labor, birth, and in the first week after birth
- In the postnatal period of infancy
- During the next 4 years

In addition, it is critical to think about what interventions are needed during each of these periods.[115,116]

It is also essential to consider what the critical impediments would be to implementing those interventions:[117]

- Which are the most difficult interventions to implement and take to scale?
- What are the key gaps in implementing them—insufficient financing, the lack of human resources, weaknesses in service delivery?
- What can be learned from the experience of those countries that have done well in reducing newborn and young child deaths?

It is also valuable to understand that the world has adopted the Every Newborn Action Plan that has five strategic objectives:[116]

- Strengthen and invest in care during the crucial period of labor, childbirth, and the first days of life
- Improve the quality of maternal and newborn care
- Reach every woman and every newborn baby and reduce inequities
- Harness the power of parents, families, and communities for change
- Count every newborn baby—improve measurement and accountability, including birth and death registration

In thinking about newborns and children who survive the neonatal period, it will also be essential to consider what causes children to get sick and die, which children get these conditions, the risk factors for these conditions, and what can be done at the least cost to address these problems. To ensure the survival and well-being of children in the postneonatal period, it will be imperative to pay particular attention to pneumonia, diarrhea, sepsis and other infections, malaria, HIV/AIDS, and soil-transmitted helminths.

The Mother-to-Be and the Mother[118]

Delaying marriage and first birth is critical in settings where women give birth as teenagers and tend to have many births with short birth intervals. In these settings, birth spacing and reducing total fertility would encourage healthier mothers and babies.

Prenatal care can help ensure that women are properly nourished and are taking prenatal micronutrient supplements. This care can also help detect problems related to hypertension or diabetes that are important to the health of the mother and the child. Mothers can also be treated during pregnancy for malaria, which can have a deleterious impact on the growth of the fetus and on child birthweight. In certain settings, measures can also be taken to help women with difficulties carrying the baby to term, seeking to avoid stillbirths and prematurity.

A substantial number of pregnant women are infected with HIV/AIDS in parts of Central and Southern Africa in particular. Prenatal care can assist in diagnosing HIV infection in a pregnant women and referring her for antiretroviral therapy for her own health and to avoid maternal-to-child transmission. Measures to prevent HIV infection among women and mothers-to-be are the most cost-effective ways to ensure that HIV is not transmitted from mothers to their children. However, if a mother is HIV-infected, then providing drug therapy to prevent transmission can also be cost-effective.[119]

It is also important to have a skilled attendant at delivery. Proper monitoring of labor and the fetus can improve pregnancy and birth outcomes. In addition, if the labor is complicated, then access to emergency obstetric care can reduce risks to both mother and child. Preventing infection is also important to the mother and child. Ensuring that the mother is vaccinated against tetanus is also critical to the prospects for child survival.[23] Early postnatal visits can also reduce neonatal deaths.[21]

The Newborn

As discussed earlier, most child deaths in the first month of life will be from the complications of prematurity, asphyxia, or sepsis. A number of cost-effective measures can be taken to address these problems. They focus on essential newborn care for all newborns, extra care for small babies, and emergency care. These measures are summarized in **Table 10-4**.[23] Low-income countries do not need to adopt expensive, high-technology solutions to reduce their neonatal death rates in the near future.

In terms of essential care of newborns, skilled attendance at delivery is crucial to save both newborn lives and the lives of mothers. It is imperative for the health of the baby, for example, that the delivery attendant cut the umbilical cord

in a hygienic manner and practice other infection controls. In addition, the baby needs to be kept warm and not bathed for the first 24 hours. The attendant should also be trained and have the equipment needed to resuscitate the baby if necessary, and efforts are under way for that to be done in the simplest possible way in low-income settings. Attendance at delivery is also an appropriate time for a trained practitioner to counsel the family about exclusive breastfeeding and recognizing the danger signs for threats to the baby's health that require immediate attention, such as pneumonia.[23]

Some babies need extra care. If the baby is born prematurely or is of low birthweight, then it is especially important that the baby be kept warm and fed properly and that any complications be managed quickly and appropriately. In high-income countries, of course, premature babies would be kept in an incubator. This option, however, rarely exists for the children of poor families in low-income countries. However, a study done in India[120] showed that the neonatal mortality rate among babies born between 35 and 37 weeks, or moderately premature babies, was reduced by 87 percent by the provision of special sleeping bags to keep the baby warm, coupled with the promotion of breastfeeding and early treatment of infections.

Another effort at keeping otherwise healthy premature and low-birthweight babies warm is kangaroo mother care (KMC). KMC involves skin-to-skin contact between a mother and her newborn, frequent and exclusive or nearly exclusive breastfeeding, and early discharge from the hospital.[121] KMC is a natural and free way to care for infants that has numerous benefits for low-birthweight and premature babies. KMC can meet a baby's needs for warmth, breastfeeding, stimulation, safety, and affection.[122] First, the baby, wearing only a diaper, is kept warm through contact with the mother's skin. Second, the skin-to-skin contact between the mother and baby enhances their psychological bond, which improves health and development. Third, the baby can nurse on demand, which helps low-birthweight babies to gain weight, among other benefits, such as protection from infection.[123] KMC should be continued at least until the baby's health is stable and the baby weighs 1.8 kilograms (4 pounds).[123] KMC can be started at a health facility and continued at home, with proper follow-up and support.[122]

Despite these efforts, some babies will become infected and will require emergency care. The question of providing antibiotics to neonates who have infections is a challenging one in many settings. In many places, only physicians are legally allowed to prescribe antibiotics. Yet, physicians may not be accessible, particularly in rural and impoverished settings that will have the highest rates of neonatal mortality.

TABLE 10-4 Interventions for Essential Newborn Care, Extra Care for Small Babies, and Newborn Emergency Care

Essential Newborn Care
- Early and exclusive breastfeeding
- Warmth provision and avoidance of bathing during the first 24 hours
- Infection control, including cord care and hygiene
- Postpartum vitamin A provided to mothers
- Eye antimicrobial to prevent ophthalmia, inflammation of the eye, or conjunctiva
- Information and counseling for home care and emergency preparedness
- Neonatal resuscitation if not breathing at birth

Extra Care for Small Babies
- Extra attention to warmth, feeding support, infection prevention and skin care, and early identification and management of complications
- Kangaroo Mother Care
- Vitamin K injection
- Monitored safe oxygen use

Emergency Care
- Providing supportive care for severe infections, neonatal encephalopathy (brain disease), severe jaundice or bleeding, seizure management, respiratory distress syndrome (RDS), and neonatal tetanus where appropriate

Data from Lawn. J. E., Zupan, J., Begkoyian, G., & Knippenberg, R. (2006). Newborn survival. In D. T. Jamison, J. G. Breman, A. R. Measham, et al. (Eds.), *Disease control priorities in developing countries* (2nd ed., pp. 531–549). Washington, DC, and New York: The World Bank and Oxford University Press; Additions made from Howson, C. P., Kinneyv, M. V., McDougall, L., Lawn, J. E., and the Born Too Soon Preterm Birth Action Group. (2012). *Born too soon: The global action report on preterm birth*. Geneva: World Health Organization.

There is evidence that community health workers can be trained to safely give antibiotics to neonates who have infections that are life-threatening.[23,120,124]

Managing Pneumonia and Diarrhea in Infants and Young Children

Pneumonia is the leading infectious killer of under-5 children and diarrhea the second-leading infectious cause of their deaths. Such deaths are almost completely unnecessary. In this light, WHO and UNICEF have recently outlined a plan to eliminate preventable deaths from pneumonia and diarrhea by 2025. They refer to this as the Integrated Global Action Plan for Pneumonia and Diarrhoea.[124]

The plan is based on the notion that children are dying needlessly of pneumonia and diarrhea because of the failure to reach them with well-known, low-cost, and highly effective interventions. A key bottleneck to reaching these children has been that such services have too often been carried out piecemeal rather than in a more integrated manner. As noted earlier, for example, only about 30 percent of children with suspected pneumonia receive appropriate antibiotics and only about 35 percent of children with diarrhea are given oral rehydration therapy.[124]

To reduce pneumonia and diarrheal deaths, the action plan suggests that national governments take an integrated approach across all government and partner organizations to deliver a series of interventions that follow the Protect, Prevent, and Treat Framework as outlined in **Figure 10-10**.

The premises of this approach are to protect children through good health practices; to prevent children from becoming ill through immunization, HIV prevention, and the provision of a healthy environment; and to treat them appropriately and at an appropriate level of quality if they do fall ill.[124]

As discussed repeatedly in the text, there are many reasons why exclusive breastfeeding until children are 6 months of age is so important, and one of them is to avoid diarrhea in settings that are not hygienic. As children move to complementary foods, a number of measures can be taken to reduce their risk of diarrheal disease. The first, of course, is to engage in better personal hygiene and more hygienic food preparation. Second, complementary foods that are fortified can help children meet their requirements for micronutrients.[11]

Some immunizations, as discussed earlier, can directly affect pneumonia and diarrhea, such as the pneumococcal vaccine, the Hib vaccine, and the rotavirus vaccine. However,

FIGURE 10-10 The UNICEF/WHO Protect, Prevent, and Treat Framework for Pneumonia and Diarrhea

PROTECT
Children by establishing good health practices from birth
- Exclusive breastfeeding for 6 months
- Adequate complementary feeding
- Vitamin A supplementation

PREVENT
Children becoming ill from pneumonia and diarrhea
- Vaccines: pertussis, measles, Hib, PCV and rotavirus
- Handwashing with soap
- Safe drinking-water and sanitation
- Reduce household air pollution
- HIV prevention
- Cotrimoxazole prophylaxis for HIV-infected and exposed children

Reduce pneumonia and diarrhoea morbidity and mortality

TREAT
Children who are ill from pneumonia and diarrhea with appropriate treatment
- Improved care seeking and referral
- Case management at the health facility and community level
- Supplies: Low-osmolarity ORS, zinc, antibiotics and oxygen
- Continued feeding (including breastfeeding)

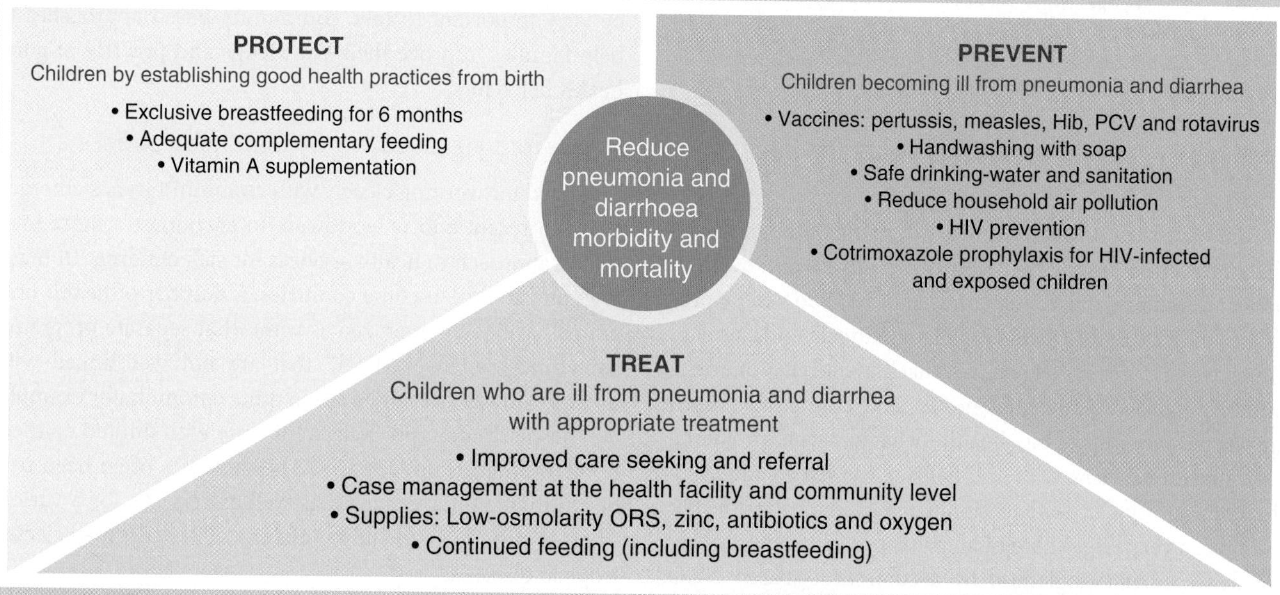

Modified from UNICEF/World Health Organization. Ending Preventable Child Deaths from Pneumonia and Diarrhoea by 2025 Geneva: World Health Organization/The United Nations Children's Fund (UNICEF); 2013, page 6.

other vaccines protect children indirectly. Ensuring that children are immunized against measles, for example, can help to reduce deaths from diarrhea. It has been estimated, in fact, that measles immunization could eliminate 6–26 percent of diarrheal deaths of children younger than 5 years.[11] Improving water supply and sanitation can be very important to reducing diarrhea in children. Unfortunately, the infrastructure to do so can be very expensive, and health benefits are gained mainly when communities adopt safer water and sanitation systems, rather than just having them adopted by individual families.[23]

When young children do get the types of diarrhea that do not require antibiotics, two very cost-effective measures can be taken to manage the illness. First is the household use of ORT. Second is supplementation with zinc, because such supplements have been shown to reduce the duration and severity of diarrhea.

Immunization

As noted throughout this chapter, immunization is a best buy for neonatal, infant, and young child health. It is also central to efforts to reduce under-5 child deaths and help ensure that children are healthy and can thrive.

As also noted earlier, there has been enormous progress in expanding the coverage of the six basic antigens as well as the newer vaccines. However, a substantial unfinished agenda of unimmunized children remains. These are children who often live in pockets in some of the largest countries in the world. Reaching these children with vaccines as soon as possible and ensuring that vaccine programs can be sustained in all regards are among the key global health challenges in the near future.

Community-Based Approaches to Improving Child Health

As you have seen throughout the text, many of the measures that are needed to reduce the burden of illness and death in neonates, infants, and young children have to do with appropriate knowledge and behavior of individuals and families. You have also read that studies that have been done in a number of places show that home- and community-based approaches to improving health behaviors and providing basic health services with the help of trained members of the community can lead to significant gains in health. For example, a very large share of all primary healthcare services are delivered in Bangladesh by a community-based NGO called BRAC.

The role of the family and community is key to newborn health. Community awareness and the engagement of women's groups have been highly effective in improving the health and survival of newborns. In one project in rural Bolivia, the involvement of local women's groups in raising awareness of maternal, fetal, and neonatal issues led to increased use of prenatal and postnatal health services, more traditional birth assistants at childbirth, and an overall 62 percent reduction of perinatal mortality. In another study in rural Nepal, working with local women's groups was key to motivating increased hygiene and health-seeking behavior, which contributed to a 30 percent reduction in neonatal mortality.[23]

In fact, a family- and community-based approach to promoting hygiene, including handwashing and umbilical cord care, keeping the newborn warm, and exclusively breastfeeding, are all important home measures that could lead to an estimated 10–40 percent reduction in neonatal mortality. Home-based supplementary feeding, using a dropper or a cup, is another important measure to ensure the survival of low-birthweight babies, who account for 60–80 percent of neonatal deaths.[23]

Table 10-5 is a summary of measures that families can take, even in low-income communities, to protect the health of their young children. You can see in the table the extent to which families, if they had better knowledge of good health practices and community support to engage in them, could promote important reductions in child morbidity and mortality. Low-income people in low- and middle-income countries are not going to have any quick increase in formal education, income, or social and political voice. Thus, it will be very important to take community-based approaches to help families improve their knowledge and practice of good health behaviors.

Integrated Management of Childhood Illness

The need for working closely with communities has emerged again in recent efforts worldwide to encourage a more integrated approach to health services for sick children. In many low- and middle-income countries, a number of health programs have been organized as somewhat separate programs, sometimes called "vertical," that are not well-linked with other health services. It has been quite common, for example, for the vaccination program to operate with limited connections to other health services. The same has often been true of family planning services, as well as services for a variety of other programs, including malaria, TB, and the neglected tropical diseases.[125]

Given the multiple factors that lead to child illness and death, however, it is widely agreed that no single child intervention is adequate to ensure a child's health. It is also agreed

TABLE 10-5 12 Key Family Health Practices

1. **Exclusive breastfeeding**: Breastfeed infants exclusively for up to 6 months. (Mothers that are HIV-positive require counseling about possible alternatives to breastfeeding.)
2. **Complementary feeding**: Starting at about 6 months of age, feed children freshly prepared energy- and nutrient-rich complementary foods, while continuing to breastfeed up to 2 years or longer.
3. **Micronutrients**: Ensure that children receive adequate amounts of micronutrients (vitamin A, iron, and zinc, in particular), either in their diet or through supplementation.
4. **Hygiene**: Safely dispose of feces, including children's feces, and wash hands after defecation before preparing meals and before feeding children.
5. **Immunization**: Take children as scheduled to complete a full course of immunizations (BCG, DPT, OPV, and measles) before their first birthday.
6. **Malaria and use of bednets**: Protect children in malaria-endemic areas by ensuring that they sleep under insecticide-treated bednets.
7. **Psychosocial development**: Promote mental and social development by responding to a child's needs for care and through talking, playing, and providing a stimulating environment.
8. **Home care for illness**: Continue to feed and offer more fluids, including breast milk, to children when they are sick. Home care for sick children includes several practices that are enumerated individually in this list of 12 key family practices, such as continuing feeding and offering more fluids, oral rehydration therapy and treatment of fever, prompt care-seeking, and compliance with a health provider's advice.
9. **Home treatment for infections**: Give sick children appropriate home treatment for infections.
10. **Care-seeking**: Recognize when sick children need treatment outside the home and seek care from appropriate providers.
11. **Compliance with advice**: Follow the health worker's advice about treatment, follow-up, and referral.
12. **Antenatal care**: Ensure that every pregnant woman has adequate antenatal care. (This includes having at least four antenatal visits with an appropriate healthcare provider and receiving the recommended doses of the tetanus toxoid vaccination. The mother also needs support from her family and community in seeking care at the time of delivery and during the postpartum and lactation period.)

Data from World Health Organization. (2004). *Family and community practices that promote child survival, growth, and development: A review of the evidence.* Geneva: World Health Organization.

that, given the interrelated factors that affect a child's health and survival, an integrated approach to managing illness is important for newborns, infants, and older children.

Integrated Management of Childhood Illness, called IMCI, is an approach that recognizes the importance of looking at the whole child and not treating one symptom or providing one intervention without looking at other possible needs. It also recognizes that care is needed at the level of overall health system, local health center, and family and community. The IMCI approach focuses on:[126]

- Improving overall health systems
- Improving the case management skills of healthcare workers
- Improving family and community health practices

IMCI is now being used in 75 countries.

A number of evaluations of IMCI efforts have taken place, revealing that:

- IMCI can improve nutritional status and reduce mortality
- IMCI is cost-effective and cost-saving, compared to alternative approaches
- IMCI leads to better worker performance[126]

However, the evaluations also revealed that it will be important to improve family and community behavior, that more support is needed for strengthening health systems to carry out needed investments, and that IMCI must be taken to scale if it is to have a significant impact on reducing child deaths.[126]

There is widespread agreement about what interventions are needed to improve child health. The key challenge to implementing such interventions, however, is not what to do, but how to do it and how to engage communities in ensuring that needed interventions are put in place effectively. There are countries, such as Sri Lanka, Cuba, and China, and states within countries, such as Kerala, in which there is widespread knowledge of appropriate health and hygiene behaviors, appropriate nutrition practices, the home management of illness, and when to seek care from health services. In Bangladesh, as you read, there has been widespread adoption of ORT, despite the low educational and income status of a large share of the population. Families and communities are the key to rapid uptake of critical measures to improve child health, and a central issue in global health today is to learn from experience about how large-scale change in health and child-caring behaviors can be promoted as quickly, effectively, and efficiently as possible.

MAIN MESSAGES

Approximately 6.3 million children around the world died in 2013 before they reached their fifth birthday. About 2.8 million, or 44 percent, died in their first 4 weeks of life. Almost 50 percent of the under-5 deaths occurred in only five countries—India, Nigeria, the Democratic Republic of Congo, Pakistan, and China.

As we learned in the vignettes that opened the chapter, the chances of survival for a newborn, an infant, and a young child are vastly different across different settings. The discrepancies within an individual country can be as wide as differences between countries. High-income countries have, on average, about 7 deaths per 1,000 live births for children younger than 5 years. However, in the poorest, least well-managed, and most conflict-ridden countries, the under-5 child mortality rate can be as high as 167 deaths per 1,000 live births, as in Angola, or 161, as in Sierra Leone.[2]

The largest cause of death of under-5 children globally is prematurity, which killed 17 percent of all of those children who died before reaching age 5 in 2013. Other conditions related to birth, such as birth asphyxia and birth trauma, were responsible for 12 percent of the deaths and congenital anomalies for 7 percent.

Pneumonia is the most important infectious killer of children who are younger than 5 years of age and is responsible for about 15 percent of their deaths. The second most important infectious cause of illness and death among children is diarrheal disease, followed by sepsis and other infections, malaria, HIV/AIDS, and measles. In Africa, malaria is the most significant killer of young children.

The social determinants of health have a major impact on the health of young children. Poverty is a significant underlying factor of morbidity and mortality among children, as is the lack of education for mothers.

Nutritional status is also a powerful determinant of whether a child lives and thrives. About 35 percent of all deaths of children under 5 years of age are related to children being undernourished. This undernourishment may stem from poor maternal nutrition, suboptimal breastfeeding, infection, or insufficient energy, protein, and key micronutrients in the child's diet.

Inadequate water and sanitation and poor hygiene practices are major risk factors for childhood illness and death. Indoor air pollution is also a major risk factor.

There are well-known, proven, and cost-effective interventions for reducing the deaths of neonates, infants, and young children. Their deaths do not stem from a failure of knowing what to do. Rather, they stem from a failure to reach all children with these interventions.

The key interventions can be oriented in a life-course approach—those important before pregnancy; during pregnancy, birth, and shortly after birth; those needed in the postneonatal period; and those most important for the young child. Among the most important interventions will be:

- Ensuring a healthy and well-nourished mother
- Prenatal care and micronutrient supplementation for the mother-to-be
- Prevention of mother-to-child transmission of HIV
- Attendance at delivery by a skilled birth attendant and referral for emergency obstetric care if needed
- Appropriate care of the newborn and referral if needed for illness
- Early and exclusive breastfeeding for 6 months
- Hygienic introduction of diverse complementary foods
- Childhood immunization
- Bednets for malaria and regular drug administration for worms
- Oral rehydration for diarrhea and early diagnosis and treatment for pneumonia

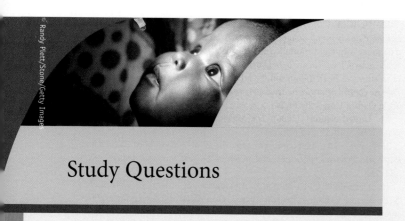

Study Questions

1. What are the most important causes of child death globally?

2. How do causes of death differ for neonates, infants, and children younger than 5 years?

3. Why are there different levels of child illness and death in different parts of the same country?

4. What is the link between nutrition and child health?

5. How does the health of young children in low-income countries vary with the income of the family?

6. How does the health of young children in low-income countries vary with the mother's level of education?

7. What is the importance to neonatal health of having a skilled birth attendant at delivery?

8. What are some of the most cost-effective interventions for saving the lives of newborns?

9. What are some of the most cost-effective interventions for saving the lives of children younger than 5 years?

10. What measures can families take, even in the absence of additional income or health services, to keep their children healthy?

REFERENCES

1. Liu, L., Oza, S., Perin, J., et al. (2015, January 30). Global, regional, and national causes of child mortality in 2000-2013, with projections to inform post-2015 priorities, an updated systematic analysis. *Lancet, 385*, 430–440.

2. World Bank. *Mortality rate, under 5 (per 1,000 live births).* Retrieved February 28, 2015, from http://data.worldbank.org/indicator/SH.DYN .MORT/countries?display=map.

3. World Health Organization. (2014). *Children: Reducing mortality (Fact Sheet No. 178).* Retrieved May 30, 2015, from http://www.who.int /mediacentre/factsheets/fs178/en/.

4. UNICEF. (2013). *Committing to child survival: A promise renewed— Progress report 2013.* New York: UNICEF.

5. World Health Organization. *Stillbirths.* Retrieved March 2, 2015, from http://www.who.int/maternal_child_adolescent/epidemiology/stillbirth/en/.

6. Lancet. (2011, April 14). *Stillbirths.* Retrieved March 2, 2015, from http://www.thelancet.com/series/stillbirth.

7. UNICEF. (2010). *Progress for children: Achieving the MDGs with equity.* New York: UNICEF.

8. Simoes, E. A. F., Cherian, T., Chow, J., Shahid-Salles, S., Laxmina-rayan, R., & John, T. J. (2006). Acute respiratory infections in children. In D. T. Jamison, J. G. Breman, A. R. Measham, et al. (Eds.), *Disease control priorities in developing countries* (2nd ed., pp. 483–497). New York: Oxford University Press.

9. World Health Organization. (2014). *Pneumonia* (Fact Sheet No. 331). Retrieved March 1, 2015, from http://www.who.int/mediacentre/factsheets /fs331/en/.

10. Keusch, G. F., Fontaine, O., Bhargava, A., et al. (2006). Diarrheal diseases. In D. T. Jamison, J. G. Breman, A. R. Measham, et al. (Eds.), *Disease control priorities in developing countries* (2nd ed., pp. 371–387). New York: Oxford University Press.

11. World Health Organization. (2014). *Malaria* (Fact Sheet No. 94). Retrieved March 1, 2015, from http://www.who.int/mediacentre/factsheets /fs094/en/.

12. Institute of Health Metrics and Evaluation. (2015). *GBD 2010 heat map.* Retrieved March 1, 2015, from http://vizhub.healthdata.org/irank /heat.php.

13. Breman, J. G., Mills, A., Snow, R. W., et al. (2006). Conquering malaria. In D. T. Jamison, J. G. Breman, A. R. Measham, et al. (Eds.), *Disease control priorities in developing countries* (2nd ed., pp. 413–431). New York: Oxford University Press.

14. World Health Organization. *HIV/AIDS mother-to-child transmission of HIV.* Retrieved March 1, 2015, from http://www.who.int/hiv/topics/mtct /en/.

15. UNAIDS. (2014). *The gap report.* Geneva: UNAIDS.

16. World Health Organization. (2015). *Measles* (Fact Sheet No. 286). Retrieved March 1, 2015, from http://www.who.int/mediacentre/factsheets /fs286/en/.

17. Brenzel, L., Wolfson, L. J., Fox-Rushby, J., Miller, M., & Halsey, N. A. (2006). Vaccine-preventable diseases. In D. T. Jamison, J. G. Breman, A. R. Measham, et al. (Eds.), *Disease control priorities in developing countries* (2nd ed., pp. 389–411). New York: Oxford University Press.

18. World Health Organization. *Soil-transmitted helminthiases.* Retrieved March 1, 2015, from http://www.who.int/gho/neglected_diseases /soil_transmitted_helminthiases/en/.

19. World Health Organization. *Intestinal worms.* Retrieved March 1, 2015, from http://www.who.int/intestinal_worms/more/en/.

20. Hotez, P. J., Bundy, D. A. P., Beegle, K., et al. (2006). Helminth infections: Soil-transmitted helminth infections and schistosomiasis. In D. T. Jamison, J. G. Breman, A. R. Measham, et al. (Eds.), *Disease control priorities in developing countries* (2nd ed., pp. 467–482). New York: Oxford University Press.

21. Lawn, J. E., Cousens, S., & Zupan, J. (2005). 4 million neonatal deaths: When? Where? Why? *Lancet, 365*(9462), 891–900.

22. UNICEF. (2015). *Neonatal mortality rates are declining in all regions but more slowly in sub-Saharan Africa.* Retrieved March 1, 2015, from http:// data.unicef.org/child-mortality/neonatal.

23. Lawn, J. E., Zupan, J., Begkoyian, G., & Knippenberg, R. (2006). Newborn survival. In D. T. Jamison, J. G. Breman, A. R. Measham, et al. (Eds.), *Disease control priorities in developing countries* (2nd ed., pp. 531–549). New York: Oxford University Press.

24. United Nations. (2006). *The Millennium Development Goals report 2006.* New York: United Nations.

25. Lawn, J. E., Blencowe, H., Oza, S., et al. (2014, May 20). Every newborn: Progress, priorities, and potential beyond survival. *Lancet, 384,* 189–205.

26. Darmstadt, G. L., Bhutta, Z. A., Cousens, S., Adam, T., Walker, N., & de Bernis, L. (2005). Evidence-based, cost-effective interventions: How many newborn babies can we save? *Lancet, 365*(9463), 977–988.

27. Black, R. E., Morris, S. S., & Bryce, J. (2003). Where and why are 10 million children dying every year? *Lancet, 361*(9376), 2226–2234.

28. UNICEF. (2005). *State of the world's children 2005.* New York: UNICEF.

29. United Nations. We can end poverty: Millennium Development Goals and beyond 2015. Retrieved December 15, 2014, from http://www .un.org/millenniumgoals/childhealth.shtml.

30. UNICEF. Immunization. Retrieved December 15, 2014, from http:// www.unicef.org/immunization/.

31. World Health Organization. (2014). Immunization coverage reaches 84%, still short of 90% goal. Retrieved December 15, 2014, from http://www .who.int/immunization/newsroom/press/immunization_coverage_july2014 /en/.

32. Bloom, D. E. (2011). The value of vaccination. In N. Curtis, A. Finn, & A. J. Pollard (Eds.), *Hot topics in infection and immunity in children: Vol. VII* (pp. 1–8). New York: Springer.

33. World Health Organization. (2014). *Global immunization data.* Geneva: WHO. Retrieved December 15, 2014, from http://www.who.int /immunization/monitoring_surveillance/global_immunization_data.pdf.

34. World Health Organization. (2013). *Global vaccine action plan 2011– 2020.* Geneva: WHO. Retrieved December 15, 2014, from http://www.who .int/immunization/global_vaccine_action_plan/GVAP_doc_2011_2020/en/.

35. Bärnighausen, T., et al. (2014). Reassessing the value of vaccines. *The Lancet Global Health, 2*(5), e251–e252. Retrieved December 15, 2014, from http://www.thelancet.com/journals/langlo/article /PIIS2214-109X%2813%2970170-0/fulltext?rss=yes.

36. Deogaonkar, R. (2012). Systematic review of studies evaluating the broader economic impact of vaccination in low and middle income countries. *BMC Public Health, 12*(1), 878.

37. Nshimirimana, D., et al. (2013). Routine immunization services in Africa: Back to basics. *Journal of Vaccines and Immunization, 1*(1), 6–12.

38. Chan, M. (2014). Beyond expectations: 40 years of EPI. *The Lancet, 383*(9930), 1697–1698. Retrieved December 15, 2014, from http://www .thelancet.com/pdfs/journals/lancet/PIIS0140673614607510.pdf.

39. World Health Organization. (2005). *Immunization coverage cluster survey. Reference manual.* Geneva: WHO. Retrieved December 15, 2014, from http://apps.who.int/iris/handle/10665/69087.

40. Demographic and Health Survey Program. (2014). *Child health.* Retrieved December 16, 2014, from http://dhsprogram.com/topics/Child -Health.cfm.

41. Wang, S., Hyde, T. B., Mounier-Jack, S., Brenzeld, L., Favine, M., Gordon, W. G., et al. (2013). New vaccine introductions: Assessing the impact and the opportunities for immunization and health systems strengthening. *Vaccine, 31,* 122–128. Retrieved December 16, 2014, from http://www .sciencedirect.com/science/article/pii/S0264410X12015927.

42. World Health Organization. (2001). *Expanded program on immunization (EPI) in the Africa region: Strategic plan of action 2001–2005.* Harare: WHO.

43. Pan American Health Organization. (2014). *About PAHO Revolving Fund: Why we need it.* Retrieved December 15, 2014, from http://www.paho.org/hq/index.php?option=com_content&view=article&id=9562&Itemid=40717&lang=en&limitstart=1.

44. Gavi, The Vaccine Alliance. *Country eligibility policy—Finance & programmatic policies.* Retrieved December 15, 2014, from http://www.gavi.org/about/governance/programme-policies/country-eligibility/.

45. Gavi, The Vaccine Alliance. *Gavi facts and figures.* Retrieved December 15, 2014, from http://www.gavi.org/about/mission/facts-and-figures/.

46. Gavi, The Vaccine Alliance. *Global immunization vision and strategy.* Retrieved December 15, 2014, from http://www.gavi.org/about/ghd/givs/.

47. Gavi, The Vaccine Alliance. (n.d.). *Investing together for a healthy future: A world free from vaccine-preventable diseases. The 2016 to 2020 investment opportunity.* Geneva: Gavi. Retrieved December 16, 2014, from http://www.gavi.org/Library/Publications/Publications-Gavi/The-2016-2020-GAVI-Alliance-Investment-Opportunity/.

48. Ryman, T., et al. (2010). Reaching Every District (RED) approach to strengthen routine immunization services: Evaluation in the African region, 2005. *Journal of Public Health, 32*(1), 18–25.

49. Arevshatian, L. (2007). An evaluation of infant immunization in Africa: Is a transformation in progress? *Bulletin of the World Health Organization, 85*(6), 449–457.

50. Cherian, T., & Okwo-Bele, J.-M. (2014). The decade of vaccines global vaccine action plan: Shaping immunization programmes in the current decade. *Expert Review of Vaccines, 13*(5), 573–575. Retrieved December 15, 2014, from http://informahealthcare.com/doi/abs/10.1586/14760584.2014.897618.

51. World Health Organization. (2013). *Global vaccine action plan 2011–2020.* Retrieved December 15, 2014, from http://www.who.int/immunization/global_vaccine_action_plan/en/.

52. World Health Organization. (2014). *Summary of WHO position papers—Recommendations for routine immunization.* Retrieved December 15, 2014, from http://www.who.int/immunization/policy/Immunization_routine_table1.pdf.

53. World Health Organization. (2014). *Children: Reducing mortality.* Retrieved December 15, 2014, from http://www.who.int/mediacentre/factsheets/fs178/en/.

54. Gavi, The Vaccine Alliance. (2012, October 1). *Department of Immunisation, Vaccines and Biologicals' estimates and projections, as of October 2012.* Retrieved December 15, 2014, from http://www.google.com/url?sa=t&rct=j&q=&esrc=s&source=web&cd=2&ved=0CCQQFjAB&url=http%3A%2F%2Fwww.gavi.org%2Flibrary%2Fpublications%2Fgavi-fact-sheets%2Fgavi-facts-and-figures%2F&ei=LnUMVeX6N_b9sATUzYKQCQ&usg=AFQjCNHfej4Prx_QKDmOEa7n8D9VQ52x-Q&sig2=iTxUdYd-rNXINv4yQ5aMvQ&bvm=bv.88528373,d.cWc&cad=rja.

55. World Health Organization. (2014, May 23). *Weekly Epidemiological Record, 89*(21), 221–236. Retrieved December 15, 2014, from http://www.who.int/wer/2014/wer8921/en/.

56. UNICEF. *Vaccine price data.* Retrieved December 15, 2014, from http://www.unicef.org/supply/index_57476.html.

57. World Health Organization. (2014). *Poliomyelitis* (Fact Sheet No. 114). Retrieved December 15, 2014, from http://www.who.int/mediacentre/factsheets/fs114/en/.

58. World Health Organization. What is vaccine derived polio? Retrieved from April 13, 2015, from http://www.who.int/features/qa/64/en/.

59. World Health Organization. (2014). *Tuberculosis* (Fact Sheet No. 104). Retrieved December 15, 2014, from http://www.who.int/mediacentre/factsheets/fs104/en/.

60. World Health Organization. *BCG vaccine.* Retrieved December 15, 2014, from http://www.who.int/biologicals/areas/vaccines/bcg/en/.

61. Gavi, The Vaccine Alliance. (2014). *GAVI Alliance progress report 2013.* Retrieved December 15, 2014, from http://gaviprogressreport.org/2013/.

62. World Health Organization. *Haemophilus influenzae type B (Hib).* Retrieved December 15, 2014, from http://www.who.int/topics/haemophilus_influenzae/en/.

63. Gavi, The Vaccine Alliance. *Pentavalent vaccine support.* Retrieved December 15, 2014, from http://www.gavi.org/support/nvs/pentavalent/.

64. Gandhi, G., et al. (2013). Projections of costs, financing, and additional resource requirements for low- and lower middle-income country immunization programs over the decade, 2011–2020. *Vaccine, 31,* B137–B148.

65. Gavi, The Vaccine Alliance. (2013). *Pneumococcal disease.* Retrieved December 15, 2014, from http://www.gavi.org/library/publications/gavi-fact-sheets/factsheet–pneumococcal-disease/.

66. Chopra, M., et al. (2013). Ending of preventable deaths from pneumonia and diarrhoea: An achievable goal. *The Lancet, 381*(9876), 1499–1506.

67. Gavi, The Vaccine Alliance. (2013). *Rotavirus disease.* Retrieved December 15, 2014, from http://www.gavi.org/library/publications/gavi-fact-sheets/factsheet–rotavirus-disease/.

68. World Health Organization. (2013, February 1). *Weekly Epidemiological Record, 88*(5), 49–64. Retrieved December 15, 2014, from http://www.who.int/wer/2013/wer8805/en/.

69. World Health Organization. (2014). *Yellow fever* (Factsheet No. 100). Retrieved December 15, 2014, from http://www.who.int/mediacentre/factsheets/fs100/en/.

70. World Health Organization. (2014). *Human papillomavirus (HPV) and cervical cancer* (Factsheet No. 380). Retrieved December 15, 2014, from http://www.who.int/mediacentre/factsheets/fs380/en/.

71. World Health Organization. (2010, December 6). *Revolutionary new meningitis vaccine set to wipe out deadly epidemics in Africa.* Retrieved December 15, 2014, from http://www.who.int/mediacentre/news/releases/2010/meningitis_20101206/en/.

72. Program for Appropriate Technology in Health. *Ending the epidemics.* Retrieved December 15, 2014, from http://www.path.org/menafrivac/overview.php.

73. Desai, S. N., & Kamat, D. (2014). Closing the global immunization gap: Delivery of lifesaving vaccines through innovation and technology. *Pediatrics in Review, 35*(7), e32–e40.

74. World Health Organization. *Immunizations, vaccines, and biologicals: Typhoid.* Retrieved December 15, 2014, from http://www.who.int/immunization/topics/typhoid/en/.

75. Thiem, V. D., et al. (2011). The Vi conjugate typhoid vaccine is safe, elicits protective levels of IgG anti-Vi, and is compatible with routine infant vaccines. *Clinical and Vaccine Immunology, 18*(5), 730–735.

76. Szu, S. C. (2013). Development of Vi conjugate—A new generation of typhoid vaccine. *Expert Review of Vaccines, 12*(11), 1273–1286.

77. Sharma, E. K. (2013, August 26). Bharat Biotech launches typhoid conjugate vaccine. *Business Today.* Retrieved December 15, 2014, from http://businesstoday.intoday.in/story/bharat-biotech-launches-typhoid-conjugate-vaccine/1/198124.html.

78. Gavi, The Vaccine Alliance. (2014, July 24). *Malaria vaccine takes first steps towards market.* Retrieved December 15, 2014, from http://www.gavi.org/Library/News/Statements/2014/Malaria-vaccine-takes-first-steps-towards-market/.

79. World Health Organization. (2014). *Immunization coverage reaches 84%, still short of 90% goal.* Retrieved December 15, 2014, from http://www.who.int/immunization/newsroom/press/immunization_coverage_july2014/en/.

80. UNICEF. *Immunization.* Retrieved December 15, 2014, from http://www.unicef.org/immunization/.

81. Tudor Hart, J. (1971). The inverse care law. *The Lancet, 297*(7696), 405–412.

82. World Health Organization. (2013, January 17). *WHO: Measles deaths decline, but elimination progress stalls in some regions.* Retrieved December 15, 2014, from http://www.who.int/mediacentre/news/notes/2013/measles_20130117/en/.

83. Schreiber, B. (2014, April). *Proposed visions and strategies for the next decade.* Presentation at the meeting of the Strategic Advisory Group of Experts (SAGE) on Immunization, Geneva, Switzerland. Retrieved January 15, 2015, from http://www.who.int/immunization/sage/meetings/2014/april/5_SAGE_April_iSC_Schreiber_Vision.pdf.

84. Gilchrist, S., et al. (2013). Lessons learned in shaping vaccine markets in low-income countries: A review of the vaccine market segment supported by the GAVI Alliance. *Health Policy and Planning, 28*(8), 838–846.

85. Lydon, P., et al. Health system cost of delivering routine vaccination in low-and lower-middle income countries: What is needed over the next decade? *Bulletin of the World Health Organization, 92*(5), 382–384.

86. Global Polio Eradication Initiative. (2004). *Strategic plan 2004–2008.* Retrieved from http://www.polioeradication.org/content/publications/2004stratplan.pdf.

87. UNICEF. *A history of global polio eradication.* Retrieved from http://www.unicef.org/immunization/files/the_history_of_polio.pdf.

88. Global Polio Eradication Initiative. (2015). *Data and monitoring.* Retrieved March 3, 2015, from http://polioeradication.org/Dataandmonitoring.aspx.

89. Kaiser Family Foundation. (2014). *The U.S. government and global polio efforts.* Retrieved from http://kff.org/global-health-policy/fact-sheet/the-u-s-government-and-global-polio-efforts/.

90. Rotary International. *Rotary's involvement in polio eradication.* Retrieved from http://www.rotaryfirst100.org/presidents/1992dochterman/polioplus.htm#.VAuOG88g_EU.

91. Modlin, J. F. (2010). The bumpy road to polio eradication. *New England Journal of Medicine, 362*(25), 2346–2349.

92. Emory University. (2013). Scientific declaration on polio eradication. Retrieved from http://vaccines.emory.edu/poliodeclaration/text.pdf.

93. John, T. J., & Vashishtha, V. M. (2013). Eradicating poliomyelitis: India's journey from hyperendemic to polio-free status. *The Indian Journal of Medical Research, 137*(5), 881–894.

94. Wassilak, S., & Orenstein, W. (2010). Challenges faced by the Global Polio Eradication Initiative. *Expert Review of Vaccines, 9*(5), 447–449.

95. 2013 Fact Sheet. (n.d.). *Measles and Rubella Initiative.* Retrieved August 10, 2014, from http://www.measlesrubellainitiative.org/wp-content/uploads/2013/07/MRI-Fact-Sheet-FINAL-JULY9.pdf

96. GBD Heatmap. (n.d.). *Institute for Health Metrics and Evaluation (IHME).* Retrieved August 13, 2014, from http://vizhub.healthdata.org/irank/heat.php

97. World Health Organization. (n.d.). Table 1: Summary of WHO Positioin Papers - Recommendations for Routine Immunization. Retrieved March 3, 2015, from http://www.who.int/immunization/policy/Immunization_routine_table1.pdf?ua=1

98. Gavi Alliance. (n.d.). *Measles vaccine.* Retrieved August 12, 2014, from http://www.gavialliance.org/support/nvs/measles/

99. Annual Report. (n.d.). *Measles & Rubella Initative.* Retrieved August 11, 2014, from http://www.measlesrubellainitiative.org/wp-content/uploads/2013/07/MRI-2012-Annual-Report.pdf

100. Pan American Health Organization (PAHO). (n.d.). *Verification of measles and rubella elimination in the Americas.* Retrieved August 12, 2014, from http://www.paho.org/hq/index.php?option=com_docman&task=doc_view&gid=19677&Itemid=

101. Six Challenges for Measles Eradication. (n.d.). *The Epidemiology Monitor.* Retrieved August 8, 2014, from http://epimonitor.net/Six_Challenges_for_Measles_Eradication.htm

102. Levine, R., & What Works Working Group. (2007). *Case studies in global health: Millions saved.* Sudbury, MA: Jones and Bartlett.

103. Henderson D. A., de Quadros, C. A., Andrus, J., Olive, J.-M., & Guerra de Macedo, C. (1992). Polio eradication from the western hemisphere. *Annual Review of Public Health, 13,* 239–252.

104. de Quadros, C. A. (2000). Polio. In J. Lederberg (Ed.), *Encyclopedia of microbiology* (2nd ed., Vol. 3, 762–772). San Diego, CA: Academic Press.

105. Gawande, A. (2004, January 12). The mop-up: Eradicating polio from the planet. *The New Yorker,* pp. 34–40.

106. Musgrove, P. (1988). Is the eradication of polio in the western hemisphere economically justified? *Bulletin of the Pan American Sanitary Bureau, 22*(1), 67.

107. Global Polio Eradication Initiative. (2003). *Progress 2003.* Retrieved May 30, 2015, from http://www.who.int/biologicals/publications/meetings/areas/vaccines/polio/2003_global_polio_%20eradication_initiative-progress.pdf?ua=1.

108. World Health Organization. (2002). *The world health report 2002: Reducing risks, promoting healthy life.* Geneva: World Health Organization.

109. West, K. P., Jr., Pokhrel, R. P., Katz, J., et al. (1991). Efficacy of vitamin A in reducing preschool child mortality in Nepal. *Lancet, 338*(8759), 67–71.

110. Rutstein, S. O., & Govindasamy, P. (2002). *The mortality effects of Nepal's vitamin A distribution program.* Calverton, MD: ORC Macro.

111. Caulfield, L. E., Richard, S. A., Rivera, J. A., Musgrove, P., & Black, R. E. (2006). Stunting, wasting, and micronutrient disorders. In D. T. Jamison, J. G. Breman, A. R. Measham, et al. (Eds.), *Disease control priorities in developing countries* (2nd ed., pp. 551–568). New York: Oxford University Press.

112. Fiedler, J. L. (1997). *The Nepal national vitamin A program: A program review and cost analysis.* Bethesda, MD: Partnerships for Health Reform Project, Abt Associates.

113. Fiedler, J. L. (2000). The Nepal national vitamin A program: Prototype to emulate or donor enclave? *Health Policy and Planning, 15*(2), 145–156.

114. Victora, C. G., Wagstaff, A., Schellenberg, J. A., Gwatkin, D., Claeson, M., & Habicht, J. P. (2003). Applying an equity lens to child health and mortality: More of the same is not enough. *Lancet, 362*(9379), 233–241.

115. Bhutta, Z. A., Das, J. K., Bahl, R., et al. for the Lancet Newborn Interventions Review Group and the Lancet Every Newborn Study Group. (2014, July 26). Can available interventions end preventable deaths in mother's newborn babies, and stillbirths, and at what cost? *Lancet, 384,* 347–370.

116. Mason, E., McDougall, L., Lawn, J. E., et al. for the Lancet Every Newborn Study Group on Behalf of the Every Newborn Steering Committee. (2014, August 2). From evidence to action to deliver a healthy start for the next generation. *Lancet, 384,* 455–467.

117. Dickson, K. E., Simen-Kapeu, A., Kinney, M. V., et al. for the Lancet Every Newborn Study Group. (2014, August 2). Every newborn: Health-systems bottlenecks and strategies to accelerate scale-up in countries. *Lancet, 384,* 438–454.

118. Unless otherwise noted, this section is based primarily on the interventions noted in Bhutta et al., Mason et al., and Dickson et al. (references 108, 109, and 110).

119. Bertozzi, S., Padian, N. S., Wegbreit, J., et al. (2006). HIV/AIDS prevention and treatment. In D. T. Jamison, J. G. Breman, A. R. Measham, et al. (Eds.), *Disease control priorities in developing countries* (2nd ed., pp. 331–369). New York: Oxford University Press.

120. Bang, A. T., Bang, R. A., Baitule, S. B., Reddy, M. H., & Deshmukh, M. D. (1999). Effect of home-based neonatal care and management of sepsis on neonatal mortality: Field trial in rural India. *Lancet, 354*(9194), 1955–1961.

121. World Health Organization. (2003). *Kangaroo mother care: A practical guide.* Geneva: WHO. Available at http://books.google.com/books?id=cTDRwoUvTnoC&printsec=frontcover&cd=1&source=gbs_ViewAPI#v=onepage&q&f=false.

122. Conde-Agudelo, A., Belizán, J. M., & Diaz-Rossello, J. L. (2007). Kangaroo mother care to reduce morbidity and mortality in low birthweight infants (Review). *The Cochrane Collaboration.* Retrieved April 23, 2011, from http://apps.who.int/rhl/reviews/CD002771.pdf.

123. Osman, N. (2009, October 13). "Kangaroo" incubation urged for Indonesia's pre-mature babies. *Jakarta Globe.* Retrieved April 23, 2011, from http://www.thejakartaglobe.com/national/kangaroo-incubation-urged-for-indonesias-premature-babies/335372.

124. UNICEF/World Health Organization. (2013). *Ending preventable child deaths from pneumonia and diarrhoea by 2025.* Geneva: World Health Organization/The United Nations Children's Fund.

125. Victora, C. G., Adam, T., Bryce, J., & Evans, D. B. (2006). Integrated management of the sick child. In D. T. Jamison, J. G. Breman, A. R. Measham, et al. (Eds.), *Disease control priorities in developing countries* (2nd ed., pp. 1117–1191). New York: Oxford University Press.

126. World Health Organization. *Integrated management of childhood illness (IMCI).* Retrieved March 2, 2015, from http://www.who.int/maternal_child_adolescent/topics/child/imci/en/.

CHAPTER **11**

Adolescent Health

LEARNING OBJECTIVES

By the end of this chapter, the reader will be able to:

- Discuss the importance of adolescent health to the global health agenda
- Review the leading causes of death and the burden of disease for adolescents
- Assess the key risk factors for those deaths and disability-adjusted life years (DALYs)
- Review the health, social, and economic consequences of key adolescent health problems
- Outline some of the main steps that could be taken to reduce the burden of disease and deaths in adolescents

VIGNETTES

Carmen is a 15-year-old girl in El Salvador. Although premarital sex is socially unacceptable in El Salvador, Carmen became sexually active at 14. When Carmen was 16, she became pregnant. As a result, she dropped out of high school and went to live with relatives in the countryside until she had her baby. It will be very difficult for Carmen to return to school, and her economic prospects have been severely damaged by getting pregnant and giving birth at such a young age.

Rachel is a 15-year-old girl in South Africa. She is one of many people her age who was born to an HIV-positive mother before South Africa made much progress in stopping mother-to-child transmission of HIV. Rachel has been taking drugs against her disease for as long a she can remember. In the last few years, however, she has found it more and more difficult to remember to take her drugs on time. She also worries constantly that her peers will know that she is HIV-positive.

John was an 18-year-old boy in Chicago, Illinois, in the United States. He had gone most of the way through high school but not completed it. There are few jobs in Chicago for young people without a high school diploma, and John spent much of his time hanging around with friends of similar background. Over time, John joined a youth gang and made some money by selling small amounts of illegal drugs, some of which he occasionally used himself. At 19, John was murdered while selling drugs on a street corner near his home, becoming one of many adolescent victims of interpersonal violence.

Rashmi is a 14-year-old girl in Punjab state in India. She is hard working and very intelligent but always feels great pressure to meet the expectations of her family and community. She worries all the time about how she can do all her chores at home, help make money for the family, do well in school, and then marry the "boy" her family will choose for her. Lately, her body has gone through a number of changes that she does not understand and she has begun to feel more and more overwhelmed about all that she has to do. In the last few months, in fact, she has found herself very happy at some times but very sad at other times. She feels like something is wrong but does not know what it is or what to do about it.

Juan was 18 when he was killed in a car crash outside Lima, Peru. Juan had just gotten his driver's license when the accident occurred at a busy intersection, where several roads came together, and the signage was confusing to those who did not know the area. Juan failed to understand that he could turn left only on the green left arrow and turned into the path of an oncoming car. The collision spun his car around and it was then hit by another car on the driver side. Juan was severely injured and died in the hospital the next day.

THE IMPORTANCE OF ADOLESCENT HEALTH

The World Health Organization defines adolescents as people between 10 and 19 years of age.[1] There are about 1.2 billion adolescents in the world, representing about one of every six people.[1] Almost 90 percent of all the adolescents in the world live in low- and middle-income countries.[2]

Adolescent health deserves special attention for several reasons. First, adolescents make up an important share of the population. Second, the burden of disease for adolescents is a unique one and needs to be addressed directly, rather than together with the needs of younger children. This is particularly so, for example, when one considers issues of sexuality and reproductive health, mental health, interpersonal violence, and road safety. Third, adolescence is a period during which important health behaviors are set and it is critical to ensure that adolescents adopt healthy behaviors. The health of future adult populations, for example, will depend, to a large extent, on whether or not adolescents drive safely, avoid excess alcohol consumption, avoid tobacco smoking, and take up healthy diets with appropriate physical activity. Finally, as shown in **Table 11-1**, there are critical links between the Millennium Development Goals (MDGs) and the health of adolescents.

This chapter examines the most critical issues in adolescent health, with a focus on low- and middle-income countries. The chapter begins by reviewing some key terms and definitions that relate to adolescents. It then examines the burden of disease for adolescents, key risk factors for those burdens, and the costs and consequences of the most important adolescent health issues. Two policy and program briefs illustrate approaches to addressing adolescent health. The chapter concludes with broader comments on how the most important health burdens among adolescents might be addressed.

TABLE 11-1 The MDGs and Adolescent Health

Goal 1: Eradicate Poverty and Hunger
Link: Poverty is both a risk factor and a consequence of poor health during adolescence. Improving the health of adolescents will enable them to grow into healthier, more productive adults. Improving the nutritional status of adolescents, many of whom are stunted or suffer from anemia, can improve both their health and the health of their children.

Goal 2: Achieve Universal Primary Education
Link: Improving the health of adolescents will have a positive impact on their enrollment and success in school.

Goal 3: Promote Gender Equality and Empower Women
Link: Improving the health of adolescent females will increase their opportunities for education, employment, income, and empowerment. These, in turn, will help to reduce the prevalence of intimate partner violence, adolescent pregnancy, and other related constraints to the health and empowerment of women.

Goal 4: Reduce Child Mortality
Link: Adolescence is a crucial developmental stage in the transition from childhood to adulthood. Efforts to improve adolescent health help ensure that the gains of efforts to reduce child mortality will be sustained. Healthy adolescents are also likely to develop into healthier parents who are better able to care for their own children.

Goal 5: Improve Maternal Health
Link: Maternal disorders are a major cause of mortality and morbidity among adolescent girls, especially in low- and middle-income countries. Reducing fertility among adolescents by promoting later marriage and childbirth, ensuring access to contraception, and strengthening obstetric care could have a significant impact on improving maternal health globally.

Goal 6: Combat HIV/AIDS, Malaria, and Other Diseases
Link: Adolescents, especially females, face especially high risks of infection with HIV. Tuberculosis (TB) is also a major killer of adolescents in sub-Saharan Africa, and malaria is a major cause of morbidity among adolescents. Reducing HIV, TB, and malaria infections among adolescents would significantly improve the health of adolescents and the general population.

Data from United Nations. Millenium Development Goals. Retrieved May 3, 2015 from http://www.un.org/millenniumgoals/

> ### TABLE 11-2   Key Terms and Definitions
>
> - The World Health Organization (WHO) defines an adolescent as a person between the ages of 10 and 19 years
> - The United Nations defines *youth* as a person between the ages of 15 and 24 years
> - The United Nations *Convention on the Rights of the Child* defines *child* as a person under the age of 18 years
>
> Data from World Health Organization. Adolescents: health risks and solutions. Retrieved May 3, 2015 from http://www.who.int/mediacentre /factsheets/fs345/en/; Data from United Nations. Definition of Youth. Retrieved May 3, 2015 from http://www.un.org/esa/socdev/documents /youth/fact-sheets/youth-definition.pdf; Data from United Nations Office of the High Commissioner for Human Rights. Convention on the Rights of the Child. Retrieved May 3, 2015 from http://www.ohchr.org/EN /ProfessionalInterest/Pages/CRC.aspx.

Key Terms and Definitions

There are a number of terms that refer to part or all of the period of adolescence. **Table 11-2** outlines the most important of such terms. It is important to note that different organizations define adolescence in different ways. Whereas many groups refer to adolescence as ages 10–19, others include young adults aged 20–24 in their consideration of adolescents. This chapter consistently defines adolescents as people 10–19 years of age.

DATA ON ADOLESCENT HEALTH

Much of the data in this chapter are taken from a major report on the health of adolescents that WHO produced in 2014.[3] Some other key data are from two *Lancet* series on adolescent health, one in 2007 and another in 2011.[4,5] Consistent with the rest of the book, some data in this chapter that refer to the burden of disease among adolescents are taken primarily from the *Global Burden of Disease Study 2010*.[6] These data are complemented, as needed, by data on particular burdens of disease, such as WHO publications on TB.

It is important to note, however, that there are important gaps in data on adolescents. Much of the focus on global health has been on children under 5 years of age and most of the available data on child health refers to that age group, as well. In addition, it is uncommon to find data for ages 10 to 19. The *Lancet* series, for example, deal with people aged 10–24. The *Global Burden of Disease Study 2010* has data on children

10 to 14 and 15 to 19 but does not have a category that aggregates those into a single category for 10- to 19-year-olds.

Moreover, although WHO has data on adolescents for high-income countries and globally, it does not show data on adolescents specifically for low- and middle-income countries. By contrast, the *Global Burden of Disease Study 2010* does include separate data for low- and middle-income countries, but that data is for a different year than the data included in the WHO report on adolescents.

ADOLESCENCE AS A TRANSITIONAL AND CRITICAL PERIOD

During the adolescent years, children undergo rapid biological, psychological, and social changes. These include hormonal changes and the onset of puberty. Psychologically, adolescence is a phase of rapid increase in cognitive and emotional development in various regions of the brain. However, the brain does not fully develop until people are about 25 years of age and, as adolescents age, they become more able to control their impulses and make more rational decisions. Younger adolescents are heavily influenced by their peers and as adolescents get older they reduce their dependence on their parents.[3,7] Some of the key changes that adolescents undergo in the physical, cognitive, social, and emotional domains are noted in **Table 11-3**.

One important point to consider about adolescence is that, in a sense, the period of adolescence has been getting longer. Puberty comes earlier for most boys and girls than it did in the past and they also marry and assume mature social roles later than was historically the case.[7]

KEY ADOLESCENT HEALTH BURDENS

Some of the most important matters concerning the health status of adolescents, particularly in low- and middle-income countries, are summarized in **Table 11-4**. The section that follows elaborates on these and other key points concerning adolescent health status.

Deaths and DALYs

As shown in **Figure 11-1**, the three leading causes of death of adolescents globally are road injury, HIV/AIDS, and self-harm. This is followed by lower respiratory infections, interpersonal violence, and diarrheal diseases. Drowning, meningitis, epilepsy, and endocrine, blood, and immune disorders are also in the top 10 causes of death. It is interesting to note that four of the leading causes of death for adolescents globally are communicable diseases that are largely preventable or treatable and that occur largely in relatively poorer countries.[3]

TABLE 11-3 Summary of Physical, Cognitive, Social, and Psychological Development in Adolescence

Changes during early adolescence—ages 10–14	
Physical Changes • Puberty, typically ages 8 to 13 in girls, 9 to 14 in boys • Muscle acquisition and growth spurts • Menstruation and breast growth (girls) • Voice deepening and facial hair growth (boys)	*Cognitive, Social, and Psychological Changes* • Self-consciousness and low self-esteem • Feelings of awkwardness or discomfort related to physical changes • Susceptible to peer pressure • Improved ability to engage in abstract thinking and introspection • Tendency to focus on the present rather than the future
Changes during late adolescence—ages 15–19	
Physical Changes • Continued physical growth, especially for boys	*Cognitive, Social, and Psychological Changes* • Increased independence and feelings of invincibility • Tendency to seek out novel and varied experiences • Increased interest in opposite-sex friendships and romantic relationships • Continued improvements in abstract thinking and introspection • Improved decision-making, critical thinking, planning skills, and moral development

Data from Office of Adolescent Health, U.S. Department of Health & Human Services. *Adolescent Development E-Learning Module*. Retrieved May 4, 2015 from http://www.hhs.gov/ash/oah/resources-and-publications/learning/ad_dev/index.html.

TABLE 11-4 Key Issues in Adolescent Health Status

- The mortality rate among adolescents is lower than among other age groups
- Road injury is the leading cause of death among adolescents, followed by HIV/AIDS, self-harm, and interpersonal violence
- Complications related to pregnancy and birth are a leading cause of death among adolescent females, ages 15–19
- Adolescent mortality rates are much higher in Africa (260.6 per 100,000 adolescents) than the global average (94.2 per 100,000 adolescents)
- The high adolescent mortality rate in Africa is driven by deaths from HIV/AIDS
- Depression is the leading cause of DALYs lost among adolescents, followed by road injuries, iron deficiency anemia, HIV, and suicide
- Injuries are a leading cause of death and DALYs, and in a majority of countries, at least 50 percent of young adolescent boys report serious injuries in the preceding year
- In some countries, up to one in three adolescents is obese
- Tobacco use is decreasing among younger adolescents in most high-income countries and in some low- and middle-income countries; however, rates of prevalence among adolescents remain high in many a range of mostly middle-income countries

Data from World Health Organization. *Health for the World's Adolescents: A second chance in the second decade*. Geneva: WHO; 2014.

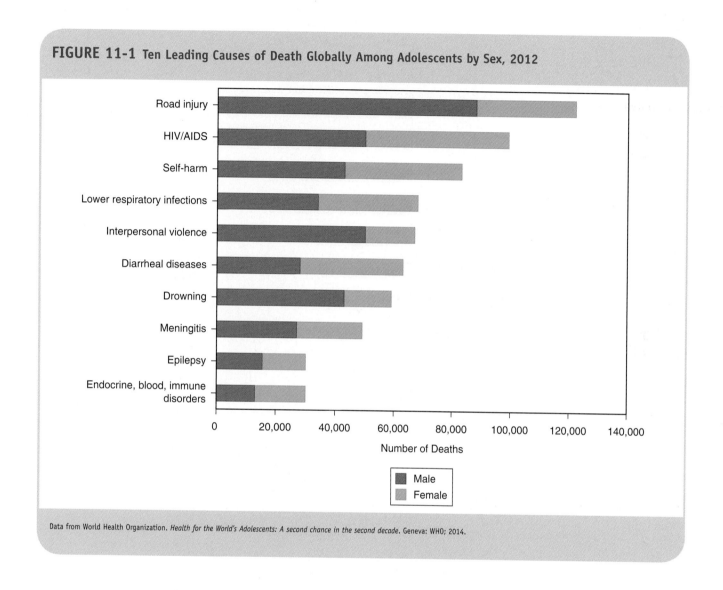

FIGURE 11-1 Ten Leading Causes of Death Globally Among Adolescents by Sex, 2012

Data from World Health Organization. *Health for the World's Adolescents: A second chance in the second decade.* Geneva: WHO; 2014.

The 10 leading causes of DALYs for adolescents globally are quite different than the 10 leading causes of deaths. In the case of DALYs, unipolar depressive disorders are first, and iron deficiency anemia, back and neck pain, anxiety disorders, and asthma all appear in the leading causes of DALYs but not in the leading causes of death.[3]

Figure 11-1 also highlights substantial differences in the patterns of death globally for males and females. The leading cause of death for males, by a significant margin, is road injury, followed by interpersonal violence, HIV/AIDS, and drowning. By contrast, the leading causes of death for females 10–19 years of age globally are HIV/AIDS, self-harm, and diarrheal diseases.

Figure 11-2 also highlights the differences in DALYs globally by sex. Road injury is the leading cause of DALYs for males, followed by unipolar depressive disorders, HIV/AIDS, and self-harm. For females, however, unipolar depression is by far the leading cause of DALYs globally, followed by iron deficiency anemia, road injury, and HIV/AIDS.[3]

The pattern of deaths also varies by country income group and by sex within those groups. **Table 11-5** shows the five leading causes of death for males and females, ages 10–14 and 15–19 for low- and middle-income countries and for high-income countries. For low- and middle-income countries, the leading cause of death among males in both age groups is road injury. However, as males age, the other two of the three leading causes move from HIV/AIDS and drowning to interpersonal violence and self-harm. In high-income countries, road injury is still the leading cause of deaths in both age groups but self-harm is the second leading cause of deaths in both age groups.

FIGURE 11-2 Ten Leading Causes of DALYs Globally Among Adolescents, by Sex, 2012

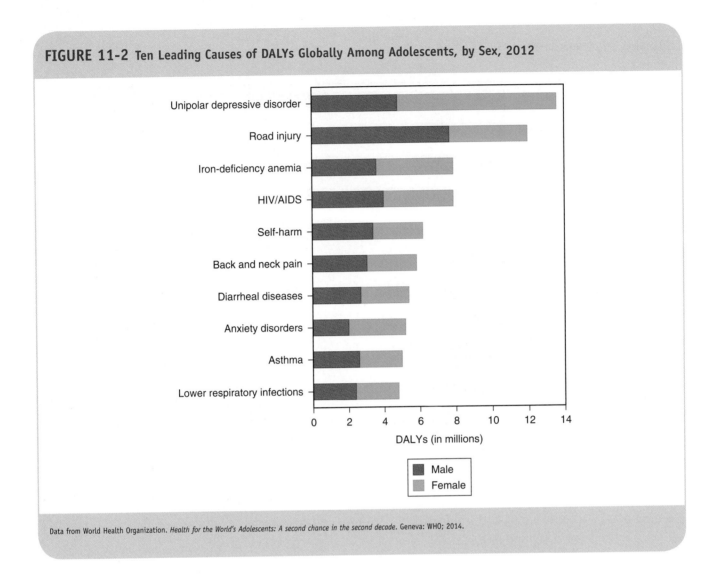

Data from World Health Organization. *Health for the World's Adolescents: A second chance in the second decade.* Geneva: WHO; 2014.

For females, the leading causes of death in low- and middle-income countries in the younger age group are mostly communicable diseases. In the older age group, however, the leading cause of death of females is self-harm. Maternal disorders are the second leading cause, reflecting adolescent pregnancy, compounded by poor nutrition and weak health services. In the high-income countries, road injury and self-harm are the two leading causes of female death in both age groups and violence becomes the third leading cause in the older age group.

The five leading causes of DALYs for males and females aged 10 to 14 and 15 to 19 in low- and middle-income countries and high-income countries are shown in **Table 11-6**. There are some important differences between the causes of DALYs in low- and middle-income countries, for 10- to 14-year-old males compared to 10- to 14-year-old males

in high-income countries. Road injury is more important in low- and middle-income countries and musculoskeletal issues and conduct disorder are in the leading causes of DALYs in high-income countries but not in low- and middle-income countries. The causes of DALYs for 10- to 14-year-old females are similar across country income groups.

For the age group 15–19, the importance of mental health disorders and road injuries is clear for males and females, in all country income groups. It is also important to note that violence is prominent in low- and middle-income countries among males and that maternal disorders are prominent in low- and middle-income countries among females.

As expected, the causes of deaths and DALYs also vary by age group, within adolescents, as one moves from being a child to being a young adult. **Figure 11-3** shows the causes of death globally for 5- to 9-year-old children; 10- to

TABLE 11-5 Five Leading Causes of Death Globally Among Adolescents, by Sex, Age Group, and Country Income Group, 2010

Low- and Middle-Income Countries		High-Income Countries	
Ages 10–14	Ages 15–19	Ages 10–14	Ages 15–19
Males	**Males**	**Males**	**Males**
1. Road injury	1. Road injury	1. Road injury	1. Road injury
2. HIV/AIDS	2. Interpersonal violence	2. Self-harm	2. Self-harm
3. Drowning	3. Self-harm	3. Drowning	3. Interpersonal violence
4. Lower respiratory infections	4. Drowning	4. Leukemia	4. Drowning
5. Forces of nature	5. Malaria	5. Congenital anomalies	5. Drug use disorders
Females	**Females**	**Females**	**Females**
1. HIV/AIDS	1. Self-harm	1. Road injury	1. Road injury
2. Lower respiratory infections	2. Maternal disorders	2. Self-harm	2. Self-harm
3. Diarrheal diseases	3. Road injury	3. Congenital anomalies	3. Interpersonal violence
4. Road injury	4. Malaria	4. Lower respiratory infections	4. Congenital anomalies
5. Malaria	5. Fire	5. Leukemia	5. Drug use disorders

Data from Institute for Health Metrics and Evaluation. Global Burden of Disease Heat Map. Retrieved May 3, 2015 from http://vizhub.healthdata.org/irank/heat.php.

14-year-old adolescents; 15- to 19-year-old adolescents; and young adults. Children 5 to 9 have low rates of death in middle- and high-income countries. Thus, globally the leading causes of death for this group are communicable diseases, such as diarrhea and pneumonia, although road injuries occur in countries of all income groups. As children age, they die less of communicable diseases and more of interpersonal violence, road injuries, and self-harm. By the time females are 15–19 in low-income countries, they face significant risks of dying of maternal causes, overwhelmingly in low-income countries.

Figure 11-4 portrays adolescent mortality rates across the WHO regions and globally, by showing the number of deaths for every 100,000 adolescents. There is clearly a strong correlation between the income group of different regions and the adolescent death rate. The death rate of adolescents in the Africa region, for example, is about 7 times that in the European region. The Eastern Mediterranean region has an adolescent death rate that is about twice the rate in the European region.

Some other key facts concerning differences within WHO regions and differences in country income groups are:[3]

- One in three deaths among adolescent males in the low- and middle-income countries in the Americas region is due to interpersonal violence.
- One in five deaths among adolescent males in the low- and middle-income countries of the Eastern Mediterranean region is due to war and conflicts.

TABLE 11-6 Five Leading Causes of DALYs, by Age Group and Sex, Globally, 2012

Ages 10–14	Ages 15–19	Ages 10–19
Males	**Males**	**Males**
1. Iron deficiency anemia	1. Road injury	1. Road injury
2. HIV/AIDS	2. Interpersonal violence	2. Unipolar depressive disorder
3. Unipolar depressive disorder	3. Self-harm	3. HIV/AIDS
4. Road injury	4. Unipolar depressive disorder	4. Interpersonal violence
5. Asthma	5. Alcohol use disorders	5. Iron deficiency anemia
Females	**Females**	**Females**
1. Unipolar depressive disorder	1. Unipolar depressive disorder	1. Unipolar depressive disorder
2. Iron deficiency anemia	2. Self-harm	2. Iron deficiency anemia
3. HIV/AIDS	3. Maternal conditions	3. HIV/AIDS
4. Diarrheal diseases	4. Anxiety disorders	4. Anxiety disorders
5. Asthma	5. Iron deficiency anemia	5. Diarrheal diseases

Data from World Health Organization. Health for the World's Adolescents: A second chance in the second decade. Geneva: WHO; 2014.

- One in six deaths among adolescent females in the South-East Asia region is due to suicide.
- One in six deaths among adolescents in the Africa region is due to HIV.
- One in five deaths among adolescents in high-income countries is due to road traffic injuries.

Risk Factors and Social Determinants

Table 11-7 shows the leading risk factors globally for DALYs for 10- to 14-year-olds and 15- to 19-year-olds. The risks of unimproved water and sanitation and iron deficiency reflect the poverty, nutritional gaps, and circumstances of home life that many adolescents face. Most of the other risks relate to the behaviors in which adolescents engage, not all of which are the most rational. Studies have shown that

TABLE 11-7 Key Attributable Risk Factors for Deaths Among Adolescents Globally, 2012

- Alcohol use
- Unsafe sex
- Lack of contraception
- Iron deficiency
- Illicit drug use
- Unsafe water, sanitation, and hygiene

Data from World Health Organization. *Health for the World's Adolescents: A second chance in the second decade.* Geneva: WHO; 2014.

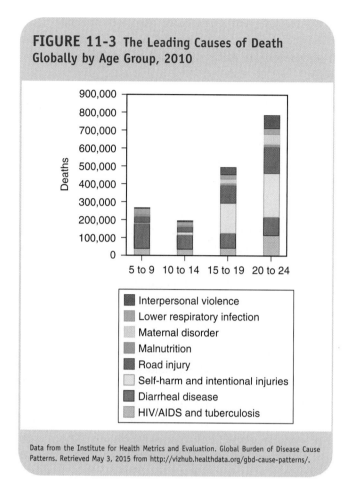

FIGURE 11-3 The Leading Causes of Death Globally by Age Group, 2010

Data from the Institute for Health Metrics and Evaluation. Global Burden of Disease Cause Patterns. Retrieved May 3, 2015 from http://vizhub.healthdata.org/gbd-cause-patterns/.

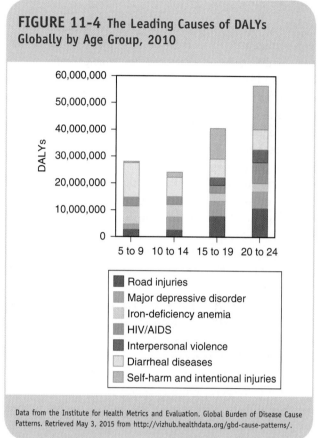

FIGURE 11-4 The Leading Causes of DALYs Globally by Age Group, 2010

Data from the Institute for Health Metrics and Evaluation. Global Burden of Disease Cause Patterns. Retrieved May 3, 2015 from http://vizhub.healthdata.org/gbd-cause-patterns/.

national wealth, income inequality, and access to education are among the most important social determinants of adolescent health.[8]

It is also important to note that the health of some populations of adolescents is more vulnerable than others. For instance, those who are marginalized due to their sexuality or ethnicity, those who live in rural areas, those who live in areas of conflict or natural disasters, and those who are incarcerated face greater risks to their health and well-being than other adolescents do.[3]

In addition, some of the differences between males and females can be attributed to gender disparities. For instance, fewer adolescent girls are enrolled in or complete secondary school and they are, therefore, less informed on health issues. Across low- and middle-income countries (excluding China), for example, only 19 percent of female adolescents have correct knowledge of HIV, compared to 30 percent of male adolescents.[5]

Young men, however, face much greater risks than women from war, interpersonal violence, and traffic accidents. In all age groups and regions, in fact, the mortality rate for adolescent males is higher than that for adolescent females, with the exception of Africa.[5] Among drivers, the risk of getting killed on the road for young men is 3 times that of their female counterparts, due to sociocultural reasons and a greater propensity for risk-taking.[9]

Clearly, the social determinants of health are exceptionally important for adolescents. National wealth, income inequality, and access to education are critical determinants of health for adolescents, as noted earlier. In addition, safe and supportive families, peers, and schools are also critical to helping adolescents develop physically, mentally, and socially. It also appears that exposure to social and other media can have an influence on adolescent behaviors and health.[8]

Additional Comments on Selected Causes of Deaths and DALYs Among Adolescents

Some of the major causes of deaths and DALYs among adolescents are elaborated upon next.

Early Pregnancy and Childbirth (Maternal Causes)

Worldwide, there are 49 births per 1,000 females aged 15–19, which amount to 11 percent of all births. Around 16 million females aged 15–19 and 2 million females under the age of 15 give birth every year, and by the age of 18, one fifth of all females have given birth. Complications from pregnancy and childbirth are the leading cause of deaths among females aged 15–19 years in many low- and middle-income countries, where 95 percent of births occur.[1] They are, for example, the leading cause of deaths in the Eastern Mediterranean region and among the top four causes in the Africa, South-East Asia and Americas regions.[3] In the WHO Africa region, where birth rates are high, adolescent females aged 15–19 are 1.5 times more likely to die compared to their male counterparts aged 15–19.[5] About 3 million girls aged 15–19 undergo unsafe abortions yearly and some of these lead to maternal death.[1]

Figure 11-5 shows the adolescent fertility rate across the World Bank regions. This figure clearly portrays the fact that adolescent fertility in sub-Saharan Africa and Latin America and the Caribbean is more than 5 times and more than 3 times, respectively, than in East Asia and Pacific. High adolescent fertility poses grave risks to young women because the risks of dying a maternal death are higher when women

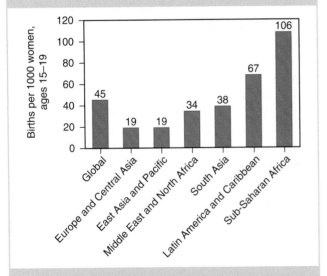

FIGURE 11-5 Adolescent Fertility, Ages 15–19, by World Bank Region and Globally, 2013

Data from the World Bank. Adolescent Fertility Rate, 2013. Retrieved May 3, 2015 from http://data.worldbank.org/indicator/SP.ADO.TFRT/countries/1W-8S-Z7-Z4-ZQ-ZJ-ZG?display=graph020406080100120.

in low resource settings, especially those who are undernourished and of short stature, give birth at young ages, with short birth intervals, in places where maternal health services are weak.

Anemia

Many young people enter adolescence having suffered from undernutrition and stunting. This is especially so in those parts of the world that are most deficient nutritionally for children, including South Asia, sub-Saharan Africa, the indigenous parts of the Americas, and the poorer and less food secure parts of other low- and middle-income regions. Iron deficiency anemia, in particular, continues to be an important part of the burden of disease for 10- to 14-year-olds. In fact, it is among the leading causes of DALYs among males and females in this age group in almost all low- and middle-income countries.[10]

HIV/AIDS and Other Sexually Transmitted Infections

It is estimated that more than 2 million adolescents are living with HIV/AIDS. In addition, although the total number of HIV-related deaths has decreased by 30 percent since its peak 8 years ago, estimates suggest that HIV/AIDS deaths among adolescents are increasing, mostly in the WHO Africa region. This could be a result of HIV-positive children who survive past childhood but may not be receiving all of the care that they require in adolescence. Among all 15- to 24-year-olds in sub-Saharan Africa, only 10 percent of men and 15 percent of women know their HIV status. In some countries, up to 60 percent of all new HIV infections occur among 15- to 24-year-olds. Adolescence is the period when most people initiate sexual activity. Adolescent girls are at special risk both biologically and socially of becoming infected with HIV. In addition, adolescents face risks of engaging in alcohol and drug use that can also lead to unsafe sexual practices and the transmission of HIV.[1]

Adolescent girls, especially in low- and some middle-income countries, face particular risks not only for HIV but also for other sexually transmitted infections. These include their immature reproductive and immune systems, gender norms that discriminate against them, age differences with male sexual partners, and pressure in some settings to engage in transactional sex or prostitution. In addition, in many high-income countries and much of sub-Saharan Africa, more than a third of adolescent girls have had sexual intercourse. Although condom use has increased in high-income countries among adolescents, data show that young women in 19 African countries used a condom in less than a third of their last sexual encounters. Given this background, most sexually transmitted infections globally occur in people younger than 25 years of age. WHO estimates that 340 million new cases of syphilis, gonorrhea, chlamydia, and trichomoniasis occur each year, and it is thought that the prevalence of sexually transmitted infections is rising in most countries.[4]

Other Communicable Diseases

Adolescent deaths and disabilities from communicable diseases like measles have decreased significantly due largely to the increased coverage of childhood vaccination. In the Africa region, between 2000 and 2012, in fact, overall deaths from communicable diseases decreased by 90 percent. However, as noted earlier, communicable diseases such as diarrhea, lower respiratory infections, and meningitis are still among the leading causes of adolescent mortality. As also shown earlier, malaria is a leading cause of DALYs for adolescents.[1]

Tuberculosis is a major cause of death for adolescents in those parts of sub-Saharan Africa where HIV/AIDS and TB have the highest prevalence rates. TB is also a major cause of adolescent death in South Asia, which also has among the highest prevalence rates of adult TB in the world.[10] The global community is now paying greater attention to the risks that young children and adolescents will get active TB disease and to their needs for effective TB treatment.

Noncommunicable Diseases

As noted earlier, the behaviors in which adolescents engage have a significant impact on their health as adults, including what and how much they eat, their levels of physical activity, and whether they drink alcohol or smoke tobacco.

Adolescents globally are increasingly eating foods high in sugar, salt, and saturated fats; and engaging in insufficient physical activity; and an increasing share of adolescents are becoming obese. In a range of countries for which there are data, fewer than one in four adolescents met the recommended guidelines on physical activity, and in some countries as many as one in three adolescents is now obese. It is especially important to note that in many countries this obesity exists side by side with a substantial share of children who suffer from underweight, stunting, and micronutrient deficiencies.[3]

In many high-income countries, the prevalence of cigarette smoking is decreasing among adolescents. In many low- and middle-income countries, however, the prevalence of cigarette smoking is increasing, as tobacco companies focus an increasing amount of attention on selling their cigarettes in these settings. The gap between male and female prevalence of cigarette smoking is also closing in some settings, as an increasing share of females smoke. **Figure 11-6** portrays the

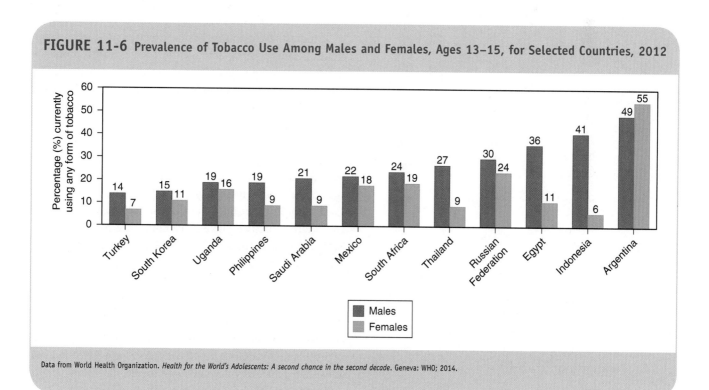

FIGURE 11-6 Prevalence of Tobacco Use Among Males and Females, Ages 13–15, for Selected Countries, 2012

Data from World Health Organization. *Health for the World's Adolescents: A second chance in the second decade.* Geneva: WHO; 2014.

prevalence of tobacco smoking among 13- to 15-year-old males and females for a selected group of countries. As shown on the figure, about 50 percent of both males and females smoke in Argentina, which has the highest prevalence for these age groups among the countries surveyed. In Indonesia about 40 percent of the males aged 13–15 smoke tobacco, although the prevalence of female smoking in Indonesia remains low.[3]

As also noted earlier, excessive drinking is a major risk factor, both directly and indirectly, for a range of health issues. Besides being a risk factor for mental health problems and a number of other conditions, alcohol consumption reduces self-control and increases risky behavior, such as unsafe sex, unsafe driving, and violence.[2] Estimates suggest that about 5 percent of all deaths of people aged 15 and 29 years of age are due to alcohol.[11] **Figure 11-7** indicates the percentage of adolescents aged 15–19 who are current drinkers, former drinkers, or lifetime abstainers, by WHO region. The figure makes clear the extent to which alcohol consumption is an important risk factor for adolescents, except in the Eastern Mediterranean and South-East Asia regions of WHO.

FIGURE 11-7 Percentage of Current Drinkers, Former Drinkers, and Lifetime Abstainers Among Adolescents Aged 15–19, by WHO Region and Globally

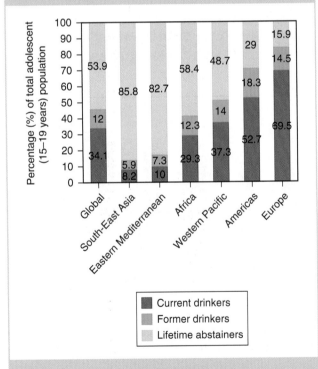

Data from World Health Organization. *Global Status Report on Alcohol and Health 2014.* Geneva: WHO; 2014.

Mental Health

Mental health is a fundamental issue for adolescents; between 10 and 20 percent of all adolescents suffer from mental health problems.[12] Depression is the leading cause of illness and disability in young people and suicide is the third most common cause of mortality.[3] Other common mental health problems among adolescents are eating and conduct disorders, anxiety, and depression. Although around half of all mental health disorders in adulthood will show symptoms by age 14, most go unnoticed and/or untreated, affecting adolescents' potential and development.[1] Those with mental disorders often face stigma, isolation, and discrimination, reducing their access to health care and education. Other risk behaviors that relate to mental health problems include violent behavior, unsafe sexual behavior, and substance abuse.[13]

The risk factors for mental health problems among adolescents are numerous and start with genetics and the health of the mother. At the earliest stages, they include having an adolescent parent, being an unintended birth, being born after a short birth interval, and having a parent who married a blood relative. They also include, for example, poor physical health and nutritional status of the child, growing up without caregivers, being orphaned, or growing up in an institution. In addition, they include exposure to harmful substances, violence, conflict, or abuse. Gender disparity, discrimination, immigrant status, or being displaced can also be a risk factor for mental health problems.[12]

Studies have also shown that experiences of school-age children can be important risks for mental health problems in adolescence and later. Beyond those mentioned already, such experiences can include being the victim of bullying, family dysfunction, pathological use of the Internet, adolescent pregnancy, and being a child soldier.[12]

Suicide, as noted earlier, deserves special mention when considering adolescent health, as well. It is among the five leading causes of deaths among adolescents 15–19 years of age in the World Bank regions of Latin America and the Caribbean, Europe and Central Asia, East Asia and Pacific, and South Asia. It is the 8th leading cause of death in the Middle East and North Africa region, and the 11th leading cause in the Africa region.[10]

Road Injuries

Road traffic injuries are the number one cause of death globally among 15- to 19-year-olds, and the second leading cause of death among adolescents 10–14 years of age.[10] Around 330 adolescents die every day and close to 400,000 young people under the age of 25 die every year from a road injury.[1] From the ages of 10 to 14 to the ages of 20 to 24, there is a sixfold increase in traffic-related deaths.[5] Many of these deaths happen in low- and middle-income countries not only among passengers in automobiles, but also among pedestrians, bicyclists, and motorcyclists.

Violence

Interpersonal violence is a leading cause of adolescent mortality, resulting in an estimated 180 deaths every day.[1] Moreover, interpersonal violence is among the five leading causes of deaths of 15- to 19-year-olds in all World Bank regions, except for sub-Saharan Africa, for which is it seventh, and South Asia, for which it is ninth. In the Latin America and the Caribbean region of the World Bank, interpersonal violence is the leading cause of death of adolescents 15 to 19 years of age.[10] Among adolescent males, around one in three deaths in the low- and middle-income countries in the WHO Americas region is attributed to violence. Thirty percent of 15- to 19-year-old girls are victims of violence by a partner.[1]

ECONOMIC AND SOCIAL CONSEQUENCES OF ADOLESCENT HEALTH ISSUES

Adolescent health issues have profound health, social, and economic consequences. First, it is clear that maintaining the health of adolescents is central to maintaining the gains that have occurred in the health of young children. More and more children are living longer and healthier lives as progress has been made, among other things, against vaccine-preventable diseases and malaria. This progress can be undone if adolescents face important health issues that take their lives away or lead to major illness or disability.

Second, the health of adolescents and behaviors in which they engage during adolescence set a foundation for their health as adults. Adolescent pregnancy can diminish the chances that a girl will complete schooling or that her child will become a well-schooled, healthy, and productive adult. Obesity during adolescence, for example, can have a permanent effect on the health and productivity of an adult. Most people who take up smoking tobacco, drinking alcohol, and using illegal drugs start such behaviors in adolescence, and these behaviors are difficult to stop as adults.

Other burdens of disease among adolescents also have substantial costs. The social and economic costs of HIV are well known, and adolescent girls are among the most at risk of being infected with HIV. Tuberculosis is a major cause of morbidity and death among adolescents in Africa, and TB leads to months of lost work, even if treated effectively. Road traffic injuries, the leading cause of deaths among adolescents

globally, can lead to substantial and long-lasting disabilities, as well as many years of life lost. Mental health issues often start in adolescence, go on for much or all of a person's life, and have enormous social and economic costs to individuals, their families, and societies.

POLICY AND PROGRAM BRIEFS

HealthWise South Africa: A Life Skills Course for Adolescents

Substance abuse and risky sexual behaviors are significant health challenges for adolescents around the world. In South Africa, where almost 18 percent of the adults are HIV-positive, these behaviors are even more serious because they increase the risk of getting infected with HIV.[14] In fact, adolescents are especially vulnerable to new HIV infections and face a particularly high incidence of HIV.[15] Key risk factors for HIV include early initiation of sexual activity, multiple sexual partners, and failure to use a condom. These risk factors also increase adolescents' risk of other sexually transmitted infections and unwanted pregnancy.

Risky sexual behavior and HIV risk are both positively correlated with substance abuse among South African adolescents. National surveys show that the prevalence for ever having used a substance was 50 percent for alcohol, 31 percent for cigarettes and 13 percent for cannabis among South African high school students.[16] Because of the strong link between substance abuse and risky sexual behaviors among adolescents, effective prevention strategies for both risk factors are essential.

HealthWise South Africa is a school-based education program designed to reduce substance abuse and risky sexual behavior among adolescents. The program was first piloted in South African high schools in 2001 and is modeled after sexual education and life skills courses taught in many American public schools. HealthWise seeks to address the myths and realities of substance abuse and empower students through lessons on self-awareness, decision making, and conflict resolution. The course also includes lessons on planning healthy leisure time activities and building positive social connections in the community.

One of the most important aspects of the HealthWise South Africa curriculum is education around condom usage. In addition to teaching students how to use condoms effectively, the curriculum teaches students where condoms can be purchased in their communities and how to negotiate condom use with their partners.

Studies have found that students who participate in HealthWise South Africa are less likely to engage in high-risk sexual behaviors or frequent drug use.[17] Students also have a greater likelihood of using a condom and increased knowledge of condom availability.[18,19] Initial positive results have increased the program's popularity, and it is now being piloted throughout Cape Town.

The initial success of HealthWise South Africa may offer the following lessons for other interventions that are oriented toward improving the sexual and reproductive health of adolescents:

- Address the emotional and psychological motivations for risk behavior
- Encourage adolescents to find alternatives to risky activities
- Recognize the classroom as an important space for health and life skills education

Cash Transfer Program for Adolescent Girls in Malawi

Malawi, one of the world's poorest countries, faces a high burden of HIV/AIDS. The adult prevalence of HIV is over 10 percent, and females, especially adolescent girls, are particularly vulnerable.[20] Women in Malawi are at highest risk of contracting HIV between ages 15 and 24 years old.[21] Interventions that reduce young women's risk of becoming infected with HIV have the potential to significantly reduce HIV prevalence in the general population.

Low educational attainment and economic dependence on men are widely understood to be important risk factors for HIV infection among adolescent girls.[22] In low-resource settings, adolescent girls often engage in transactional sex with older men to pay for school fees and other day-to-day expenses. Cash transfer programs have the potential to reduce the incentive for adolescent girls to engage in such risky transactional sex and ultimately reduce the number of new HIV infections among young women.

In the rural Zomba district of Malawi, a randomized trial was conducted to assess the effect of a cash transfer program on HIV prevalence among young women. Over 1,000 young, unmarried women (ages 13–22 years) participated in the program. Half of them were randomly assigned to receive conditional cash transfers, with school attendance required to receive payments. The other half received unconditional cash transfers and did not have to attend school to receive their payments. Those who were going to get payments were randomly assigned by lottery to receive monthly payments ranging from $1 to $5. Participants completed behavioral risk assessments at baseline and 12 months later. Eighteen months after baseline, their HIV status was tested.

After the 18-month program, participants of the cash transfer program had a significantly lower HIV prevalence rate of 1.2 percent, compared to 3.0 percent in the control group who got no cash transfer payment. The study also showed that there was no significant difference in the effect between the conditional and unconditional cash transfer programs. This suggests that, where monitoring school attendance is difficult, even unconditional cash transfers can have the desired effect on health. The program also found that the cash transfers significantly reduced the number of sexual encounters girls had, especially with older men. This evidence supports the notion that cash transfers can reduce HIV prevalence by reducing the need for young women to engage in transactional sex with older men.

In response to this study and other similar studies in the region, conditional cash transfer programs are being scaled up significantly in Malawi. UNAIDS and the World Bank have pledged funds to help the Malawian government expand its existing cash transfer program. Similar efforts are also being expanded in neighboring countries, including South Africa, Botswana, and Kenya.[23]

The conditional cash transfer program in Malawi highlights the importance of helping to address the underlying causes of risk behavior, such as economic need. It also suggests that unconditional cash transfer programs may be as effective as conditional cash transfer programs.

BROAD-BASED MEASURES TO IMPROVE ADOLESCENT HEALTH IN LOW- AND MIDDLE-INCOME COUNTRIES

Adolescents are a unique group, with a particular burden of disease related to a specific set of risk factors. It is critical, therefore, that policymakers pay particular attention to the adolescent period and take a life-course perspective to it, seeing it as one stage in a series of age categories that people pass through as they go through life. It will also be important that policymakers collect data specific to adolescents, breaking it down into early adolescence, 10–14 years, and later adolescence, 15–19 years. This would provide an enhanced basis for analyzing and acting on adolescent health issues. Evidence also suggests that approaches to improving adolescent health will be more effective if adolescents are given opportunities to voice their needs to identify programs to address them.[7]

The importance of social determinants to the well-being of adolescents also argues for a broad-based approach to addressing their health needs. Thus, it will be important for policymakers to take an approach to adolescent health that integrates interventions at the community, family, and school levels. It will also be critical to enhance educational opportunities, especially for girls, and to manage the economy in ways that promote employment for the large numbers of adolescents making their way into the labor force in many countries.[8]

Health authorities lack control over many of the factors that concern road traffic injuries and morbidity and mortality from interpersonal violence. Those responsible for road safety will need to take measures that can address the risks for adolescent drivers, including, for example, improving licensing requirements, taking a stepwise approach to their driving rights, and enforcing drunk driving laws. Governments will also need to take measures to promote home and school environments that reduce the risks of adolescent violence, such as promoting better child nutrition, better parental caring behaviors, and welcoming school environments. Gun control can also reduce adolescent violence.[8]

There are also a number of measures that health systems can take to help address adolescent health issues. First, by adopting universal health coverage, health systems can reduce the barriers to care that many adolescents face. Second, health systems can take measures to be more adolescent friendly. They can train providers in the needs of adolescents and create settings that encourage adolescents to seek care. Health authorities can also lead efforts within countries to enact and enforce laws that reduce risk to adolescents, such as those concerning road safety and the use of tobacco, alcohol, and drugs. Many health systems have focused adolescent health almost exclusively on sexual and reproductive health. However, such services need to expand their focus and address a broader range of health concerns.[3]

Health interventions in specific areas also need to take into account the particular needs of adolescents. Efforts to promote family planning and reduce maternal deaths, for example, must pay attention to early marriage, adolescent pregnancy, and short birth intervals among young mothers. Efforts to reduce new HIV infections among adolescents will have to take into account, among other things, the early sexual debut of many adolescents, multiple sexual partners, transactional sex among young females, access of adolescents to condoms, and the risks that alcohol and substance abuse pose for unsafe sexual practices. In addition, policies on alcohol and tobacco must always include efforts to limit sales to minors.

WHO has developed guidelines for health services and interventions that can address the health needs and risks that adolescents face. The recommended services are summarized in **Figure 11-8**. These services and interventions are meant to complement the broader approach taken to reduce risk, reduce harm, and treat adolescent health problems in specific areas.[3] WHO guidelines for offering support and treatment for tobacco cessation for adolescents, for example, must be seen in the context of efforts to tax tobacco, prohibit the advertising of tobacco products, reduce the number of places that people can smoke, and prohibit the sale of tobacco to minors. Thus, the figure also includes some comments on the broader policy measures that are needed in specific areas.

MAIN MESSAGES

The health of adolescents is critical to the global health agenda. Adolescents constitute an important part of the population in all countries. In addition, the health of adolescents is central to preserving the gains made in child health. It is also central to laying a solid foundation for the health of future adults.

A specific focus on adolescent health is essential because adolescents are neither children nor adults and because adolescence is a time of rapid biological and psychological change. Adolescents go through hormonal and other changes, become more influenced by peers and less by family, and may engage in risk-taking behaviors until they are able to exercise more rational control over their impulses and emotions.

In addition, adolescents have a unique burden of disease. Younger adolescents, especially in low- and middle-income countries, continue to fall ill and die from preventable or treatable communicable diseases, such as diarrhea, pneumonia, malaria, meningitis, and HIV/AIDS. Older adolescent girls, especially in low-income countries, face serious risks of dying from maternal causes and from contracting HIV. There is also a substantial burden of anemia. Increasingly, however, as the burden of communicable diseases is reduced, more and more adolescents, in all parts of the world, face a burden of disease dominated by road injuries, depression, interpersonal violence, and suicide. It is also important to note that, side by side with continuing high prevalence of childhood underweight and micronutrient deficiencies, an increasing share of the world's adolescents are overweight and obese.

The risk factors for the communicable diseases that affect adolescents are well known and include, among other things, poor nutrition; inadequate water, sanitation, and hygiene; and poor coverage of immunization and other health services. Early pregnancy is also an important risk factor for maternal morbidity and mortality. Social determinants of health, such as poverty, abuse, living in rural areas, poor family educational attainment, and gender discrimination are key to understanding the burden of disease among many adolescents. Peer relationships, living with conflict or the aftermath of disasters, and having few economic options are

FIGURE 11-8 Key Health Services and Interventions for Improving Adolescent Health

HIV

- Promote greater adolescent awareness about HIV and the importance of later sexual debut, limited partners, and correct and consistent condom use
- HIV testing and counselling
- Voluntary medical male circumcision in countries with generalized HIV epidemics
- Prevention of Mother-to-Child Transmission
- Anti-Retroviral Therapy
- Contraceptive information and services

Sexual and Reproductive Health/Maternal Health

- Care in pregnancy, childbirth, and postpartum period for adolescent mother and newborn infant
- Contraception
- Prevention and management of sexually transmitted infections
- Safe abortion care

Mental Health

- Community-based approaches to diagnosis, psychosocial support, and referral of complex cases
- Management of conditions specifically related to stress
- Management of emotional disorders
- Management of behavioral disorders
- Management of adolescents with developmental disorders
- Management of other significant emotional or medically unexplained complaints
- Management of self-harm/suicide

Substance Use

- Establish and enforce an appropriate minimum age for purchase and consumption of alcoholic beverages
- Assessment and management of alcohol use and alcohol use disorders
- Assessment and management of drug use and drug use disorders
- Screening and brief interventions for hazardous and harmful substance use during pregnancy

Road Injuries

- Develop and implement policies to prevent intoxicated driving
- Set blood alcohol concentration (BAC) limits to less than 0.05g/dl for the general population and less than 0.02 g/dl for young/novice drivers
- Graduated licensing programs for young/novice drivers

Nutrition

- First, childhood measures to reduce infection, ensure food security, and ensure good nutritional status of adolescents
- Intermittent iron and folic acid supplementation
- Health education of adolescents, parents, and caregivers regarding healthy diet
- BMI-for-age assessment

Physical Activity

- Health education of adolescents, parents, and caregivers regarding physical activity

Tobacco Control

- Raise tobacco taxes and prohibit tobacco sales to minors
- Encourage total elimination of smoking and tobacco smoke in public places
- Implement other key measures of WHO convention on tobacco

Integrated Management of Common Conditions

- Management of common complaints and conditions
- Assessment of home, education, employment, eating, activity, drugs, sexuality, safety, suicide/depression

Immunization

- Tetanus
- Human papillomavirus
- Measles
- Rubella
- Meningococcal infections
- Japanese encephalitis
- Hepatitis B
- Influenza

Data from the author and World Health Organization. *Health for the World's Adolescents A second chance in the second decade. 2014*; http://apps.who.int/adolescent/second-decade/. Accessed May 1, 2015.

also important determinants of the health and well-being of adolescents and whether or not they engage in tobacco use, alcohol abuse, unsafe sex, risky driving, or suffer from mental health issues.

The consequences of poor adolescent health to individuals, families, and societies are immense. An unhealthy adolescent is unlikely to have a healthy and productive adulthood. In addition, adolescents may fall ill with conditions, such as mental health, alcohol, or substance abuse disorders that can go on for many years and will be costly to themselves and to society.

There are a number of measures that can be taken to address adolescent health issues. At the broadest levels of society, it will be important to promote education to the secondary level for females as well as males. Investing in water, sanitation, and hygiene will also be fundamental. Economic policies that encourage job creation and productive employment for the large numbers of adolescents who will enter the job market will also be essential.

Health systems can also take a number of institutional steps to better address adolescent health needs. They need to train their staff to pay attention to the unique burdens of disease and needs of adolescents. They need to improve their collection of data that is specific to adolescents. It will also be important that specific health programs, such as for TB or HIV, focus particular attention on adolescents, the risk factors for their getting active TB disease or becoming infected with HIV, and measures that could be taken to reduce the specific risks for these diseases that adolescents face. Moving to universal health coverage can also help to reduce the barriers that many adolescents face to accessing health services, as would ensuring that such health services are friendly to adolescents.

Other specific interventions could also be made to reduce the burden of disease among adolescents. Improving licensing requirements for driving, taking a stepwise approach to adolescent driving, and stricter enforcement of drunk driving laws can reduce road traffic injuries among adolescents. Keeping girls in school longer, improving knowledge about reproductive health and family planning, and enhancing access to family planning and maternal health services could reduce the burden of reproductive health burdens among adolescents. Taking a community-based approach to mental health issues, with specific attention to adolescents, psychosocial support and referral for difficult cases could help to reduce the high burden of mental health conditions and suicide among adolescents.

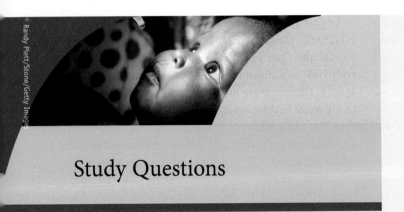

Study Questions

1. Why is specific attention to the health of 10- to 19-year-olds needed?

2. What are the leading burdens of disease among adolescents globally?

3. How do these burdens vary between sexes and between low-income and high-income countries?

4. How do they vary between younger adolescents and older adolescents?

5. What are the most important social determinants of the health of adolescents?

6. What are some of the most important health and social consequences of health issues among adolescents?

7. What could be done to reduce the burden of reproductive health issues among adolescents?

8. What could be done to reduce the burden of road injuries among adolescents?

9. What could be done to reduce the burden of mental health conditions among adolescents?

REFERENCES

1. World Health Organization. (2014). *Adolescents: Health risks and solutions* (Fact Sheet No. 345). Retrieved May 1, 2015, from http://www.who.int/mediacentre/factsheets/fs345/en/.

2. Gore, F. M., Bloem, P. J., Patton, G. C., et al. (2011, June 18). Global burden of disease in young people aged 10–24 years: A systematic analysis. *Lancet, 377*(9783), 2093–2101.

3. World Health Organization. (2014). *Health for the world's adolescents: A second chance in the second decade.* Geneva: World Health Organization. Retrieved May 1, 2015, from http://apps.who.int/adolescent/second-decade/.

4. Bearinger, L. H., Sieving, R. E., Ferguson, J., & Sharma, V. (2007, March 27). Global perspectives on the sexual and reproductive health of adolescents: Patterns, prevention, and potential. *Lancet, 369,* 1220–1231.

5. Patton, G. C., Coffey, C., Cappa, C., et al. (2012, April 25). Health of the world's adolescents: A synthesis of internationally comparable data. *Lancet, 379,* 1665–1675.

6. Lancet. *Global Burden of Disease Study 2010.* Retrieved May 4, 2015, from http://www.thelancet.com/global-burden-of-disease.

7. Sawyer, S. M., Afifi, R. A., Bearinger, L. H., et al. (2012, April 25). Adolescence: A foundation for future health. *Lancet, 379,* 1630–1640.

8. Viner, R. M., Ozer, E. M., Denny, S., et al. (2012, April 25). Adolescence and the social determinants of health. *Lancet, 379,* 1641–1652.

9. World Health Organization. (2007). *Youth and road safety.* Geneva: World Health Organization.

10. Institute of Health Metrics and Evaluation. (2015). *GBD 2010 heat map.* Retrieved May 5, 2015, from http://vizhub.healthdata.org/irank/heat.php.

11. World Health Organization. (n.d.). *School and youth health promotion.* Retrieved May 5, 2015, from http://who.int/school_youth_health/en/.

12. Kieling, C., Baker-Henningham, H., Belfer, M., et al. (2011, October 17). Child and adolescent mental health worldwide: Evidence for action. *Lancet, 378,* 1515–1525.

13. World Health Organization. (n.d.). *Child and adolescent mental health.* Retrieved May 5, 2015, from http://www.who.int/mental_health/maternal-child/child_adolescent/en/.

14. UNICEF. (2013). *Getting to zero: HIV in Eastern and Southern Africa.* Retrieved April 21, 2015, from http://www.unicef.org/esaro/Getting-to-Zero-2013.pdf.

15. Simbayi, L. C., Shisana, O., et al. (2012). *South African national HIV prevalence, incidence and behaviour survey.* Retrieved April 21, 2015, from http://www.hsrc.ac.za/en/research-data/view/6871.

16. Wegner, L., Flisher, A. J., Caldwell, L. L., et al. (2008). Healthwise South Africa: Cultural adaptation of a school-based risk prevention programme. *Health Education Research, 23*(6), 1085–1096.

17. Tibbits, M. K., et al. (2011). Impact of HealthWise South Africa on polydrug use and high-risk sexual behavior. *Health Education Research, 26*(4), 653–663.

18. Coffman, D. L., Smith, E. A., Flisher, A. J., & Caldwell, L. L. (n.d.). *Effects of HealthWise South Africa on condom use self-efficacy.* Retrieved April 21, 2015, from http://54.172.146.51/sites/default/files/promising_practices/g3p_docs/Coffman%20Condom%20Efficacy%20PREV322R2.pdf.

19. Smith, E. A., Palen, L., Caldwell, L L., Flisher, A. J., et al. (2008). Substance use and sexual risk prevention in Cape Town, South Africa: An evaluation of the HealthWise Program. *Prevention Science, 9*(4), 311–321.

20. UNAIDS. (2013). *HIV and AIDS estimates (2013): Malawi.* Retrieved April 21, 2015, from http://www.unaids.org/en/regionscountries/countries/malawi.

21. Misiri, H., Edriss, A., Aalen, O., & Dahl, F. (2012). Estimation of HIV Incidence in Malawi from cross-sectional population based sero-prevalence data. *Journal of International AIDS Society, 15*(1), 14.

22. Baird, S. J., Garfein, R. S., McIntosh, C. T., & Özler, B. (2012). Effect of a cash transfer programme for schooling on prevalence of HIV and herpes simplex type 2 in Malawi: A cluster randomised trial. *Lancet, 379,* 1320–1329.

23. UNAIDS. (2014). *Scaling up cash transfer for HIV prevention among adolescent girls and young women.* Retrieved April 21, 2015, from http://www.unaids.org/en/resources/presscentre/featurestories/2014/august/20140818cash-transfers.

CHAPTER **12**

Communicable Diseases

By the end of this chapter the reader will be able to:

- Discuss the determinants of selected communicable diseases, including emerging and reemerging infectious diseases and antimicrobial resistance
- Understand key concepts concerning the prevention, transmission, and treatment of those diseases
- Review the costs and consequences of communicable diseases of importance
- Outline some of the most important examples of successful interventions against communicable diseases
- Understand key challenges to the future prevention and control of these diseases

VIGNETTES

Henrietta was a 35-year-old Kenyan mother of four who lived in Mombasa. Over the last 4 months, Henrietta was barely able to digest her food, had frequent bouts of diarrhea, and had been losing weight. She worried about having AIDS. Henrietta went to a local clinic where she was tested and found to be HIV-positive. She had been infected by her husband, who was a long-distance truck driver.

Maria was 33 years old and lived in the mountains of Peru. For some time, she had not been feeling well. She often had a fever, was coughing a lot, and had night sweats. Maria had tuberculosis (TB) earlier and worried that this might be TB again. Maria was correct. In fact, this time she had drug-resistant TB, which would be difficult and expensive to treat and might not be curable. When Maria was sick the first time, she started her prescribed 6 months of treatment. However, because she felt much better after the first 2 months of drugs, she did not take the rest of them.

Wole was 4 years old and lived in southwestern Nigeria. He had flulike symptoms, a fever, and a headache. His mother suspected he might have malaria but decided she would see if he got better before taking him to the doctor. In another few days, however, Wole was much sicker and weaker. He was also dizzy and, shortly thereafter, lapsed into a coma. His mother rushed him to the local health center but he died within a few hours. Unfortunately, Wole had the most virulent form of malaria.

Sanjay was 18 months old and lived in Lucknow, India. His mother was a day laborer and his father was a rickshaw driver. They lived in a hut in a large slum with little access to water and no sanitation. Sanjay was below the normal height and weight for his age and looked only 12 months old. Over the past year, Sanjay had six bouts of severe diarrhea.

THE IMPORTANCE OF COMMUNICABLE DISEASES

Communicable diseases are immensely important to the global burden of disease and in 2010 accounted for about 31 percent of all deaths and 40 percent of all disability-adjusted life years (DALYs) in low- and middle-income countries.[1] In 2013, it was estimated that HIV/AIDS killed about 1.5 million people.[2] That same year, TB was also responsible for about 1.5 million deaths,[3] diarrhea killed almost 800,000 children under 5 years of age,[4] and malaria killed about 550,000 people.[5] Parasitic infections also account for an enormous burden of disease and disability. In addition, the world faces important threats from emerging and reemerging infectious diseases and from antimicrobial resistance.

Communicable diseases are the most important burden of disease in sub-Saharan Africa, where they make up almost 50 percent of the total DALYs.[1] They are also especially important in South Asia, where they make up about 22 percent of total DALYs.[1] These diseases disproportionately affect the poor. Better-off people have the knowledge and income to protect themselves from diseases spread by unsafe water. They do not live in the crowded circumstances that can spread TB, and they also protect themselves as much as possible against malaria. In addition, they immunize their children against vaccine-preventable diseases at rates that are much higher than poor people do.

Communicable diseases are also of enormous economic consequence. These diseases constrain the physical and mental development of infants and young children and reduce their future economic prospects. The impacts of HIV, TB, malaria, and the neglected tropical diseases on adult productivity are also exceptionally large. In addition, the direct and indirect costs of treatment for an infected person are often a substantial share of their income, causing them to borrow money or sell their already limited assets and forcing them to sink into poverty. High rates of communicable diseases are also impediments to the investment needed to spur economic growth. The appearance of an emerging infectious disease or the reemergence of a disease can cause billions of dollars in lost income for individuals, communities, and countries.

Much of the burden of communicable diseases is avoidable because many of these diseases can easily be prevented or treated. Vaccines are an extremely cost-effective way to prevent a number of communicable diseases in children. The safe use of water can reduce the burden of diarrhea and certain parasitic diseases. There are inexpensive, safe, and effective treatments for TB, malaria, and many parasitic infections. Unfortunately, these technologies are not sufficiently used in low- and middle-income countries, especially by the poor. In addition, the more rational use of antibiotics could reduce the development of antimicrobial resistance.

Given their importance and their impact on the poor, the communicable diseases are of immense relevance to the Millennium Development Goals (MDGs), as noted in Table 12-1.

This chapter introduces the reader to some of the major communicable diseases and their associated burden of morbidity, disability, and mortality in low- and middle-income countries. It will also outline how selected communicable diseases can be controlled. The chapter then presents a number of briefs and case studies on efforts to address communicable diseases. The chapter concludes by reviewing some of the key challenges the world faces in the control of these diseases.

TABLE 12-1 Key Links Between Communicable Diseases and the MDGs

Goal 1: Eradicate Extreme Hunger and Poverty
Communicable diseases are associated with high rates of morbidity and mortality that can immiserate people. Communicable diseases can be part of a cycle of disease and malnutrition. In addition, communicable diseases reduce one's ability to work, thereby decreasing productivity and household income.

Goal 2: Achieve Universal Primary Education
Enrollment, attendance, and performance of children in schools is closely linked with health status. Communicable diseases are the leading cause of illness among the poor in sub-Saharan Africa and especially important among the poor in South Asia, as well.

Goal 4: Reduce Child Mortality
Lower respiratory infections, diarrheal diseases, HIV/AIDS, and malaria are among the leading causes of death of children under 5 years of age in low- and middle-income countries.

Goal 5: Improve Maternal Health
Malaria can cause anemia and mortality in pregnant women and is an important cause of poor maternal outcomes. HIV also has deleterious effects on pregnancy.

Goal 6: Combat HIV/AIDS, Malaria, and Other Diseases
Reducing the burden of communicable diseases is at the core of meeting this development goal.

Goal 8: Develop a Global Partnership for Development
The most important communicable diseases are being addressed through public–private partnerships or through product-development partnerships, such as Roll Back Malaria; Stop TB Gavi; the Global Fund to Fight AIDS, TB, and Malaria; the Global Polio Eradication Initiative; the Global Alliance for TB Drug Development; the Malaria Vaccine Initiative; and the International Partnership on Microbicides.

Data from United Nations. Millennium Development Goals. Available at: http://www.un.org/millenniumgoals/goals. Accessed July 11, 2006.

This chapter focuses on emerging and reemerging infectious diseases and antimicrobial resistance, HIV/AIDS, TB, malaria, and a set of parasitic and bacterial infections often referred to as "neglected tropical diseases." The chapter will not comment on bio-terrorism. Pneumonia is treated in the chapter on child health, because it is an especially important cause of morbidity and mortality for young children in low- and middle-income countries.

This chapter is only introductory. Communicable diseases are a very important topic about which an exceptional amount of material has been written. Those interested in gaining a deeper understanding of these diseases are encouraged to read some of the materials cited in this chapter.

KEY TERMS, DEFINITIONS, AND CONCEPTS

As you begin to explore communicable diseases in greater detail, there are a number of terms and concepts with which you should be familiar. These are defined in **Table 12-2**. It is also important to note that a communicable disease is a disease that is transmitted from an animal to another animal, an animal to a human, a human to another human, or a human to an animal. Transmission can be direct, such as through respiratory means, or indirect through a vector, such as a mosquito in the case of malaria. Most people use the term *communicable disease* in a manner that is synonymous with *infectious disease*. However, others prefer to speak separately about diseases caused by infectious agents, such as TB, and those caused by parasites, such as hookworm. This chapter generally uses the term *communicable disease* to refer to both infectious and parasitic diseases. However, because it is common to refer to "emerging and reemerging *infectious* diseases," that term will also be used when appropriate.

As we examine the basic concepts concerning communicable diseases, it is also important to know how such diseases can be spread. This is shown in the following list, which includes examples of diseases spread in each manner:

- *Foodborne:* Salmonella, *Escherichia coli, Entamoeba histolytica*
- *Waterborne:* Cholera, rotavirus
- *Sexual or bloodborne:* Hepatitis, HIV
- *Vector-borne:* Malaria, onchocerciasis
- *Inhalation:* Tuberculosis, influenza, meningitis
- *Nontraumatic contact:* Anthrax
- *Traumatic contact:* Rabies

In addition, it is critical to understand the ways in which communicable diseases can be controlled. These are noted in the following list of examples of control measures that may be used against the given diseases. The reader should note, however, that a number of different control measures are taken against many diseases.

- *Vaccination:* Smallpox, polio, measles, diphtheria, pertussis, tetanus, hepatitis B, yellow fever, meningitis, influenza
- *Mass chemotherapy:* Onchocerciasis, hookworm, lymphatic filariasis
- *Vector control:* Malaria, dengue, yellow fever, onchocerciasis, West Nile virus
- *Improved water, sanitation, hygiene:* Diarrheal diseases
- *Improved care seeking, disease recognition:* Maternal health, neonatal health, diarrheal disease, respiratory disease
- *Case management (treatment) and improved caregiving:* Diarrheal disease, respiratory disease, HIV/AIDS, TB
- *Case surveillance, reporting, and containment:* Avian influenza, meningitis, cholera
- *Behavioral change:* HIV, sexually transmitted infections, Guinea worm, Ebola virus

---

TABLE 12-2 Communicable Disease Definitions

- **Case**—An individual with a particular disease.
- **Case fatality rate**—The proportion of persons with a particular condition (cases) who die from that condition.
- **Control (disease control)**—Reducing the incidence and prevalence of a disease to an acceptable level.
- **Elimination (of disease)**—Reducing the incidence of a disease in a specific area to zero.
- **Emerging infectious disease**—A newly discovered disease.
- **Eradication (of disease)**—Termination of all cases of a disease and its transmission globally.
- **Parasite**—An organism that lives in or on another organism and takes its nourishment from that organism.
- **Reemerging infectious disease**—An existing disease that has increased in incidence or has taken on new forms.

Data from Centers for Disease Control and Prevention. Reproductive Health Glossary. Availabe at: http://www.cdc.gov/reproductivehealth/Data_Stats/Glossary.htm. Accessed April 15, 2007; Dowdle, WR. The Principles of Disease Elimination and Eradication. Available at: http://www.cdc.gov/mmwr/preview/mmwrhtml/su48a7.htm. Accessed December 27, 2010.

A final concept of exceptional importance when discussing communicable diseases is the concept of *drug resistance*. This refers to the extent to which infectious and parasitic agents develop an ability to resist drug treatment.

NOTE ON THE USE OF DATA IN THIS CHAPTER

It is important to note the data sources for this chapter. Most of the data are taken from the World Health Organization (WHO). However, other data are from organizations such as UNAIDS, Roll Back Malaria, and the Global Network on Neglected Tropical Diseases. These data are complemented by data on the burden of disease and risk factors from the *Global Burden of Disease Study 2010.*

THE BURDEN OF COMMUNICABLE DISEASES

Communicable diseases accounted in 2010 for about 31 percent of total deaths and about 40 percent of total DALYs in low- and middle-income countries.[1] **Table 12-3** summarizes the major causes of death from communicable diseases for the world and for low- and middle-income countries.

The relative importance of communicable diseases, compared to noncommunicable diseases and injuries, varies considerably by region. **Figure 12-1** indicates the share of total deaths by region that is represented by communicable diseases. Figure 12-1 further highlights the fact that South Asia and sub-Saharan Africa have the highest burden of deaths from communicable diseases, relative to other causes of death. However, communicable diseases are the largest cause of death only in sub-Saharan Africa.

The relative importance of specific communicable diseases to the burden of disease also varies by region. HIV/AIDS is of particular importance in sub-Saharan Africa, as is malaria. The neglected diseases are also much more important in sub-Saharan Africa than in any other region.

The burden of specific communicable diseases varies by age group. Diarrheal disease, malaria, lower respiratory infections, and measles are most important for young children. The heaviest burden of HIV/AIDS and TB are in people who are 15 to 59 years old, although there is also a substantial TB burden for people older than that. In **Table 12-4**, one can see the leading causes of deaths from communicable diseases in low- and middle-income countries, by broad age group.

There are relatively small differences in the distribution of deaths from communicable diseases between males and females in low- and middle-income countries. However, it

TABLE 12-3 Leading Causes of Death from Selected Communicable Diseases, 2010, by Number of Deaths in Thousands

Condition	World	Low- and Middle-Income Countries
Lower Respiratory Conditions	2,814	2,341
HIV/AIDS	1,465	1,370
Diarrheal Diseases	1,446	1,413
Tuberculosis	1,196	1,150
Malaria	1,170	1,170
Measles	125	125

Data from Institute for Health Metrics and Evaluation (IHME). (2013). GBD Heat map. Seattle, WA: IHME, University of Washington. Retrieved December 29, 2014, from http://vizhub.healthdata.org/irank/heat.php.

FIGURE 12-1 Deaths from Communicable Diseases, as Percent of Total Deaths, by World Bank Region and for High-Income Countries, 2010

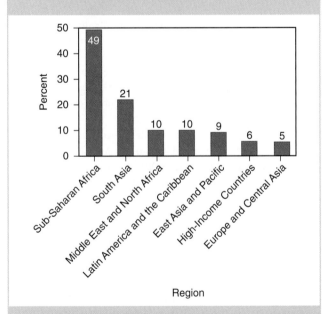

Data from Institute for Health Metrics and Evaluation (IHME). GBD Compare. Seattle, WA: IHME, University of Washington, 2013. http://vizhub.healthdata.org/gbd-compare. Accessed December 29, 2014.

TABLE 12-4 Leading Causes of Death in Low- and Middle-Income Countries by Broad Age Group, 2010, as Percentage of Total Deaths

Under-5		Ages 5–14		Ages 15–49	
Cause	Percent of Total Deaths (%)	Cause	Percent of Total Deaths (%)	Cause	Percent of Total Deaths (%)
Lower respiratory infections	12.5	Diarrheal diseases	7.9	HIV/AIDS	12.8
Preterm birth complications	12.4	HIV/AIDS	7.5	Road injury	8.2
Malaria	10.0	Road injury	6.9	Tuberculosis	5.3
Diarrheal diseases	9.9	Malaria	6.7	Self-inflicted injuries	4.8
Sepsis and other infections	7.6	Lower respiratory infections	6.6	Ischemic heart disease	4.7
Neonatal encephalopathy	7.4	Typhoid and paratyphoid fevers	5.2	Interpersonal violence	3.8
Other neonatal disorders	5.2	Drowning	4.9	Cerebrovascular disease	3.5
Congenital anomalies	4.9	Meningitis	3.8	Lower respiratory infections	3.1
Protein-energy malnutrition	4.0	Congenital anomalies	2.4	Maternal disorders	3.1
Meningitis	3.0	Protein-energy malnutrition	2.3	Malaria	2.8

The IHME data for 15–19 year olds diverges in important ways from WHO data, especially regarding the importance of cerebrovascular disease in IHME data. Please consult Chapter 11 for WHO data.
Data from Institute for Health Metrics and Evaluation (IHME). (2013). GBD compare. Seattle, WA: IHME, University of Washington. Retrieved December 29, 2014, from http://vizhub.healthdata.org/gbd-compare.

TABLE 12-5 Leading Causes of Death in Low- and Middle-Income Countries by Sex, 2010, as Percentage of Total Deaths

Males		Females	
Cause	Percent of Total Deaths (%)	Cause	Percent of Total Deaths (%)
Ischemic heart disease	10.2	Cerebrovascular disease	11.3
Cerebrovascular disease	9.8	Ischemic heart disease	9.8
Chronic obstructive pulmonary disease	6.2	Lower respiratory infections	6.3
Lower respiratory infections	5.6	Chronic pulmonary obstructive disorder	5.9
Road injury	3.9	Diarrheal diseases	4.1
Tuberculosis	3.3	HIV/AIDS	3.6
HIV/AIDS	3.3	Diabetes mellitus	3.2
Diarrheal diseases	3.1	Malaria	3.0
Trachea, bronchus, and lung cancers	2.8	Tuberculosis	2.4
Malaria	2.8	Preterm birth complications	2.1

Data from Institute for Health Metrics and Evaluation (IHME). (2013). GBD compare. Seattle, WA: IHME, University of Washington. Retrieved December 29, 2014, from http://vizhub.healthdata.org/gbd-compare.

is consistently the case that TB generally affects males more than females, although TB is among the leading killers of women ages 15 to 49 in parts of sub-Saharan Africa, South Asia, Europe and Central Asia, and Andean Latin America.[6] It is also true that the HIV/AIDS epidemic is being increasingly feminized and that HIV/AIDS now ranks higher as a cause of death for women than it is for men. These facts are illustrated in **Table 12-5**.

THE COSTS AND CONSEQUENCES OF COMMUNICABLE DISEASES

The economic and social costs of communicable diseases are very high. First, these diseases constrain the health and development of infants and children, often by having an impact on their schooling and on their productivity as adult workers. Second, stigma and discrimination against people with HIV, those with TB, and those with a variety of other debilitating communicable diseases, such as leprosy and lymphatic filariasis, are strong and pervasive. Third, adults who suffer from the diseases discussed in this chapter suffer substantial losses in productivity and income. Fourth, families spend considerable sums of money trying to treat these illnesses. Fifth, high rates of communicable diseases in any country reduce investments in that country's development. Finally, as noted earlier, emerging and reemerging infectious diseases can have enormous economic consequences, far in excess of their impact on health.

THE LEADING BURDENS OF COMMUNICABLE DISEASES

The sections that follow examine emerging and reemerging infectious diseases and antimicrobial resistance, HIV, TB, malaria, diarrhea, and neglected tropical diseases. The chapter reviews the nature and magnitude of each of these causes, as well as who is affected by them, their risk factors, their social and economic consequences, and what can be done to address these problems in cost-effective ways. The chapter also discusses future challenges in addressing the most important communicable diseases.

Emerging and Reemerging Infectious Diseases and Antimicrobial Resistance

The Burden of Emerging and Reemerging Infectious Diseases

Throughout human history, new diseases have appeared periodically, sometimes wreaking substantial damage. The first recorded epidemic of the bubonic plague, for example, was in the 6th century. More recently, new diseases have emerged, such as the Ebola virus in 1976, HIV in the 1980s, severe acute respiratory syndrome (SARS) in the 1990s, and H5N1 influenza, commonly called "bird flu," which first appeared in humans in 2003. These new diseases are referred to as "emerging infectious diseases."[7,8] Some examples of emerging infectious diseases are shown in **Table 12-6**. It is important to note that some diseases, like those in the table, have infected only a limited number of people, while some other diseases that have emerged, such as HIV, have infected tens of millions of people.

Even as new diseases have emerged, some existing diseases have spread more widely in areas in which they had already been present, have spread to places in which they had not appeared before, or have taken on new forms. These diseases are referred to as "reemerging infectious diseases."[7,8] In recent years, there have been outbreaks of a number of reemerging infectious diseases, including West Nile virus in the Western Hemisphere; dengue fever, which spread from South America to the Caribbean and into the United States; cholera in South America, and Ebola in West Africa. Some examples of reemerging infectious diseases are given in **Table 12-7**.

Resistant forms of disease can emerge or reemerge when bacteria, parasites, and viruses are altered through mutation, natural selection, or the exchange of genetic material among strains and species.[9] The development of resistance is a natural phenomenon; however, it can be sped up by human action, as discussed further later in this chapter. It can also develop and spread faster than would otherwise be the case because of human inaction—the failure to address it in timely and effective ways. It took only a few years after penicillin was introduced, for example, before strains of bacteria that were susceptible to penicillin had become resistant to it. The drug of choice for malaria for many years, chloroquine, can no longer be used in most places, because the malaria there is resistant to it. **Table 12-8** shows when a sample of resistant strains of bacteria, viruses, and parasites were first detected.

Emerging and reemerging infectious diseases are excellent examples of critical health issues that are truly global. They can arise anywhere and at any time. They can spread, sometimes rapidly, within and across countries. Different countries, with the help of various international organizations and networks, have to work together in technically sound ways, and sometimes urgently, if the problem of these diseases is to be addressed effectively.

In fact, the threat of emerging and reemerging infectious diseases is continuous and has been called "a perpetual challenge."[7] One study examined 335 events related to emerging and reemerging infectious diseases that had occurred between 1940 and 2004.[10] This analysis revealed that about 60 percent of these events were related to zoonoses—the spread of infection from animals to humans. The study also indicated that most of those events came from wildlife and that wildlife were related to an increasing share of emerging and reemerging infections over time. About 23 percent were related to vector-borne diseases that are spread by arthropods, such as mosquitoes, ticks, or fleas. The Global Outbreak Alert and Response Network (GOARN) verified 578 outbreaks in 132 countries that occurred just between 1998 and 2001.[11]

The problem of drug resistance is also substantial. It is estimated that in 2013 about 480,000 people globally developed multidrug-resistant TB.[12] There is also resistance to all of the drugs that treat malaria. A study in Uganda showed that 100 percent of the samples of *Shigella*, a bacterium that causes diarrhea, were resistant to a drug that had been commonly used to treat it.[13] In addition, methicillin-resistant *Staphylococcus aureus*, commonly known as MRSA, which used to be of concern mainly in hospital settings, has now spread to the community in many countries.

The U.S. Institute of Medicine (IOM) carried out important assessments of emerging and reemerging infectious diseases in 1992 and 2003.[14] The IOM highlighted the most important factors that contribute to the emergence and reemergence of infectious diseases, which are summarized in **Table 12-9**.

It is clear that changes in these factors and change in their relationship with one another have been linked to the emergence and reemergence of infectious diseases. Change in the environment and land use, for example, can have a major impact on disease emergence. This could include the well-known example of Lyme disease in the suburban United States, as housing has pushed up against deer populations and deer ticks have spread Lyme disease to humans. The emergence of Ebola virus as populations have pushed up against tropical rain forests also shows the potential impact of environmental change on the emergence of disease. The increasing amounts of travel and commerce in food and

TABLE 12-6 Selected Examples of Emerging Infectious Diseases

Year of Outbreak	Disease	Place	Source
1967	Marburg	Germany and Yugoslavia	Centers for Disease Control and Prevention. *Known cases and outbreaks of Marburg hemorrhagic fever, in chronological order.* Retrieved February 26, 2015, from http://www.cdc.gov/vhf/marburg /resources/outbreak-table.html.
1976	Ebola	Zaire (Democratic Republic of Congo)	Centers for Disease Control and Prevention. *Known cases and outbreaks of Ebola hemorrhagic fever, in chronological order.* Retrieved February 26, 2015, from http://www.cdc.gov/vhf/ebola/outbreaks /history/chronology.html.
1993	Cryptosporidiosis	Milwaukee, United States	MacKenzie, W., Hoxie, N., Proctor, M., et al. (2004). A massive outbreak in Milwaukee of cryptosporidium infection transmitted through the public water supply. *New England Journal of Medicine, 331,* 161–197.
1993	Hantavirus	New Mexico, Arizona, Colorado, and Utah, United States	Centers for Disease Control and Prevention. *Tracking a mystery disease: Highlights of the discovery of hantavirus pulmonary syndrome.* Retrieved February 26, 2015, from http://www.cdc .gov/hantavirus/hps/history.html.
1996	Variant Creutzfeldt-Jakob disease (vCJD; mad cow disease)	United Kingdom	Centers for Disease Control and Prevention. New Variant CJD: Fact Sheet. Retrieved July 13, 2015, from http://www.cdc.gov/media/pressrel/fs020418 .htm.
1997	H5N1 (avian influenza)	Hong Kong, China	World Health Organization. Media centre. Fact sheet. *Avian Influenza.* Retrieved July 13, 2015, from http://www.who.int/mediacentre/factsheets /avian_influenza/en/.
1999	Nipah virus	Malaysia and Singapore	Centers for Disease Control and Prevention. *Nipah Virus (NiV).* Retrieved February 26, 2015, from http://www.cdc.gov/vhf/nipah/.
2002	SARS	China	Centers for Disease Control and Prevention. *Frequently asked questions about SARS.* Retrieved February 26, 2015, from http://www.cdc.gov/sars /about/faq.html.
2012	Middle East Respiratory Syndrome (MERS)	Arabian Peninsula	Centers for Disease Control and Prevention. *Middle East Respiratory Syndrome (MERS).* Retrieved January 1, 2015, from http://www.cdc.gov /coronavirus/MERS/about/index.html.

Data from Centers for Disease Control and Prevention. Middle East Respiratory Syndrome (MERS). Retrieved January 1, 2015, from http://www.cdc.gov /coronavirus/MERS/about/index.html.

TABLE 12-7 Selected Examples of Reemerging Infectious Diseases

Year of Outbreak	Disease	Place	Source
1994	Plague	India	Centers for Disease Control and Prevention. *International notes update: Human plague—India, 1994.* Retrieved August 31, 2010, from http://www.cdc.gov/mmwr/preview/mmwrhtml/00032992.htm.
1997	Cholera	Peru	World Health Organization. *1998—Cholera in Peru.* Retrieved August 31, 2010, from http://www.who.int/csr/don/1998_02_25/en/index.html.
1998	Rift Valley fever	Ethiopia	Food and Agriculture Organization of the United Nations. *Flare-up of Rift Valley Fever in the Horn of Africa.* Retrieved August 31, 2010, from http://www.fao.org/newsroom/en/news/2007/1000473/index.html.
2003	Human monkeypox	Texas, United States	Centers for Disease Control and Prevention. *Questions and answers about Monkeypox.* Retrieved August 31, 2010, from http://www.cdc.gov/ncidod/monkeypox/qa.htm.
2009	Dengue	Florida, United States	Centers for Disease Control and Prevention. *Locally acquired dengue—Key West, Florida, 2009–2010.* Retrieved August 31, 2010, from http://www.cdc.gov/mmwr/preview/mmwrhtml/mm5919a1.htm.
2014	Ebola	West Africa	World Health Organization. *Ebola virus disease fact sheet.* Retrieved January 1, 2015, http://www.who.int/mediacentre/factsheets/fs103/en/.

Data from Centers for Disease Control and Prevention. International Notes Update: Human Plague—India, 1994. Available at: http://www.cdc.gov/mmwr/preview/mmwrhtml/00032992.htm. Accessed August 31, 2010. World Health Organization. 1998—Cholera in Peru. Available at: http://www.who.int/csr/don/1998_02_25/en/index.html. Accessed August 31, 2010. Food and Agriculture Organization of the United Nations. Flare-up of Rift Valley Fever in the Horn of Africa. Available at: http://www.fao.org/newsroom/en/news/2007/1000473/index.html. Accessed August 31, 2010. Centers for Disease Control and Prevention. Monkeypox: Questions and Answers. Available at: http://www.cdc.gov/ncidod/monkeypox/qa.htm. Accessed August 31, 2010. Centers for Disease Control and Prevention. Locally Acquired Dengue—Key West, Florida, 2009–2010. Available at: http://www.cdc.gov/mmwr/preview/mmwrhtml/mm5919a1.htm. Accessed August 31, 2010. World Health Organization. Ebola virus disease fact sheet. Available at: http://www.who.int/mediacentre/factsheets/fs103/en/. Accessed January 1, 2015.

other goods also have the potential to spread communicable diseases more rapidly than ever. Improvements in technology may yield many benefits. Yet, they might also create the conditions for the emergence of disease, such as Legionnaire's disease in the cooling towers of air conditioners.[15]

The factors that contribute to the development of drug resistance are well known. They include:[16,17]

- The increasing use of drugs
- Poor prescribing and dispensing practices
- Inappropriate use of the drugs by prescribers, dispensers, and patients
- Failure of patients to take appropriate doses of drugs

- The use of counterfeit or poor quality drugs that do not contain the appropriate level of therapeutic ingredients
- Too much use of antibiotics in agriculture, cattle and poultry raising, and fish farming
- Weak health systems, with poor laboratory capacity to diagnose disease and test for drug susceptibility

Some of the factors that might contribute to the more rapid spread of resistant forms of disease include:[16,18,19]

- Weak infection control in healthcare settings
- Poor sanitation and hygiene
- A lack of surveillance, leading to late detection of the disease

TABLE 12-8 Selected Examples of Drug Resistance, by Disease

Disease	Resistant Drug	Place	Description	Source
HIV	Any first-line drug	New York City, New York, United States	Primary resistance was 24.1% in 2003–2004.	Nugent, R., Back, E., & Beith, A. (2010, June 14). *The race against drug resistance*. Retrieved August 31, 2010, from http://www.cgdev.org/content/publications/detail/1424207.
		United Kingdom	Primary resistance was 19.2% in 2003.	Nugent et al.
Malaria	Chloroquine	Iran	Median failure rate in the presence of *Plasmodium falciparum* was 72.5% in 1996–2004.	Nugent et al.
		Ecuador	Median failure rate in the presence of *P. falciparum* was 85.4% in 1996–2004.	Nugent et al.
	Sulfadoxine-pyrimethamine	Philippines	Median failure rate in the presence of *P. falciparum* was 42.6% in 1996–2004.	Nugent et al.
		Myanmar	Median failure rate in the presence of *P. falciparum* was 27.8% in 1996–2004.	Nugent et al.
Multidrug-resistant tuberculosis (MDR-TB)	At least isoniazid and rifampicin	New York City, New York, United States	In this outbreak in the early 1990s, 1 in 10 cases of TB was MDR-TB.	Global Alliance for TB Drug Development. *Multidrug-resistant TB*. Retrieved February 26, 2015, from http://www.tballiance.org/why/mdr-xdr.php.
		Russia	16.3% of TB cases in Russia were MDR-TB in 2007–2008.	World Health Organization. *Multidrug and extensively drug-resistant TB (M/XDR-TB): 2010 Global report on surveillance and response*. Retrieved February 26, 2015, from http://www.who.int/tb/features_archive/m_xdrtb_facts/en/.

TABLE 12-8 Selected Examples of Drug Resistance, by Disease (*continued*)

Methicillin-resistant *Staphylococcus aureus* (MRSA)	Beta-lactams (methicillin and other common antibiotics such as oxacillin, penicillin, and amoxicillin)	Colombia	Over 50% of *S. aureus*–infected individuals carried resistant strains in 2006.	Nugent et al.
		Japan	Over 50% of *S. aureus*–infected individuals carried resistant strains in 2006.	Nugent et al.
Pneumonia	Penicillin	Israel, Poland, Romania, Spain	Over 25% of *S. pneumoniae* isolates were resistant in 2002.	Nugent et al.
		France	Over 53% of *S. pneumoniae* isolates were resistant in 2002.	Nugent et al.
	Erythromycin	Vietnam	92% resistance rate in 2001.	Nugent et al.
		Taiwan	86% resistance rate in 2001.	Nugent et al.

Data from Nugent, R., Back, E., & Beith, A. (2010). Center for Global Development. The Race Against Drug Resistance. Retrieved August 31, 2010, from http://www.cgdev.org/content/publications/detail/1424207; Global Alliance for TB Drug Development. Drug-Resistant TB. Retrieved August 31, 2010, from http://www.tballiance.org/why/mdr-tb.php; World Health Organization. Multidrug and Extensively Drug-Resistant TB (M/XDR-TB): 2010 Global Report on Surveillance and Response. Retrieved April 29, 2011, from http://www.who.int/tb/features_archive/world_tb_day_2010/en/index.html.

TABLE 12-9 Key Factors Contributing to the Emergence and Reemergence of Infectious Diseases

Microbial adaption and change
Human susceptibility to infection
Climate and weather
Changing ecosystems
Economic development and land use
Human demographics and behavior
Technology and industry
International travel and commerce
Breakdown of public health measures
Poverty and social inequality
War and famine
Lack of political will
Intent to harm

Data from Smolinski MI, Hamburg MA, Lederberg J, eds. Microbial Threats to Health. Washington DC: The National Academies Press; 2004:4–7.

It is important to highlight that weaknesses in public health measures or breakdowns in public health services can also contribute in a number of ways to the emergence and reemergence of infectious diseases, including the development and spread of drug resistance. During the Ebola outbreak in West Africa in 2014 and 2015, for example, already weak health systems were even less able to combat communicable diseases such as malaria. In addition, from the end of World War II until the advent of HIV, there was an increasing sense in high-income countries that "infectious diseases had been conquered."[20] As a consequence, many countries scaled back their attention to such diseases, including TB. This reduction of attention to TB was associated, for example, with a resurgence of TB and drug-resistant TB in a number of settings, such as in New York City in the late 1980s.[20]

The Consequences of Emerging and Reemerging Infectious Diseases

The costs of emerging and reemerging diseases have varied considerably but have sometimes been very large, as shown in **Table 12-10**. In each of these cases, there were direct costs of caring for those affected, such as the costs of hospitalization. In addition, there were substantial indirect costs. The 1991 cholera epidemic in Peru, for example, led to a decline in people's social activities and their normal expenditures and had a major impact on the local economy. It also led to a substantial decline in tourism in a country in which this sector plays an important role. The plague in India in 1994 led to a significant short-term decline in trade and commerce between India and the rest of the world. The U.K. government had to kill livestock to eliminate the possibility of mad cow disease and to convince a world that would not eat beef from the United Kingdom that this beef would be safe in the future. SARS led to a worldwide fear of a pandemic and to major reductions in trade, travel, and commerce between parts of Asia and the rest of the world. SARS also had an impact on the economy of Canada, after travelers received a warning from WHO about the risk of SARS in that country.[8] The World Bank estimated that the Ebola outbreak in 2014 in West Africa could cause the economies of Guinea, Liberia, and Sierra Leone to grow by 2.1, 3.4, and 3.3 percent less than they would have grown in the absence of Ebola.[21]

It is important to note that these costs are not in proportion to deaths from these events. Between 1990 and 1998, for example, only 41 people died in the United Kingdom of mad cow disease.[8] Although SARS generated great fears, only 774 deaths were caused by this disease.[22] Ebola had infected about 22,000 people in Guinea, Liberia, and Sierra Leone and had killed about 8,600 people by the middle of January 2015. It had also had extensive social and economic impacts. The costs of these events appear to be related to the fear of possible spread rather than the actual morbidity and mortality caused by the disease.

The costs and consequences of drug resistance are also very high. The average cost of treating a case of drug-resistant TB has been estimated in one study to be about 175 times the cost of treating a case that is susceptible to first-line drugs.[16] WHO has recently noted that the average costs of treating drug-susceptible TB in high-burden countries ranged from about $100 to $500, whereas the costs of treating drug-resistant TB ranged from around $9,000 to $49,000.[3] The lowest cost of curing a patient of malaria with artemisinin-based combination therapy (ACT) is about 10 times the cost of curing a patient with chloroquine.[23] The cost of treating someone for certain infections with amoxicillin/clavulanic acid can be 25 to 60 times more expensive than treating them with penicillin. In addition, people are sicker longer and sometimes die, as health providers try to find drugs to which these diseases are susceptible. Moreover, the use of some drugs actually encourages the development of resistance to other drugs, making it harder to treat some conditions.[16]

Addressing Emerging and Reemerging Infectious Diseases

In some respects, the development of emerging and reemerging infectious diseases, including antimicrobial resistance, is inevitable, given that it partially arises as a result of natural processes. On the other hand, we do have control over some of the factors that help to drive the development of these

TABLE 12-10 Selected Examples of the Economic Costs of Emerging and Reemerging Infectious Diseases

Disease	Country	Year(s)	Cost
Cholera epidemic	Peru	1991	$771 million
Plague	India	1994	$1.7 billion
Mad cow disease	United Kingdom	1990–1998	$30 billion
Anthrax	United States	2001	$1 billion
SARS	Asia	2003	$30 billion

Data from World Health Organization. Infectious Diseases Across Borders: The International Health Regulations. Geneva: WHO; 2007.

diseases. In principle, for example, population pressure on the environment could be reduced and land use planning could limit destruction of animal habitats. In practice, however, these approaches will require substantial change in the way people live and will not occur unless incentives are in place and reasonable alternatives exist. There are also many ways we can more appropriately use drugs. The use of drugs can also be decreased when they are not needed.[10,24]

Thus, even as people work both within and across countries to change some of the structural factors that drive the emergence and reemergence of infectious diseases, they can take more immediate actions to reduce these threats and the threat of antimicrobial resistance. Some measures to address these problems will have to be taken within nations but others will require international action.

The foundation for strengthening the capacity to address emerging and reemerging infectious diseases has to focus on "highly sensitive national surveillance systems, public health laboratories that can rapidly detect outbreaks caused by emerging and reemerging infections, and mechanisms that permit timely containment."[8] This must also be coupled with the willingness of countries to share information about disease outbreaks in a timely manner with other countries. There is also a need for global coordination of these efforts.

Disease surveillance is based on GOARN, a network of existing disease surveillance networks established in 2000.[25] Those who participate in it include an array of technical institutions, networks, and organizations that can contribute information to the global network, such as United Nations agencies, the International Federation of Red Cross and Red Crescent Societies, and Doctors Without Borders. WHO coordinates the network, building on the resources of its participants.

WHO published an updated version of the International Health Rules (IHR) in 2005.[25] The IHR laid out a framework that is intended to guide national and global efforts at strengthening surveillance capacity and the national and global capacity to respond to outbreaks. They make provisions for generating and reviewing information about disease outbreaks from a variety of sources, including both official sources and information from nonstate actors. This approach is meant to broaden the potential sources of information about outbreaks and overcome risks that would be posed by states that do not want to share information in a timely manner about disease outbreaks within their own country.

National action and global cooperation on disease surveillance and response were tested during an outbreak of H1N1 swine flu in Mexico in 2009, which was thought to pose a serious risk of becoming a global pandemic. In this case, the Mexican government did report the outbreak to WHO in a timely manner, there was a rapid global response coordinated by WHO, and a vaccine was developed quickly against this virus. However, when a pandemic did not come about, there was some criticism of WHO for exaggerating the risks that this outbreak posed.[26] Nonetheless, it appears that the response of Mexico in this case was considerably more helpful to the world than the long delay that China had in notifying the world about its SARS outbreak in 2003.

National and global capacity was also tested during the 2014 and 2015 Ebola outbreak in West Africa. In this case, Guinea, Liberia, and Sierra Leone were unable to respond adequately, given the weak governance and health systems in those countries. In addition, the international community appeared to respond very slowly and long after assistance should have first been provided. The reasons for this will continue to be examined, but the poor international response appears to have stemmed, among other things, at least partly from budget and staff cuts to the appropriate units of WHO in Geneva and weaknesses in the Africa office of WHO.[27]

In many ways, global efforts to address drug resistance have been inadequate. There has been some progress in addressing resistance on a disease-by-disease basis, such as efforts to better diagnose, track, and treat drug-resistant TB or drug-resistant malaria. There have also been countries, particularly in Europe, that have sought to reduce the use of antibiotics. Nonetheless, the world has continued to fail to establish a well-coordinated mechanism that can work across countries and diseases to address, in a coherent and effective manner, the factors that drive the development of drug resistance.[16] Some believe that this is a critical failure that places the world at grave risk of additional threats from resistant forms of disease and a real risk of running out of antibiotics and other drugs that can effectively address such diseases.

The Center for Global Development in Washington, DC convened a Drug Resistance Working Group from 2007 to 2010. The final report of the group made a number of recommendations about how the world might more forcefully move against drug resistance. These are shown in **Table 12-11**.

WHO prepared a major report on antimicrobial resistance that was published in 2012.[28] WHO proposed that, to better combat antimicrobial resistance, countries should adopt a policy package that would include:[29]

- A comprehensive national plan that would be financed, would engage civil society, and for which the government would be accountable
- Improved surveillance and laboratory capacity
- Uninterrupted access to essential medicines of assured quality

TABLE 12-11 Key Recommendations from the Center for Global Development Drug Resistance Working Group on Addressing Drug Resistance

- Improve surveillance by collecting and sharing resistance information across networks of laboratories.
- Establish an expert technical working group to develop, maintain, and monitor global standards for postmarketing drug quality and ensure that publicly funded drug procurement requires adherence to this standard.
- Create a new partnership of associations of medicine providers, regulators, and others involved in the drug supply chain to promote quality-assured provision of drugs, with accreditation of suppliers and better information to consumers.
- Strengthen national drug regulatory authorities in low- and middle-income countries.
- Catalyze research and development of resistance-fighting technologies by creating a web-based marketplace for the sharing of research in this area.

Data from Nugent R, Beck E, Beith A. The Race Against Drug Resistance. Washington DC: Center for Global Development; 2010.

- The regulation and promotion of rational use of medicines, including in animal husbandry
- Improved infection control
- The fostering of innovation in the fight against resistance

The Lancet also established an infectious disease commission, which issued in 2013 a major study of antimicrobial resistance. The commission suggested a plan of action against drug resistance that included the need for:[30]

- Studies of the economic burdens of drug resistance
- A global surveillance system for resistance
- Better regulation and stricter monitoring of prescribing practices for antibiotics
- Enhanced education of the public of the dangers of overprescribing antibiotics
- The phaseout of the use of antibiotics for animal husbandry
- The development of new models for research and development on antibiotics
- Improved governance of antibiotics, both nationally and globally

Future Challenges

An important question concerns the extent to which diseases are emerging and reemerging more rapidly than before, given the pace of changes in our environment and the increasing globalization of travel, trade, and transport. A detailed analysis of this question concluded that between 1940 and 2004, the number of occurrences of emerging and reemerging infectious diseases did increase over time and peaked in the 1980s, probably in association with the spread of HIV.[7,10] In addition, when considering measures to address emerging and reemerging infectious diseases, it is critical to remember that, for diseases that spread from human to human, there may be only a limited window for action after an outbreak begins if a pandemic is to be averted.[8] There is also a growing concern about the potential impact of the recent economic crises in the United States and Europe on the ability or willingness of governments to fund critical public health services. This is despite the fact that the potential economic consequences of possible disease outbreaks should make them more willing, rather than less willing, to address such threats during times that are already economically distressed.

Indeed, the factors that contribute to the emergence and reemergence of infectious diseases are becoming more prominent in some places. Infectious disease specialists predict that in the face of rapidly evolving and adapting pathogens, continued population growth, popular encroachment into areas with forests and wildlife, and climate change, new diseases will emerge and already known diseases will reemerge at an increasing pace.[31,32]

In addition, these tendencies will be exacerbated by poverty, environmental degradation, war, or the lack of effective public health interventions. Public health specialists also believe that the world must be vigilant about the possibility that a major pandemic could arise from a newly emerging or reemerging infectious disease. This could be the case, for example, with H5N1 influenza if that virus developed the ability to spread more efficiently from human to human.[10,20,24]

The development of drug resistance is also accelerating and spreading to places where it has not been prevalent before.[17] This stems partly from the growing use of antibiotics in low- and middle-income countries, as some of them have witnessed significant economic growth and increasing levels of education. It also reflects, however, that this increasing use is taking place in environments in which the other drivers of resistance have not yet been managed effectively.[16]

Of course, once drug-resistant forms of bacteria, viruses, or parasites do develop, they can spread more easily than ever, given the extent to which people travel, for example.[19]

In addition, the behaviors in which people engage can also have an important bearing on the spread of resistant forms of microbes, such as people's failure to adhere to drug regimens or their use of poor quality drugs.

The problem of drug resistance is also compounded by the limited number of new anti-infective drugs that are under development and the speed with which even new drugs become subject to resistance.[16] In addition, there has been insufficient research and development for drugs to combat some of the most important burdens of disease for the poor in low- and middle-income countries, including those for which there is increasing resistance. Until recently, for example, almost all of the existing TB drugs were at least 40 years old.

HIV/AIDS

The Burden of HIV/AIDS

Rarely has a single pathogen had a greater impact on the human condition than HIV. Some of the basic facts about HIV/AIDS are presented in **Table 12-12**. HIV is a virus that can be spread through:

- Unprotected sex—primarily vaginal and anal intercourse
- Mother-to-child transmission, during birth or through breastfeeding
- Blood, including by transfusion, needle sharing, or accidental needle stick
- Transplantation of infected tissue or organs

TABLE 12-12 HIV/AIDS Basic Facts: 2013

Number of people living with HIV/AIDS: 35.0 million

Number of pregnant women living with HIV: 1.5 million

Prevalence among adults 15–49: 0.8%

Number of new HIV infections: 2.1 million

Children under 15 newly infected with HIV: 240,000

Global distribution of new infections: 1.5 million in the WHO Africa Region, 116,000 in the South-East Asia Region, 160,000 in the Region of the Americas, 100,000 in the Western Pacific Region, 140,000 in the European Region

Number of HIV-related deaths: 1.5 million

Number of HIV-positive people being treated with antiretroviral therapy (ART): 12.9 million

Proportion of all adults living with HIV receiving ART: 38%

Proportion of all children living with HIV receiving ART: 24%

UNAIDS fast track targets: By 2020, have only 500,000 new infections per year and "90-90-90" (90% of people living with HIV knowing their status, 90% of people who know their status being treated, and 90% of those being treated having a suppressed viral load)

Data from World Health Organization. (2014). Global update on the health sector response to HIV. Retrieved January 7, 2015, from http://apps.who.int/iris/bitstr eam/10665/128494/1/9789241507585_eng.pdf?ua=1; Prevalence estimate from World Health Organization. Global Health Observatory. Retrieved January 7, 2015, from http://www.who.int/gho/hiv/epidemic_status/prevalence/en/; Estimates for the proportion of adults and children receiving ART from UNAIDS and targets from UNAIDS. Fast track ending the AIDS epidemic by 2030. (2015). http://www.unaids.org/sites/default/files/media_asset/JC2686_WAD2014report_en.pdf.

Being an uncircumcised male increases the risk of acquiring HIV. Females are also at greater biological and social risk than males of being infected with HIV. Having a sexually transmitted disease also increases the risk of HIV infection.

The efficiency with which the virus is transmitted varies. The virus is spread most efficiently from exposure to infected blood products and through the sharing of infected needles. There is a 90 percent probability of being infected by a transfusion of blood from an HIV-positive person.[33] The efficiency of transmission is also relatively high from sharing needles with an HIV-infected person. Sexual transmission depends on the type of sexual act and whether the HIV-positive person is male or female. Male-to-female transmission is higher than female-to-male transmission. The risk of unprotected receptive anal intercourse is about 30 times greater than it is for receptive or insertive vaginal intercourse.[33]

HIV attacks the human immune system. The time from becoming infected until one is diagnosed with AIDS varies. However, without treatment for HIV, about half of those infected will be diagnosed with AIDS in 10 years. Infectiousness is high during the initial period of infection and also increases as the immune system weakens and in the presence of other sexually transmitted infections.[34]

As the immune system of an HIV-positive person deteriorates, that person will suffer from a variety of what are called opportunistic infections, because they take advantage of the person's compromised immunity. As their disease reaches a fairly advanced state, HIV-positive people who are not on antiretroviral therapy may fall ill with TB, herpes infections, a variety of cancers, and an array of significant communicable diseases such as toxoplasmosis and cryptococcal meningitis, which has become a major killer of those infected with HIV.[33]

The main routes of transmission of HIV vary by location. In the first phases of the epidemic in high-income countries and in Brazil, HIV was largely spread through unprotected sex among men who have sex with men. In sub-Saharan Africa, the disease has been spread overwhelmingly through unprotected sex between men and women, especially among those engaging in high-risk behaviors, such as sex workers and their clients and men engaging in sex with multiple female partners. In China, the epidemic was originally centered in a group of people who received transfusions from blood that had been infected with the blood of HIV-positive people. From there, it spread largely through sex between men and women but also through injecting drug use. In Russia and much of the former Soviet Union, the epidemic is driven by injecting drug users who are HIV-positive and who share needles. The epidemic is spreading from them to other groups largely through unprotected sex.

When HIV first appears in a population, it is generally concentrated in certain key populations, such as sex workers, men who have sex with men, and injecting drug users. These groups were earlier referred to as "groups engaging in high risk behaviors," "high-risk groups," or "most at risk populations." If the virus is controlled in these groups, then the spread to the general population can be limited. However, if it is not controlled, then the epidemic becomes more widespread in the general population and prevalence can be quite high. Cambodia has an epidemic that is concentrated. South Africa and Zimbabwe, for example, have epidemics that have broadly spread in the population.

It is estimated that about 35 million people worldwide were infected with the HIV virus in 2013 and that about 1.5 million people that year suffered AIDS-related deaths.[35] It is also estimated that about 2.1 million people were newly infected with HIV in 2013.[35] About 32 million of the 35 million infections were among adults and about 3.3 million among children. Fifty-five percent of the adults who are infected are females. Of the 1.5 million AIDS-related deaths in 2013, 1.4 million were among adults. With about 25 million infections, sub-Saharan Africa has about 70 percent of total infections worldwide and about 80 percent of the AIDS-related deaths.[35]

The prevalence of HIV varies considerably by region and by country. The prevalence rate of HIV by country is shown in **Figure 12-2**.

The region with the highest prevalence rate of HIV/AIDS is sub-Saharan Africa, where 4.7 percent of the adults 15–49 years of age are HIV-positive. The region with the next highest adult prevalence rate is Eastern Europe and Central Asia,[35] at 0.7 percent. Relatively high rates of HIV/AIDS are found in central and southern Africa, as high as 26 percent in Swaziland and 23 percent in Lesotho and Botswana. South Africa has an adult prevalence rate of about 18 percent. Outside of sub-Saharan Africa, there are only a few countries with HIV prevalence over 1 percent, including Haiti, Belize, Guyana, Suriname, Djibouti, and Thailand.[35]

Thirty-nine percent of new HIV infections in 2012 were among those ages 15 to 24.[36] They also occur among infants due to maternal-to-child transmission. In the high-income countries, efforts have been made to address maternal-to-child transmission, and there are almost no such cases any longer. In the highest prevalence countries, maternal-to-child transmission continues, although there has been important progress in reducing it. In fact, the number of children newly infected fell by about 35 percent between 2009 and 2012.[35]

The number of new HIV infections peaked globally in 1999. The number of new infections among adults in low- and middle-income countries fell by 30 percent between

FIGURE 12-2 HIV Prevalence by Country, 2013

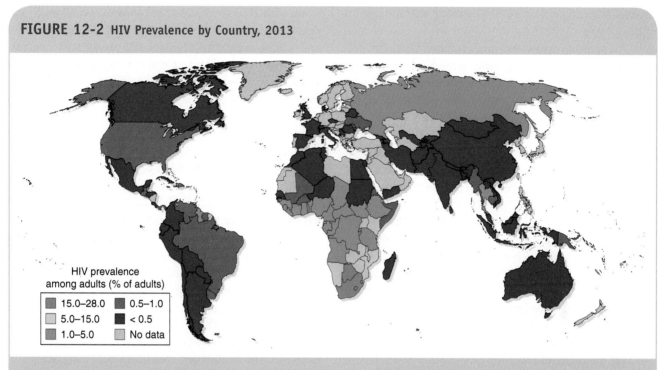

HIV prevalence
among adults (% of adults)

- 15.0–28.0
- 5.0–15.0
- 1.0–5.0
- 0.5–1.0
- < 0.5
- No data

Data from UNAIDS. AIDSinfo: HIV prevalence among adults. Retrieved January 28, 2015, from http://www.unaids.org/en/dataanalysis/datatools/aidsinfo; The United States prevalence estimate from UNAIDS. United States: HIV and AIDS Estimates (2012). Retrieved January 28, 2015, from http://www.unaids.org/en/regionscountries/countries/unitedstatesofamerica/; The Argentina estimate is from UNAIDS. Argentina: HIV and AIDS Estimates (2012). Retrieved January 28, 2015, from http://www.unaids.org/en/regionscountries/countries/argentina/; The France estimate is from UNAIDS. France: HIV and AIDS Estimates (2012). Retrieved January 28, 2015, from http://www.unaids.org/en/regionscountries/countries/france/; The Canada estimate is from UNAIDS. HIV and AIDS Estimates (2012). Retrieved January 29, 2015, from http://www.unaids.org/en/regionscountries/countries/canada/; The Russian estimate is from World Health Organization. World Health Statistics. France: World Health Organization, 2011. The Chinese estimate is from UNAIDS. HIV in China: Facts & Figures.

2001 and 2012. Moreover, rates of HIV among adults declined by over 50 percent between 2001 and 2012 in 26 low- and middle-income countries. However, the rates of new infection are growing in Eastern Europe and Central Asia and in the Middle East and North Africa.[35]

The *Global Burden of Disease Study 2010* indicated that HIV was the sixth leading cause of death for all age groups globally but the second leading cause of death in sub-Saharan Africa. For people aged 15–49 in sub-Saharan Africa, HIV was the leading cause of death. HIV was the fifth leading cause of DALYs globally, the second for all age groups in sub-Saharan Africa, but the first for people aged 15–49 in sub-Saharan Africa.[37]

HIV Treatment

The global community has made a commitment to trying to ensure that all people with HIV are placed on treatment as soon as they become clinically eligible, which WHO defined in its 2010 guidelines as having a CD4 cell count below 350, revised in 2013 to 500.[38] In the last decade, there has been an enormous amount of progress in getting people with HIV on treatment. By the end of 2012, about 9.7 million people were

on treatment, of whom 1.6 million were placed on treatment in 2012.[38] Using the 2010 guidelines as a benchmark, 61 percent of all persons in low- and middle-income countries who were eligible for treatment were on treatment.[35] However, if one uses the 2013 guidelines as a benchmark, then only 34 percent of the eligible adults in low- and middle-income countries are being treated. In addition, there have been persistent gaps in the coverage of pregnant women, men, and children.[35]

The Costs and Consequences of HIV

HIV has significant social and economic consequences, especially in high prevalence countries in sub-Saharan Africa, which go beyond its impact on morbidity and mortality. HIV affects family cohesion, business, trade, labor, the armed forces, agricultural production, education systems, governance, public services, and even national security.

In the absence of treatment, a person infected with HIV will eventually become sicker, progress to full-blown AIDS, and suffer from a variety of opportunistic infections, as noted previously. As this happens, the person becomes less able to work, loses part or all of his or her income, and becomes dependent on others for care. The caretaker may also lose his or her income.

This cycle has caused enormous economic losses to individuals and their families, especially in sub-Saharan Africa. A study done in Tanzania, for example, indicated that men with AIDS lost an average of 297 days of work over an 18-month period, and women lost an average of 429 days of work over that same period, which implies that these women were essentially unable to attend to any of their normal tasks.[39] A study in Thailand showed that families that suffered from AIDS lost an average of 48 percent of their income as a result of their illness.[40]

Another important consequence of HIV is the creation of a large number of orphans, defined as an individual 15 years old or younger who has lost one or both parents to the disease. UNICEF estimated in 2012 that there were close to 19 million "AIDS orphans."[41] Despite efforts by many families to care for their relatives, many orphans do not have anyone with whom to live and may resort to living on the street, where they are at risk of falling into commercial sex or crime.

Like a number of other communicable diseases, HIV is a highly stigmatized condition. HIV, however, has a special stigma because people in many societies believe that people acquire HIV by engaging in behaviors that society does not sanction, such as men having sex with men, commercial sex work, or injecting drug use. Understanding the notion of stigma and discrimination against people with HIV/AIDS is central to understanding the epidemic.

In fact, over the course of the epidemic, stigmatization of HIV/AIDS in many societies has led to an unwillingness to allow people with HIV to attend schools or be employed, get health care, live in certain places, or even live with their families. Stigma has also been a major constraint to people's getting tested or treated for HIV. It has also complicated prevention efforts in some settings by driving underground some of the very people it is important to reach, such as sex workers and injecting drug users.

For the poorest countries, the direct cost of AIDS treatment is very expensive compared to per capita income and per capita health expenditure, even at the reduced prices for those drugs that have been agreed upon globally. In 2014, the lowest price available for first-line therapy by low- and middle-income countries was about $140 per patient per year.[42] A study of the costs of antiretroviral therapy to reduce maternal-to-child transmission found that the median cost in low-income countries per case of maternal-to-child transmission averted was about $800.[43] Although these costs are dramatically lower than before, many of the lowest-income countries that are providing antiretroviral therapy to people living with HIV spend less per capita on health each year than the costs of HIV treatment.[44] Thus, it will be difficult for low-income countries with high HIV prevalence to support the costs of such treatment without considerable and sustained external assistance.[45] This question is explored later in this chapter in the policy and program brief on the long-term costs and financing of HIV/AIDS.

Many studies have been done on the potential impact of HIV on the economic growth of different countries. Some of these have helped convince governments that failure to address HIV early could result in lower economic growth of their country. Overall, the early studies suggested that HIV would have a large impact on the economic growth of high-prevalence countries in Africa, largely because HIV tends to strike people in their most productive years.[39] The higher the prevalence and the more families use their savings to help pay for the costs of illness, the more likely HIV will have a negative impact on the growth of per capita income.[46] Although these arguments make sense intuitively, there are very few recent studies that have tried to examine how rates of economic growth for different countries would have changed if they had lower rates of prevalence of HIV/AIDS.

Addressing the Burden of HIV/AIDS

Despite considerable and increasing efforts, there is not yet either a preventive or therapeutic vaccine for HIV. In the absence of such a vaccine, halting the spread of HIV will have to focus on the prevention of new infections.

Several countries had earlier prevention efforts that were considered successful, such as Cambodia, Thailand, and Uganda. Studies of the success of HIV/AIDS programs suggest that such successes have consistently been associated with a number of factors related to strong political leadership, commitment, and open communications, including:[33]

- Sustained political leadership at the highest levels
- Involvement of a broad range of civil society efforts to address HIV/AIDS, including opinion leaders and religious leaders
- Broad-based programs to change social norms in the population
- Open communication about HIV/AIDS and related sexual matters
- Programs to reduce stigma and discrimination

In addition, we also know that to be successful, efforts to address HIV/AIDS need to include:[33]

- Good epidemic surveillance
- Information, education, and communication
- Voluntary counseling and testing

- Condom promotion
- Screening and treatment for sexually transmitted infections
- Prevention of mother-to-child transmission through antiretroviral treatment and avoiding pregnancy
- Voluntary male medical circumcision
- Interventions that target populations that transmit the virus from high-risk to low-risk populations
- Prevention of bloodborne transmission through blood safety, harm reduction for injecting drug users, and universal precautions in healthcare settings.

In addition, these efforts should be linked with pre-exposure prophylaxis in selected populations. They should also be linked with efforts now being promoted globally to ensure that by 2020:[47]

- 90 percent of the people with HIV will know their HIV status
- 90 percent of those with HIV will be receiving anti-retroviral therapy
- 90 percent of those being treated will have suppressed viral loads.

At the same time, countries need to continue to address stigma and discrimination against HIV-affected people.

Additional comments follow on some of the interventions noted previously.

First, the approach to prevention will need to vary with the nature of the epidemic. In low-level and concentrated epidemics, some of the focus can be on changing the behaviors of those who engage in high-risk behaviors. The approach to prevention in a more generalized epidemic, however, will need to be broader.[33] Unfortunately, many countries have failed to align their investments in addressing HIV with the nature of their epidemics. In Asia, for example, 90 percent of the funds spent on youth were spent earlier on low-risk youth, who made up only 5 percent of the new infections.[48]

Second, there is an increasing understanding that prevention efforts have to include a combination of approaches, with different weight given to different activities, depending on the nature of the epidemic. These efforts will have to combine education and behavior change; biomedical approaches, such as male medical circumcision and drug therapy; and structural approaches, including measures such as improving income-earning opportunities and food security to reduce the risk of women engaging in transactional sex.

Education and behavior change efforts must focus on increasing correct knowledge of HIV, increasing the demand for HIV testing, later sexual debut, fewer sexual partners, and correct and consistent condom usage when engaging in high-risk sex. These activities are especially important in key populations, including sex workers and their clients and men who have sex with men.

These behavior change interventions need to be accompanied by efforts at harm reduction for injecting drug users. These are efforts to encourage the use of clean needles among injecting drug users, through needle exchange programs. They also include opioid substitution therapy to try to wean addicts off heroin.

There has also been increasing attention paid to trying to stem mother-to-child transmission of HIV. The most cost-effective measure to reduce mother-to-child transmission of HIV is to avoid unwanted pregnancies of HIV-positive women through contraception. Providing antiretroviral therapy to pregnant women infected with HIV in accordance with the WHO 2013 guidelines is also cost-effective.[49] If done properly, it can essentially eliminate mother-to-child transmission, whereas in the absence of such treatment, about one third of HIV-positive pregnant women will give birth to a baby who is HIV-positive.[50]

There is evidence that circumcised males are 40–60 percent less likely to be infected with HIV than uncircumcised males.[51] A number of voluntary medical male circumcision efforts are now under way as a component of HIV/AIDS prevention activities. Kenya has made important progress in this area and it will be important to learn from this and other experiences about the most cost-effective approaches to scaling up voluntary male medical circumcision in different settings.[52]

Ensuring that the blood supply is safe and free of the HIV virus, among other infectious agents, is cost-effective and must be a high priority in all settings.

As noted earlier, there has been substantial progress in low- and middle-income countries in placing HIV-infected people on antiretroviral therapy. Once patients are under treatment, it is exceptionally important that they take all of their drugs exactly as prescribed in order to avoid developing resistance and to stay as healthy as possible. If the drugs are discontinued because of interrupted supply, poor compliance by the patient, or poor performance of the health system, resistance may develop and the patient may require more expensive second-line drugs. Those infected with drug-resistant strains of HIV can also infect other people with those strains.

Overall, effective HIV/AIDS therapy depends on individuals accessing counseling and testing, a definitive HIV test, a clinical diagnosis of the patient, a laboratory assessment of the individual's immune status with a CD4 cell count, patient adherence to their drug regimen, sound patient nutrition, and sound and continuous monitoring and evaluation of the patient.

Critical Challenges in HIV/AIDS

A number of critical challenges constrain the fight against HIV/AIDS. First has been the difficulty of finding an HIV vaccine. Given the fact that there are about 1.5 million new infections a year, it is important to continue the search for a vaccine.[53] The search for a safe and effective microbicide must also continue.[54]

Second, although there has been a reduction in HIV incidence globally, the number of new infections annually suggests that it is essential that greater attention be paid to the prevention of such infections. More countries need to focus on prevention, with the political leadership and commitment that has been linked to the HIV success stories to date. We also need to ensure that countries invest in the most cost-effective approaches to prevention in their setting. As long as pregnant women continue to be infected, it is important to continue to scale up prevention of mother-to-child transmission. Greater attention must also be paid to the reduction of stigma among the most stigmatized groups, including men who have sex with men and injecting drug users.

The efforts to offer universal antiretroviral treatment for those eligible will continue. However, this work will confront weak health systems and a lack of trained health workers as it expands further. Successful early treatment of HIV reduces the patient's viral load to an imperceptible level, stems their transmission of HIV, and reduces the likelihood that the patient will contract a number of opportunistic infections, such as TB. Thus, it will be important to diagnose people as early as possible after they are infected, place them on treatment as early in their infection as possible, and ensure that their treatment is effective. This is part of a strategy that is increasingly thought of as treatment as prevention and part of the 90-90-90 goals noted earlier.[47]

Financing treatment, especially in low-income, high-prevalence countries in which there continues to be a substantial number of new infections, will be very difficult and require sustained external support for many years. This highlights the need to continue at every level to reduce the price of antiretroviral therapy as far as possible both for first line and second line treatment regimens.

Improving the management of TB and HIV co-infection will also be essential. This is discussed further in the section on TB that follows.

Tuberculosis

The Burden of Tuberculosis

Some of the basic facts concerning TB are noted in **Table 12-13.**

TABLE 12-13 TB Basic Facts: 2013

Number of people living with TB: 11.0 million

Number of new TB cases: 9.0 million

Number of TB deaths: 1.5 million

Proportion of new cases with multidrug-resistant TB: 3.5%

Estimated number of new multidrug-resistant TB cases, among notified patients: 300,000

Global distribution of prevalence by WHO region: 41% in South-East Asia, 21% in the Western Pacific Region, 25% in Africa, 9% in the Eastern Mediterranean Region, 4% in Europe, and 3% in the Americas

India had 24% of all global cases and China had 11%

Target of the Global Plan to Stop TB: By 2025, 75% reduction in TB deaths, compared with 2015 and also halve the TB incidence rate (to less than 55 TB cases per 100,000 population)

Data from WHO. Global tuberculosis report 2014. Retrieved January 6, 2015, from http://www.who.int/tb/publications/global_report/gtbr14 _main_text.pdf?ua=1.

Tuberculosis is caused by the bacteria *Mycobacterium tuberculosis*, and it is spread through aerosol droplets. People breathe in the TB bacteria that is transmitted from other people who are ill with tuberculosis disease. Tuberculosis can affect all organs of the body, but in about 80 percent of cases the infection is in the lungs.[12,55]

To get TB, one has to be exposed to someone with the disease. The likelihood of exposure is greater if you are living with people with active pulmonary TB disease, especially in crowded circumstances, such as slum dwellings or prisons. Homeless people are also more susceptible to becoming ill with TB. Conditions that weaken the immune system also make one more susceptible to developing active TB disease.[55,56]

An untreated person with active pulmonary TB can infect 10 to 15 people annually. About two-thirds of those with active TB disease will die of the disease if not treated properly. Pulmonary TB can be spread from person to person, but people with TB in other organs (extrapulmonary TB) generally do not spread TB. Active TB is characterized by a persistent cough for more than 3 weeks, decreased appetite, general weakness, and profuse night sweats.[12,55]

Not everyone infected with TB bacteria becomes sick with it. Rather, the TB remains latent in the bodies of about 90 percent of those infected and they will not develop TB disease. People with latent TB do not spread TB to others. About one-third of the world's population is infected with TB. It is estimated that the infection will break down to cause active TB in about 10 percent of those people, especially if the person is immune-compromised.[12] This could occur because of malnutrition, HIV infection, use of immune-suppressing drugs, or illness such as diabetes, or some cancers. Smoking is also a risk factor for TB disease.[12,56]

The relationship between TB and HIV is a very important public health issue. The *lifetime* risk of developing active TB for a person who is *not* infected with HIV is 10 percent. If a person is HIV-positive, however, the *annual* risk of developing active TB is much greater. People living with HIV, in fact, are about 30 times more likely to get TB than people who are HIV-negative. HIV is also associated with a higher proportion of TB that is not pulmonary, compared to TB that is not linked to HIV.[12]

The recommended approach for diagnosing drug-susceptible pulmonary TB in low- and middle-income countries has been bacteriology, either smear microscopy or culture examination. However, there is now an additional method drawing on bacteriological samples, which is rapid and can detect drug-susceptible or rifampicin-resistant disease: Xpert™ MTB/RIF. This test uses molecular techniques and is more sensitive and more specific than sputum smear microscopy. Diagnosing TB in HIV-positive people and children may require other clinical diagnostic processes, as does extrapulmonary TB, that are not discussed here.[3,12,57]

There are about 9 million new cases of TB each year. Africa has the highest estimated incidence rate with 280 new cases each year per 100,000 population. More than half of the new cases in the world, however, occur in the WHO regions of South-East Asia and the Western Pacific. In addition, India accounts for about 24 percent of all new cases and China 11 percent. About 60 percent of all new cases are among men.[3] Exposure and susceptibility are associated with gender-differences in TB burden, but there is variability in relative burden by sex in different age groups and in different settings.[6] Nonetheless, TB is also a leading killer of women, with more than 500,000 female deaths attributed to TB annually. In addition, about 80,000 HIV-negative children per year die of TB.[3]

Of the 9 million people who developed TB in 2013, about 1.1 million, or 13 percent, were HIV-positive. Eighty percent of these people were in the Africa region. However, the number of deaths associated with TB/HIV co-infection has been declining, as an increasing proportion of those with HIV have been placed on antiretroviral treatment, as discussed in the earlier section on HIV.[3]

In the 2010 study of the global burden of disease, TB was the 10th most important cause of death worldwide for all age groups and both sexes.[37] Seventy-five percent of the TB infections and deaths occur in the most productive age group—those who are 15 to 54 years old.[3,12] TB was the sixth leading cause of deaths for all age groups in sub-Saharan Africa in 2010 and the third leading cause of death among people in sub-Saharan Africa aged 15–49. TB was the 13th leading cause of DALYs globally among all age groups but the fifth leading cause of DALYs globally among those aged 15–49. For men in sub-Saharan Africa, TB was the fourth leading cause of DALYs.[37]

As the world has expanded its efforts against both TB and HIV, the incidence of TB has fallen by about 1.5 percent per year between 2000 and 2013. In addition, the TB mortality rate has dropped by about 45 percent between 2000 and 2013. TB prevalence also fell during that period by 41 percent. Global targets for TB include reduction in incidence, prevalence, and mortality. These are falling in all WHO regions. However, they are not falling fast enough to meet global targets in the Africa, Eastern Mediterranean, or European regions.[3]

There has been an increase in TB infections that are resistant to one or more TB drugs. These forms of TB are called drug-resistant TB, multidrug-resistant TB (MDR-TB), and extensively drug-resistant TB (XDR-TB). Almost 5 percent of the TB cases that were detected worldwide in 2013 were estimated to be multidrug resistant.[3] WHO defines multidrug resistant TB as "resistance to isoniazid and rifampicin, with or without resistance to other first-line drugs."[58] WHO defines extensively drug-resistant TB as "resistance to at least isoniazid and rifampicin, and to any fluoroquinolone, and to any of the three second-line injectables (amikacin, capreomycin, and kanamycin)."[58]

An underlying cause for the development of resistant forms of TB is the failure to complete TB treatment, as was the case for Maria in one of the opening vignettes. However, it is also possible to be infected with drug-resistant TB directly from another person. Drug-resistant strains are found in many countries and are difficult and expensive to treat. Drug resistance is especially important in countries in which drug regulation and TB programs are weak or have fallen into disarray, such as Eastern Europe, and the greatest burdens of drug resistant TB today are in Eastern Europe, China, and India.[3] In 2006, a number of cases of XDR-TB were found in South Africa among HIV patients, and 52 of 53 patients died within 25 days, despite being on HIV treatment. This caused considerable alarm in the public health community.[58]

The Costs and Consequences of TB

The cost of TB to families, communities, and countries is very high, given the large number of people who are sick with TB, the relatively long course of the illness, and the losses people face when they do have TB. A study of TB in India suggested that those sick with TB lost about 3 months of wages, spent an amount equal to about one quarter of national income per capita on care and treatment, and took on debts to pay for this care that were equal to about 10 percent of per capita income.[59] A similar study in Bangladesh indicated that those sick with TB lost 4 months of wages.[60] A Thai study showed that TB patients spent more than 15 percent of their annual wages on TB, 12 percent of them took out bank loans to help make up for the costs of their illness, and 16 percent sold part of their property to finance the costs of dealing with their illness.[61] A recent study found that TB patients lost about 60 percent of their individual annual income and 40 percent of household income due to TB and that falling ill with TB could be financially catastrophic to many families.[61]

There are also significant social costs associated with TB. Because of the stigma associated with TB, females who fall ill with TB in some parts of the world may be shunned by their families. In one Indian study, 15 percent of the women with TB faced familial rejection.[63] In another Indian study, 8 percent faced rejection.[58]

A study of the macroeconomic impact of TB suggested that the economic growth of a country is inversely correlated with the rate of TB. Every increase of 10 percent in the incidence of TB was associated with lower annual economic growth of 0.2–0.4 percent.[64] A study of the economic costs of TB in the Philippines indicated that the annual economic loss due to morbidity and premature mortality from TB was equal to almost $150 million. In addition, the cost to the Philippines of treating all of the expected cases of TB would be between $8 million and $29 million.[65]

Addressing the Burden of TB

A vaccine for TB called Bacillus Calmette–Guérin (BCG) is a standard part of the Expanded Program of Immunization for Children. The vaccine reduces severe TB in children, but because children are not important transmitters of TB and due to variable efficacy of the vaccine in different settings, the vaccine has little impact on the overall incidence or prevalence of TB.[66] Rather, the control of TB depends on effective treatment of active tuberculosis. In many respects, implementing a poor TB program is worse than having no TB program at all because a poor TB program can give rise to drug-resistant TB by enabling the use of drugs without quality of care.

WHO recommends a 6-month regimen for drug-susceptible disease that includes four drugs—isoniazid, rifampin, pyrazinamide, and ethambutol—for the first 2 months and then isoniazid and rifampin for the following 4 months.[67]

Once an active case of TB is identified, appropriate drugs are required in adequate supply for 6 months. Patient adherence with the TB regimen is required for effective therapy and patient-centered supportive supervision, and enablers are needed throughout the course of treatment. Part of this effort has focused on ensuring that someone, other than a family member, ensures that the TB patient takes their drugs. Healthcare workers, nongovernmental organization (NGO) staff, and community volunteers and leaders, such as teachers, religious leaders, and other community members, can support patients in treatment.[3]

Treating active drug-susceptible TB through an organized quality-assured care program is highly cost-effective, with fairly recent studies showing the cost ranging from $5 to $50 per DALY averted in most regions. The cost of treating a TB case, in fact, can be as low as $100 in a number of low-income countries, such as India and Myanmar. BCG is cost-effective in reducing severe cases of childhood TB in high prevalence settings. As noted in the section on antimicrobial resistance, the cost of treating drug-resistant TB can approach $50,000 per patient.[66]

The Management of TB/HIV Co-Infection

As noted in the section on HIV/AIDS, TB is an opportunistic infection of HIV. As the immune system of an HIV-positive person declines, TB is one of the diseases that can develop. This is especially so in populations where many people have latent TB. In addition, TB has been the leading cause of death of adults who are HIV-positive and not on antiretroviral therapy, although, as discussed in a policy brief later in the chapter, cryptococcal meningitis may now be responsible for more deaths of HIV-positive people in Africa than TB.

WHO recommends a number of measures to prevent and manage TB and HIV co-infection. These are generally referred to as "scaling up the three *Is*". They include:

- intensified case finding to ensure that all of those who are HIV-positive are tested for TB and all of those with TB are tested for HIV;

- giving isoniazid, an antibiotic, to people with HIV to help prevent their getting TB;
- enhancing infection control in healthcare settings so that TB does not spread among those who are infected with HIV.

There are still substantial gaps in many countries in managing TB/HIV co-infection in conjunction with these guidelines.[68,69]

Challenges in TB Prevention and Care

WHO has developed a new End TB Strategy, building on two previous global TB strategies from 1995 to 2015. The new strategy seeks to end the global TB epidemic by 2035, with a 95 percent reduction in TB deaths and a drop in incidence to 10 per 100,000 people. It also calls for the elimination of catastrophic costs for TB–affected families by 2020.

The strategy is based on expanding TB prevention and care through a focus on high-impact interventions in a patient-centered way, working with a wider array of public and private partners, pursuing policy shifts associated with universal health coverage, social protection and poverty alleviation, and pursuing basic research, development of new tools, and operational research. The strategy acknowledges the urgent need for better diagnostics and ways of treating latent TB. It also highlights the need for safer and easier drug regimens for active TB disease, as well as a new vaccine, to drive down deaths and incidence much more rapidly.[70]

Indeed, although there has recently been progress in improving TB diagnostics, one critical challenge in TB is the need to develop more effective vaccines, inexpensive and rapid diagnostics for all forms of TB, and drug therapy that will lessen the duration of treatment and the number of pills that patients have to take. A related challenge is to ensure that new tools, such as new diagnostics, are put into use and scaled up as rapidly as possible.

In some regions there also remains the need to diagnose more of those with TB, and in some regions, particularly Eastern Europe and Central Asia, there is a need to cure a larger share of those who are treated, with low treatment success heavily linked to the large burden of undetected drug-resistant disease. The MDR-TB response is underfunded, leaving a low capacity to diagnose cases, as well as ensure immediate and full quality treatment even if diagnosed.[3]

A considerable amount of TB diagnosis and treatment is carried out in the private sector, and often with very poor quality, such as using nonstandard drug regimens and little or no patient follow-up, and excessive diagnostic test charges. Improving TB diagnosis and treatment will require further

efforts at linking all providers of TB diagnosis and treatment with national TB control programs. There has been some important progress in this direction, but there remain enormous gaps for public–private partnerships to reach global targets, especially in Asia.[3]

There are still major gaps in the implementation of the WHO guidelines on the collaborative treatment of TB and HIV. Significant improvements are needed in a number of settings to strengthening collaboration between TB and HIV programs so that WHO guidelines can be put more firmly in place in all countries.[3]

The End TB Strategy also emphasizes the importance of further linking TB efforts with the strengthening of health systems and their coverage. This includes the improvement of laboratory services and infection control and further integrating TB care in at primary level, especially community-based care. The strategy also highlights the importance of promoting more community-based approaches to information and education about TB and the increased involvement of patients, communities, and civil society in TB efforts.[3]

Putting the new strategy in place will require additional financial and technical resources.[3] The fight against TB could face important challenges in finding the needed financial resources in the present global environment.

Malaria

The Burden of Malaria

Some basic facts about malaria are presented in **Table 12-14**.

Malaria is caused by parasites in the genus *Plasmodium*, five species of which infect humans: *P. falciparum*, *P. vivax*, *P. ovale*, *P. malariae*, and *P. knowlesi*. These parasite species exist in different proportions in different regions of the world. For example, *P. falciparum* dominates in Africa, *P. vivax* occurs in temperate zones, and *P. ovale* is found in South Asia and tropical Africa.[71] *P. knowlesi* is the least common form and primarily affects macaques. However, it can also infect humans, especially in forested areas of Southeast Asia.[72] Malaria is spread by the bite of the female *Anopheles* mosquito. Essentially, the mosquito carries the parasite from an infected person to an uninfected person.

In 2014, 97 countries had ongoing transmission of malaria and about half of all people in the world lived in places at risk of malaria. In addition, there were thought to be about 200 million cases of malaria in the world in 2014. About 80 percent of the cases occurred in Africa, 12 percent in Southeast Asia, and 5 percent in the Eastern Mediterranean region of WHO. Almost 550,000 people died of malaria in 2013. About 90 percent of the deaths were in Africa, and

TABLE 12-14 Malaria Basic Facts: 2013

Number of people at risk of malaria infection: 3.2 billion

Number of malaria cases: 198 million

Number of malaria-related deaths: 548,000

Global distribution of cases in selected WHO regions: 82% in Africa, 12% in South-East Asia, 5% in the Eastern Mediterranean Region

Burden of malaria-related deaths: 90% in Africa; 78% occurred in children under 5 years of age

Proportion of households owning at least one insecticide-treated bed net: 67%

Number of people protected through indoor residual spraying: 123 million

Roll Back Malaria Objectives: Reduce global malaria deaths to near zero by end of 2015; Reduce global malaria cases by 75% from 2000 levels by end of 2015; Eliminate malaria by the end of 2015 in 10 new countries (since 2008) and in the WHO European Region

Progress Towards Objectives: Azerbaijan and Sri Lanka reported 0 indigenous cases for the first time and 11 other countries maintained 0 cases

Data from WHO Global Malaria Program. *World malaria report 2014*. Retrieved January 6, 2015, from http://www.who.int/malaria/publications /world_malaria_report_2014/wmr-2014-no-profiles.pdf.

almost 80 percent of those who died were children under 5 years of age, almost all of them in Africa.[73]

Malaria is the 10th leading cause of death for all ages and both sexes globally. However, it is the third leading cause of death globally among children under 5 years of age. For the sub-Saharan Africa region, malaria is the leading cause of death for all age groups and for those under 5 years of age. In terms of DALYs, malaria is the sixth leading cause among all age groups and the fourth leading cause among those under 5 years of age.[37] For all age groups globally, malaria made up about 2.2 percent of all deaths. About 10 percent of all deaths of those under 5 globally, however,

were attributed to malaria. In sub-Saharan Africa, almost 20 percent of all deaths of children under 5 years of age were attributed to malaria.[1] Malaria is the leading cause of DALYs in sub-Saharan Africa among all age groups. It is also the leading cause of DALYs for children under 5 years of age in sub-Saharan Africa.[37]

The most important risk factor for malaria is being bitten by mosquitoes that carry the malaria parasite. This risk varies with the feeding habits of various species of mosquitoes, the climate, and the time of year. Some people have a degree of immunity to malaria from having grown up in malarial zones, and the risks of contracting malaria increase if one does not have such immunity.[71]

Pregnant women who contract malaria are at high risk of giving birth to low birthweight children. Malaria in pregnancy is also associated with spontaneous abortion, stillbirth, premature delivery, and severe anemia in the mother and the baby.[74] It was estimated in a 2006 study that 45 million pregnancies occurred annually in malaria-endemic areas of Africa and 23 million occur in high malaria transmission areas. It was also suggested that 3 to 15 percent of African mothers suffered severe anemia, accounting for 10,000 malaria-related anemia deaths per year. It was further estimated that globally, malaria would cause about 30 percent of low birthweight in newborns and between 75,000 and 200,000 infant deaths per year.[71]

The Costs and Consequences of Malaria

The cost of malaria at the family level is substantial because individuals often have malaria up to five times per year. In one study in Ghana, for example, there were 11 cases of malaria per household, per year, on average.[40] These same studies showed that individuals lost one to five work days per episode of malaria, that the indirect cost of dealing with their illness was greater than the direct costs of treatment, and that each episode of malaria probably cost an adult about 2 percent of his annual income.[40] In many African countries, malaria typically accounts for 30 percent or more of outpatient visits and hospital admissions for children under 5 years of age.[75]

It is estimated that $12 billion is lost annually due to malaria in Africa alone.[75] Roll Back Malaria suggests that the economic costs of malaria in countries with a high malaria burden is a loss of about 1.3 percent of GDP per year. One study suggested that a 10 percent reduction in malaria was associated with a 0.3 percent increase in economic growth. Clearly, malaria in sub-Saharan Africa is a deterrent to trade, business development, tourism, and foreign investment.[76,77]

Addressing the Burden of Malaria

Despite many years of effort, there is still no vaccine against malaria. However, there is widespread agreement on the key interventions required to roll back malaria. These include:

- Prompt treatment of those infected, based on confirmed diagnosis
- Intermittent preventive therapy for pregnant women
- Long-lasting insecticide-treated bednets for people living in malarial zones
- Indoor residual spraying of the homes of people in malarial zones

Appropriate treatment of malaria is essential to reduce malaria morbidity and mortality. If people with malaria are treated promptly, then mosquitoes that bite them will not carry malaria to another person. Drugs such as chloroquine, Fansidar (sulfadoxine and pyrimethamine), and mefloquine were used earlier as standard treatments for malaria in different settings. However, they faced growing levels of drug resistance.

WHO today recommends artemisinin-based combination therapies (ACT) for treating uncomplicated malaria caused by *P. falciparum* and for treating *P. vivax* infections that are not responsive to chloroquine.[78] The use of ACT has grown from only 11 million courses of treatment in 2005 to almost 400 million courses of treatment in 2013. In addition, pregnant women are being treated with intermittent preventive therapy from between 18 and 24 weeks of their pregnancy through delivery, to improve birth outcomes for both mothers and children, as noted earlier.[79]

Treatment of malaria should be based on a confirmed diagnosis, traditionally through a microscopic examination of a blood smear, but which was often not done. A rapid diagnostic device was developed to make it easier to test for malaria in low-resource settings, and the use of these kits has become widespread, growing from almost 90 million in 2010 to almost 320 million in 2013. It was estimated that almost 200 million microscopic examinations were done to diagnose malaria in 2013, of which about 120 million were in India alone.[73]

The use of long-lasting insecticide-treated bednets is another important pillar of malaria control. Bednets, impregnated with a biologically safe insecticide, are being widely distributed for free and sold by governments, donors, and the private sector. It is estimated that over 200 million bednets were distributed in 2014, a major increase over the 70 million distributed in 2012.[73] About 44 percent of the people at risk are estimated to be sleeping under bednets, an increase from only 2 percent in 2004.[5]

Spraying the inside of homes, or indoor residual spraying, is also important. Only about 3.5 percent of the population at risk of malaria globally and 7 percent of the people at risk in Africa are thought to have been covered with such spraying in 2013.[5,73] Four classes of insecticide are approved by WHO for indoor residual spraying. Pyrethroids have been the insecticide of choice for spraying but DDT is also approved for such efforts. Assessments are made to examine resistance to the insecticides and the need to rotate insecticides to slow the development of resistance to them. Particular attention is also being paid to potential environmental risks of the insecticides.[80]

Reducing the number of mosquitoes that carry malaria at the community level relies on effective communication and commitment by local leaders, the identification of breeding sites, and the availability of appropriate larvicides and/or tools to drain potential breeding sites. However, reducing the number of mosquitoes, called source reduction, is particularly difficult in Africa because the vector, *Anopheles gambiae*, is ubiquitous and breeds in all types of standing water.[71]

Challenges in Addressing Malaria

The global goals for malaria include:

- Reducing global malaria cases from 2000 levels by 75 percent in 2015
- Reducing global malaria deaths to zero by 2015
- Eliminating malaria in 8 to 10 countries by 2015
- Eliminating malaria in the European region by 2015

The global plan for addressing malaria also includes the goal of long-term eradication of malaria, through progressive elimination in different countries.[5]

It is clear from the data given earlier on the number of cases and on the number of deaths that there has been enormous progress against malaria recently. It is also clear that much of this stems from the concerted efforts of countries and their global partners to ensure better diagnosis and treatment and greater use of bednets, indoor residual spraying, and intermittent treatment of pregnant women.

Nonetheless, a number of efforts will need to be expanded and improved to meet global goals and, ultimately, to eliminate malaria from an increasing number of countries. Achieving key goals will require, first, the scaling up of key interventions for prevention. This includes trying to ensure 100 percent coverage for people at risk with long-lasting insecticide-treated bednets, indoor residual spraying, and intermittent therapy for pregnant women. Progress in these areas will have to include not only the dissemination of bednets but also greater efforts at behavior change to ensure that families actually use the nets properly when they have them.

There are also substantial gaps in the diagnosis and treatment of malaria, with many cases diagnosed without confirming the presence of malaria by microscopy or a rapid diagnostic test. In addition, many of those who suffer from malaria are not given the right medicine or not given medicine in a timely manner, which can result in death.[5]

A substantial share of those diagnosed with and treated with malaria seek care in the private sector. The quality of those private services is often inadequate and people may be given inappropriate or counterfeit drugs. Improving the speed and quality of diagnosis and treatment will require that national malaria programs find effective ways of working with private medical providers in almost all countries in Africa.

Better diagnostics could also be helpful. In addition, the continuous development of new drugs to fight malaria is also critical, given the speed with which malaria has developed resistance to other drugs and the limited number of drugs that now work effectively against malaria. Five countries have now shown resistance to ACT and there are no new proven drugs available to combat malaria.[5]

There is growing resistance to the insecticides used for indoor residual spraying. It will be extremely important to monitor that resistance. Forty-nine countries have now reported resistance to at least one class of insecticides, and 39 countries have reported resistance to two classes of drugs.[5]

There has been some progress in the development of a malaria vaccine; however there is not yet an approved vaccine. A safe, effective, and affordable vaccine could make major inroads against malaria.

It will also be important to continue to engage in research and learn what works in cost-effective ways in different settings. Efforts are now under way, for example, to see if relatively small pockets of malaria in countries nearing elimination could be addressed through selective seasonal drug therapy.[81]

Diarrheal Disease

The Burden of Diarrheal Disease

WHO defines diarrhea as: "the passage of three or more loose or liquid stools per day (or more frequent passage than is normal for the individual)."[4] Diarrhea is caused by certain bacteria, viruses, and/or parasites that are transmitted by contaminated water or food through the fecal–oral route, such as *Shigella* sp., *Salmonella* sp., *Cholera vibrio*, rotavirus, and *Escherichia coli*. Diarrheal disease agents can be spread by dirty utensils, dirty hands, or flies. Poor recognition of the extent of illness, failed home care, and lack of knowledge about simple therapies increase the severity of diarrhea.[82]

Diarrheal diseases most significantly impact the poor, especially children in low- and middle-income countries. Poor housing, crowding, lack of safe water and sanitation, cohabitation with domestic animals, lack of refrigeration for food storage, and poor personal and community hygiene all contribute to the transmission of diarrheal disease agents. In addition, poor nutrition contributes to poor immunity and increases the frequency and severity of diarrhea. Diarrhea causes severe dehydration and a loss of body water and can kill infants and young children very quickly.[82]

Diarrheal disease mortality has decreased significantly in the past 30 years, from an estimated 4.6 million deaths in the 1980s to 760,000 deaths in 2013.[4] This decline has largely been due to improved nutrition of infants, better disease recognition by families and healthcare providers, improved care seeking, appropriate use of oral rehydration therapy, increasing rates of coverage of the measles vaccine, and the growing use of the rotavirus vaccine.

Nonetheless, the burden of diarrheal disease remains very substantial. Diarrhea is a major cause of death and sickness for children younger than 5 years. WHO estimated in 2013 that there were about 1.7 billion cases of diarrheal disease every year.[4] WHO also estimated that children under 3 years of age in low- and middle-income countries suffer on average about 3 episodes of diarrhea annually, although rates vary worldwide.[4]

Diarrheal diseases are the cause of about 10 percent of all deaths of children under 5 in low- and middle-income countries, sub-Saharan Africa, and South Asia. Diarrheal diseases are the fourth leading cause of death for under-5 children in low- and middle-income countries. These diseases are the third leading cause of DALYs among under-5 children. In sub-Saharan Africa and in South Asia, diarrheal diseases are the third leading cause of death and the third leading cause of DALYs.[37]

Addressing the Burden of Diarrhea

There are five major disease prevention strategies for diarrhea. Perhaps most effective is the promotion of exclusive breastfeeding for 6 months. This is advantageous to the child and mother because the child receives both maternal antibodies and a nutritious and uncontaminated meal. Mothers benefit from an increased birth interval and a healthier child. The second prevention intervention is improved complementary feeding, introduced with breastfeeding after 6 months. The third is rotavirus immunization. WHO estimated in 2012 that rotavirus was the cause of about 450,000 deaths of children under 5 years of age in 2008, before the vaccine began to be more widely used in low- and middle-income countries.[83] The next strategy is increased measles immunizations. Data indicate a clear link between measles immunization and reduced incidence and deaths from diarrhea. If measles coverage is increased, especially in Africa, then the burden of diarrheal disease will decline. The fifth prevention strategy is improving access to safe water supply and sanitation. Clean water and appropriate sanitation will reduce the incidence of diarrheal disease. Furthermore, proper handwashing can reduce diarrhea incidence by 3 percent.[84] Ensuring that an increasing share of children have sufficient levels of vitamin A by raising supplementation rates is also important.[85]

Three case management interventions can significantly reduce the severity and mortality of diarrheal disease. The use of oral rehydration therapy (ORT) is the most cost-effective case management intervention, especially if home-made solutions are administered. Earlier estimates suggested that although the use of ORT had expanded globally, only about 49 percent of the diarrhea cases worldwide ere managed with ORT or home fluids.[82] Related to this, it was also estimated that zinc supplementation during an acute diarrhea episode for 10 to 14 days during and after diarrhea could prevent 300,000 deaths per year.[86] Third, antibiotics can be given for bloody diarrhea, primarily caused by *Shigella* infection. However, delivering this intervention where it is most needed may depend on careful training of nonphysician healthcare personnel because most low-income and many middle-income countries do not have enough physicians living in places where they are most needed.[82]

Neglected Tropical Diseases[87]

The Burden of Neglected Tropical Diseases

More than 1 billion people are infected with one or more of the neglected tropical diseases (NTDs).[88] These 13 diseases, shown in **Table 12-15**, are the most common afflictions of the world's poorest people.

NTDs have a terrible impact on health, impede child growth and development, harm pregnant women, and often cause long-term debilitating illnesses. They cause an extraordinary amount of ill health, disability, and disfigurement and are often deadly. As a result, those who suffer from NTDs are frequently shunned by their families and their communities. In addition, people with these diseases are often unable to work productively, leading to enormous economic losses for them, their families, and the nations in which they live.

Despite their significance, relatively little financial support was provided until recently to address NTDs, compared to the burden of ill health they cause. This is especially regrettable because significant progress has been made to control or eliminate some of the NTDs, including Chagas disease, lymphatic filariasis, onchocerciasis, and leprosy. It is also lamentable because a rapid-impact package of four drugs that

---

TABLE 12-15 Selected Neglected Tropical Diseases, Ranked by Prevalence

Ascariasis (roundworm)
Trichuriasis
Hookworm infection
Schistosomiasis
Lymphatic filariasis (elephantiasis)
Onchocerciasis (river blindness)
Trachoma
Chagas disease
Leishmaniasis
Leprosy
Human African trypanosomiasis
Buruli ulcer
Dracunculiasis

Compiled by the author from WHO Factsheets on individual diseases. Retrieved July 17, 2015 from http://www.who.int/neglected_diseases/diseases/en/.

---

can simultaneously treat the seven most common NTDs for about 50 cents per year is available.[89] Given the exceptional amount of good health that can be gained in the fight against NTDs for such a small amount of money, an important global challenge is to spread the rapid-impact package as quickly as possible to all of the places where it can be of benefit.

The NTDs shown in Table 12-15 are 13 parasitic and bacterial infections that affect about one in six people in the world and about 500 million children.[90] Seven of these diseases are especially important, given the large number of people affected by them and the manner in which they can be addressed. A number of infections related to intestinal worms, which are called "soil-transmitted helminths," affect an extraordinary number of people. These include roundworm (ascariasis), which affects more than 1 billion people worldwide; as well as whipworm (trichuriasis) and hookworm, each of which affects over 700 million people.[90] The four other most common NTDs are schistosomiasis (snail fever), affecting about 200 million people; lymphatic filariasis (elephantiasis), which affects 120 million people; blinding trachoma, affecting more than 40 million people; and onchocerciasis (river blindness), which affects about 26 million people.[90]

A number of diseases kill more people than NTDs do. However, some estimates suggest that NTDs result in as many DALYs annually as would be caused by malaria,[91] largely because of the extent to which the NTDs make people sick for long periods of time and the manner in which they cause long-lasting disabilities.

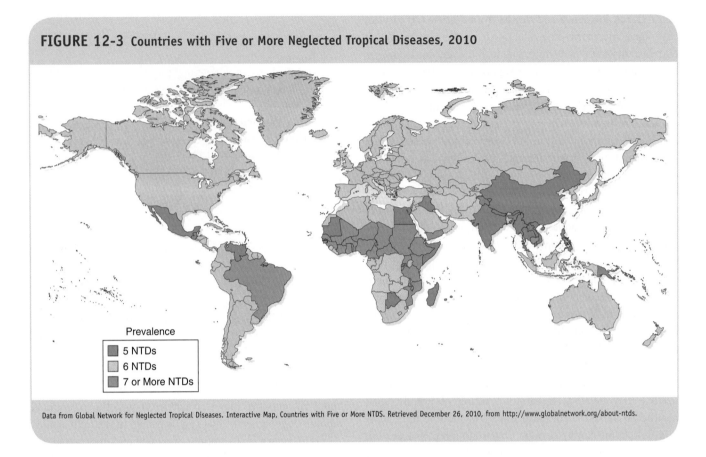

FIGURE 12-3 Countries with Five or More Neglected Tropical Diseases, 2010

Prevalence
- 5 NTDs
- 6 NTDs
- 7 or More NTDs

Data from Global Network for Neglected Tropical Diseases. Interactive Map, Countries with Five or More NTDS. Retrieved December 26, 2010, from http://www.globalnetwork.org/about-ntds.

Figure 12-3 shows the global distribution of NTDs. Seven different NTDs can be found in a number of countries, mostly in Africa, but also including Brazil and Cambodia. Six of the common NTDs are found in many countries in sub-Saharan Africa, and five NTDs can be found in many of the other low- and middle-income countries of Africa, Asia, and Latin America.

NTDs are diseases of poverty, affecting nearly everyone in the "bottom billion" of the world's poorest people. NTDs are especially prevalent in subtropical and tropical climates. Women and children who live in unhygienic environments with limited access to clean water and sanitary methods of waste disposal face the biggest threat of NTDs. Pregnant women also face special risks from some NTDs, as discussed later in this section. People engaged in farming are particularly susceptible to NTDs because of their close contact with soil, which can harbor many of the parasites and worms that cause NTDs. People who live in Africa and rely on rivers for drinking and bathing are also more likely to be affected by certain NTDs, such as onchocerciasis. Individuals whose labor or domestic chores are centered on freshwater sources are also more likely to contract NTDs.[92]

In addition, the burden of the worm diseases concerns not only being infected but also the number of worms in the body. Children of preschool age have the greatest number of worms. In addition, the prevalence of intestinal worms in many school-aged children in the highest burden countries is exceptionally high. In 2009, for example, it was estimated that over 75 percent of the school-age children in Rwanda were infected with soil-transmitted helminths.[93]

Without going into too much detail, it is valuable to understand how some of the most common NTDs are transmitted and some of their most important clinical manifestations:[92]

- The *soil-transmitted helminths* have very similar life cycles. Humans ingest the eggs of the worms. The eggs hatch into larvae, which travel to different parts of the body, depending on the type of worm. The worms might feed on food from the human host or attach themselves to the intestinal lining and live off the blood of the host. Eggs pass from the human host in feces and can then be picked up by others who will get infected.
- *Schistosomiasis* is caused by a liver fluke. People with schistosomiasis release fluke eggs in their urine

or feces. The flukes infect freshwater snails. When humans swim, bathe, or work in water with infected snails, the fluke can penetrate their skin. One form of fluke manifests itself in the intestinal tract and liver and another in the urinary tract; both can cause severe disease.

- The cycle of transmission for *lymphatic filariasis* is very different from that for the helminthic infections. In this case, mosquitoes bite infected humans and pick up the larvae, which develop inside the mosquito and migrate to the insect's mouth. When this mosquito bites a human, it transmits the hatched larvae into the skin. Larvae can survive in the lymphatic system for up to 6 years, and when they die, they cause the severe disfigurement associated with lymphatic filariasis.

- The black fly that causes *onchocerciasis* goes through a similar process. Infected flies carry the larvae from person to person through bites in the skin. These become adult worms, and the females release millions of small larvae into the body.

- *Trachoma* is caused by bacteria that lead to a discharge in the eye. It is transmitted when someone comes in contact with the discharge, usually by touch. However, flies can also spread the disease from person to person.

The Consequences of the Neglected Tropical Diseases

NTDs can have debilitating social and economic consequences as well as a major impact on the health and well-being of those infected. On the clinical side, for example, trachoma can lead to redness and swelling of the eye, sensitivity to light, corneal scarring, and eventually permanent blindness. Schistosomiasis is associated with painful and/or bloody urination, bloody diarrhea, enlargement of the liver and/or spleen, and liver cancer; it is also the most deadly of the NTDs. Lymphatic filariasis is well known for the remarkable swelling it can cause in the limbs and genitals. Onchocerciasis leads to skin problems and blindness.

The helminthic infections are generally associated with abdominal pain, loss of appetite, malnutrition, diarrhea, and anemia. In addition, chronic helminthic infection in children can limit the physical and mental development of the child. Pregnant women with hookworm are at high risk of giving birth to low birthweight babies, of birthing babies who fail to thrive, and of having poor milk production. In addition, pregnant women with anemia, commonly caused by hookworm in low-income countries, are three and a half times more likely to die during childbirth than women who are not anemic. This risk is especially significant, because

one quarter to one-third of pregnant women in sub-Saharan Africa are infected with hookworm.[94] Whipworm also can lead to severe growth retardation in children.

NTDs by themselves not only have enormous effects on individuals but also worsen the effects of other major infectious diseases or make individuals more susceptible to them. Recent studies have shown that many people have one or more NTDs at the same time as they have HIV/AIDS or malaria, which worsens the intensity of those diseases. In addition, helminthic infections may serve as important factors in the transmission of HIV.[95] Genital schistosomiasis in females may develop into lesions that increase susceptibility to becoming infected with HIV.[96] Neglected tropical diseases are also associated with the onset of some chronic noncommunicable diseases, such as the bladder cancer associated with urinary schistosomiasis.[97]

Social stigma is a major consequence of the NTDs. Many of the NTDs cause disability and disfigurement, resulting in individuals being shunned by their families and their communities. When not treated, for example, leprosy can cause terrible skin lesions that have been stigmatized since biblical times. Few health conditions are as stigmatizing as the swelling of limbs and genitalia that can result from lymphatic filariasis. Individuals who are stigmatized are less likely to leave their homes to seek diagnosis and treatment. Social stigma is particularly demoralizing for young women because they are often left unmarried and unable to work, in settings where the social value of a woman has much to do with her marital status.

NTDs also have a major impact on the productivity of individuals and the economic prospects of communities and nations. Children are disproportionately affected by NTDs and often suffer long-term consequences from them. In some areas, hookworm infection in school-age children contributes to drops in school attendance by over 20 percent, and poor school attendance and poor school performance reduce future earnings. In fact, hookworm has been shown to reduce future wage-earning capacity in some affected areas by up to 43 percent.[98]

NTDs adversely affect economic productivity at the individual, family, community, and national levels. NTDs lead to important losses in income that cause some families to sell assets to try to stay financially solvent. In addition, regions severely affected by onchocerciasis often cannot be used effectively for economic activities such as farming, because families that try to live in these areas are at risk of being blinded by the disease. Trachoma alone has been shown to contribute annually to an estimated $2.9 billion loss in productivity worldwide.[99]

Addressing the Neglected Tropical Diseases

Despite the many people still affected by NTDs, there has been considerable progress in the fight against a number of them. Onchocerciasis was eliminated as a public health problem in 10 countries in West Africa and Guinea worm is nearing eradication, as a result of a global effort that focused on health education and teaching people to filter their water through finely woven cloth. In fact, the number of Guinea worm cases fell from more than 3.5 million in 1986 in 20 countries to 126 cases in 4 countries at the end of 2014.[100]

In 1997, WHO developed a strategy known as SAFE (surgery, antibiotics, face washing, environmental change) to combat trachoma worldwide. As a result of this program, trachoma prevalence has been reduced globally from 149 million cases in 1997 to 41 million cases today.[90] The program was particularly effective in Morocco, where the SAFE strategy was the first to be tested at the national level. Through the donation of over $72 million worth of drugs by Pfizer to treat trachoma, as well as interventions to improve environmental hygiene, the prevalence of trachoma declined by an extraordinary 99 percent.[101] Trachoma in Morocco is discussed further in this chapter in one of the case studies.

Lymphatic filariasis has been controlled in 13 countries that are now in a surveillance phase of the disease.[102] This was accomplished by the annual administration of appropriate drugs to all of the people of an affected area, usually by working closely with communities. Two pharmaceutical companies, Merck and Pfizer, have donated drugs for the program against lymphatic filariasis. In its first 8 years alone, the Global Program to Eliminate Lymphatic Filariasis made significant progress in preventing the disease. An estimated 6.6 million newborns were saved from acquiring lymphatic filariasis during this period, and 9.5 million people previously infected with overt manifestations of the disease were protected from developing severe disease.[103] Since 2000, when the Global Program for the Elimination of Lymphatic Filariasis was established, the number of people infected by the disease annually has dropped by 43 percent.[102]

In addition, a better foundation has been set globally, as well as within some countries, for dealing more effectively and on a broader scale with NTDs. This builds upon work done by a variety of partnerships, including the Global Alliance to Eliminate Lymphatic Filariasis, the African Programme for Onchocerciasis Control, and the Partnership for Parasite Control. The Global Network for Neglected Tropical Diseases, for example, has been established at the Sabin Vaccine Institute to help develop more coherent, effective, and efficient approaches to NTD control. The Global Network is composed of a number of member organizations that deliver treatments on the ground, including the founding members, The Liverpool School of Tropical Medicine, Earth Institute at Columbia University, Helen Keller International, the International Trachoma Initiative, the Schistosomiasis Control Initiative at Imperial College, and the Task Force for Global Health. The Global Network works to build advocacy, policy, and resource mobilization efforts to support members and local governments in implementing NTD control programs.[92,104]

The successes against NTDs thus far suggest that considerable additional progress can be made, rapidly and at relatively low cost, to combat the exceptional number of cases of NTDs that remain worldwide. However, further progress is likely to require concerted action in a number of areas, including scaling up the rapid-impact package, focusing on deworming, integrating NTD control with other programs, developing new technologies to address NTD control, and moving forward with political will.

It is essential to quickly scale up the rapid-impact package referred to earlier, to address the seven most common NTDs. The package includes a combination of four of six drugs: albendazole or mebendazole, praziquantel, ivermectin or diethylcarbamazine, and azithromycin (see **Table 12-16**).

Pharmaceutical companies, including Eisai, GlaxoSmithKline, Johnson & Johnson, Merck KGaA, Pfizer, and Sanofi donate the drugs used to implement the rapid impact package. In sub-Saharan Africa, the projected overall cost of the program is about 50 cents per person per year, which would be a best buy in global health, given its low cost and large impact on public health.

Following the lessons of the onchocerciasis program and others, the rapid-impact package can be implemented rapidly with the help of medicine distributors who are chosen from among members of the affected communities. They are brought into the program through social mobilization activities. These efforts bring together key actors from the public and private sector in a partnership and seek to involve affected communities in the design, implementation, and monitoring of the program.[105] This type of community-directed treatment for onchocerciasis with ivermectin has proven particularly successful in rural Africa, where treatment was extended in 2010 alone to 76 million people.[106] In fact, a study done in 2008 showed that community-directed interventions are much more effective than conventional delivery approaches, which have less community participation, in combating most communicable diseases in sub-Saharan Africa.[105]

Periodic deworming of young children is also a best buy in global health and should be a major focus of attention.[107] Deworming is the single most cost-effective means to improve school attendance. There is also historical evidence

TABLE 12-16 NTD Treatment for Selected Endemicity Scenarios

Medicine Set	Endemicity Scenario				Recommended Combination of Medicines
	STH	LF	SCH	ONCHO	Medicines
A	✓	✓	✓	✓	ALB + IVM + PZQ
B	✓	✓		✓	ALB + IVM
C	✓	✓	✓		ALB + DEC + PZQ
D	✓	✓			ALB + DEC
E	✓				ALB/MBD

ALB = albendazole; DEC = diethylcarbamazine; IVM = ivermectin; LF = lymphatic filariasis; MBD = mebendazole; ONCHO = onchocerciasis; PZQ = praziquantel; SCH = schistosomiasis; STH = soil-transmitted helminths

Note: The Rapid Impact Package would also include azithromycin to treat trachoma.

Data from Weaver, Sankara D. The ABCs of NTDs. Presentation at the USAID Mini-University, September 12, 2008.

that deworming improves children's cognitive skills and their potential to learn and leads to greater literacy and higher productivity among adults.[108] In addition, recent studies have shown that deworming children may significantly reduce the burden of malaria, because children infected with ascariasis are twice as likely to get severe malaria as children who are not infected.[109]

Moreover, there are considerable opportunities, in regions of high prevalence of malaria and HIV/AIDS, for effectively integrating NTD treatment programs with existing HIV and malaria control programs. This integration could help to reduce the burden of NTDs and the burden of HIV/AIDS and malaria, while contributing to improving the cost-effectiveness of all of the programs. This is especially important because hookworm and schistosomiasis often worsen the effects of malaria.[110] The distribution of bednets and treatment for NTDs such as onchocerciasis and lymphatic filariasis could also help to control malaria. Such a program led to a substantial improvement in the use of bednets in central Nigeria, where insecticide-treated bednet distribution was combined with mass drug administration for treatment of lymphatic filariasis and onchocerciasis.[111]

Future Challenges

As we look to the longer run, it is also important to invest in the search for new technologies that could help to address NTDs in more effective and efficient ways. With

the assistance of the Bill & Melinda Gates Foundation and private donors, work is under way by the Vaccine Development Program at the Sabin Vaccine Institute to develop both hookworm and schistosomiasis vaccines. A safe and effective hookworm vaccine, particularly one that would confer life-long immunity, would eliminate the need to provide medicine for deworming twice a year to all children living in affected areas, which is a substantial undertaking. The development of a vaccine for schistosomiasis is also being carried out by the Institut Pasteur.

It is also critical to develop new drugs to combat the NTDs. The world is now dependent on only four drugs to address the seven most common NTDs. There is resistance to some of the drugs, and more extensive use of them could lead to additional resistance. Developing drugs that can combat the NTDs more effectively than the present drugs continues to be a goal of considerable importance.[112]

At the same time as countries seek to prevent and treat NTDs through programs of mass drug administration or treatment of specific diseases, they need to work with communities to address the underlying risks for NTDs. For the seven most common NTDs, these risks overwhelmingly relate to the unsanitary living conditions of the poor. It will remain important for people to better understand the importance of good hygiene, to have better access to safe water and sanitary disposal of human waste, and to eliminate worm and parasite breeding sites. In the long run, progress in all of these directions will help to reduce the burden of NTDs and sustain reductions. Unfortunately, however, these developments are not likely to take place quickly. The fastest and most cost-effective route to reducing the burden of NTDs will be to implement the rapid-impact package as quickly as possible.

POLICY AND PROGRAM BRIEFS

Five policy and program briefs follow to illustrate some of the key points noted in this chapter. Two concern emerging and reemerging infectious diseases—one on chikungunya fever and the other on Ebola virus. The next one concerns *Cryptococcus* disease, which has become one of the leading causes of death of people infected with HIV. The fourth is about an effort by a nongovernmental organization in India to address TB more effectively and efficiently. The fifth brief concerns a public–private partnership to improve the control of drug-resistant TB. The last is a summary of some important findings concerning the long-term costs of HIV/AIDS and how they might be met both globally and at the level of countries with different burdens of disease and different income levels.

Chikungunya Fever

Chikungunya fever is a mosquito-borne disease caused by chikungunya virus. *Aedes aegypti* and *Aedes albopictus* mosquitoes are responsible for spreading the virus.[113] These mosquitoes transmit chikungunya by feeding on a person already infected with the virus. Whereas outbreaks of chikungunya virus are usually found in Africa, Southeast Asia, India, and islands in the Indian Ocean, the increasing presence of *Aedes* mosquitoes in the Caribbean, Europe, and America make many regions susceptible to the virus and able to maintain the virus within their local populations.

The virus was first detected in humans in 1952 after a minor chikungunya virus outbreak in Tanzania.[113] No major outbreaks of the virus were recorded until 2004, when two coastal communities in Kenya—Lamu Island and Mombasa—experienced large chikungunya epidemics.[113] The first outbreak on Lamu Island was initially thought to be due to malaria, but eventually testing determined chikungunya to be the cause. The attack rate on Lamu Island was 75 percent, meaning that 13,500 of 18,000 of the island's residents were infected.[114]

The 2004 epidemics in Kenya spread to islands of the Indian Ocean. In La Réunion, for example, it was estimated that 255,000 individuals were infected with the virus. The overall attack rate in La Réunion was estimated to be 35 percent in mid-2006.[115] In 2006, India experienced a chikungunya outbreak with an official estimate of 1.3 million cases. Infected individuals traveling in and out of India spread

the virus to Italy, where 197 cases of the virus were documented.[116] By the end of March 2014, the disease spread to the Western Hemisphere, with more than 15,000 suspected cases reported in the Caribbean.[117] **Figure 12-4** shows the areas of the world now at risk of chikungunya.

Although outbreaks of chikungunya virus have spread dramatically, the clinical presentation of the disease has remained consistent. The symptoms include headache, back pain, nausea, vomiting, rash, high fever, and severe joint pain and typically last for 10 days.[117] The virus can also lead to chronic symptoms in which patients experience severe joint pain, fatigue, and depression for up to 2 years after the onset of the disease.[117] The frequency of chronic symptoms among people with chikungunya virus depends on the time between symptom onset and follow-up. In La Réunion, 80 to 93 percent of patients reported chronic symptoms, in India 49 percent of patients reported chronic symptoms, and in South Africa 12 to 18 percent of patients reported chronic symptoms.[113] Still, death from the virus is extremely rare. For example, India reported 1.39 million cases of the virus in 2006 with no attributable deaths. La Réunion Island reported that out of the 266,000 cases of chikungunya, 254 were fatal. Thus, the case-fatality rate in La Réunion was only about 1/1000.[118]

Although chikungunya can affect men and women of all ages, the groups most at risk for developing a severe form of the disease are newborns and people over the age of 65. In addition, those living in tropical and subtropical climates and in areas that depend on water storage containers are at greater risk for contracting the virus, as *Aedes* mosquitoes rely on pools of water to lay their eggs.[119]

Although transmitting chikungunya during pregnancy is rare, fetuses that develop chikungunya during pregnancy are typically asymptomatic at birth and then develop fever, pain, rash, and swelling. The highest risk for transmitting chikungunya to the developing fetus occurs between the onset of labor and childbirth. The transmission rate during this period of pregnancy is as high as 49 percent.[113] Infants infected during labor experience more severe forms of chikungunya than the average person, with symptoms that include neurologic disease, hemorrhagic symptoms, and myocardial disease. Infants who suffer from neurologic disease often develop long-term mental disabilities as they mature.[113]

Individuals over the age of 65 have a 50 times higher mortality rate from the disease compared to younger adults (less than 45 years of age). Adults over the age of 65 have a higher frequency of underlying diseases, which decreases immunologic responses to chikungunya.[113] During the La Réunion outbreak in 2006, the only deaths due to the

FIGURE 12-4 Countries and Territories Where Chikungunya Cases Have Been Reported (as of July 1, 2014)

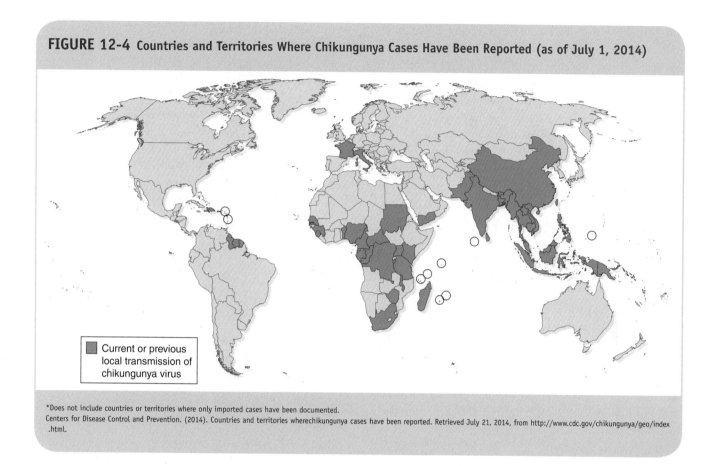

Current or previous
local transmission of
chikungunya virus

*Does not include countries or territories where only imported cases have been documented.
Centers for Disease Control and Prevention. (2014). Countries and territories wherechikungunya cases have been reported. Retrieved July 21, 2014, from http://www.cdc.gov/chikungunya/geo/index
.html.

virus were reported among older people.[120] Although older people living in areas without piped water are likely to be more at risk of contracting chikungunya, the virus can be extremely dangerous to the immunologically compromised and to those over age 65.

The two main vectors for transmitting the virus, *Aedes albopictus* and *Aedes aegypti,* both use water-filled breeding sites to reproduce and thrive in areas lacking piped water.[119] *Aedes albopictus* typically lives in habitats containing coconut husks, cocoa pods, bamboo stumps, tree holds, and rock pools. Habitats such as these are most often found in tropical and subtropical areas of the world.[116] *Aedes aegypti* also relies on water to lay its eggs but often occupies urban areas with or without vegetation. Thus, its major production places are human-made water containers and tree holes.[121]

Chikungunya virus is dramatically expanding its geographical range for three main reasons. First, chikungunya virus can establish itself in places far from the original site of infection because it can be maintained locally in a mosquito–human–mosquito cycle. For example, in 2007, the virus spread from India to Italy after someone was infected with

the disease in India and traveled back home to Italy. In Italy, the local mosquitoes picked up the virus from the traveler and transmitted the disease. During the outbreak in Italy, 197 cases were reported.[119]

Second, distant populations are also at risk for developing the virus because *Aedes* mosquitoes, the principal vectors of the disease, are present all over the world. For instance, both strains are present in the Americas, where the virus has not been widespread.[113] *Aedes aegypti* will be the most important vector in urban areas that have not yet come in contact with the virus, whereas *Aedes albopitcus* will play a more significant role in temperate areas and areas where the disease is already well established.[113]

Third, it is believed that once exposed to the virus, individuals will develop long-lasting immunity that will protect them against reinfection.[113] Thus, lack of exposure to the virus puts people at greater risk for contracting the disease and sustaining viral transmission.

The economic and social consequences resulting from chikungunya include strains on existing healthcare systems and public health infrastructure as well as long-term direct and productivity costs for those infected. Chikungunya epidemics can burden healthcare systems and hospitals—especially when the healthcare system has never encountered the virus and when hospitals have limited resources. For example, the 2005 outbreak in La Réunion resulted in substantial economic losses. Medical expenses were estimated at $59 million, with 60 percent due to direct medical costs.[114] Expenditure on medical consultations accounted for 47 percent, hospitalizations 32 percent, and drugs 19 percent of the direct medical costs.[114] The costs related to care for outpatients and inpatients were $120 and $2,700, respectively. The costs for those hospitalized were equal to about 12 percent of gross domestic product (GDP) per capita.[114]

Many rural villages use antibiotics as part of their treatment of chikungunya virus. However, antibiotics are ineffective against the virus. Taking antibiotics in response to chikungunya virus will only create resistance to the antibiotics. In Mallela, India, 65 percent of patients were treated with antibiotics.[120] Thus, it appears that irresponsible use of medicines and more broadly lack of education about the disease might also contribute to significant economic and potential health costs from the virus. Chikungunya virus is also associated with a loss of productivity. In Mallela, approximately 8.9 working days per case were lost as a result of the virus.[120]

In order to prevent the spread of the virus, household, national, and global plans should be employed to prevent mosquito bites, improve the efficiency and effectiveness of healthcare systems in responding to outbreaks, and establish control systems to stop the spread of the virus to new regions of the world.

The most important prevention technique is to stop mosquito bites. Mosquito bites can be avoided by sleeping under an insecticide-treated bednet, staying away from artificial light at night, using insect repellant, and wearing long sleeves and pants.[113] Patients can also avoid being bitten by reducing the number of mosquito habitats coming from natural and artificially filled water containers.[113]

On a national level, a number of steps should be considered by healthcare facilities to prepare for a chikungunya outbreak. These include creating a triage system to facilitate the flow of patients, developing ways to identify the introduction of the virus within a surveillance system, educating public health officials about the threat of the virus, and developing institutional plans to address disease surveillance.[113] After the virus has been introduced into an area, healthcare institutions should activate existing plans to respond to the outbreak. Healthcare institutions must work with the ministry of health to ensure rapid and frequent communication within healthcare facilities and to address staffing, bed capacity, durable supplies, and continuation of essential medical services.[113] Chikungunya surveillance should be built upon existing surveillance of the dengue virus.[121]

From a global perspective, the World Health Organization has responded by formulating evidence-based outbreak management plans and delivering technical support and guidance to countries for the effective management of outbreaks and cases. WHO has also provided training on clinical management, diagnosis, and vector control at the regional level.[113] In addition, the Pan American Health Organization (PAHO) along with the Division of Vector-borne Diseases of the U.S. Centers for Disease Control and Prevention created a working group that convened in Lima, Peru to discuss the threat this virus represents and to examine measures that might be taken to mitigate this threat.[113] The organizations created guidelines intended to increase awareness about the threat of chikungunya and the necessary control to prevent the spread of chikungunya in each member country.[113] Countries around the world should work together to establish control systems and educate the media, the public, and officials about the disease, the mode of transmission, the need for symptomatic and supportive treatment, and effective control measures.

The Ebola Outbreak of 2014 and 2015

Background

Ebola hemorrhagic fever is caused by the Ebola virus. From its emergence in 1976 until January 2015, Ebola had infected around 25,000 people, all of whom were in Africa, were exposed to someone who acquired the disease in Africa, or were involved in a laboratory accident.[122] As of January 31, 2015, 42.6 percent of those ever infected died of the disease (10,848 deaths).[123,124] However, in some outbreaks the case fatality ratio has been as high as 90 percent. Although there are five types of Ebola virus, only three have been responsible for human outbreaks: *Zaire ebolavirus*, *Sudan ebolavirus*, and *Bundibugyo ebolavirus*.[122]

Ebola is characterized by flulike symptoms, diarrhea, vomiting, and massive hemorrhaging. The incubation period ranges from 2 to 21 days, although symptoms usually begin 8 to 10 days after infection.[125] The disease is transmitted by exposure to bodily fluids such as blood, saliva, vomit, diarrhea, or semen. However, the disease cannot be transmitted prior to the onset of symptoms. There is no specific cure and no tested vaccine for Ebola.

The populations affected have traditionally been medical workers and poor, rural residents of the Democratic Republic of the Congo (DRC), Uganda, South Sudan, the Republic of the Congo (ROC), and Gabon. In previous outbreaks 10–25 percent of the cases have been medical workers. Of the 2,348 cases prior to 2014, 41 percent were in the DRC, 25 percent in

Uganda, 14 percent in South Sudan, 10 percent in the ROC, and 9 percent in Gabon.[122]

Many believe the main risk factor for initial infection to be exposure to sick or dead animals, in particular bats and primates in the forest. Fruit bats are thought to be the natural host of the virus.[126] Once an outbreak has begun, the risk factors for infection include direct contact with symptomatic patients at home or using improper safety procedures in medical facilities.

Since 1976, there have been 35 distinct outbreaks of Ebola. The first outbreak occurred in northwestern DRC, centered around the Yambuku mission. Another large outbreak occurred in the DRC in 1995, infecting 315 individuals and killing 81 percent of those ill.[122] Roughly one-fourth of those infected were healthcare workers.[127] During the first outbreak of Ebola in 1976, 26.7 percent of the cases were infected by accidental needle stick or by reuse of unsanitized needles used on other Ebola patients. Person-to-person transmission accounted for 46.9 percent of the cases. Much of the person-to-person transmission occurs during the process of caring for sick family members or during funeral procedures in which individuals are in close contact with the deceased.[128]

The West African Outbreak of 2014

The 2014 West African outbreak of Ebola is the largest outbreak ever of the disease. As of January 27, 2015, there were 22,124 cases and 8,829 deaths.[129] This is the first outbreak of Ebola seen in West Africa and the first to affect major urban centers. The viral strain is *Zaire ebolavirus* and is very closely related to strains previously seen in the DRC and Gabon.[130]

The outbreak was initially reported in Guinea on March 24, 2014. As of January 31, 2015, Nigeria, Senegal, Spain, the United States, the United Kingdom, Mali, Sierra Leone, and Liberia had also been affected.[124] By early February 2015, however, transmission was ongoing only in Sierra Leone, Liberia, and Guinea. The case fatality ratio of around 40 percent was less than in previous outbreaks.

Among other international partners, the primary actors in the outbreak response were the health ministries of the affected countries, the U.S. Centers for Disease Control and Prevention (CDC), the World Health Organization, the United Nations (UN), Médecins Sans Frontières (MSF), and UNICEF.

Epidemic Control

Based on previous outbreaks, the best practices for control include community education about safe home care and burial practices, proper hospital safety and sanitation procedures, case management and isolation, laboratory confirmation of cases, and active disease surveillance.

Control efforts for this outbreak were largely consistent with these practices. On August 8, 2014, roughly 8 months after the first case was believed to have occurred and 5 months after the first cases were reported, WHO assigned the Ebola outbreak its highest threat level: public health emergency of international concern.[131] The CDC also deployed staff to all affected countries and MSF provided 302 international staff and hired 3,600 local staff at eight Ebola case-management centers.[132] The governments of Sierra Leone, Liberia, and Guinea all instituted travel restrictions and border closures to neighboring countries.

Such efforts had little effect on the outbreak until October 2014 when the overall epidemic hit its peak.[133] The number of cases from then until January 2015 steadily dropped; the week of January 18, 2015 to January 25, 2015 was the first time since June 2014 that the weekly incidence of cases was less than 100.[134] Liberia especially saw a drop in cases, having only four during that same week.[133]

The initial failure of control efforts can be attributed to four challenges in this region: poor public health surveillance and border control, lack of medical personnel and supplies, lack of coordination in response, and lack of regional experience and education about the disease. In addition, many believe the international response was late and initially insufficient.

Beginning in 2007, 194 WHO member states instituted the revised International Health Regulations (IHR) in order to coordinate and develop countries' detection and response capabilities for infectious diseases such as Ebola.[135] However, 80 percent of the ratifying countries, including those affected in this outbreak, have not yet met their IHR responsibilities.[136] Such inaction on IHR principles affected active case finding and border control. WHO estimates that the actual case count has been 2–4 times higher than that reported, simply because mobilizing resources for case finding has been so challenging.[137] In addition, although border screening and travel bans were enforced, 34 percent of the new cases, as of September 2014, were still occurring in the cross-border region of Sierra Leone, Liberia, and Guinea, indicating a high level of border permeability.[138]

As with previous bouts of Ebola, healthcare staff were particularly affected, making up around 10 percent of the fatalities. Supplies of personal protective equipment and clinic capacity were also grossly inadequate in most areas.[139] Although MSF had eight Ebola treatment centers with a total capacity of 650 beds, the organization reported that it had reached its operational limit numerous times throughout the outbreak. Many individuals thus remained home for care instead of waiting in line at a treatment center. UNICEF provided crucial medical resources; however, the procurement of such supplies was hindered by the speed with which they could be produced.[140] In addition, airline travel bans and travel restrictions by countries without ongoing transmission, such as the United States, prevented such supplies from more easily getting into the affected countries. (WHO does not endorse such travel restrictions.)

Furthermore, the lack of education about the disease helped to drive the epidemic. Some families continued to perform burial ceremonies at home; this was responsible for nearly 60 percent of the cases in Guinea.[139] Also, due to a lack of confidence in allopathic medicine and the government, several communities rioted or denied access to healthcare workers. Out of fear of further spread, some violently threatened medical staff and "set free" isolated patients in hospitals.[141]

Meeting Future Challenges

On August 28, 2014, WHO organized its plan for the end of the outbreak in 6–9 months in its *Ebola Response Roadmap*. The tenets of this plan were reiterated in the UN STEPP Strategy from September 2014, which set the primary goals as stop the outbreak, treat the infected, ensure essential services, preserve stability, and prevent outbreaks in unaffected countries.[142]

From November 2014 to the end of January 2015, the incidence rate of disease declined. Given this changing epidemiology, which defies most previous estimates, on January 21, 2015, the United Nations Office for the Coordination of Humanitarian Affairs released an updated strategy for January–June 2015. This new strategy built upon STEPP. It aimed to reallocate resources in order to prioritize treatment and safe burial practices in areas with high ongoing transmission and to enforce contact tracing in areas with lower risk.[142] Since December 17, 2014, MSF has also been carrying out clinical trials for a new drug, favipiravir, from its treatment center in Guéckédou, Guinea. Such a drug, if effective, could have an impact on this and future outbreaks of Ebola.[143]

However, prevention of such a situation in the future is more dependent on ameliorating the fundamental causes of Ebola outbreaks: poor education, poor sanitation, and unsafe burials. As the epidemic wanes in Liberia, cases continued in Guinea and Sierra Leone. Liberia's recent success illustrates the action needed to prevent outbreaks in the future. It is believed that Liberia, which saw a dramatic drop in cases in mid-October 2014, could have benefitted from an earlier receipt of foreign resources due to an earlier spike in cases. This enabled the hiring of more safe burial teams and medical staff. Others believe that the concentration of cases in Monrovia, the capital, meant that the epidemic affected a more educated population than the outbreaks in Sierra Leone and Guinea, where cases have primarily been in rural and less educated populations.[144] The response of the Liberian people to the epidemic has revolved around community engagement and education. Behaviors changed much more rapidly than in Sierra Leone and Guinea, enabling a steep drop in the country's burden of Ebola.

Cryptococcosis: A New Leading Cause of Death in Patients with HIV

Background

Cryptococcosis is an opportunistic infection caused by the fungus *Cryptococcus* that results in respiratory illness or meningitis, including symptoms such as headache, fever, neck pain, vomiting, altered mental status, and sometimes death.[145] *Cryptococcus* fungus is present in soil types across the world and generally enters the body by being inhaled and infecting the lungs or the brain. However, the fungus cannot be spread from person to person.[145]

Cryptococcosis is a deadly illness that is growing in incidence worldwide, especially in HIV-positive adults in low-income countries, where access to antiretroviral medication is limited. Over 900,000 people worldwide fall ill with cryptococcal meningitis each year, two-thirds of whom will die after 3 months of infection.[146] Cryptococcal disease accounts for between 13 percent and 44 percent of deaths in HIV-infected cohorts in resource-limited countries, surpassing tuberculosis as the leading cause of death in some areas.[147]

Whereas almost all people with healthy immune systems can fight off this fungal infection without experiencing illness, immunocompromised people, such as adults with untreated HIV/AIDS, are at increased risk for cryptococcosis.[148,149] HIV co-infection further complicates cryptococcal treatment, as introduction of antiretroviral drugs in a patient with untreated or newly treated cryptococcal infection can actually cause the fungal disease symptoms to worsen, a condition known as immune reconstitution inflammatory syndrome (IRIS).[150,151] Sub-Saharan Africa, which is home to many people with untreated HIV infection, is the region most affected by cryptococcosis, accounting for 70 percent of cases.[146]

The Problem

Cryptococcosis is a debilitating and often deadly illness that reduces productivity and cuts short the lives of HIV-positive people in low-income settings. Though a test for *Cryptococcus* exists, a high share of patients with cryptococcal infection do not receive prompt diagnosis and treatment.[152] Undiagnosed and untreated cryptococcal disease is extremely costly in both human and economic terms, disproportionately affecting low- and middle-income countries. The case fatality rate of cryptococcal disease in South Africa is between 35 and 65 percent, more than double or triple the rate in high-income countries.[153]

The cost of treating a person with cryptococcal meningitis who is admitted to a hospital in South Africa is estimated to be over $2,800.[154] However, a simple dipstick test, called the cryptococcal antigen lateral flow assay, or CrAg LFA, could save lives and reduce costs.[154] This rapid and inexpensive test for *Cryptococcus* can detect the pathogen before symptoms develop and in time for effective use of antifungal treatment.[155]

Available Solutions and Response

The burden of cryptococcal disease is steadily increasing; yet available inexpensive diagnostic and treatment technologies are not in widespread use.[151] The World Health Organization recommends testing for and treating cryptococcosis in all HIV-positive populations with CD4 cell counts less than 100.[156] This screening is critical for identifying who should be administered appropriate treatment, such as amphotericin-B or fluconazole antifungal medication.[157] A study in Uganda has shown that implementation of CrAg LFA testing for people with CD4 cell counts < 100 would be extremely cost-effective, costing only $1.57 per DALY averted, making testing for *Cryptococcus* much cheaper than the estimated to $20 to $100 per DALY averted for tuberculosis testing programs.[158–160] A cost-effectiveness study in Vietnam confirmed the value of cryptococcal screening programs in Asia, suggesting that the cost per life year gained was similar to that of tuberculosis testing programs, in the range of $119 to $190.[161,162] Fluconazole, a first choice antifungal drug, is available to low- to middle-income countries for free via Pfizer's Diflucan Partnership Program.[163] Despite this, potent fungicidal drugs are often unavailable in low-resource, high-endemicity regions.[164] Based on this evidence and the WHO guidelines, South Africa has proposed a clinical treatment procedure for the country's cryptococcal screening program, including recommendations on CrAg LFA screening for persons with CD4 cell count less than 100 and subsequent testing and antifungal therapy as needed.[165]

Looking Forward

The WHO and South African cryptococcal disease testing guidelines are only a few years old, and no reliable data is available on what proportion of HIV-positive people worldwide are actually being screened for *Cryptococcus* or treated for it appropriately. Countries must quickly scale up implementation of these testing and treatment guidelines in order to avoid significant deaths due to opportunistic infection in HIV/AIDS patients.

A Comprehensive Approach to Tuberculosis: Operation ASHA and the Last-Mile Pipeline

Background

For many years, India has had the largest number of TB cases of any country in the world. The Indian government took important steps to address TB in 1993 when it established the Revised National Tuberculosis Control Program (RNTCP) based on the WHO DOTS model. An evaluation of the program in 2004, however, still found that default rates were 15 percent across the nation and TB centers were not distributed in a manner consistent with need. Furthermore, very little data existed nationwide regarding MDR-TB rates, though estimates projected 3.4 percent of new TB cases to be MDR-TB cases.[166] Despite progress in addressing TB over the last 2 decades, India's TB program still faces enormous challenges. Nongovernmental organizations like Operation ASHA are building public–private partnerships with the government to try to bridge some of the most important gaps in program quality and coverage.[167]

The Intervention

In 2006, Operation ASHA launched its first TB treatment center in a Hindu temple located in Sangam Vihar, a slum in southern Delhi with a population of roughly 500,000. Since then, with support from the government and various individual donors, ASHA has been able to expand its program and provide rigorously monitored treatment regimens for people with TB.

Each treatment center in the organization's model consists of two primary points of contact: a community DOTS provider (CDP) and a counselor. Operation ASHA found local community members who were highly involved in the community, like social workers, shopkeepers, and priests, to serve as CDPs for each center. The CDP manages the treatment center and ensures that medications have been received from local district hospitals.

Counselors are local community members trained to recognize the symptoms of TB and implement DOTS. Counselors travel throughout communities to detect possible new cases and collect sputum samples for testing. If a patient is found to be positive, a local hospital physician gives the patient a prescription. Counselors then revisit the homes of those diagnosed with TB and seek to sign with the patient an agreement that the patient will take all their drugs as intended for 6 months and that the counselor will monitor their drug treatment. Each day, patients come to pick up their medication from the treatment center. If they miss a day of their treatment, counselors follow up the next day to ensure that patients stick to their treatment regimens.[168]

In addition, Operation ASHA's direct connection with communities has become a pipeline for comprehensively enhancing the health of the populations it serves. Counselors also advise families on other health issues like malnutrition and family planning. Based on the needs assessments of villages, counselors can then recommend that ASHA provide additional health services. Since 2006, for example, ASHA has distributed over 600,000 simple analgesics, iron tablets, protein supplements, oral rehydration packets, and contraceptives, as well as 4,000 blankets, free of cost to people in the communities that it serves.[169]

In March 2010, ASHA also launched a pilot biometrics-based treatment delivery scheme. The system, known as eCompliance, gives counselors a netbook, fingerprint reader, and cell phone. New TB patients are enrolled by registering their fingerprints, and records of treatment regimens are kept in a netbook database. Central electronic medical records are also kept. The system also generates messages when patients miss a day of treatment so counselors can follow up and ensure that patients comply with their regimens.[168,170]

The Impact

In South Delhi alone, where Operation ASHA began, the death rate for tuberculosis decreased by the end of ASHA's first year from 6 percent to 2.5 percent of patients in treatment. The detection rate of TB-positive patients also increased in ASHA centers by 2009 from 82 per 100,000 people in 2005 to 160 per 100,000 by 2009.[167] Operation ASHA has brought down default to 3.2 percent in its centers, as opposed to the 11.75 percent default rate observed by other organizations working in South Delhi. Studies have also shown that eCompliance pilots have reduced default rates from 3 percent to 1.5 percent in the 78 centers using the system. Operation ASHA's success in India has also led to expansions into Cambodia.[171] As of 2014, 6.1 million individuals were covered by Operation ASHA's 245 centers spread across 3,000 villages in India and two provinces in Cambodia. More than 5 million of these 6.1 million individuals previously had minimal or no access to TB treatment.[168]

Costs and Financing

Having established an early public–private partnership with the Indian government, ASHA serves as an extension of the government's TB compliance centers, especially after business hours. Whereas government TB compliance centers operate during normal business hours, Operation ASHA

hires local individuals like shopkeepers in order to extend business hours for patients' convenience. ASHA receives roughly 80 percent of its funding from the government, with additional support from individual donors. For every Indian rupee ASHA invests in its patients, the government provides roughly 6 rupees in the form of diagnostics and medication. Operation ASHA also trains local individuals, like shopkeepers, to be counselors and establishes centers within existing buildings, like shops, to keep rent costs down.[172] Both of these factors make ASHA an extremely cost-effective model for compliance. Treating TB patients for the entire 6 months of treatment costs ASHA only $25, as opposed to the $300 cost typically incurred by comparable NGOs.[168]

Lessons Learned

From its initial launch in 2006, Operation ASHA's approach was rooted in the community to ensure that treatment centers were run by local community members, had flexible hours, and were within walking distances for patients. This emphasis on the community made Operation ASHA's target populations more willing to trust ASHA and comply with treatment. The organization has invested in local capacity building through its CDPs and counselors and by doing so, has created a functioning model to monitor DOTS implementation.[172] Rates of attrition among ASHA's staff are low, and employment through ASHA provides local CDPs and counselors with a source of income. Although ASHA's funding primarily is derived from individual donors and the government, it is a promising innovation in TB treatment compliance programs.

ASHA's example also demonstrates the potential value of public–private partnerships. ASHA receives its medications and diagnostics primarily through the support of local government hospitals but is then able to reach the last mile of delivery by connecting directly with communities. Above all, ASHA has brought care to its patients' doorsteps and has used its direct pipeline into communities as a means of addressing other health issues, as well. Although little data exists on the financial stability of ASHA's current model or the impact of its approach to care, its efforts have been deemed innovative and it continues to show promise as a scalable model for addressing the needs of TB patients in a number of settings.

Public–Private Partnerships for Addressing Drug-Resistant Tuberculosis[173]

Eli Lilly is a major pharmaceutical firm. It was founded in 1862 and is based in Indianapolis, Indiana, in the United States. Like a number of major corporations, Lilly has a program of corporate social responsibility (CSR), in which it tries to go beyond its normal corporate activities to be directly helpful to the larger community.

Lilly's flagship CSR program is the Lilly MDR-TB Partnership. This public–private initiative was established in 2003 to help confront the deadly global epidemic of MDR-TB. The partnership, which encompasses global health and relief organizations, academic institutions, and private companies, has adopted a broad-based approach to tackle the complex interwoven medical, social, and economic challenges posed by TB. It mobilizes over 20 global healthcare partners on five continents to share resources and knowledge to confront TB and MDR-TB. The partnership is funded to spend $135 million over 9 years.

The partnership was launched to support WHO's goal of treating 20,000 MDR-TB patients annually by 2010, a goal that was met 3 years early. Lilly first supplied drugs at concessionary prices to MSF, Partners in Health (PIH), and WHO. Lilly then embarked on a program to provide knowledge and financial assistance to reputable pharmaceutical manufacturers in China, India, Russia, and South Africa—the countries most severely affected by MDR-TB—so they can manufacture drugs against MDR-TB in their own countries at a reasonable price.

Understanding that TB cannot be conquered by medicine alone, the partnership tries to address TB from a number of perspectives. First, for example, the Lilly MDR-TB Partnership has implemented community-level programs in over 80 countries to raise awareness about MDR-TB, increase access to treatment, ensure correct completion of treatment, and empower patients by eliminating the stigma of the disease. These programs include a comprehensive media campaign to try to ensure that TB-related messages reach patients and their families, communities, healthcare workers, and policymakers.

The partnership also trains healthcare workers to recognize, treat, monitor, and prevent the further spread of MDR-TB. Training materials and courses have been designed to ensure that the knowledge learned is passed on to peers, furthering the quality of patient care. In addition, workplace toolkits and training programs allow companies to adopt policies and procedures to detect TB and properly treat and care for their workers.

The partnership also undertakes a number of efforts at the global level. It works with policymakers, for example, to raise awareness about the toll that TB takes on the global population and encourage new initiatives to curb the spread of MDR-TB. In addition, Lilly created the Lilly TB Drug Discovery Initiative. This is a not-for-profit partnership that will draw on the global resources of its partners, including

medicinal libraries—information on different chemical compounds used in making drugs—donated by Lilly, to pioneer research on the development of new drugs against TB that will require a shorter course of therapy than the existing drugs.

So far, the Lilly MDR-TB Partnership has met a number of its aims, including:

- Training of healthcare practitioners, including thousands of nurses, doctors, and hospital managers, through online courses and in-person workshops. For example, the International Council of Nurses has trained more than 1,000 nurses on TB and MDR-TB in more than a dozen countries in their Lilly-supported Training of Trainers program. Each of these nurses has gone on to train other nurses in their workplace, resulting in over 19,000 nurses trained on TB and MDR-TB to date.
- Continued transfer of Lilly drug technologies to seven partners to increase the local supply of drugs at affordable prices.
- Distribution of TB workplace toolkits to help organizations rapidly implement TB control programs to thousands of companies worldwide. Representatives of more than 1,500 organizations in India and South Africa have been directly trained on the use of the toolkit.
- Providing valuable input and support into the development and implementation of regional and national TB programs in the four countries hardest hit by MDR-TB (China, India, Russia, and South Africa).

These efforts have produced a number of valuable outcomes to date, including lower death rates, higher cure rates, better adherence to treatment, and increased TB and MDR-TB awareness.

The Long-Term Costs and Financing of HIV/AIDS

In 2008, an international consortium of partners, called aids2031, was established to examine the future of HIV/AIDS. The consortium was especially interested in understanding the trajectory of the epidemic to 2031—50 years after the virus was discovered—under various scenarios. The idea of taking such a long-term view of the epidemic was that it would allow countries and their partners to better understand how measures they take or fail to take today can affect the course of their epidemic in the long run.

Nine international and multidisciplinary working groups were established to carry out the work of aids2031. One of them was charged with examining the long-term costs and financing of HIV/AIDS.[174] This Costs and Financing Working Group was asked to estimate the long-term costs and financing of HIV/AIDS using different scenarios, so that policymakers and stakeholders could make more appropriate policy choices in the short and medium run for addressing their epidemics as effectively and efficiently as possible. The working group was led by the Results for Development Institute, a think tank based in Washington, DC.

In particular, the Costs and Financing Working Group sought to answer the following questions:

- What would it cost to address the epidemic under various scenarios over the next 2 decades?
- What factors would be the most important drivers of the costs?
- How can governments, donors, and stakeholders use scarce resources most effectively and efficiently to prevent more infections, keep more people alive, and protect and nurture AIDS orphans?
- How can HIV/AIDS efforts be financed in the future, and in what ways should that financial burden be shared among individuals, their countries, development partners, and private and philanthropic organizations?

The Working Group on Costs and Financing carried out its work on three levels. First, it prepared a global estimate of costs and financing broadly across a number of countries. In collaboration with partners in Cambodia and South Africa, the working group then examined the long-term costs and financing of HIV/AIDS efforts in greater detail in each of those countries. These case studies sought to apply and validate at the national level the costing, priority setting, and financial mobilization tools that had been developed by aids2031 through its global work. In addition, it was hoped that the country case studies would provide valuable information for stakeholders in Cambodia and South Africa and provide valuable lessons for other countries, as well.

Global View

The analysis of the estimated global cost of AIDS was led by the Results for Development Institute. The aids2031 project estimated that globally, between 2009 and 2031, HIV/AIDS will cost between $397 billion and $722 billion, depending on the policy choices that governments and donors adopt.[175] Four different scenarios were considered to estimate this projected cost: current trends, rapid scale-up, hard choices, and structural change.[175]

If the current trends continue, the number of new HIV infections in 2031 drops only slightly to 2.1 million while costing $490 billion. Rapid scale-up would include 80 percent coverage of most interventions, save 7 million lives, avert 14.2 million infections, and cost $722 billion. On the other hand, the hard choices scenario is the most cost-effective approach and focuses on a small number of cost-effective activities, costing $397 billion. The hard choices option is estimated to result in more HIV/AIDS-related deaths than under the rapid scale-up scenario, but deaths would be significantly lower than with the current trends. The structural change option would cost $579 billion and is estimated to have the greatest impact in reducing future spread of the infection, with 1.2 million people newly infected with HIV in 2031.[175]

The working group forecasted the availability of funds to fight AIDS. Currently, over half of the funding sources are from domestic expenditures; however, AIDS programs rely heavily on external funding, especially in low-income countries. The working group found that middle-income countries with a low burden of HIV/AIDS will eventually be able to take on the costs of their HIV/AIDS response. Middle-income countries with a high burden of HIV/AIDS will be able to address HIV/AIDS over the next 10 years if there is a rapid scale-up, matched by outside funds. However, low-income countries with a high burden of disease will remain dependent on external support to be able to address the high cost of HIV/AIDS.[175]

Cambodia Case Study

The Cambodia case study was led by the Cambodian National Center for HIV/AIDS, Dermatology, and Sexually Transmitted Infections (NCHADS), working in close collaboration with staff from the Ministry of Economy and Finance. Cambodia was selected as an example of a low-prevalence, low-income country. In addition, Cambodia was potentially an especially valuable case study because it had made enormous progress against the epidemic, bringing new infections down from about 16,000 a year in 1998 to almost 2,000 a year in 2009. However, the financing of its HIV/AIDS program was 90 percent dependent on Cambodia's development partners, and it appeared that these partners would not sustain this level of financing much longer.

The Cambodian study team developed six scenarios to explore the epidemiologic consequences of different policy choices, what each scenario would cost, and how Cambodia's HIV/AIDS program could be financed in the future to maximize desired outcomes at the lowest cost. These scenarios ranged from trying to engage in the best possible level of coverage as fast as possible, the best coverage scenario, to a worst case scenario, in which Cambodia would not be able to continue even its present levels of coverage of key program activities. They also included a current coverage scenario and scenarios in which Cambodia sharply focused on the most at-risk populations, as well as expanded coverage to reduce mother-to-child transmission of HIV, called the hard choice 1 and hard choice 2 scenarios.[176] The study team also included a structural change scenario to examine how political, social, and economic changes could affect the epidemic and reduce risk for certain populations.

Overall, the analysis indicated that the current HIV/AIDS program in Cambodia is likely to lead to further declines in HIV prevalence and incidence over the next 2 decades. In fact, all scenarios for HIV incidence, except the worst case scenario, have a downward trend. However, even in the best coverage scenario, Cambodia would still have 1,000 new HIV infections per year. In the worst case scenario, in which coverage of interventions falls from current levels, Cambodia could have as many as 3,800 new HIV infections per year, which would represent a reversal of the significant gains achieved in Cambodia.

The key findings related to costs are that HIV/AIDS resource requirements will continue to increase over the next 2 decades. Cumulative financial needs vary between $1.3 billion and $2.2 billion over the next 2 decades, depending on the path taken by the Cambodian HIV/AIDS program.[176] However, the outcomes from these two choices are not substantially different. Thus, Cambodia will need to focus on getting the best value for money from its HIV/AIDS program by focusing HIV/AIDS investments on those areas that are most cost-effective. This may lead to an approach similar to that of the hard choice scenarios, for example, with attention, as well, to key elements in the structural change scenario. It will also be valuable for Cambodia to focus on further enhancing the efficiency of its HIV/AIDS program by taking steps such as improving the efficiency of its training and supervision programs, reducing the costs of laboratory supplies and equipment, and increasing the quality of the drug treatment program even as it seeks to reduce costs of drugs.[176]

The Cambodian HIV/AIDS program has been very dependent on external financing, and there is substantial risk that such financing will be reduced. Assuming that donor assistance would eventually decline from 90 percent to 50 percent, three scenarios for development assistance were examined: the optimistic scenario, gradually reducing funding to 50 percent in 2025; the moderate scenario, reducing funding to 50 percent by 2020; and the pessimistic scenario, rapidly reducing funding to 50 percent in 2015. The optimistic scenario would result in an annual funding gap of $9 million, whereas the pessimistic scenario would result in an annual gap of $21 million.[176] Over the longer term, Cambodia

should be able to meet the costs of its HIV/AIDS program through increasing fiscal space for HIV/AIDS that will come with economic growth. However, if Cambodia's development partners withdraw financing from the HIV/AIDS program too quickly, Cambodia could face substantial difficulty in making up the deficit in the short term.

South Africa Case Study

South Africa was selected as a case study because of its exceptionally high rate of prevalence of HIV, the large number of new infections annually, the enormous costs associated with treating all of those infected with AIDS, and the need to better understand how those costs would be financed. At the time, South Africa had the largest number of HIV-infected people of any country, about 5.7 million, and almost half a million new infections per year. South Africa represented a high-prevalence, middle-income country, the study of which could have lessons for a number of other countries. The South Africa study was conducted by the Centre for Economic Governance and AIDS in Africa (CEGAA), working in close collaboration with the South African Ministry of Health and the South African Ministry of Finance.

The aids2031-South Africa project aimed to estimate the influence of political will, available resources, rate of behavioral change, and implementation capacity on the magnitude, nature, costs, and impacts of the national response to HIV/AIDS in South Africa.[177] Three scenarios were developed to explore the financial and epidemiologic consequences of different policy choices: hard choices; narrow NSP (national strategic plan), and expanded NSP.[178]

The analysis showed that the estimated costs from now until 2031 under the narrow NSP, or the current national approach, are $88 billion, with the number of new infections falling only slightly to 350,000 per year.[177] If the expanded NSP option is pursued, total costs may rise to $102 billion over the next 20 years, but the number of infections would fall dramatically to 200,000 annually. Under the hard choices scenario, only the most cost-effective prevention activities would be expanded, decreasing the number of new infections to about 225,000 per year, a scenario whose cumulative costs were estimated at $79 billion.[177] In the coming years, the hard choices and expanded NSP scenarios offer better alternatives to addressing AIDS than the current national strategic plan. The hard choices scenario could lower the number of infections at a lower cost, although it would not halve the number of new infections as the more expensive expanded NSP scenario might.[177]

It will be necessary for South Africa to step up current HIV/AIDS prevention strategies, carefully manage spending and expansion of antiretroviral therapy, address the impending HIV/AIDS financing gap, and improve cost analysis and monitoring, leading to fewer HIV infections in the future and lower costs to address HIV/AIDS in the next 2 decades.[177] Stepped-up prevention strategies include the widespread implementation of proven effective tools, such as male circumcision, condom promotion, and prevention of mother-to-child transmission. Investment in social change programs that focus on high-risk and vulnerable populations may also result in greater reductions in new HIV infections.[177] The number of ART patients is expected to increase to 2 or 3 million over the next decade. In South Africa, treatment accounts for approximately two-thirds of the current HIV/AIDS spending. It will be necessary for South Africa to carefully manage spending related to treatment services, investing in personnel and infrastructure to meet the increased need for treatment. The cost of addressing HIV/AIDS is expected to increase twofold over the next few years, requiring an effective financial mobilization strategy by the government. It will be necessary to increase domestic financing, while filling in funding gaps with external support sources such as the U.S. President's Emergency Plan for AIDS Relief (PEPFAR) or the Global Fund. In order to assist with the budgeting process, it is recommended that facility- and project-based cost estimates be determined and made available in a database. Cost-effectiveness studies of prevention interventions are needed to pursue the most cost-effective approaches and to inform key policy decisions.[177]

CASE STUDIES

The control of communicable diseases remains challenging. However, important progress has been made against many of these diseases as noted throughout the chapter. Given the exceptional importance of communicable diseases in low-income countries, this chapter includes four case studies. One of them examines the efforts of Thailand to address sexually transmitted diseases and HIV/AIDS. Another discusses China's attempt to control TB through DOTS. The last two cases concern NTDs, one on Chagas disease in Latin America and another on trachoma in Morocco. Those interested in more detail on the NTD cases can consult *Millions Saved: Proven Successes in Global Health.*[178]

Preventing HIV/AIDS and Sexually Transmitted Infections in Thailand

Background

In Thailand, approximately 1 in every 60 persons is infected with HIV/AIDS and 75,000 children have been orphaned by AIDS.[179,180] Between 1989 and 1990, HIV among sex workers tripled, from 3.1 percent to 9.3 percent, and a year later reached 15 percent. Over the same period, the proportion of male conscripts already infected with HIV when tested upon entry to the army at age 21 rose sixfold, from 0.5 percent in 1989 to 3 percent in 1991.[180]

The Intervention

In 1989, Dr. Wiwat Rojanapithayakorn, director of a regional office for communicable disease control in Thailand's Ratchaburi province, sought to curb AIDS by making sex in brothels safe, going well beyond the government's approach of raising awareness through mass advertising and education campaigns. Knowing that he could be effective only with political support, he sought the cooperation of the provincial governor. The steep rise in AIDS persuaded the governor to acquiesce, even though prostitution is illegal in Thailand and the government's intervention could imply that it tolerated or even condoned it.

A program was launched with one straightforward rule for all brothels in Ratchaburi: no condom, no sex. Until then, brothels had been reluctant to insist that their clients use condoms for fear of losing them to other establishments where condoms were not required. However, with condoms mandatory in all brothels, the competitive disincentive to individual workers and brothels was removed. Health officials, with the help of the police, held meetings with brothel owners and sex workers to provide them with information and free condoms. Men seeking treatment for sexually transmitted infections (STIs) were asked to name the brothel they had last visited, and health officials would then visit the establishment to provide more information. This pilot program had dramatic results, bringing down STIs in Ratchaburi within just a few months.[181] In 1991, the National AIDS Committee, chaired by Prime Minister Anand Panyarachun, adopted this 100 percent condom program at the national level.

The Impact

Condom use in brothels nationwide increased from 14 percent in early 1989 to more than 90 percent by June 1992.[182] An estimated 200,000 new infections were averted between 1993 and 2000. New STI cases fell from 200,000 in 1989 to 15,000 in 2001, and the rate of new HIV infections fell fivefold between 1991 and 1993–1995.[183] Such dramatic results have raised questions about their accuracy, as well as about their real causes, but independent studies have found the program to be genuinely effective.

The program did little to encourage the use of condoms in casual but noncommercial sex. Interventions among injecting drug users also did not expand to the national level, and the prevalence of HIV among this group is now as high as 50 percent.[184]

Costs and Benefits

Total government expenditure on the AIDS program remained steady at approximately $375 million from 1998 to 2001, representing 1.9 percent of the health budget. Of this, 65 percent was spent on treatment and care.

Lessons Learned

The success of the program is due, in part, to the sheer scale and level of organization of the sex industry in Thailand, assisting officials in tracing and coopting brothel owners. Thailand also had a good network of STI services within a well-functioning health system, providing treatment and advice, as well as crucial data for decision makers both at the baseline and when the program took effect. Cooperation among health authorities, governors, and the police was critical to success. Strong leadership from the prime minister, backed by significant financial resources, also made swift action possible. Maintaining Thailand's remarkable results in slowing the AIDS epidemic needs continued vigilance. Due to the high cost of treating STIs, the HIV prevention budget declined by two-thirds between 1997 and 2004.[185] Although the Thai experience provides no blueprint for other countries with very different starting conditions, it does demonstrate that targeted strategies and political courage can effect change in deeply entrenched behaviors.

Controlling TB in China

Background

Although China established a national tuberculosis program in 1981, inadequate financial support hindered its success. In 1991, with $58 million from the World Bank, China embarked on the largest informal experiment in TB control in history: the 10-year Infectious and Endemic Disease Control project in 13 of its 31 mainland provinces.[186] The project adopted the DOTS (directly observed therapy, short course) strategy. Individuals demonstrating TB symptoms were referred to county dispensaries, where they received free diagnosis and treatment. Village doctors were given financial incentives for enrolling patients and completing their treatment. Efforts were also made to strengthen the institutions involved with the establishment of a national tuberculosis project office and a tuberculosis control center. Quarterly reports were submitted by each county to the province, the central government, and the National Tuberculosis Project Office, which strengthened monitoring and quality control.

Impact

China achieved a 95 percent cure rate for new cases within 2 years of adopting DOTS, and a remarkable cure rate of 90 percent for those who had previously undergone unsuccessful treatment.[187] The number of people with TB declined by over 37 percent between 1990 and 2000, and 30,000 TB deaths were prevented each year. More than 1.5 million patients were treated, leading to the elimination of 836,000 cases of pulmonary TB.[188]

Costs and Benefits

The program cost $130 million. The World Bank and WHO estimated that successful treatment was achieved at a cost of less than $100 per person. One healthy life was saved for an estimated $15 to $20, with an economic rate of return of $60 for each dollar invested.[189]

Lessons Learned

The success of China's program can be attributed to strong political commitment, leadership, adequate funding, and a sound technical approach delivered through a relatively strong health system. It was found that DOTS could be scaled up rapidly without sacrificing quality. Free diagnosis and treatment served as an effective incentive for patients, and incentives for doctors to diagnose and complete treatment also worked well. However, the overall rate of case detection proved disappointing, mainly due to the inadequate referral of suspected TB cases from hospitals to TB dispensaries; hospitals charging for services had no incentive to refer patients to dispensaries where services were provided for free.[190] In addition, patients at hospitals often abandoned treatment prematurely. Despite the program's success, TB remains a deadly threat in China, and efforts continue to maintain cure rates, as well as to expand DOTS coverage to the remaining population.

Controlling Chagas Disease in the Southern Cone of South America

Background

Chagas disease, or American trypanosomiasis, was Latin America's most serious parasitic infection in the early 1990s. Endemic in all seven countries of the southern cone, it caused an estimated 16 to 18 million infections and 50,000 deaths each year. In Brazil alone, it was estimated that over a 2-year period the economic costs of the disease were almost $240 million and that $750 million would have been needed to treat its main health effects.[191]

The Intervention

The disease is named after Carlos Chagas, the Brazilian doctor who first described it in 1909 and subsequently discovered its cause: the parasite *Trypanosoma cruzi*. The parasites are found in the feces of "kissing bugs" that live within house walls in poor, rural areas and emerge at night to suck human blood. The parasites enter the bloodstream when insect bites are rubbed or scratched or when food is contaminated. They can also enter via infected blood or be transmitted from mother to fetus.

The first phase of the disease, the acute phase, is marked by fever, malaise, and swelling, and can sometimes be fatal, especially in young children. But most cases enter the second, chronic phase when the parasite damages vital body organs, resulting in heart failure, stomach pain, constipation, and swallowing difficulties that can lead to malnutrition.[192] One third of cases are fatal.

In the absence of a vaccine or cure, control efforts needed to focus on eliminating the vector and screening the blood supply. Early attempts at control included methods such as dousing house walls with kerosene or scalding water or enclosing and filling houses with cyanide gas. The introduction of synthetic insecticides offered a more plausible solution, and spraying campaigns began in several countries in the 1950s and 1960s. Brazil launched a national eradication campaign in 1983, involving nationwide spraying and volunteer schemes. Brazil's early success demonstrated the technical feasibility of vector control. However, it also highlighted the need for regional efforts against border-crossing insects, and the need for sustained political commitment.[193]

In 1991 a new control program called INCOSUR (Southern Cone Initiative to Control/Eliminate Chagas) was launched to bolster national resolve and prevent cross-border reinfestations. Led by the Pan American Health Organization (PAHO), the initiative was jointly adopted by Argentina, Bolivia, Brazil, Chile, Paraguay, Uruguay, and later, Peru. The countries financed and managed their own programs but met annually to share operational aims, methods, and achievements. Intercountry technical cooperation agreements fostered the sharing of information among regional scientists and governments, with additional scientific support from a network of researchers in 22 countries. Between 1992 and 2001, more than 2.5 million homes were sprayed. Canisters that release insecticidal fumes when lit were also provided. Houses were improved to eliminate hiding places for insects, adobe walls were replaced with plaster, and metal roofs were constructed. The screening of blood donors for the parasite is now virtually universal in 10 South American countries.[194]

Impact

Incidence in the seven INCOSUR countries fell by an average of 94 percent by 2000. Overall, the number of new cases on the continent fell from 700,000 in 1983 to fewer than 200,000 in 2000.[195] The number of deaths each year from the disease

was halved from 45,000 to 22,000. By 2001, disease transmission was halted in Uruguay, Chile, and large parts of Brazil and Paraguay. Surveys indicate an improved sense of well-being, domestic pride, and security. Central America and the Amazon region remain the next major challenges.

Costs and Benefits

Financial resources for INCOSUR, provided by each of the seven countries, have totaled more than $400 million since 1991. The intervention is considered among the most cost-effective interventions in public health, at just $37 per DALY averted in Brazil.[195]

Lessons Learned

Chris Schofield, a researcher at the London School of Hygiene and Tropical Medicine, attributes INCOSUR's success to three factors: it was big and designed to reach a definitive end point; it had a simple, well-proven technical approach; and it gained political continuity from a close coordination between researchers and governments. Alfredo Solari, Uruguay's former minister of health, mentions four elements of success: peer pressure from neighboring countries in an exercise dealing with border-crossing insects; commitment by all participating countries, backed by international organizations like PAHO and WHO; an international technical secretariat at PAHO that verified surveillance, shared information about progress, processed certification requests, and organized annual meetings; and a favorable economic and institutional environment that allowed resources for expensive national health programs. Sustaining the achievements of INCOSUR will require vigilance, because premature curtailment of active surveillance against the disease could lead to disease resurgence.

Controlling Trachoma in Morocco

Background

Trachoma is the second leading cause of blindness, after cataracts, and the number one cause of preventable blindness in the world. Although it has been eliminated in North America and Europe, trachoma still afflicts more than 41 million people in 57 countries, especially in hot, dry regions where access to clean water, sanitation, and health care is limited.[99,196] In Morocco, trachoma was once widespread, but in the 1970s and 1980s, treatment with antibiotics lowered its incidence in urban areas. A 1992 survey found that 5.4 percent of Moroccans still suffered from trachoma, mainly in five rural provinces in the southeast, where 25,000 people showed a serious decline in vision, 625,000 needed treatment for inflammatory trachoma, and 40,000 urgently required surgery.

The Intervention

Caused by the bacterium *Chlamydia trachomatis*, trachoma is highly contagious, spreading mainly among children through direct contact with eye and nose secretions, infected clothing, and fluid-seeking flies. Transmission of the disease is rapid in overcrowded conditions of poor hygiene and poverty. In endemic areas, prevalence rates in children ages 2 to 5 years can reach 90 percent.[197] Women are infected at a rate two to three times that of men because of their close contact with children. Repeated trachoma infections can lead to a painful in-turning of the eyelash, which can cause blindness.

In 1991, Morocco formed the National Blindness Control Program (NBCP) with several international and other agencies to eliminate trachoma by 2005. Between 1997 and 1999, this program implemented a pilot strategy to treat trachoma, developed by the Edna McConnell Clark Foundation, called SAFE (surgery, antibiotics, face washing, and environmental change). SAFE differed from earlier approaches by emphasizing behavioral and environmental change, in addition to medication. Under this four-part strategy, a quick and inexpensive surgery to prevent blindness was provided for large numbers of patients in small towns and villages. Antibiotics were used to treat infection and prevent scarring. Face washing, especially among children, was promoted through an education campaign. Living conditions and community hygiene were improved by constructing latrines, drilling wells, storing dung away from flies, and providing health education.[198]

In the mid-1990s, Pfizer discovered Zithromax (azithromycin), a one-dose cure to replace the 6-week course of tetracycline that had been used for treatment, ensuring a higher compliance rate. Pfizer donated the drug for Morocco, as well as for a number of other countries, through the International Trachoma Initiative (ITI), a private–public partnership that it forged along with the Clark Foundation.

Impact

Between 1999 and 2003, the SAFE strategy led to a 75 percent decline in trachoma in Morocco. Overall, the prevalence of active disease in children under 10 was reduced by 90 percent since 1997.[197,198]

Costs and Benefits

The Moroccan government provided most of the financing for the program. ITI supplemented this with several grants, and UNICEF contributed $225,000. Pfizer's donation of tens of millions of dollars' worth of Zithromax (azithromycin) to Morocco and other countries represents one of the largest donations of a patented drug in history.

Lessons Learned

Government commitment to the program was critical to its success, in addition to the array of effective interventions. Four key factors were also listed by ITI: the program was based on solid scientific evidence; it was locally organized and, therefore, responded well to local circumstances; it fit within a broader agenda of health promotion, disease control, and health equity; and treatment was closely linked with prevention and the development of a strong public health infrastructure. ITI and its many partners have helped ensure that Morocco's success with SAFE, like the disease that it has nearly eliminated, is contagious.

FUTURE CHALLENGES TO THE CONTROL OF COMMUNICABLE DISEASES

A number of challenges constrain efforts to address the burden of the most important communicable diseases. Some of these relate to the need for countries to cooperate to combat communicable diseases. Some concern the ability of weak health systems in low- and middle-income countries to tackle communicable diseases effectively and efficiently. Others relate to the issues raised by specific diseases.

First, it is imperative to enhance political commitment to the prevention and control of these diseases. Sustained political support at the highest levels is essential if progress is to be made against HIV/AIDS, and this is also true for the other leading causes of communicable disease. Countries will be successful in acting against these diseases only if they make them a real priority both politically and financially.

Second, the underlying causes of communicable diseases in low- and middle-income countries relate to poverty, people's lack of empowerment, people's lack of knowledge of appropriate health behaviors, and a lack of access to basic infrastructure such as safe water, sanitation, and health services. These issues will take many years to address in most low-income countries. Ways must be found in the short and medium term to work with communities to overcome some of these constraints, such as through community-based water supply and sanitation schemes and community-based distribution of drugs for neglected diseases.

It is likely that health systems in many low- and middle-income countries will continue to be weak for many years, as well. This suggests that efforts to address communicable diseases will also have to be based on partnerships with a variety of actors. These include communities, religious groups and other nongovernmental organizations, the private sector, and government. The great successes in the control of communicable diseases to date have all been built upon the foundation of public–private partnerships. The polio eradication effort includes, for example, a remarkable amount of public–private collaboration, as does the campaign against onchocerciasis. It is especially important that these actors work together in the future across an array of diseases and health systems issues and not just on individual diseases. Moreover, only by involving private providers of a variety of types can many diseases, such as TB and malaria, be addressed, because those providers are already so involved in service delivery.

Strengthening the surveillance of disease at the local, national, and global levels is also fundamental to effective disease control. A competent body of public health professionals needs to be responsible for managing surveillance networks. Appropriate laboratory infrastructure must be an essential part of any improved surveillance efforts. Continuous sharing of surveillance information within and across countries is necessary to prepare for special problems, to know when they arise, and to respond to them effectively.

The lack of adequately trained and appropriately deployed human resources for health will also remain an issue, especially in low-income countries. There will not be enough personnel, the incentives for their performance will be lacking, and the personnel who do exist will largely be available only in the larger cities for some time to come. Thus, it will be important to have the lowest level of worker possible handle various health services so that scarce higher-level workers can focus on those things they alone can do.

The challenge of financing enhanced efforts in the control of communicable diseases will also be formidable. Without major changes in their spending patterns and rapid economic growth, many low- and middle-income countries will not be able to pay for the expanded efforts needed to combat the major communicable diseases. Rather, they will have to depend for some time on financial assistance from the high-income countries and private sector partners. Nonetheless, there is room in many communicable disease control programs to improve efficiency and effectiveness, by focusing on the most cost-effective approaches.

Scientific and technical challenges also remain. There is no effective vaccine for any of the diseases that are the focus of this chapter, except for rotavirus for some forms of diarrhea. Drug resistance is a constant issue in HIV/AIDS, a threat in the control of diarrhea and some parasitic infections, and a major issue in the control of TB and malaria. It is imperative that new drugs be developed that can prevent or overcome such resistance at the same time as the world makes better progress in the more rational use of antibiotics.

Another challenge will be the need to develop models in low- and middle-income countries to provide chronic care of people with HIV/AIDS. Most health service efforts in low-income countries focus on acute care. The treatment of HIV with antiretroviral therapy creates the possibility that people who are HIV-positive can have full and productive lives for many years. However, it also means that countries with very weak health systems that are mostly accustomed to treating acute illnesses will have to develop effective and efficient models for treating some people for many years of their life. Such platforms might be able to serve noncommunicable diseases as well.

Another important issue is how low-income and resource-poor countries will be able to financially sustain the progress that they do make in HIV treatment and several other areas related to the prevention and control of communicable diseases. Successful efforts to prevent and control these diseases will reduce prevalence and, ultimately, reduce the demands on the health system. As the prevalence of hookworm declines, for example, countries will be able to spend less money for hookworm treatment programs. However, the demands on health systems for treatment for HIV/AIDS will continue to be great for many years to come. Low- and middle-income countries with high HIV prevalence will have to plan carefully how AIDS treatment can be financed in the future. This is especially important because once people start taking antiretroviral therapy, it is imperative that they continue to take it.

Monitoring and evaluation is an essential tool of public health programming. If the world is to make progress against the most important communicable diseases and continue to learn what is most cost-effective in addressing these diseases, then it is important to enhance the quality of monitoring and evaluation of health investments. All activities require a monitoring and evaluation component to track project progress, estimate cost-effectiveness of the effort, and assess the impact of the activities that are being financed.

MAIN MESSAGES

In 2010 communicable diseases accounted for about 31 percent of total deaths and 40 percent of DALYs in low- and middle-income countries. These diseases are especially prevalent in sub-Saharan Africa but they also take a major toll in South Asia. The burden of communicable diseases is similar for men and women, but the HIV/AIDS epidemic is taking an increasing toll on women and TB generally affects men more than women.

Emerging and reemerging infectious diseases and antimicrobial resistance represent grave threats to public health, in all countries. Emerging and reemerging infectious diseases have the potential to do great economic damage to individual countries and the international community, vastly in excess of their direct impact on morbidity and mortality. Enhancing global cooperation on disease surveillance and on action against these diseases is essential for the effective identification and control of emerging and reemerging infectious diseases. Substantial efforts will be needed by individual countries and globally to promote more rational use of antibiotics and better quality of antibiotics, if the development of resistant forms of bacteria, viruses, and parasites is to be slowed down.

HIV/AIDS is an especially important burden, but the number of HIV/AIDS cases is declining. About 35 million people are now infected with HIV; in 2013 about 1.5 million people died from the disease, and another 2.1 million were infected with it that same year.

The HIV/AIDS epidemic is helping to fuel TB. About one-third of the world is infected with TB, and there are approximately 9 million new cases of active TB disease in the world every year. Both HIV and TB mostly affect people in their productive years.

Malaria kills about 550,000 million people a year, mostly young children in Africa. It also causes a huge burden of morbidity because cases of malaria are so common and people may get more than one case a year. Malaria also poses very substantial risks to pregnant women. Diarrhea is an especially important burden of disease for children, as well, and is also responsible for about 760,000 child deaths a year. A number of parasitic and infectious diseases, referred to as "neglected tropical diseases" pose an exceptional burden of disease, again largely in sub-Saharan Africa and South Asia. The worm *Ascaris*, for example, infects more than 1 billion people worldwide. Trichuris and hookworm infect 800 million and 700 million, respectively.

The economic and social consequences of the communicable diseases are very considerable. Diarrhea and worms can cause children to fail to develop properly, delay their entry into and performance in school, and reduce their productivity as adults. HIV/AIDS, TB, and malaria also greatly affect adult productivity. The direct and indirect costs of these diseases to individuals and families are very high and often cause people to borrow money, sell their limited assets, and fall below the poverty line. There is good evidence that high levels of malaria are an impediment to economic growth in low-income countries in Africa.

Addressing HIV/AIDS will require expanding a combination of investments tailored in different countries to the nature of their epidemics. Strong political leadership, focusing on the groups most at risk, and addressing the needs of "bridge populations" are parts of successful prevention efforts. Other key parts of prevention are maintaining a clean blood supply, testing and counseling, and condom promotion, in connection with efforts to delay sexual debut and reduce the number of sexual partners. It is also important to stem the transmission of HIV from mother to child. Male circumcision programs are now being expanded. An increasing number of people are being treated for HIV worldwide, and efforts are under way to meet 90-90-90 targets by 2020—to ensure that 90 percent of those with HIV know their status, to ensure that 90 percent of them are treated, and to ensure that 90 of those treated have suppressed viral loads. Effective treatment reduces transmission and reduces the burden of opportunistic infections, such as TB. The earlier people are put on treatment after becoming infected, the fewer people they will infect with HIV.

The mainstay of efforts to address TB has been DOTS, which stands for directly observed therapy, short-course. This is a very cost-effective way of treating TB. The global goal is to eliminate TB as a public health problem by 2035. This will require, among other things, expanded efforts at early diagnosis and appropriate treatment with high quality drugs; treatment of all people with TB; vaccination of children with BCG; and enhanced efforts at managing TB/HIV co-infection. The aim is to link these efforts with greater involvement of communities, improved regulatory frameworks, and improved efforts to address the social determinants of disease. While important progress has been made with traditional tools of diagnosis and new diagnostic tools are being increasingly used, it will also be important to develop improved diagnostics, a more effective TB vaccine, and more effective and shorter course drug regimens.

Malaria can be addressed through prompt diagnosis and treatment, intermittent treatment of pregnant women, the use of insecticide-treated bednets, and indoor residual spraying. Proper treatment to avoid the development of resistance is central to efforts in TB, HIV, and malaria.

The burden of diarrhea can be reduced through immunization against rotavirus and measles and supplementation with zinc. Oral rehydration therapy is a cost-effective way of managing diarrhea in infants and children. The best approach to diarrhea, of course, would be to try to avoid it through improved hygiene. Better access to safe water and sanitation will also help to reduce the burden of diarrhea and some of the parasitic and bacterial infections that make up the neglected diseases. In the short run, however, there is a package of mass drug administration and drug therapy that can be integrated with other disease control efforts to reduce the burden of the NTDs in a cost-effective way.

The challenge of addressing the burden of communicable diseases effectively is substantial. They are mostly diseases of poverty that also reflect a lack of access to safe water and sanitation, poor knowledge of appropriate health behaviors, and a lack of health services that are geared to meet the highest priority needs. In addition, several of these diseases are highly stigmatized, efforts to control them must be carried out in countries with weak health systems, and considerably more financing is needed for these efforts than has been available. Nonetheless, there has been major, and sometimes exceptional, progress in the last 40 years in addressing smallpox, onchocerciasis, Guinea worm, and a number of vaccine-preventable diseases in children. The lessons from those experiences suggest that it is possible, through concerted efforts and partnerships and greatly enhanced disease surveillance efforts, to continue making such progress.

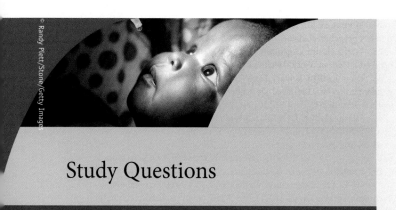

Study Questions

1. What are the most important communicable diseases in terms of deaths in low- and middle-income countries? In terms of DALYs?

2. In what regions will the deaths from HIV/AIDS be most important? In what regions will malaria be most important?

3. What is driving the HIV epidemic in Russia? In sub-Saharan Africa?

4. In sub-Saharan Africa, what would be the most cost-effective measures to try to prevent further transmission of the HIV virus? What approach would you take to prevention in South Asia, and why would it differ from what you would do in sub-Saharan Africa?

5. What groups are especially at risk for malaria? What steps would you take to try to reduce the burden of malaria?

6. What is DOTS? What are the key focuses of this approach? Why has it been more effective than previous approaches to TB control?

7. If relatively few people die as a direct result of parasitic diseases, why are they so important?

8. What are the concerns about drug resistance for malaria and TB? How can resistance be kept to a minimum?

9. Why is it important to develop a vaccine for HIV?

10. What are the drivers of antimicrobial resistance? What measures could a country take to try to reduce the development of resistance?

REFERENCES

1. Institute of Health Metrics and Evaluation. (2010). *GBD compare.* Retrieved January 31, 2015, from http://vizhub.healthdata.org/gbd-compare/.

2. UNAIDS. (2014). *Global statistics.* Retrieved January 31, 2015, from http://www.unaids.org/sites/default/files/media_asset/20140716_FactSheet_en.pdf.

3. World Health Organization. (2014). *Global tuberculosis report 2014.* Geneva: World Health Organization.

4. World Health Organization. (2013). *Diarrhoeal disease* (Fact sheet No. 330). Retrieved January 31, 2015, http://www.who.int/mediacentre/factsheets/fs330/en/.

5. World Health Organization. (2014). *World malaria report 2014.* Geneva: World Health Organization.

6. World Health Organization. *Tuberculosis and gender.* Retrieved December 22, 2010, from http://www.who.int/tb/challenges/gender/en.

7. Fauci, A. S. (2005). *2005 Robert H. Ebert memorial lecture. Emerging and re-emerging infectious diseases: The perpetual challenge.* New York: Milbank Memorial Fund.

8. Heymann, D. L. (2005). Emerging and re-emerging infectious diseases from plague and cholera to Ebola and AIDS: A potential for international spread that transcends the defences of any single country. *Journal of Contingencies and Crisis Management, 13*(1), 29–31.

9. Heymann, D. (2008). Emerging and re-emerging infections. In W. Kirch (Ed.), *Encyclopedia of public health.* New York: Springer.

10. Jones, K. E., Patel, N. G., Levy, M. A., et al. (2008, February 21). Global trends in emerging infectious diseases. *Nature, 451*, 990–993.

11. Heymann, D. L. (2002). The microbial threat in fragile times: Balancing known and unknown risks. *Bulletin of the World Health Organization, 80*(3), 179.

12. World Health Organization. (2015). *Tuberculosis* (Fact Sheet No. 104). Retrieved July 4, 2015, from http://www.who.int/mediacentre/factsheets/fs104/en.

13. Centers for Disease Control and Prevention. (1998). Preventing emerging infectious diseases: A strategy for the 21st century. *MMWR Morbidity and Mortality Weekly Report, 47*(No. RR-15), 1–14.

14. National Institutes of Health. (2009). *Microbial evolution and co-adaptation: A tribute to the life and scientific legacies of Joshua Lederberg. Workshop summary.* Institute of Medicine Forum on Microbial Threats. Washington, DC: National Academies Press.

15. Cohen, M. L. (2000). Changing patterns of infectious diseases. *Nature, 406*, 762–767.

16. Nugent, R., Beck, E., & Beith, A. (2010). *The race against drug resistance.* Washington, DC: Center for Global Development.

17. Okeke, I. N., Bhutta, Z. A., Duse, A. G., et al. (2005). Antimicrobial resistance in developing countries. Part I: recent trends and current status. *The Lancet Infectious Diseases, 5*(8), 481–493.

18. Okeke, I. N., Bhutta, Z. A., Duse, A. G., et al. (2005) Antimicrobial resistance in developing countries. Part II: strategies for containment. *The Lancet Infectious Diseases, 5*(9), 568–580.

19. Laxminarayan, R., Bhutta, Z. A., Duse, A., et al. (2006). Drug resistance. In D. T. Jamison, J. G. Breman, A. R. Measham, et al. (Eds.). *Disease control priorities in developing countries* (2nd ed., pp. 1031–1051). Washington, DC: The World Bank.

20. Snowden, F. M. (2008). Emerging and reemerging diseases: A historical perspective. *Immunological Reviews, 225*, 9–26.

21. World Bank. (2014). *The economic impact of the 2014 Ebola epidemic.* Washington, DC: The World Bank.

22. Centers for Disease Control and Prevention. (n.d.). Severe Acute Respiratory Infection (SARS). Frequently Asked Questions about SARS. Retrieved July 5, 2015 from http://www.cdc.gov/sars/about/faq.html.

23. Médecins Sans Frontières. (2003). *Q&A: ACT NOW to get malaria treatment that works to Africa.* Retrieved February 2, 2015, http://www.msf.org/article/qa-act-now-get-malaria-treatment-works-africa.

24. Morens, D. M., Folkers, G. K., & Fauci, A. S. (2008). Emerging infections: A perpetual challenge. *The Lancet Infectious Diseases, 8*(11), 710–719.

25. World Health Organization. (2005). *International health regulations* (2nd ed.). Geneva: World Health Organization.

26. Lynn, J. (2010, January 12). WHO to review its handling of H1N1 flu pandemic. *Reuters.* Retrieved December 29, 2010, from http://www.reuters.com/article/idUSTRE5BL2ZT20100112.

27. Salaam-Blyther, T. (2014). *U.S. and international health responses to the Ebola outbreak in West Africa.* Washington, DC: Congressional Research Service.

28. World Health Organization. (2012). *The evolving threat of antimicrobial resistance: Options for action.* Geneva: World Health Organization.

29. Leung, E., Weil, D. E., Raviglione, M., & Nakatani, H., on behalf of the World Health Organization World Health Day Antimicrobial Resistance Technical Working Group. (2011). The WHO policy package to combat antimicrobial resistance. *Bulletin of the World Health Organization, 89*, 290–292.

30. Laxminarayanan, R., Duse, A., Wattal, C., et al. (2013). Antibiotic resistance—The need for global solutions. *The Lancet Infectious Diseases, 13*(12), 1057–1098. doi: 10.1016/S1473-3099(13)70318-9.

31. Mackey, T. K., & Liang, B. A. (2012). Threats from emerging and re-emerging neglected tropical diseases (NTDs). *Infection Ecology and Epidemiology, 2.* doi: 10.3402/iee.v2i0.18667.

32. Dash, A. P., Bhatia, R., Sunyoto, T., & Mourya, D. T. (2013). Emerging and re-emerging arboviral diseases in Southeast Asia. *Journal of Vector Borne Diseases, 50*, 77–84.

33. Bertozzi, S., Padian, N. S., Wegbreit, J., et al. (2006). HIV/AIDS prevention and treatment. In D. T. Jamison, J. G. Breman, A. R. Measham, et al. (Eds.), *Disease control priorities in developing countries* (2nd ed., pp. 331–370). New York: Oxford University Press.

34. Chin, J. (Ed.). (2000). *Control of communicable diseases manual* (17th ed.). Washington, DC: American Public Health Association.

35. UNAIDS. (2014). *Global report: UNAIDS report on the global AIDS epidemic 2014.* Geneva: World Health Organization.

36. UNAIDS. (2013). *Global Report UNAIDS report on the global AIDS epidemic 2013.* Geneva. UNAIDS.

37. Institute of Health Metrics and Evaluation. (2010). *GBD 2010 heatmap.* Retrieved February 3, 2015, http://vizhub.healthdata.org/irank/heat.php.

38. UNAIDS. (2013). *AIDS by the numbers.* Geneva: UNAIDS.

39. Brown, L. R. (1997). *The potential impact of AIDS on population and economic growth rates.* Retrieved November 22, 2006, http://ideas.repec.org/p/fpr/2020br/43.html.

40. Russell, S. (2004). The economic burden of illness for households in developing countries: A review of studies focusing on malaria, tuberculosis, and human immunodeficiency virus/acquired immunodeficiency syndrome. *American Journal of Tropical Medicine and Hygiene, 71*(2 Suppl), 147–155.

41. UNICEF. (2013). *Towards an AIDS-free generation—Children and AIDS: Sixth stocktaking report, 2013.* New York: UNICEF.

42. Medicins San Frontiers Access Campaign. (n.d.). Untangling the web of antiretroviral price reductions, 17th edition. Retrieved May 24, 2015, from http://www.msfaccess.org/sites/default/files/MSF_UTW_17th_Edition_4_b.pdf.

43. Galarraga, O., Wirtz, V., Figueroa-Lara, A., et al. (2011). Unit costs for delivery of antiretroviral treatment and prevention of mother to child transmission of HIV: A systematic review for low- and middle-income countries. *Pharmacoeconomics, 29*(7), 579–599.

44. World Bank. (2015). *Health expenditure per capita (current US$).* Retrieved February 2, 2015, from http://data.worldbank.org/indicator/SH.XPD.PCAP.

45. Resch, S., Ryckman, T., & Hecht, R. (2015). Funding AIDS programmes in the era of shared responsibility: An analysis of domestic spending in 12 low- and middle-income countries. *The Lancet Global Health, 3*(1), e52–e61.

46. Ainsworth M., & Over, M. (1994). AIDS and African development. *World Bank Research Observer, 9*(2), 203–240.

47. UNAIDS. (2014). *90-90-90 an ambitious treatment target to help end the AIDS epidemic*. Geneva: UNAIDS.

48. UNAIDS. (2010). *UNAIDS report on the global AIDS epidemic*. Geneva: UNAIDS.

49. World Health Organization. *Mother-to-child transmission of HIV*. Retrieved February 5, 2015, from http://www.who.int/hiv/topics/mtct/en/.

50. World Health Organization. (2010). *Guidelines on HIV and infant feeding 2010*. Geneva: World Health Organization.

51. Centers for Disease Control and Prevention. (2008). *Male circumcision and risk for HIV transmission: Implications for the United States*. Retrieved February 27, 2015, from http://stacks.cdc.gov/view/cdc/13545/.

52. Dickson, K. E., Tran, N. T., Samuelson, J. L., Njeuhmeli, E., Cherutich, P., et al. (2011) Voluntary medical male circumcision: A framework analysis of policy and program implementation in Eastern and Southern Africa. *PLoS Med*, 8(11), e1001133. doi: 10.1371/journal.pmed.1001133.

53. International AIDS Vaccine Initiative. Retrieved February 5, 2015, from http://www.iavi.org/.

54. International Partnership on Microbicides. Retrieved February 5, 2015, from http://www.ipmglobal.org/.

55. Centers for Disease Control and Prevention. (2015). *Basic TB facts*. Retrieved February 3, 2015, from http://www.cdc.gov/tb/topic/basics/.

56. Centers for Disease Control and Prevention. (n.d.). *Tuberculosis basic TB facts*. Retrieved May 26, 2015, from http://www.cdc.gov/tb/topic/basics/risk.htm.

57. World Health Organization. (2012). *Tuberculosis: Drug resistant tuberculosis: Frequently asked questions*. Retrieved May 26, 2015, from http://www.who.int/tb/challenges/mdr/tdrfaqs/en/.

58. Centers for Disease Control and Prevention. *Extensively drug-resistant tuberculosis (XDR TB)—Update*. Retrieved November 19, 2006, http://www.cdc.gov/tb/topic/drtb/xdrtb.htm.

59. Chand, N., Singh, T., Khalsa, J. S., Verma, V., & Rathore, J. S. (2004). A study of socio-economic impact of tuberculosis on patients and their family. *Chest*, 126(4), 832S.

60. Croft, R. A., & Croft, R. P. (1998). Expenditure and loss of income incurred by tuberculosis patients before reaching effective treatment in Bangladesh. *International Journal of Tuberculosis and Lung Disease*, 2(3), 252–254.

61. Tanimura, T., Jaramillo, E., Weil, D., Raviglione, M., & Lonnroth, K., Financial Burden for tuberculosis patients in low- and middle-income countries: A systematic review. *European Respiratory Journal*, 43, 1763–1775.

62. Kamolratanakul, P., Sawert, H., Kongsin, et al. (1999). Economic impact of tuberculosis at the household level. *International Journal of Tuberculosis and Lung Disease*, 3(10), 869–877.

63. Rajeswari, R., Balasubramanian, R., Muniyandi, M., Geetharamani, S., Thresa, X., & Venkatesan, P. (1999). Socio-economic impact of tuberculosis on patients and family in India. *International Journal of Tuberculosis and Lung Disease*, 3(10), 869–877.

64. Grimard, F., & Harling, G. (2004). *The impact of tuberculosis on economic growth*. Paper presented at the Northeast Universities Development Consortium Conference, Montréal, Quebec. Retrieved November 22, 2006, from http://neumann.hec.ca/neudc2004/fp/grimard_franque_aout_27.pdf.

65. Peabody, J. W., Shimkhada, R., Tan, C., Jr., & Luck, J. (2005). The burden of disease, economic costs and clinical consequences of tuberculosis in the Philippines. *Health Policy and Planning*, 20(6), 347–353.

66. Dye, C., & Floyd, K. (2006). Tuberculosis. In D. T. Jamison, J. G. Breman, A. R Measham, et al. (Eds.), *Disease control priorities in developing countries* (2nd ed., pp. 289–312). New York: Oxford University Press.

67. World Health Organization. (2010). *Guidelines for the treatment of tuberculosis* (4th ed.). Geneva: World Health Organization.

68. World Health Organization. *WHO policy on collaborative TB/HIV activities guidelines for national programmes and other stakeholders*. Geneva: World Health Organization.

69. World Health Organization. (n.d.). *Scaling up the three Is for TB/HIV*. Retrieved May 26, 2015, from http://www.who.int/hiv/topics/tb/3is/en/.

70. World Health Organization. (2014). *The end TB strategy*. Geneva: World Health Organization.

71. Breman, J. G., Mills, A., Snow, R. W., & Mulligan, J.-A. (2006). Conquering malaria. In D. T. Jamison, J. G. Breman, A. R. Measham, et al. (Eds.), *Disease control priorities in developing countries* (2nd ed., pp. 413–432) New York: Oxford University Press.

72. Jaap, J. vH., Rutten, M., Koelewijn, R., et al. (2009). Human *Plasmodium knowlesi* infection detected by rapid diagnostic tests for malaria. *Emerging Infectious Diseases*, 15(9), 1478–1480.

73. Roll Back Malaria. (2014). *Key malaria facts*. Retrieved February 3, 2015, from http://www.rollbackmalaria.org/keyfacts.html.

74. World Health Organization. *Malaria. Malaria in pregnant women*. n.d. Retrieved July 5, 2015 from http://www.who.int/malaria/areas/high_risk_groups/pregnancy/en/

75. World Health Organization. *10 facts on malaria*. Retrieved February 3, 2015, from http://www.who.int/features/factfiles/malaria/malaria_facts/en/index8.html.

76. USAID. (2011). *The President's Malaria Initiative: Fifth annual report to Congress*. Retrieved February 28, 2015, from http://www.pmi.gov/docs/default-source/default-document-library/pmi-reports/pmi_annual_report11.pdf.

77. Roll Back Malaria Partnership. *Economic costs of malaria*. Retrieved November 22, 2006, from http://www.rbm.who.int/cmc_upload/0/000/015/363/RBMInfosheet_10.htm.

78. World Health Organization. (n.d.). *Malaria: Overview of malaria treatment*. Retrieved May 26, 2015, from http://www.who.int/malaria/areas/treatment/overview/en/.

79. World Health Organization. (2014). *WHO policy brief for the implementation of intermittent preventive treatment of malaria in pregnancy using sulfadoxine-pyrimethamine*. Geneva: World Health Organization.

80. President's Malaria Initiative. *Indoor residual spraying*. Retrieved February 3, 2015, from http://www.pmi.gov/how-we-work/technical-areas/indoor-residual-spraying.

81. World Health Organization. (2012). *WHO policy recommendation: Seasonal malaria chemoprevention (SMC) for* Plasmodium falciparum *malaria control in highly seasonal transmission areas of the Sahel sub-region in Africa*. Geneva: World Health Organization.

82. Keusch, G. T., Fontaine, O., Bhargava, A., & Boschi-Pinto, C. (2006). Diarrheal diseases. In D. T. Jamison, J. G. Breman, A. R. Measham, et al. (Eds.), *Disease control priorities in developing countries* (2nd ed., pp. 371–388) New York: Oxford University Press.

83. World Health Organization. (2012). *Estimated rotavirus deaths for children under 5 years of age: 2008, 453,000*. Retrieved February 6, 2015, from http://www.who.int/immunization/monitoring_surveillance/burden/estimates/rotavirus/en/.

84. Huttly, S. R., Morris, S. S., & Pisani, V. (1997). Prevention of diarrhoea in young children in developing countries. *Bulletin of the World Health Organization*, 75, 163–174.

85. UNICEF and The World Health Organization. (2009). *Diarrhoea: Why children are still dying and what can be done*. New York: UNICEF.

86. Black, R. E. (2003). Zinc deficiency, infectious disease, and mortality in the developing world. *Journal of Nutrition*, 133(5 Suppl 1), 1485S–1489S.

87. This section of the chapter is adapted with permission from Skolnik, R., & Ahmed, A. (2010). *Ending the neglect of neglected tropical diseases*. Washington, DC: Population Reference Bureau.

88. World Health Organization. *Neglected tropical diseases*. Retrieved December 14, 2009, from http://www.who.int/neglected_diseases/en.

89. Global Network Neglected Tropical Diseases. *The solution*. Retrieved February 9, 2015, from http://www.globalnetwork.org/solution.

90. Global Network Neglected Tropical Diseases. *The 7 most common NTDs*. Retrieved July 4, 2015, from http://www.globalnetwork.org/neglected-tropical-diseases/fact-sheets.

91. Musgrove, P., & Hotez, P. J. Turning neglected tropical diseases into forgotten maladies. *Health Affairs, 28*(6), 1691–1706.

92. Global Network for Neglected Tropical Diseases. *About.* Retrieved February 28, 2015 from http://www.globalnetwork.org/about.

93. The Access Project. Neglected Tropical Diseases Control Program. Retrieved December 15, 2009, from http://www.theaccessproject.com/index .php/about/ntd.

94. Brooker, S., Hotez, P. J., & Bundy, D. A. P. (2008). Hookworm-related anemia among pregnant women: A systematic review. *PLoS Neglected Tropical Diseases, 2*(9), e291.

95. Hotez, P. J., Brindley, P. J., Bethany, J. M., et al. Helminth infections: The great neglected tropical diseases. *Journal of Clinical Investigation, 118*(4), 1311–1321.

96. Kjetland, E. F., Ndhlovu, P. D., Gomo, E., et al. (2006). Association between genital schistosomiasis and HIV in rural Zimbabwean women. *AIDS, 20*(4), 593–600.

97. Hotez, P. J., & Daar, A. S. (2008). The CNCDs and the NTDs: Blurring the lines dividing noncommunicable and communicable chronic diseases. *PLoS Neglected Tropical Diseases, 2*(10), e312.

98. Global Network for Neglected Tropical Diseases. *Hookworm.* Retrieved February 28, 2015, from http://www.globalnetwork.org/hookworm.

99. Global Network for Neglected Tropical Diseases. *Trachoma.* Retrieved July 4, 2015, from http://www.globalnetwork.org/trachoma.

100. The Carter Center. (2015). *Guinea worm disease: Worldwide case totals.* Retrieved February 9, 2015, from http://www.cartercenter.org/health /guinea_worm/case-totals.html.

101. International Trachoma Initiative. *What is trachoma?* Retrieved April 30, 2011, from http://www.trachoma.org/world's-leading-cause-preventable-blindness.

102. World Health Organization. (2014). *Lymphatic filariasis* (Fact Sheet No. 102). Retrieved February 9, 2015, from http://www.who.int/mediacentre /factsheets/fs102/en/.

103. Molyneux, D. H. (2009). 10 years of success in addressing lymphatic filariasis. *Lancet, 373*(9663), 529–530.

104. Global Network for Neglected Tropical Diseases. *Founding partners.* Retrieved February 9, 2015, from http://www.globalnetwork.org /founding-partners.

105. World Health Organization. (2008). *Community-directed interventions for major health problems in Africa.* Geneva: World Health Organization.

106. World Health Organization. (2015). *Onchocerciasis* (Fact Sheet No. 374). Retrieved February 9, 2015, from http://www.who.int/mediacentre /factsheets/fs374/en/.

107. Copenhagen Consensus Center. Retrieved December 15, 2009, from http://www.copenhagenconsensus.com/Home.aspx.

108. Evidence Action. (n.d.). *Deworm the world initiative: The evidence for deworming.* Retrieved May 26, 2015, from http://www.evidenceaction .org/dewormtheworld/.

109. Hotez, P. J., Molyneux, D. H., Fenwick, A., Ottesen, E., Ehrlich Sachs, S., & Sachs J. D. (2006). Incorporating a rapid-impact package for neglected tropical diseases with programs for HIV/AIDS, tuberculosis, and malaria. *PLoS Medicine, 3*(5):e102. doi:10.1371/journal.pmed.0030102.

110. Hotez, P. J., & Molyneux, D. H. (2008). Tropical anemia: One of Africa's greatest killers and a rationale for linking malaria and neglected tropical disease control to achieve a common goal. *PLoS Neglected Tropical Diseases, 2*(7), e270.

111. Hopkins, D. R., Eigege, A., Miri, E. S., et al. (2002). Lymphatic filariasis elimination and schistosomiasis control in combination with onchocerciasis control in Nigeria. *American Journal of Tropical Medicine and Hygiene, 67*(3), 266–272.

112. Geraghty, J. (2009). Expanding the biopharmaceutical industry's involvement in fighting neglected diseases. *Health Affairs, 28*(6), 1774–1777.

113. Preparedness and response for chikungunya virus. (2011). *PAHO, 1,* 1–131. Retrieved July 17, 2014, from the Pan American Health Organization database.

114. Soumahoro, M., Hanslik, T., Pelat, C., Atsou, K., Gazere, B., Boelle, P., et al. (2011). The chikungunya epidemic on La Réunion Island in 2005–2006: A cost-of-illness study. *PLoS Neglected Tropical Diseases, 5*(6), e1197.

115. Sissoko, D., Malvy, D., Ezzedine, K., Renault, P., Moscetti, F., Ledrans, M., et al. (2009). Post-epidemic chikungunya disease on Reunion Island: Course of rheumatic manifestations and associated factors over a 15-month period. *PLoS Neglected Tropical Diseases, 3*(3), e389.

116. World Health Organization. (2011). *Chikungunya* (Fact Sheet No. 327). Retrieved July 19, 2014, from http://www.who.int/mediacentre /factsheets/fs327/en/.

117. National Center for Emerging and Zoonotic Infectious Diseases. (2014). *Chikungunya: Information for the general public.* Retrieved July 17, 2014, from http://www.cdc.gov/chikungunya/pdfs/CHIKV_FACT%20 SHEET_CDC_General%20Public_cleared.pdf.

118. Mavalankar, D., Shastri, P., Bandyopadhyay, T., Parmar, J., & Ramani, K. V. (2008, March). Increased mortality rate associated with chikungunya epidemic, Ahmedabad, India. *Emerging Infectious Diseases, 4*(3). Retrieved February 28, 2015, from http://wwwnc.cdc.gov/eid/article/14/3/07-0720.

119. National Center for Emerging and Zoonotic Infectious Diseases. *Dengue and the* Aedes aegypti *mosquito.* Retrieved July 21, 2014, from http:// www.cdc.gov/dengue/resources/30jan2012/aegyptifactsheet.pdf.

120. Seyler, T., Hutin, Y., Ramanchandran, V., Ramakrishnan, R., Manickam, P., & Murhekar, M. (2010). Estimating the burden of disease and the economic cost attributable to chikungunya, Andhra Pradesh, India, 2005–2006. *Transactions of the Royal Society of Tropical Medicine and Hygiene, 104*(2), 133–138.

121. Centers for Disease Control and Prevention. (2012). *Aedes aegypti Aedes albopictus.* Retrieved from http://www.cdc.gov/dengue /resources/30Jan2012/comparisondenguevectors.pdf.

122. Centers for Disease Control and Prevention. *Outbreaks chronology: Ebola virus disease.* Retrieved January 31, 2015, from http://www.cdc.gov /vhf/ebola/resources/outbreak-table.html.

123. World Health Organization. (2014). *Ebola virus disease* (Fact Sheet No. 103). Retrieved September 4, 2014, from http://www.who.int /mediacentre/factsheets/fs103/en/.

124. Centers for Disease Control and Prevention. *2014 Ebola outbreak in West Africa.* Retrieved January 31, 2015, from http://www.cdc.gov/vhf/ebola /outbreaks/2014-west-africa/index.html.

125. Centers for Disease Control and Prevention. *Signs and symptoms.* Retrieved January 31, 2015, from http://www.cdc.gov/vhf/ebola/symptoms /index.html.

126. Leroy, E., Kumulungui, B., Pourrut, X., Rouquet, P., Hassanin, A., Yaba, P., et al. (2005). Fruit bats as reservoirs of Ebola virus. *Nature, 438,* 575–576.

127. Centers for Disease Control and Prevention. (2014). *Infection control for viral haemorrhagic fevers in the African health care setting.* Retrieved January 31, 2015, from http://www.cdc.gov/vhf/abroad/vhf-manual.html.

128. Breman, J. G., Piot, P., Johnson, K. M., White, M. K., Mbuyi, M., Sureau, P., Heymann, D. L., et al. (1978). The epidemiology of Ebola haemorrhagic fever in Zaire, 1976. In S. R. Pattyn (Ed.), *Ebola virus haemorrhagic fever* (pp. 103–124). Amsterdam: Elsevier/North-Holland. Retrieved September 4, 2014, from http://www.itg.be/internet/ebola/pdf /EbolaVirusHaemorragicFever-SPattyn.pdf.

129. Centers for Disease Control and Prevention. (2015). *Ebola outbreak in West Africa—Case counts.* Retrieved January 31, 2015, from http://www.cdc .gov/vhf/ebola/outbreaks/2014-west-africa/case-counts.html.

130. Baize, S., Pannetier, D., Oestereich, L., Rieger, T., Koivogui, L., Magassouba, N., et al. (2014). Emergence of Zaire Ebola virus disease in Guinea— Preliminary report. *New England Journal of Medicine, 371*(15). Retrieved January 31, 2015, from http://www.nejm.org/doi/pdf/10.1056/NEJMoa1404505.

131. World Health Organization. (2014, August 8). *Statement on the meeting of the International Health Regulations Emergency Committee regarding the 2014 Ebola outbreak in West Africa.* Retrieved January 31, 2015, from http:// www.who.int/mediacentre/news/statements/2014/ebola-20140808/en/.

132. Médecins Sans Frontières. *Ebola.* Retrieved September 4, 2014, from http://www.doctorswithoutborders.org/our-work/medical-issues/ebola.

133. European Centre for Disease Prevention and Control. (2015). *Epidemiological situation.* Retrieved February 1, 2015, from http://www.ecdc.europa.eu/en/healthtopics/ebola_marburg_fevers/Pages/epidemiological-situation.aspx.

134. World Health Organization. (2015, January 28). *Ebola situation report—28 January 2015.* Retrieved February 1, 2015, from http://apps.who.int/ebola/en/ebola-situation-report/situation-reports/ebola-situation-report-28-january-2015.

135. World Health Organization. (2008, January 1). *International health regulations (2005).* Retrieved September 7, 2014, from http://www.who.int/ihr/9789241596664/en/.

136. Levine, M. (2014, July 17). WHO can't fully deal with Ebola outbreak, health official warns. *The Los Angeles Times.* Retrieved September 7, 2014, from http://www.latimes.com/world/africa/la-fg-who-ebola-20140718-story.html.

137. World Health Organization. (2014). *Ebola response roadmap.* Retrieved from http://apps.who.int/iris/bitstream/10665/131596/1/EbolaResponseRoadmap.pdf?ua=1.

138. European Centre for Disease Prevention and Control. (2014). *Rapid risk assessment: Outbreak of ebola virus disease in West Africa. Fourth update.* Retrieved from http://ecdc.europa.eu/en/publications/Publications/Ebola-virus-disease-west-africa-risk-assessment-27-08-2014.pdf.

139. World Health Organization. (2014, August 12). *WHO Director-General briefs Geneva UN missions on the Ebola outbreak.* Retrieved September 4, 2014 from http://www.who.int/dg/speeches/2014/ebola-briefing/en/.

140. UNICEF. (2014). *Ebola virus disease: Personal protective equipment and other ebola-related supply update.* Retrieved from http://www.unicef.org/supply/index_75984.html.

141. Nossiter, A. (2014, July 27). Fear of Ebola breeds a terror of physicians. *The New York Times.* Retrieved from http://www.nytimes.com/2014/07/28/world/africa/ebola-epidemic-west-africa-guinea.html?_r=0.

142. United Nations Office for the Coordination of Humanitarian Affairs. (2015). *Ebola outbreak: Updated overview of needs and requirements for January–June 2015.* Retrieved from http://reliefweb.int/sites/reliefweb.int/files/resources/updated_overview_of_needs_and_requirements_for_january-june_2015_0.pdf.

143. Médecins Sans Frontières. (2014, December 29). *Clinical trial for potential Ebola treatment starts in MSF clinic in Guinea.* Retrieved from http://www.doctorswithoutborders.org/article/clinical-trial-potential-ebola-treatment-starts-msf-clinic-guinea.

144. Onishi, N. (2015, January 31). As Ebola ebbs in Africa, focus turns from death to life. *The New York Times.* Retrieved from http://www.nytimes.com/2015/02/01/world/as-ebola-ebbs-in-africa-focus-turns-from-death-to-life.html?emc=edit_th_20150201&nl=todaysheadlines&nlid=67361508.

145. Centers for Disease Control and Prevention. (2013). *Cryptococcal meningitis: A deadly fungal disease among people living with HIV/AIDS.* Retrieved February 28, 2015, from http://www.cdc.gov/fungal/pdf/at-a-glance-508c.pdf.

146. Park, B. J., Wannemuehler, K. A., Marston, B. J., Govender, N., Pappas, P. G., & Chiller, T. M. (2009). Estimation of the current global burden of cryptococcal meningitis among persons living with HIV/AIDS. *AIDS, 23*(4), 525–530. doi: 10.1097/QAD.0b013e328322ffac.

147. French, N., Gray, K., Watera, C., Nakiyingi, J., Lugada, E., Moore, M., et al. (2002). Cryptococcal infection in a cohort of HIV-1-infected Ugandan adults. *AIDS, 16*(7), 1031–1038.

148. D'Souza, C. A., Kronstad, J. W., Taylor, G., Warren, R., Yuen, M., Hu, G., et al. (2011). Genome variation in *Cryptococcus gattii,* an emerging pathogen of immunocompetent hosts. *mBio, 2*(1), e00342-00310. doi: 10.1128/mBio.00342-10.

149. Rodriguez-Cerdeira, C., Arenas, R., Moreno-Coutino, G., Vasquez, E., Fernandez, R., & Chang, P. (2014). Systemic fungal infections in patients with human immunodeficiency virus. *Actas Dermo-Sifiliográficas, 105*(1), 5–17. doi: 10.1016/j.adengl.2012.06.032.

150. Perfect, J. R., Dismukes, W. E., Dromer, F., Goldman, D. L., Graybill, J. R., Hamill, R. J., et al. (2010). Clinical practice guidelines for the management of cryptococcal disease: 2010 update by the Infectious Diseases Society of America. *Clinical Infectious Diseases, 50*(3), 291–322. doi: 10.1086/649858.

151. Boulware, D. R., Meya, D. B., & Muzoora, C. (2013). ART initiation within the first 2 weeks of cryptococcal meningitis is associated with higher mortality: A multisite randomized trial. Paper presented at the 20th Conference on Retroviruses and Opportunistic Infections, Atlanta, GA.

152. Perfect, J. R. (2013). Fungal diagnosis: How do we do it and can we do better? *Current Medical Research and Opinion, 29*(Suppl 4), 3–11. doi: 10.1185/03007995.2012.761134.

153. Lessells, R. J., Mutevedzi, P. C., Heller, T., & Newell, M. L. (2011). Poor long-term outcomes for cryptococcal meningitis in rural South Africa. *South African Medical Journal, 101*(4), 251–252.

154. Rajasingham, R., Meya, D. B., & Boulware, D. R. (2012). Integrating cryptococcal antigen screening and pre-emptive treatment into routine HIV care. *Journal of Acquired Immune Deficiency Syndromes, 59*(5), e85–e91. doi: 10.1097/QAI.0b013e31824c837e.

155. Parkes-Ratanshi, R., Wakeham, K., Levin, J., Namusoke, D., Whitworth, J., Coutinho, A., et al. (2011). Primary prophylaxis of cryptococcal disease with fluconazole in HIV-positive Ugandan adults: A double-blind, randomised, placebo-controlled trial. *Lancet Infectious Diseases, 11*(12), 933–941. doi: 10.1016/S1473-3099(11)70245-6.

156. World Health Organization. (2013). *HIV/AIDS: 8.1 Prevention, screening, and management of common coinfections. Consolidated ARV guidelines, 2013.* Retrieved from http://www.who.int/hiv/pub/guidelines/arv2013/coinfection/prevcoinfection/en/index5.html.

157. Southern African HIV Clinicians Society. (2013). Guideline for the prevention, diagnosis and management of cryptococcal meningitis among HIV-infected persons: 2013 update. *Southern African Journal of HIV Medicine, 14*(2), 76–86.

158. Dowdy, D. W., Steingart, K. R., & Pai, M. (2011). Serological testing versus other strategies for diagnosis of active tuberculosis in India: A cost-effectiveness analysis. *PLoS Med, 8*(8), e1001074. doi: 10.1371/journal.pmed.1001074.

159. Vassall, A., van Kampen, S., Sohn, H., Michael, J. S., John, K. R., den Boon, S., et al. (2011). Rapid diagnosis of tuberculosis with the Xpert MTB/RIF assay in high burden countries: A cost-effectiveness analysis. *PLoS Med, 8*(11), e1001120. doi: 10.1371/journal.pmed.1001120.

160. Meya, D. B., Manabe, Y. C., Castelnuovo, B., Cook, B. A., Elbireer, A. M., Kambugu, A., et al. (2010). Cost-effectiveness of serum cryptococcal antigen screening to prevent deaths among HIV-infected persons with a CD4+ cell count < or = 100 cells/microL who start HIV therapy in resource-limited settings. *Clinical Infectious Diseases, 51*(4), 448–455. doi: 10.1086/655143.

161. Smith, R. M., Nguyen, T. A., Ha, H. T. T., Thang, P. H., Thuy, C., Lien, T. X., et al. (2013). Prevalence of cryptococcal antigenemia and cost-effectiveness of a cryptococcal antigen screening program—Vietnam. *PLoS One, 8*(4). doi: ARTN e62213.

162. Burgos, J. L., Kahn, J. G., Strathdee, S. A., Valencia-Mendoza, A., Bautista-Arredondo, S., Laniado-Laborin, R., et al. (2009). Targeted screening and treatment for latent tuberculosis infection using QuantiFERON-TB Gold is cost-effective in Mexico. *International Journal of Tuberculosis and Lung Disease, 13*(8), 962–968.

163. Pfizer. (2014). *Diflucan® Partnership Program.* Retrieved from http://www.directrelief.org/focus/disease-prevention/hivaids/diflucan-partnership-program/.

164. Sloan, D. J., & Parris, V. (2014). Cryptococcal meningitis: Epidemiology and therapeutic options. *Clinical Epidemiology, 6,* 169–182. doi: 10.2147/CLEP.S38850.

165. The South African Cryptococcal Screening Initiative Group. (2012). Phased implementation of screening for cryptococcal disease in South Africa. *South African Medical Journal, 102*(12), 914–917.

166. Sachdeva, K. S., Kumar, A., Dewan, P., Kumar, A., & Satyanarayana, S. (2012). New vision for Revised National Tuberculosis Control Programme

(RNTCP): Universal access—"Reaching the un-reached." *Indian Journal of Medical Research, 135*(5), 690–694. Retrieved from http://www.pubmed-central.nih.gov/articlerender.fcgi?artid=3401704&tool=pmcentrez&rendertype=abstract.

167. Pai, M., Yadav, P., & Anupindi, R. (2014). Tuberculosis control needs a complete and patient-centric solution. *The Lancet Global Health, 2*(4), e189–e190. doi:10.1016/S2214-109X(14)70198-6.

168. Anupindi, R. (2014). *Operation ASHA: An effective, efficient, and scalable model for tuberculosis treatment.* Retrieved from http://globalens.com/casedetail.aspx?cid=1429339.

169. Schwab Foundation for Social Entrepreneurship. *Shelly Batra.* Retrieved October 9, 2014, from http://www.schwabfound.org/content/shelly-batra.

170. Bhatnagar, N., Sinha, A., Samdaria, N., & Gupta, A. (2012). Biometric monitoring as a persuasive technology?: Ensuring patients visit health centers in India's slums. *Persuasive Technology. Design for Health and Safety,* 169–180.

171. Operation ASHA. (n.d.). Retrieved October 9, 2014, from http://healthmarketinnovations.org/program/operation-asha.

172. Operation ASHA. (2012). *Operation ASHA: Fighting tuberculosis worldwide.* Retrieved from http://www.opasha.org/.

173. The Lilly MDR-TB Partnership. Retrieved August 12, 2010, from http://www.lillymdr-tb.com; and personal communications with Karen Van der Westhuizen and Patrizia Carlevaro of the Eli Lilly Corporation.

174. aids2031 Costs and Financing Working Group. (2010). *Costs and choices: Financing the long-term fight against AIDS.* Washington, DC: Results for Development Institute.

175. Hecht, R., Stover, J., Bollinger, L., Muhib, F., Case, K., & de Ferrant, D. (2010). Financing of HIV/AIDS programme scale-up in low-income and middle-income countries, 2009–31. *Lancet, 376,* 1254–1260.

176. Saphonn, V., Chhorvann, C., Sopheab, H., Luyna, U., & Seilava, R. (2010). *The long-run costs and financing of HIV/AIDS in Cambodia.* Washington, DC: Results for Development Institute.

177. Guthrie, T., Ndlovu, N., Muhib, F., Hecht, R., & Case, K. (2010). *The long-run costs and financing of HIV/AIDS in South Africa.* Cape Town, South Africa: Centre for Economic Governance and AIDS in Africa.

178. Levine, R. (2004). *Millions saved: Proven successes in global health.* Washington, DC: Center for Global Development.

179. UNAIDS. (2002). *AIDS epidemic update (December).* Geneva: UNAIDS.

180. Centers for Disease Control and Prevention. *Global AIDS Program, country profiles: Thailand.* Retrieved February 6, 2004, from http://www.cdc.gov/nchsp/od/gap/countries/thailand.htm.

181. UNAIDS. (2000). *Evaluation of the 100% Condom Programme in Thailand.* Geneva: UNAIDS, in collaboration with the Ministry of Public Health, Thailand. Document 00.18E.

182. Rojanapithayakorn, W., & Hanenberg, R. (1996). The 100% condom programme in Thailand. *AIDS, 10*(1), 1–7.

183. Celentano, D., Nelson, K., Lyles, C., et al. Decreasing incidence of HIV and sexually transmitted diseases among young Thai men: Evidence for success of the HIV/AIDS control and prevention program. *AIDS, 12*(5), F29–F36.

184. Chitwarkorn, A. (2004). HIV/AIDS and sexually transmitted infections in Thailand: Lessons learned and future challenges. In J. P. Narain (Ed.), *AIDS in Asia: The challenge continues* (pp. 141–157). New Delhi: Sage.

185. UNAIDS. (2004). *Report on the global AIDS epidemic.* Geneva: UNAIDS.

186. China Tuberculosis Control Collaboration. (1996). Results of directly observed short-course chemotherapy in 112,842 Chinese patients with smear-positive tuberculosis. *Lancet, 347,* 358–362.

187. World Health Organization Regional Office for the Western Pacific. (2002). *DOTS for all: Country reports.* Geneva: World Health Organization.

188. Zhao, F., Zhao, Y., & Liu, X. (2003). Tuberculosis control in China. *Tuberculosis, 85,* 15–20.

189. The World Bank. (2002). *Implementation completion report for the China Infectious Diseases Control Project.* Washington, DC: The World Bank.

190. Chen, X., Zhao, F., Duanmu, H., Wan, L., Wang, X., & Chin, D. P. (2002). The DOTS strategy in China: Results and lessons after 10 years. *Bulletin of the World Health Organization, 80*(6), 430–436.

191. World Health Organization. (1991). *Control of Chagas disease. Report of a WHO expert committee* (WHO Technical Report Series: 811). Geneva: World Health Organization.

192. Centers for Disease Control and Prevention. *Chagas disease. Provider fact sheet.* Retrieved April 29, 2011, from http://www.cdc.gov/parasites/chagas/resources/factsheet.pdf.

193. Dias, J. C. P., Silveira, A. C., & Schofield, C. J. (2002). The impact of Chagas disease control in Latin America—a review. *Memorias do Instituto Oswaldo Cruz, 97,* 603–612.

194. Schmunis, G. A., Zicker, F., Cruz, J., & Cuchi, P. (2001). Safety of blood supply for infectious diseases in Latin American countries, 1994–1997. *American Journal of Tropical Medicine and Hygiene, 65,* 924–930.

195. Moncayo, A. (2003). Chagas disease: Current epidemiological trends after interruption of vectorial and transfusional transmission in the southern cone countries. *Memorias do Instituto Oswaldo Cruz, 98*(5), 577–591.

196. Kumaresan, J., & Mecaskey, J. (2003). The global elimination of blinding trachoma: Progress and promise. *American Journal of Tropical Medicine and Hygiene, 69*(5 Suppl), S24–S28.

197. Mecaskey, J., Knirsch, C., Kumaresan, J., & Cook, J. (2003). The possibility of eliminating blinding trachoma. *Lancet, 3,* 728–734.

198. West, S. (2003). Blinding trachoma: Prevention with the SAFE strategy. *American Journal of Tropical Medicine and Hygiene, 69*(5 Suppl), S18–S23.

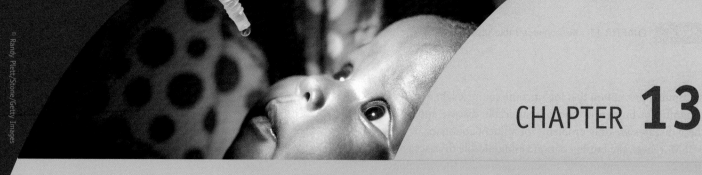

CHAPTER **13**

Noncommunicable Diseases

LEARNING OBJECTIVES

By the end of this chapter the reader will be able to:

- Describe the burden of noncommunicable diseases worldwide
- Discuss the most important risk factors for the burden of non-communicable diseases
- Outline the costs and consequences of noncommunicable diseases, tobacco use, alcohol use disorders, mental health disorders, and vision and hearing loss
- Review measures that can be taken to address the burden of noncommunicable diseases in cost-effective ways
- Describe some successful cases of dealing with noncommunicable diseases

VIGNETTES

Roberto was 45 years old and lived in Bogota, Colombia. He had a government desk job and had been overweight for most of his adult life. He got little exercise. He had read about increasing rates of diabetes in Colombia but still thought this was largely a disease of people in rich countries. Last year, Roberto started feeling thirsty all the time, had dry mouth, and felt weak after exertion. He went to his doctor who diagnosed him as having type II diabetes.

Shanti was 35 years old and lived in Sri Lanka. She had grown up in a village, had worked hard on her family's small farm, and had been healthy for all of her adult life. She had two children and had not had any problems during either pregnancy. During a recent visit to the local health center, however, the doctor discovered that Shanti had high blood pressure. The doctor talked with Shanti about changing her diet and also prescribed medication for her. The medicine she needs is not expensive but, unfortunately, Shanti has to take this medicine for the remainder of her life.

Alexei was 47 years old and lived in Moscow, Russia. Alexei had been smoking one pack of cigarettes a day since he was 16 years old. He heard on television and on the radio about the bad effects that cigarettes have on health. Urged by his children to stop smoking, he tried unsuccessfully on several occasions to quit. Over the last few months, Alexei developed a continuous cough and was often short of breath. Alexei had lung cancer.

Lai Ying was a factory worker who lived in Guandong Province, China. Until recently she had been a happy and healthy young woman. Lately, however, Lai Ying had felt very unhappy, did not feel like getting out of bed in the morning, did not want to go to work, and had no energy when she was at work. Lai Ying's family noticed that she was not eating properly and that she was not herself. However, they thought she was having a difficult time at work or with a boyfriend and that she would soon be fine. After some months of this behavior, Lai Ying committed suicide by taking an overdose of sleeping pills.

THE IMPORTANCE OF NONCOMMUNICABLE DISEASES

Noncommunicable diseases (NCDs) are of immense and growing importance worldwide. In fact, the burden of non-communicable diseases is greater than the burden of communicable diseases in low- and middle-income countries, as well as in high-income countries. Only in sub-Saharan Africa is the burden of communicable diseases higher than that of noncommunicable diseases.[1] This contradicts some people's continuing perception that low-income countries do not face a significant burden of noncommunicable disease and that these diseases are only problems for affluent countries.

Moreover, the burden of noncommunicable diseases will increase in low- and middle-income countries as they develop economically, become more integrated with the global economy, urbanize, and age. WHO estimates that the burden of noncommunicable diseases in sub-Saharan Africa will almost equal by 2020 the burden of communicable, maternal, perinatal, and nutritional disorders (Group I disorders).[2] Among the most important of the noncommunicable health conditions that low- and middle-income countries face are cardiovascular disease, cancer, mental disorders, musculoskeletal disorders, diabetes, and chronic respiratory disease.[1]

The risk factors for noncommunicable diseases relate in significant ways to lifestyle, much of which is within people's control. This chapter discusses, for example, the importance of diet, physical activity, tobacco use, and alcohol use to the onset of certain noncommunicable diseases. By engaging in appropriate health behaviors, it is possible for people to considerably reduce the risk of getting heart disease, some cancers, or diabetes.

Some noncommunicable diseases can be prevented at relatively low cost, but these diseases are often very expensive to treat. It is possible, for example, to significantly reduce the chances of getting lung cancer by making a modest investment in smoking cessation therapy and by quitting smoking. By contrast, the cost of treating lung cancer through drugs and surgery is considerably more.

This chapter focuses on noncommunicable diseases. It pays particular attention to cardiovascular disease, cancer, diabetes, and mental disorders because of their important and growing contribution to the global burden of disease, including in low- and middle-income countries. It also covers vision and hearing loss, because of the large amount of disability they cause and the extent to which they will become more common causes of disability in the future. Because of the importance of tobacco and alcohol as risk factors for noncommunicable diseases, the chapter also contains specific sections on these topics.

The chapter first introduces you to definitions of selected health conditions. It then examines the burden of noncommunicable diseases and the risk factors for those diseases. Following that, it comments on some of the most important costs and consequences of those diseases. It then reviews what steps can be taken to address the burden of noncommunicable diseases in cost-effective ways and discusses several examples of successful efforts to prevent and deal with noncommunicable diseases. The chapter concludes with comments on some of the future challenges that must be addressed if the burden of noncommunicable diseases is to be reduced.

KEY DEFINITIONS

Communicable diseases are illnesses caused by an infectious agent that spreads from a person or an animal to another person or animal. Noncommunicable diseases are, in many respects, the opposite of communicable diseases. First, they cannot be spread from person to person by an infectious agent, even if they might be associated with one. Second, they tend to last a long time. Third, they can be very disabling, can seriously impair the ability of people to engage in day-to-day activities, and often lead to death if they are not treated appropriately.

The terms *chronic disease* and *degenerative disease* are often used interchangeably with noncommunicable disease. In this text, however, we shall consistently use the term *noncommunicable disease*. The most recent studies of the burden of disease include the following under noncommunicable diseases: cardiovascular and circulatory diseases; neoplasms (cancers); musculoskeletal disorders; diabetes, urogenital, blood, and endocrine diseases; mental and behavioral disorders; chronic respiratory diseases; neuropsychiatric disorders, such as epilepsy, and Alzheimer's disease; digestive diseases; cirrhosis of the liver; and other noncommunicable disorders, including sense organ disorders, such as hearing loss, glaucoma, or cataracts, and skin disorders.[1]

You are already familiar with most of the terms used in this chapter; however, a few key terms with which you may be less familiar are defined in **Table 13-1**.

A NOTE ON DATA

This chapter includes data on both deaths and disability-adjusted life years (DALYs) for the most common noncommunicable diseases. An important part of the data in the chapter, therefore, is based on the *Global Burden of Disease Study 2010* that was published in 2013 and its related publications and website. Much of the other data used in this chapter comes from the World Health Organization (WHO).[2-4] The chapter also takes data from studies of specific diseases and efforts that countries are making to reduce the burden of noncommunicable diseases.

THE BURDEN OF NONCOMMUNICABLE DISEASES

Cardiovascular Disease

Ischemic heart disease caused about 7 million deaths in 2010 and is the leading specific cause of death globally for

TABLE 13-1 Key Terms and Definitions

Blood glucose—Blood sugar, the main source of energy for the body.

Body mass index (BMI)—Body weight in kilograms divided by height in meters squared (kg/m²).

Cancer—One of a large variety of diseases characterized by uncontrolled growth of cells.

Cardiovascular disease—A disease of the heart or blood vessels. This term encompasses both ischemic heart disease and stroke.

Cholesterol—A fatlike substance that is made by the body and is found naturally in animal-based foods such as meat, fish, poultry, and eggs.

Diabetes—An illness caused by poor control by the body of blood sugar.

Hypertension—High blood pressure, with a reading of 140/90 or greater.

Ischemic heart disease—A disturbance of the heart function due to inadequate supply of oxygen to the heart muscle.

Obesity—A BMI equal to or greater than 30

Overweight—A BMI equal to or greater than 25 but less than 30

Stroke—Sudden loss of function of the brain due to clotting or hemorrhaging.

Data from Global Cardiovascular Infobase. Glossary. Retrieved April 14, 2007, from http://www.cvdinfobase.ca/cvdbook/En/Glossary.htm; National Institutes of Health. Obesity, Physical Activity, and Weight-Control Glossary. Retrieved April 14, 2007, from http://win.niddk.nih .gov/publications/glossary.htm; WHO. Obesity and Overweight. February 15, 2015, from http://www.who.int/mediacentre/factsheets/fs311/en/.

all age groups and both sexes.[5] Stroke was the second leading cause of death globally among all age groups and for both sexes in 2010 and was responsible for about 6 million deaths.[5] Together, ischemic heart disease and stroke, generally referred to in burden of disease studies as cardiovascular disease (CVD), made up almost 25 percent of all deaths globally in 2010.[1]

In low- and middle-income countries, stroke was the leading cause of death in 2010 and was responsible for about 10.5 percent of deaths among all age groups and for both sexes. Ischemic heart disease was the second leading cause of death in these countries and responsible for about 10 percent of deaths among all age groups and both sexes in 2010.[1,5]

Ischemic heart disease is the largest cause of death among all age groups for both sexes in all regions, except East Asia and the Pacific, where stroke is a higher cause of death, and in sub-Saharan Africa, where communicable diseases still predominate. Together, ischemic heart disease and stroke make up about 54 percent of all deaths in Europe and Central Asia and about 30 percent of all deaths in East Asia and the Pacific but only about 7 percent of the total deaths in sub-Saharan Africa.[1] CVD rates are higher in Eastern Europe than in Western Europe, although the rates of CVD are falling in some Eastern European countries. The highest rates of CVD are in the former Soviet Union, where they contributed to declines in life expectancy.[6]

Ischemic heart disease was the leading cause of DALYs globally among all age groups and both sexes in 2010, and stroke was the third leading cause of DALYs. For high-income countries, however, ischemic heart disease was the leading cause of DALYs and stroke second. For low- and middle-income countries, ischemic heart disease was the third leading cause and stroke was the fifth leading cause.[5]

Between 1990 and 2010 noncommunicable diseases became more predominant as the leading causes of deaths for all age groups and both sexes globally and for low-, middle- and high-income countries. Over that same period, noncommunicable diseases also became more prominent as causes of DALYs globally and for low-, middle-, and high-income countries.[7]

In 2008, WHO published projections of the burden of disease until 2030. These projections suggested that by 2030, ischemic heart disease and cerebrovascular disease combined will be:[8]

- The second leading cause of DALYs in low-income countries, behind perinatal conditions but ahead of unipolar depressive disorders
- The largest cause of DALYs by a substantial margin in lower-middle-income countries, ahead of unipolar depressive disorders
- The leading cause of DALYs in upper-middle-income countries and almost 3 times more DALYs than the next cause of burden, HIV/AIDS
- The leading cause of DALYs in high-income countries, with 30 percent more DALYs than the next leading cause, which is unipolar depressive disorders

Given limited access to prevention programs or appropriate treatment, deaths from CVD generally occur earlier in low- and middle-income countries than in high-income countries. In India, for example, CVD occurs in people at younger ages more than in high-income countries. Whereas in high-income countries only about 22 percent of CVD deaths are in people under 70 years of age, in India, about 50 percent of the CVD deaths occur in people under 70.[9]

To help get a better understanding of the importance of CVD to the burden of disease, **Table 13-2** shows the burden of deaths and DALYs worldwide and by regions that are associated with CVD, compared to some of the other leading causes of death and DALYs, including diabetes, cancer, TB, HIV, and malaria.

TABLE 13-2 Deaths and DALYs from Leading Causes, by World Bank Region, Low- and Middle-Income Countries, High-Income Countries, and Globally, 2010, as Percentage of Total Deaths and DALYs

Region	Stroke	Diabetes	Cancer	TB	HIV/AIDS	Malaria
East Asia and Pacific						
Deaths	19	3	22	2	<1	<1
DALYs	8	3	13	2	1	<1
Europe and Central Asia						
Deaths	20	<1	15	<1	2	<1
DALYs	9	2	10	1	2	<1
Latin America and the Caribbean						
Deaths	9	5	16	<1	2	<1
DALYs	3	3	8	<1	2	<1
Middle East and North Africa						
Deaths	12	3	10	<1	<1	<1
DALYs	5	3	5	<1	<1	<1
South Asia						
Deaths	6	2	7	4	1	<1
DALYs	2	2	4	3	1	<1
Sub-Saharan Africa						
Deaths	4	1	4	4	12	13
DALYs	1	<1	2	2	10	13
Low- and Middle-Income Countries						

TABLE 13-2 Deaths and DALYs from Leading Causes, by World Bank Region, Low- and Middle-Income Countries, High-Income Countries, and Globally, 2010, as Percentage of Total Deaths and DALYs (*continued*)

Region	Stroke	Diabetes	Cancer	TB	HIV/AIDS	Malaria
Deaths	11	3	12	3	3	3
DALYs	4	2	6	2	4	4
High-Income Countries						
Deaths	10	3	27	<1	<1	<1
DALYs	4	3	17	<1	1	<1
Global						
Deaths	11	2	15	2	3	2
DALYs	4	2	8	2	3	3

Note: The source of this data refers to low- and middle-income countries as developing countries.

Data from Institute for Health Metrics and Evaluation (IHME). (2013). GBD compare. Seattle, WA: IHME, University of Washington. Retrieved February 15, 2015, from http://vizhub.healthdata.org/gbd-compare. Accessed February 15, 2015.

Some of the risk factors for cardiovascular disease are modifiable and some are not. Men have a higher risk of heart disease than women who are premenopausal, but postmenopausal women have the same risk of cardiovascular disease as men. In addition, men and women have similar risks of stroke. The medical history of one's family is also significant. If a male relative had coronary heart disease before 55 years of age or a female relative before 65 years of age, then one has a higher risk of heart disease. Ethnicity is also relevant, as people with African or Asian ancestry have higher risks than other groups. Aging also increases risk, with the risk of a stroke doubling every 10 years after age 55.[10]

Other risk factors are modifiable—one can change them by changing behavior. These include hypertension, which is the biggest risk factor for strokes and a major risk factor for heart disease. Tobacco use is also a major risk factor for CVD, with higher risks for women and those who started smoking early and smoke a lot. High levels of cholesterol, which are linked to a diet high in saturated fats and the lack of physical activity, are also risks. The lack of physical activity is a risk for obesity that in turn is a risk for diabetes, which doubles your risk of CVD. Excess alcohol consumption is also associated with heart disease.[10]

Social factors can be important risks for CVD. There is good evidence that higher risks of CVD are associated, for example, with poverty, stress, and being isolated socially. Depression is also an important risk factor for CVD.[10]

Diabetes

There are several types of diabetes. The two most common are called type I and type II diabetes. Type I diabetes is thought to be an autoimmune disorder that attacks and destroys the cells in the pancreas that produce insulin. Without insulin, the body is not able to use glucose (blood sugar) for energy. To treat the disease a person must inject insulin, follow a diet plan, exercise daily, and test blood sugar several times a day.[11]

Type I diabetes usually begins before the age of 30. This type of diabetes was previously known as insulin-dependent diabetes mellitus or juvenile diabetes.[11] Type II diabetes was previously known as noninsulin-dependent diabetes mellitus or adult-onset diabetes. Type II diabetes is the most common form of diabetes mellitus, present in about 90–95 percent of all diabetics. People with type II diabetes produce insulin; however, they either do not make enough insulin or their bodies do not efficiently use the insulin they do make.[11]

FIGURE 13-1 Diabetes Prevalence Rate Among Adults in International Diabetes Federation Regions, 2014

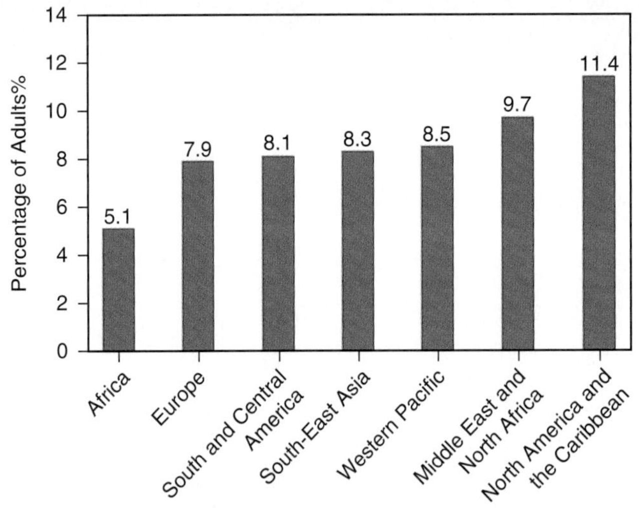

Data from International Diabetes Federation. (2013). IDF Diabetes Atlas, 6th ed. Brussels, Belgium: Author.

The International Diabetes Federation estimated that 382 million people and 8.3 percent of adults worldwide had diabetes in 2013.[12] As shown in **Figure 13-1**, the prevalence rate of diabetes varies across International Diabetes Federation regions, from a high of 11.4 percent of the population in North America and the Caribbean to a low of 5.1 percent in Africa.

The rate of diabetes also varies by country. The highest rates are to be found in the island nations of the Western Pacific, where around a quarter to a third of all people have diabetes. The Middle East also has very high rates, with a number of countries, such as Kuwait, Saudi Arabia, and Qatar having about 25 percent of their adults with diabetes.[12]

The global burden of disease study estimated that diabetes was the 9th leading cause of death worldwide in 2010 among all age groups and both sexes and that about 1.3 million people died of diabetes in 2010. Diabetes was the 8th leading cause of death in high-income countries and the 10th leading cause of death in low- and middle-income countries. About 80 percent of all deaths from diabetes are in low- and middle-income countries.[5]

Diabetes has a number of important and costly complications. Among the most common are eye problems that can cause blindness, kidney problems, circulatory problems that can result in amputation of the lower extremities, stroke, and coronary heart disease. About two-thirds of the people with diabetes have some disability, compared to less than one third of the people without diabetes.[13] Diabetes was the 8th leading cause of DALYs in high-income countries in 2010 and the 16th leading cause in low- and middle-income countries.

The prevalence of diabetes worldwide is increasing at a rapid rate, mostly associated with the rapid increase in the amount of obesity in the world.[14] Some students of global health now refer to diabetes as an "epidemic." **Table 13-3** shows, by International Diabetes Federation regions, the number of people by region with diabetes in 2013, the number projected in 2035, and the percentage increase that is projected for each region over the period 2013 to 2035.

As evident from the table, the numbers are projected to double in Africa and the Middle East and North Africa, increase by about half to about 60 percent in the other low- and middle-income regions, and by a quarter to a third in the high-income regions.[12] These projections, in fact, indicate that almost 600 million people will have diabetes in 2035, with about 80 percent of those continuing to be in today's low- and middle-income countries.

TABLE 13-3 Diabetes Mellitus, 2013 Estimates of Prevalence and 2035 Projections of Prevalence, by IDF Region

IDF Region	2013 Estimates (Millions)	2035 Projections (Millions)	Projected Increase
Africa	19.8	41.4	109%
Middle East and North Africa	34.6	67.9	96%
South-East Asia	72.1	123.0	71%
South and Central America	24.1	38.5	60%
Western Pacific	138.2	201.8	46%
North America and Caribbean	36.7	50.4	37%
Europe	56.3	68.9	22%
World	381.8	591.9	55%

Data from International Diabetes Federation. (2013). *IDF diabetes atlas* (6th ed.). Burssels, Belgium: IDF.

The risk factors for type I diabetes are still being studied. However, type I diabetes is associated with a family history of diabetes. In addition, "environmental factors, increased weight and height development, increased maternal age at birth, and exposure to some viral infections" have also been linked to developing type I diabetes.[12] Type II diabetes is also associated with a family history of diabetes. In addition, it is associated with diet and physical inactivity, obesity, insulin resistance, ethnicity, and increasing age.[12,15] In high-income countries, less-educated and lower-income individuals have higher rates of diabetes than better-educated and wealthier people.[16]

Cancer

Cancer is a unique challenge because there are many forms of cancer and each may have different characteristics concerning who they affect, their risk factors, and how they can be prevented and treated.

Globally, all forms of cancer made up about 15 percent of all deaths for all age groups and both sexes in 2010. This would make cancers the second leading cause of death after cardiovascular disease. However, all forms of cancer combined led to more deaths than either ischemic heart disease or stroke when considered separately.[1]

Globally, all forms of cancer made up 7.6 percent of all DALYs in 2010. This was the second leading cause of DALYs next to CVD. However, as with deaths, all forms of cancer when taken together led to more DALYs than either ischemic heart disease or stroke.[1]

According to GLOBOCAN, the database of the International Agency for Cancer Research, there were 14.1 million new cancer cases in 2012 and 8.2 million cancer-related deaths. This compares with 12.7 million new cases and 7.6 million deaths in 2008. Prevalence estimates for 2012 show that there were 32.6 million people, 15 years or older, alive and who had a cancer diagnosed in the previous 5 years.[17]

The most commonly diagnosed cancers worldwide in 2012 were those of the lung (1.8 million, 13.0 percent of the total), breast (1.7 million, 11.9 percent), and colorectum (1.4 million, 9.7 percent). The most common causes of cancer death were cancers of the lung (1.6 million, 19.4 percent of the total), liver (0.8 million, 9.1 percent), and stomach (0.7 million, 8.8 percent).[17]

Table 13-4 shows WHO data on the leading causes of cancer globally, for the world, for more developed regions and for less developed regions.

The number of deaths caused by different types of cancers is shown in **Table 13-5**.

Cancers of the breast and cervix have had a striking increase in the recent past. In fact, breast cancer is the leading cause of cancer death currently in low- and middle-income countries and also the leading cause of cancer death for women globally. In 2012, 1.7 million women were diagnosed

TABLE 13-4 Leading Causes of Cancer for the World, More Developed Regions and Less Developed Regions, Number of Cases in Thousands, 2012

	Type of Cancer	Cases	Type of Cancer	Cases	Type of Cancer	Cases	Type of Cancer	Cases	Type of Cancer	Cases	Type of Cancer	Cases
World	Lung	1,825	Breast	1,671	Colorectum	1,361	Prostate	1,095	Stomach	952	Liver	782
More Developed Regions	Breast	788	Lung	758	Prostate	742	Colorectum	737	Stomach	275	Liver	134
Less Developed Regions	Lung	1,066	Breast	883	Stomach	677	Liver	648	Colorectum	624	Cervical	445

Data from International Agency for Research on Cancer, WHO. GLOBOCAN 2012: Estimated cancer incidence, mortality, and prevalence worldwide in 2012. Retrieved February 15, 2015, from http://globocan.iarc.fr/Pages/fact_sheets_cancer.aspx.

TABLE 13-5 Leading Causes of Cancer Deaths, by World Bank Region and for High-Income Countries, Number of Deaths in Thousands, 2010

Region	Cancer Type	Deaths	Cancer Type	Deaths	Cancer Type	Deaths	Cancer Type	Deaths	Cancer Type	Deaths	Cancer Type	Deaths
East Asia and Pacific	Trachea, bronchus, and lungs	618	Liver	461	Stomach	333	Colorectal	194	Esophageal	191	Breast	87
Europe and Central Asia	Trachea, bronchus, and lungs	132	Colorectal	79	Stomach	75	Breast	50	Pancreatic	33	Liver	23
Latin America and the Caribbean	Trachea, bronchus, and lungs	67	Stomach	54	Colorectal	48	Prostate	47	Breast	38	Liver	30
Middle East and North Africa	Trachea, bronchus, and lungs	22	Liver	17	Stomach	16	Breast	14	Brain	10	Colorectal	10
South Asia	Trachea, bronchus, and lungs	114	Stomach	81	Esophageal	77	Breast	61	Other Pharynx	56	Cervical	49
Sub-Saharan Africa	Liver	45	Cervical	45	Esophageal	24	Stomach	24	Breast	23	Trachea, Bronchis, and Lungs	20
High-Income Countries	Trachea, bronchus, and lungs	512	Colorectal	300	Stomach	163	Breast	159	Pancreatic	148	Prostate	139

Data from Institute for Health Metrics and Evaluation (IHME). GBD Heatmap. Seattle, WA: IHME, University of Washington, 2013. http://vizhub.healthdata.org/irank/heat.php. Accessed February 15, 2015.

with breast cancer globally, reflecting a 20 percent increase in the breast cancer incidence rate since 2008. There are about 528,000 new cases of cervical cancer each year. The effects of cervical cancer are most notable in sub-Saharan Africa, and 70 percent of the global burden of cervical cancer falls in low- and middle-income countries.[17]

The global burden of cancer has continued to grow as more people in more places continue to live longer and the burden of communicable diseases decreases in these populations. Although cancer is common everywhere, the types of cancer most prevalent in a region can depend on environmental factors and standard of living.[18] Generally, worldwide trends show that in low- and middle-income countries, the economic and societal shift toward lifestyles typical of high-income countries leads to a rising burden of cancers associated with reproductive, dietary, and hormonal risk factors. As income levels increase, cancers for which sedentary behavior or high fat consumption is a risk factor tend to increase as a proportion of all cancers.[19] Increases in breast cancer in low-income countries will be largely due to changes in reproductive practices, with women choosing to have fewer children, have their first pregnancy later in life, and breastfeed for a shorter period.[20]

Although cancer incidence has been increasing in most regions of the world, there are obvious inequalities between rich and poor countries. Incidence rates remain highest in higher-income regions due to average longer life spans, but mortality is relatively much higher in lower- and middle-income developed countries, likely due to a lack of early detection and access to treatment facilities. For example, breast cancer incidence has reached more than 90 new cases per 100,000 women annually in Western Europe, a high-income region, compared with 30 per 100,000 in Eastern Africa, a low-income region. However, breast cancer mortality rates in these two regions are almost identical, at about 15 per 100,000.[19]

Moreover, many low- and middle-income countries face a double burden of cancer due to cancers caused by infectious agents combined with cancers associated with behavioral risks. The situation in high-income countries is more nuanced, depending on the country. Incidence for some cancer types, including prostate, colorectum, and female breast is increasing in several countries.[20] However, some countries have decreasing mortality trends. In the United States, cancer mortality decreased by 23 percent in men and 15 percent in women between 1990 and 2008. Decreasing mortality trends can largely be attributed to changing smoking habits, especially in men.

In both high- and low-income countries, men and women are both affected by cancer. Certain cancers have higher incidence rates in women, like breast cancer, and

TABLE 13-6 Prevalence and Mortality of Cervical Cancer, by WHO Region and for Low- and Middle-Income and High-Income Countries, Number of Deaths in Thousands, 2012

Region	Cases	Deaths
World	528	266
Africa	92	57
Americas	83	36
Eastern Mediterranean	15	8
Europe	67	28
South-East Asia	175	94
Western Pacific	94	43
Low- and middle-income countries	445	230
High-income countries	83	35

Data from International Agency for Research on Cancer (IARC). GLOBOCAN

others affect men and women equally. Certain reproductive cancers, such as cervical cancer or prostate cancer, are specific to men or women. Although men and women of all ages are at risk for developing cancer, this risk increases with age. Cancer has a higher incidence in older individuals above 65 years due to more prolonged exposure to environmental risk factors and to the accumulation of genetic change. Moreover, the incidence of cancer tends to be higher in urban regions because of the differences in lifestyle and increased risk of exposure to carcinogens.[21]

There are many risk factors for cancer and they vary by the type of cancer (see **Table 13-7**). Some cancers are associated with tobacco use, such as lung and esophageal cancers. Tobacco use is one of the greatest risk factors for cancer in general. Tobacco is most directly linked to lung cancer, but using tobacco can also indirectly increase the risk of other cancers such as prostate and breast cancers. Alcohol is associated with liver, upper digestive tract, breast, and colorectal cancers, whereas diets high in red and processed meats and low in fiber have been associated with colorectal cancer. Obesity is a risk factor for breast (postmenopausal), colorectal, endometrium,

TABLE 13-7 Leading Risk Factors by Cancer Type

Cancer	Leading Risk Factors
Breast	Genetic predisposition, radiation exposure, alcohol, obesity (postmenopausal)
Cervical	HPV
Colorectal	Diets high in red meat and low in fiber; alcohol (men)
Liver	Hepatitis B virus, hepatitis C virus, schistosomiasis, alcohol
Lung	Tobacco use, asbestos exposure, air pollution
Pancreatic	Alcohol, obesity
Skin	UVA/UVB exposure

Data from World Health Organization (WHO). 2014. Cancer Prevention. Retrieved August 4, 2014, from http://www.who.int/cancer/prevention/en/.

kidney, esophageal, and pancreatic cancers. Similarly, low physical activity can be a major risk factor for colon, breast, and endometrial cancers.[20]

Other cancers are associated with infectious agents. Liver cancer, for example, is associated with the hepatitis B virus, cervical cancer is associated with the human papillomavirus, and stomach cancer is associated with the bacteria *Helicobacter pylori*. Liver cancer is also associated with schistosomiasis, a parasitic worm that is also called "bilharzia," which infects more than 200 million people worldwide.[22] There are also numerous environmental and occupational carcinogens, such as asbestos, which was the cause of lung cancer in many roofing workers in the United States, for example.

WHO projections made in 2008 suggest that in 2030 cancers will be among the 10 leading causes of DALYs only in the high-income countries.[23]

Mental Disorders

One of the major categories of noncommunicable diseases in the *Global Burden of Disease Study 2010* is mental and behavioral disorders. This includes a number of mental disorders such as unipolar depressive disorders, anxiety disorders, bipolar affective disorder, and schizophrenia. The category also includes behavioral disorders such as alcohol use disorders, drug use disorders, and pervasive development disorders. Together, mental and behavioral disorders are very important to the burden of disease, causing about 7.4 percent of all DALYs in low- and middle-income countries in 2010.[1] Covering a wide range of such disorders, however, is beyond the scope of this chapter, and it will, therefore, cover only selected mental disorders.

Four mental disorders contribute the largest share to the burden of mental disorders. These are unipolar depressive disorders, which will be referred to here as depression, schizophrenia, anxiety disorders, and bipolar affective disorder. These conditions are defined briefly in **Table 13-8**.

Only a low burden of deaths is directly associated with mental disorders. Estimates of the global burden of disease for 2010, however, indicate that these four most common mental disorders contribute just over 5 percent of the total DALYs in low- and middle-income countries, about equal to the burden of HIV and TB combined or the burden of ischemic heart disease.[1] Depression alone is estimated to be associated with 3 percent of the DALYs globally for both sexes and all age groups.[1]

The *Global Burden of Disease Study 2010* suggests that there is a substantial difference between the burden of these disorders in low- and middle-income countries, in which they represent about 4.5 percent of DALYs and in high-income countries, in which they represent about 8 percent of DALYs. That same study suggests that globally, women also suffer substantially more DALYs related to these disorders than men do, about 7.2 percent, compared to 4.6 percent.[1]

TABLE 13-8 Key Mental Health Terms and Definitions

Bipolar disorder—A serious mood disorder characterized by swings of mania and depression

Depression—A mental state characterized by feelings of sadness, loneliness, despair, low self-esteem, and self-reproach

Panic disorders—An anxiety disorder characterized by attacks of acute intense anxiety

Schizophrenia—A mental illness, the main symptoms of which are hallucinations, delusions, and changes in outlook and personality

Data from Ohio Psychological Association. Psychological Glossary. Retrieved April 14, 2007, from http://www.ohpsych.org/Public /glossary.htm; The Royal College of Psychiatrists. Diagnoses or Conditions. Retrieved April 14, 2007, from http://www.rcpsych.ac.uk /healthadvice/moreinformation/definitions/diagnosesorconditions.aspx.

It is also essential to examine how the burden of disease from mental disorders varies by age group. Mental and behavioral disorders, as they are categorized in the global burden of disease study, are the largest cause of DALYs for the 15- to 49-year-old age group, globally, in high-income countries and in low-income countries.[1] In fact, looking at specific causes for this age group globally, major depressive disorder is the 4th leading cause of DALYs, self-harm is 6th, and anxiety disorder is 10th. For high-income countries, major depressive disorders are the second leading cause of DALYs and self-harm is fourth.[5] Mental health disorders take a particular toll on adolescents aged 15 to 19 years. Major depressive disorders are the 2nd leading cause of DALYs, self-harm, 4th, and panic anxiety, 5th for both sexes in this age group.[5]

One reason for the large burden of these conditions is the substantial number of people who suffer mental disorders. Another is that mental disorders start at relatively young ages, they go on for a long time, they are often not cured, and they, therefore, produce large amounts of disability. There is also some mortality, largely from suicide, that is associated with mental disorders.

There are only limited data on the burden of mental disorders from low- and middle-income countries. Nonetheless, earlier studies suggest that when assessing the burden of these four disorders per million people, South Asia has the highest rate of depression among all regions. The rate of depression is fairly consistent across better-off regions, somewhat lower in East Asia and Pacific, and only about half as high in sub-Saharan Africa as in Europe and Central Asia.[24] The rates of schizophrenia range from about 1,600 DALYs per million people in Europe and Central Asia to about 2,100 DALYs per million people in East Asia and Pacific.[24] Bipolar disorder ranges from 1,400 DALYs per million people in Europe and Central Asia to 1,830 DALYs per million people in the Middle East and North Africa.[24] The range for panic disorders is very narrow, with all regions clustering in the range of 700 to 800 DALYs per million people.[24]

The WHO 2008 projections of the burden of disease to 2030 by country income group suggest that unipolar depressive disorders will grow in importance in all income groups and be exceptionally important as a share of the total burden of disease in the future. They are projected, for example, to become almost 6 percent of total DALYs in low-income countries and the second leading cause of the burden of disease. They would be over 6 percent in lower-middle-income countries and the highest cause and about 6 percent in upper-middle-income countries and the third highest cause. The projections also suggest that unipolar depressive disorders will be over 8 percent of the burden of disease in high-income countries in 2030.[8]

There appear to be both genetic and nongenetic risk factors for mental disorders. It is clear that women suffer from depression more than men, as noted earlier. Early childhood abuse, violence, and poverty may be important environmental risk factors for depression. However, there is still very little definitive evidence on the risk factors for schizophrenia, depression, bipolar disorder, or panic disorders.[24]

Vision and Hearing Loss

Vision Loss

The aging of populations globally and continued improvements in life expectancy will increase the importance of vision and hearing loss as causes of the burden of disease. It will also shift the types of problems that cause visual impairment.

The major reasons for vision loss are refractive disorders, such as near- and farsightedness and astigmatism, which is responsible for 43 percent of vision loss; unoperated cataract, which is responsible for 33 percent of vision loss; and glaucoma, which is responsible for 2 percent of vision loss. The leading cause of blindness is unoperated cataracts. Blindness can also be caused, among other things, by glaucoma, vitamin A deficiency, and rubella. Some blindness also has parasitic and infectious causes, such as trachoma and onchocerciasis, although the number of people who are blind because of these causes has declined as progress has been made against these diseases.[25] Diabetes-related eye disease can also cause blindness. Over 80 percent of vision loss can be prevented or cured.

WHO estimates that 285 million people were visually impaired in 2014, of whom 39 million were blind and 246 million had low vision. About 90 percent of those who suffer visual impairment live in low- and middle-income countries. About 65 percent of those who suffer visual impairment are over 50 years of age. About 19 million children also suffer such impairment, and 12 million of them have refractive errors that could be corrected with appropriate services.[25]

The *Global Burden of Disease Study 2010* suggests that visual impairment was responsible for about 0.8 percent of all DALYs in 2010. The study also indicated that visual impairment was responsible for about 0.95 percent of DALYs in high-income countries and 0.75 percent of DALYs in low- and middle-income countries. This burden of DALYs would be similar to that for asthma or kidney disease.[1]

The main risk factors for visual impairment are poverty, gender, age, and a lack of access to health services. Cigarette smoking is also a risk factor for cataracts and glaucoma. Women are disproportionately affected by visual impairment, largely a function of constraints to their accessing appropriate preventive and curative care.[26]

WHO 2008 projections of the burden of disease to 2030 suggest that refractive errors will be the leading cause related to visual impairment in the future. These are projected to be in the top 10 causes of the burden of disease in low-, upper-middle-, and high-income countries in 2030, with between 2.5 percent and 3.5 percent of the total burden of disease.[8]

Hearing Loss

WHO estimates that in 2014 about 360 million people in the world had hearing loss that was disabling. This was equal to about 5 percent of the world's population and was made up of 328 million adults and 32 million children.[27] About 80 percent of them had adult-onset hearing loss and about 20 percent had childhood-onset hearing loss.[21] About one-third of people over 65 years of age are affected by disabling hearing loss.[27] More males have suffered hearing loss than females, probably a result of exposure to noise.[27]

The global burden of disease study for 2010 indicated that 0.64 percent of DALYs globally could be attributed to deafness and hearing loss. The corresponding figures were 0.61 percent for low- and middle-income countries and 0.78 percent for high-income countries. The global figure is a similar burden to that for osteoarthritis but more than that for schizophrenia.[1]

Childhood-onset hearing loss is related to congenital conditions, infection of the ear, or complications of other diseases, such as meningitis. Adult-onset hearing loss is related to exposure to noise and chemicals, as well as to aging. Poverty, poor hygiene, a failure to get vaccinated, and other causes that contribute to children getting infections are also risk factors for hearing loss.[26]

WHO 2008 projections of the burden of disease to 2030 suggest that adult-onset hearing loss will be in the top 10 causes of the burden of disease in all country income groups. It will range from about 2.6 percent of the total burden of disease in low-income countries to just over 4 percent of the total burden of disease in high-income countries.[8]

Tobacco Use

Tobacco is such an important risk factor for cardiovascular disease, cancer, and diabetes that it bears specific mention of its own. Globally and for all ages and both sexes, tobacco is the third leading attributable risk factor for death. Tobacco is also the third leading risk factor for death in low- and middle-income countries and in high-income countries. Tobacco holds the same ranking as a risk factor for DALYs.[5]

It is estimated that about 5 million deaths annually are associated with the use of tobacco, of which about half are in low-income countries.[28,29] It is also estimated that 1 in 5 males over 30 and 1 in 20 females over 30 who die worldwide die of tobacco-related deaths.[28,29] Ultimately, one-half to two-thirds of those who smoke will die of causes related to tobacco.[28] In addition, half of all tobacco-related deaths occur among people ages 35 to 69.[28] The most common tobacco-related deaths are from CVD; diseases of the respiratory system, such as emphysema; and cancers. Tobacco use can also increase the risk of getting TB or dying from it, as well as substantially increase the risk of becoming diabetic.[29]

Most tobacco is used through smoking either cigarettes or *bidis*, which are hand-rolled cigarettes used largely in South Asia. It is estimated that about 1.5 billion people smoke worldwide.[29] Of countries that participated in a recent review of tobacco prevalence by WHO, Russia had the highest rate of smoking prevalence at about 39 percent of all adults. Indonesia was the second highest with 34.8 percent of adults smoking. The lowest rate of the countries surveyed was Nigeria, with 3.9 percent prevalence.[29]

In all regions of the world, men smoke more than women do (see **Table 13-9**). This is most pronounced in

TABLE 13-9 Smoking Prevalence, by Sex, in World Bank Regions, High-Income Countries, and Globablly, 2011

Region	Females	Males
East Asia and Pacific	3	48
Europe and Central Asia	22	40
Latin America and Caribbean	12	26
Middle East and North Africa	3	35
South Asia	4	29
Sub-Saharan Africa	7	37
High-income countries	22	37
Global	7	37

Data from World Bank. World Bank data: Smoking prevalence. Retrieved February 18, 2015, from http://data.worldbank.org/indicator/SH.PRV.SMOK.MA/countries/1W-Z4?display=graph.

low-income countries, in which relatively small shares of women smoke. Prevalence for men was estimated earlier to vary from 29 percent in sub-Saharan Africa to 63 percent in East Asia and Pacific. The rates for women were estimated to vary from 5 percent in East Asia and Pacific and the Middle East and North Africa to 24 percent in Latin America and the Caribbean.[28] The highest rate of smoking prevalence among males is 67 percent in Indonesia. Russia has the second highest rate of prevalence, at just over 60 percent. Of the countries surveyed, the lowest rates of smoking among women were 0.4 percent in Uruguay and 0.5 percent in Egypt.[29]

The extent to which people take up smoking varies not only by sex but also by socioeconomic status and level of educational attainment. The higher the socioeconomic status and the higher the level of education, the less likely a person is to smoke. Most people who smoke start when they are teens. In addition, it is important to note that tobacco is physically addictive and once one starts to smoke, it is difficult to stop.[30]

In some countries, such as Canada, Poland, Thailand, the United Kingdom, the United States, and Uruguay, the use of tobacco has been declining. However, usage is increasing among men in low- and middle-income countries and among women in all regions. Unless steps are taken to stop the spread of tobacco use, we are likely to see continued growth in CVD and cancers related to smoking. CVD and cancers related to smoking are often avoidable, and the overwhelming majority will occur in today's low- and middle-income countries.[29]

Alcohol

Alcohol is a major public health problem. Alcohol use disorders constitute an important burden of disease, making up about 0.7 percent of all DALYs globally, about 0.6 percent in low- and middle-income countries, and more than 1.5 percent in high-income countries. Globally, this is similar to the burden of anxiety disorders and drug use disorders.[5] In addition, alcohol use disorders are the ninth leading attributable risk factor for deaths globally, the ninth leading risk factor in low- and middle-income countries, and the sixth leading risk factor in high-income countries. Alcohol is the fifth leading attributable risk factor for DALYs globally, the fifth in high-income countries, and the eighth in low- and middle-income countries.[5] In addition, it is valuable to note that among men, the DALYs attributable to alcohol use disorders in 2010 was estimated to be 1.9 percent in Western Europe, 2.0 percent in Central Europe, and 3.3 percent in Eastern Europe.[1]

High-risk drinking is defined as drinking 20 grams or more per day of pure alcohol for a woman and 40 grams a day for a man.[31] This is equal to about one quarter of a bottle

of wine for a woman and one-half a bottle of wine for a man. High-risk drinking may also be defined to include the total amount that is consumed, the frequency with which it is consumed, and the extent to which one engages in binge drinking.

High-risk drinking has a negative effect on people's health in a number of ways. Among other things, it increases the risks for hypertension, liver damage, pancreatic damage, hormonal problems, and heart disease.[31] In addition, alcohol intoxication is associated with accidents, injuries, accidental death, and a variety of social problems, including the first sexual encounters of teens, unprotected sex, and intimate partner violence. It is also possible to become dependent on alcohol, which has a number of negative psychological and physical consequences. Moreover, fetal alcohol syndrome is associated with low birthweight babies who are at risk of developmental disabilities.

The prevalence of high-risk drinking varies by region. It has been estimated that men in Europe and Central Asia have the highest rates of high-risk drinking: about 21 percent between ages 45 to 59. People in the Middle East and North Africa have the lowest rates, which are reported to be very low. South Asia also has a very low prevalence of high-risk drinking.[29] The prevalence rate of high-risk drinking also varies by age, with fewer people engaging in high-risk drinking after age 60 than at younger ages. In each region, high-risk drinking is higher among men than women, except in South Asia.[31]

There is very little evidence about the determinants of high-risk drinking, especially in low-income settings. Studies done in high-income countries suggest that lower socioeconomic status and lower educational attainment are risk factors for drinking to the level of intoxication.[31]

THE COSTS AND CONSEQUENCES OF NONCOMMUNICABLE DISEASES, TOBACCO USE, ALCOHOL USE DISORDERS, AND VISION AND HEARING LOSS

The Costs of Noncommunicable Diseases Broadly

The economic costs of noncommunicable diseases are substantial and are growing, given the increasing burden of cardiovascular disease and diabetes. These costs include the direct costs of treating noncommunicable diseases, which by their nature require many years of treatment. They also include indirect costs that result from lost productivity. These are also very substantial, given that noncommunicable diseases often start at relatively younger ages, often cause substantial disability, and can persist for many years.

In addition, many actors in the global health arena previously carried out their work as if high-income countries faced the burden and costs of noncommunicable diseases and low- and middle-income countries faced only the burden and costs of communicable diseases. However, in light of the increasing amount of noncommunicable diseases in low- and middle-income countries, it is clear that these countries do not have the luxury of facing *either* communicable *or* noncommunicable diseases. Rather, even low-income countries now *simultaneously* face the burden and costs of communicable diseases, noncommunicable diseases, and injuries. Some additional comments follow on the costs and consequences of noncommunicable diseases.

A study conducted in 2007 estimated the economic costs of selected noncommunicable diseases in 23 low- and middle-income countries. In those countries, the selected diseases make up 80 percent of the noncommunicable burden. This study noted that men in low- and middle-income countries are 56 percent more likely to die at the same age of such causes than men in high-income countries, and women are 86 percent more likely to die at the same age than women in high-income countries of these causes. The study further concluded that these countries would lose $84 billion in economic production between 2006 and 2015 alone, as a result of the large and growing burden of noncommunicable diseases.[32]

The World Economic Forum commissioned a study in 2011 on noncommunicable diseases in low- and middle-income countries. That study concluded that the cumulative output lost to these conditions in low- and middle-income countries over the next 2 decades would be $47 trillion. The study also suggested that low- and middle-income countries would bear an increasing share of the costs of these diseases in the future.[33]

A more recent study examined the costs of noncommunicable diseases in China and India from 2012 to 2030. This study concluded that China would face costs of $27.8 trillion and India, $6.2 trillion. These costs would largely be driven in both countries by the costs of CVD, mental health, and respiratory diseases. The costs in China would be substantially greater than in India largely because of the much larger share of the population in China that would be older, and since China is further along the epidemiological transition than India.[34]

A study done on the costs of NCDs in the Eastern Caribbean island states found that patients suffering from noncommunicable diseases spent on average 36 percent of their annual household income on care for their disease.[35] A policy and program brief is included later in the chapter on the costs of noncommunicable diseases in the Pacific Island states.

Cardiovascular Disease

Only a small number of studies have been done on the direct and indirect costs of CVD in low- and middle-income countries. A study conducted in South Africa suggested that the direct costs of treating cardiovascular disease were about 25 percent of all healthcare expenditures, which was equal to between 2 and 3 percent of GDP in that country.[36] The indirect costs of cardiovascular disease on the economy are likely to be substantial, given the relatively low age at which such diseases affect people in many countries.

Diabetes

It is estimated that the direct costs of treating diabetes vary between 2.5 percent and 15.0 percent of health expenditures in different countries, depending on the prevalence of disease and the extent and costs of the treatment available.[12] Given the level of development of different low- and middle-income regions, it is likely that the Latin America and Caribbean region has the highest expenditure on diabetes per capita and sub-Saharan Africa the lowest such expenditures.[12]

The indirect costs of diabetes in low- and middle-income countries are substantial, partly reflecting the fact that many people in those countries live with diabetes without proper treatment and, therefore, suffer from disability and related losses in productivity. In fact, the direct and indirect costs of diabetes are likely to grow in all regions as the number of people with diabetes increases, as noted earlier. The brief on the Pacific Islands later in the chapter highlights the fact that those countries now face costs as high as $39,000 per year per patient for diabetes related dialysis.[37]

Mental Disorders

There are relatively few reliable data on the direct and indirect costs of mental disorders. In addition, the studies that have been done largely refer to high-income countries. Nonetheless, they are indicative of the large and usually unappreciated costs of mental illness in all countries. A study done in the United States estimated that the direct and indirect costs of mental illness were equal to about 2.5 percent of gross national product (GNP), and a similar study done in Europe estimated that the costs of mental illness there were between 3 and 4 percent of GNP.[38] Studies done in Canada, the United Kingdom, and the United States showed that about half of the total costs of mental illness were direct costs and about half were indirect costs. These indirect costs are so substantial for mental illness that one study done in the United States estimated almost 60 percent of the productivity losses that come from illness, accidents, or injuries are linked with mental illness.[38] Studies done in the United States and the United Kingdom showed, in addition, that workers suffering from depression lost 40 to 45 days of work in a year as a result of their illness.[38] A policy and program brief on mental disorders later in the chapter highlights of the exceptionally high costs of mental disorders in low- and middle-income countries.

Hearing and Vision Loss

Unfortunately, very little information is available about the economic costs of vision and hearing loss, especially in low- and middle-income countries. This is despite the large number of DALYs attributed to them now and the growing number of DALYs that will be associated with them as populations age. The limited information that is available refers mostly to the United States. A study done in 1995, for example, suggested that the economic cost to the United States from vision loss was almost $40 billion annually, of which about 60 percent was direct costs and 40 percent indirect costs.[39] Another study, published in 2006, estimated that the annual economic loss from major vision disorders in the United States was about $35 billion, of which about $16 billion was direct medical costs, about $11 billion other direct costs, and about $8 billion in productivity losses.[40] A comprehensive review of the existing literature on hearing loss in low- and middle-income countries was published in 2010. It did not indicate either country or global estimates of the economic costs of hearing loss; however, it did indicate some of the costs that would be associated with hearing loss, for which economic costs could be calculated, including:[41]

- Constraints to the formal education of children with hearing loss, with its attendant consequences on their employment and earning prospects
- The number of school days missed by children with disabilities
- The costs of additional medical visits associated with children with disabilities
- The high cost of education for students with hearing loss
- The difficulties of adults with hearing loss in finding and keeping employment
- Income levels for people with hearing loss that can be 45 percent of the levels of people without hearing loss, even in high-income countries

Tobacco Use

Calculating the costs of smoking to an economy can be very complicated.[42] The simplest way to do so is to calculate gross costs, which include all the costs associated with smoking-related diseases. Studies on the costs of smoking have largely focused on the costs of smoking in the high-income countries. These studies suggested that the gross costs of smoking

to various high-income economies range from 0.1–1.1 percent of GDP and that the costs to low- and middle-income countries might be just as high.[42] The prevalence rates of smoking are increasing among women everywhere and among men in low-income countries. We should expect, therefore, that the economic costs of smoking in those countries will increase for some time. In fact, it is estimated that 70 million people died of smoking-related causes between 1950 and 2000 and that, if present trends in tobacco use continue, an additional 150 million people will die of smoking-related causes between 2000 and 2025. Of course, the economic costs of this will be great.[43]

Alcohol Use Disorders

For the economic costs of alcohol use disorders, as for many other issues, there are relatively few data for low- and middle-income countries. Excessive alcohol use, as discussed earlier, is linked with health problems of the drinker. In addition, it is linked with violence and injuries caused by the drinker, such as when driving while intoxicated. When calculating the economic costs of excessive alcohol drinking, therefore, one has to take account of the costs of health care for the user and for others whose injuries or health condition were caused by the user. The indirect costs of excessive alcohol drinking will include the productivity losses of the drinker and people hurt by the drinker because of excessive drinking. The limited studies that have been done on the costs of alcohol abuse can only be considered indicative because they did not follow any standard methodology. However, they all reveal substantial costs of alcohol abuse, as a share of GDP:[44]

> Canada: 1.1 percent
> France: 1.4 percent
> Italy: 5.6 percent
> New Zealand: 4.0 percent
> South Africa: 2.0 percent

A 2009 study examined the economic costs attributable to alcohol in four high-income countries and two middle-income countries. The costs were greater than 1 percent of GDP in all countries. The highest costs were found in the United States, at 2.7 percent of GDP, and South Korea, at 3.3 percent of GDP.[45]

ADDRESSING THE BURDEN OF NONCOMMUNICABLE DISEASES

There are also relatively few data available about cost-effective investments to address the burden of noncommunicable diseases in low- and middle-income countries, except, perhaps, for tobacco. However, there is an increasing amount of information about efforts to address these issues in high-income countries and a growing body of information on dealing with these issues in low- and middle-income countries. Although the circumstances in high-income countries may be quite different from those in low- and middle-income countries, the efforts undertaken to date may provide some useful lessons for low- and middle-income countries as they seek to prevent the burden of noncommunicable diseases from developing further. In considering how to address noncommunicable diseases, it is important to note that some interventions can be made at the level of the population, whereas others are based on personal contact with an individual.[28]

The section that follows first includes comments on approaches to addressing NCDs broadly.

The second set of comments examines some key risk factors for NCDs, including tobacco, alcohol, hypertension, and obesity. Further comments are then offered on diabetes, cancer, mental disorders, and hearing and vision loss.

Addressing Noncommunicable Diseases Broadly

The United Nations convened a high-level meeting on non-communicable diseases in September 2011. This meeting resulted in an international political commitment to trying to reduce the burden of NCDs by 25 percent by the year 2025.[46] This meeting highlighted the idea that all countries, including today's low- and middle-income countries, must take measures now to reduce the burden of noncommunicable diseases. This includes efforts that can reduce the burden of NCDs for those already afflicted by them, as well as efforts to prevent the burden of NCDs from growing.

The final declaration of the meeting indicated a number of steps that countries could take to address their burden of NCDs, including:[47]

- Focusing on prevention and the main risk factors of tobacco, alcohol, dietary risks, and the lack of physical activity
- Engaging all government parties in the battle against NCDs
- Increasing funding to address NCDs

The declaration further noted that countries should:[47]

- Take multisectoral, cost-effective approaches to addressing NCDs
- Speed action on the measures indicated in the Framework Convention on Tobacco
- Implement WHO recommended approaches to diet, physical activity, alcohol, and the marketing of unhealthy foods to children

- Promote cost-effective measures to reduce salt, sugar, and saturated fats in foods and eliminate trans fats in food
- Promote vaccination against the infectious causes of NCDs, such as the vaccines against hepatitis B and the human papilloma virus

The declaration from the meeting also highlighted a number of measures that should be taken to strengthen the ability of health systems to monitor NCDs and to act on them effectively, such as enhancing universal health coverage and improving access to affordable medicines.[47]

The declaration also highlighted the conclusions of an international action group on NCDs that published its findings in April 2011, with the aim of influencing the outcome of the high-level meeting. That group based the selection of its proposed actions on a number of criteria, including that the actions would have a solid evidence basis, could lead to a substantial reduction in premature deaths and disability, would be low cost and cost-effective, and would be politically and financially feasible. On this basis, the group suggested that countries should immediately begin to take the following actions in the five priority areas that are noted:

- Tobacco: Accelerate the implementation of the Framework Convention on Tobacco Control
- Salt: Promote greater popular awareness and voluntary action by the food industry to reduce salt consumption
- Obesity, unhealthy diet, and physical inactivity: Promote greater knowledge and take measures on taxes, food labeling, food subsidies, and food marketing to reduce overconsumption and the consumption of unhealthy fats, and to encourage greater consumption of fresh fruits and vegetables and of physical activity
- Harmful alcohol intake: Increase alcohol taxes, ban advertising, and restrict sales
- Cardiovascular disease: Promote the use of proven drugs for high-risk individuals[48]

As a follow-up to the high-level meeting, the World Health Assembly, the governing body of WHO, endorsed in May 2013 the Global NCD Action Plan 2013–2020. The action plan includes a number of voluntary global targets as noted in **Table 13-10**. The action plan also contains a number of indicators for each of the targets. The Global NCD Action Plan also lays out a series of evidence-based, cost-effective measures that are best buys in addressing the burden of NCDs. The most important of these are shown in **Table 13-11**.

TABLE 13-10 Global NCD Action Plan Voluntary Global Targets

Framework Element	Target
Mortality and Morbidity	
Premature mortality from noncommunicable disease	A 25% relative reduction in the overall mortality from cardiovascular diseases, cancer, diabetes, or chronic respiratory diseases
Behavioral Risk Factors	
Harmful use of alcohol	At least 10% relative reduction in the harmful use of alcohol, as appropriate, within the national context
Physical inactivity	A 10% relative reduction in prevalence of insufficient physical activity
Salt/sodium intake	A 30% relative reduction in mean population intake of salt/sodium
Tobacco use	A 30% relative reduction in prevalence of current tobacco use in persons aged 15+ years
Biological Risk Factors	
Raised blood pressure	A 25% relative reduction in the prevalence of raised blood pressure or contain the prevalence of raised blood pressure, according to national circumstances
Diabetes and obesity	Halt the rise in diabetes and obesity
National Systems Response	
Drug therapy to prevent heart attacks and strokes	At least 50% of eligible people receive drug therapy and counseling (including glycemic control) to prevent heart attacks and strokes
Essential noncommunicable disease medicines and basic technologies to treat major noncommunicable diseases	An 80% availability of the affordable basic technologies and essential medicines, including generics, required to treat major noncommunicable diseases in both public and private facilities

Data from WHO. Global Action Plan: for the prevention and control of noncommunicable diseases, 2013–2020. Geneva; 2013.

The section that follows elaborates on steps that countries can take to address the key risk factors for the most significant NCDs. The section also comments on steps that can be taken to address mental disorders and vision and hearing loss.

Tobacco Use

The Framework Convention on Tobacco, agreed upon in 2003, outlines the measures that countries have agreed to undertake to reduce both the demand for and the supply of tobacco.[49] WHO then elaborated on these measures by outlining the Mpower program for tobacco control, which consists of six elements:[50]

- Monitor tobacco use and prevention policies
- Protect people from tobacco smoke
- Offer help to quit tobacco use
- Warn about the dangers of tobacco use
- Enforce bans on tobacco advertising, promotion, and sponsorship
- Raise taxes on tobacco

The following comments elaborate on these points.

TABLE 13-11 Selected Policy Measures in the Global NCD Action Plan

Objective	Selected Policy Measure
Tobacco use	Reduce affordability of tobacco products by increasing tobacco excise taxes Create by law completely smoke-free environments in all indoor workplaces, public places, and public transport Warn people of the dangers of tobacco and tobacco smoke through effective health warnings and mass media campaigns Ban all forms of tobacco advertising, promotion, and sponsorship
Harmful use of alcohol	Regulating commercial and public availability of alcohol Restricting or banning alcohol advertising and promotions Using pricing policies such as excise tax increases on alcoholic beverages
Physical inactivity and unhealthy diet	Reduce salt intake Replace trans fats with unsaturated fats Implement public awareness programs on diet and physical activity
Cardiovascular disease and diabetes	Drug therapy (including glycemic control for diabetes mellitus and control of hypertension using a total risk approach) and counseling to individuals who had a heart attack or stroke and to persons with high risk (greater than 30%) of a fatal and nonfatal cardiovascular event in the next 10 years Acetylsalicylic acid for acute myocardial infarction
Cancer	Prevention of liver cancer through hepatitis B immunization Prevention of cervical cancer through screening (visual inspection with acetic acid or Pap smear if cost-effective), linked with timely treatment of precancerous lesions

Data from WHO. Global Action Plan: for the prevention and control of noncommunicable diseases, 2013–2020. Geneva; 2013.

Evidence suggests a number of steps can be taken to reduce the use of tobacco. Almost all countries tax cigarettes; however, low- and middle-income countries tend to tax cigarettes at lower rates than do high-income countries. Public demand for cigarettes is sensitive to price, and the poorer the country, the more price increases will affect demand. Studies conducted in low- and middle-income countries indicate that a 10 percent increase in cigarette taxes can lead to an 8 percent reduction in the demand for cigarettes. Under these circumstances, taxing cigarettes would be an effective policy for reducing cigarette consumption.[28] Smuggling is a significant issue when countries raise tobacco taxes. However, there is evidence that 10 percent greater expenditure on efforts to reduce smuggling can lower smuggling by 5 percent and tobacco consumption by 2 percent.[29]

For countries where there is weak government enforcement of laws, it will be more difficult to enforce restrictions on smoking; however, an increasing number of countries are undertaking these measures. Studies suggest that countries that can enforce legal restrictions can reduce the number of cigarettes smoked between 5 and 25 percent and can reduce smoking uptake by about 25 percent.[28] The effectiveness of these actions is likely to be enhanced in settings in which there are also strong social norms against smoking.

There is also evidence from high-income countries that consumption of cigarettes can be reduced by about 6 percent through a total ban on cigarette advertising, which is another step that low- and middle-income countries should consider.[28] Countries should also provide the public with information about the negative effects of smoking tobacco. There is evidence from high-income countries that such efforts led to short-term reduction in cigarette consumption of between 4 and 9 percent and long-term declines of between 15 and 30 percent.[28]

High-income settings that have had the biggest impact on reducing tobacco consumption have undertaken comprehensive tobacco control programs that generally included efforts to prevent young people from starting smoking, encouraging all smokers to quit smoking, reducing exposure to passive smoking, and eliminating disparities in smoking among different population groups by helping those most at risk to reduce tobacco consumption.[28] It remains critically important to stop people from taking up smoking; however, in order to reduce tobacco-related deaths in the near future, it is essential to reduce consumption among those already smoking. Preventing young people from taking up smoking will have an impact on tobacco-related deaths only in the more distant future. There is evidence that brief counseling sessions by medical providers can double quit rates by about 4 to 8 percent. Medications that aid quitting tobacco smoking can triple the rates of quitting by 8 to 12 percent.[29]

Alcohol

Despite the high burden of disease and economic costs that are related to excessive drinking of alcoholic beverages, very few countries have embarked on coherent efforts to reduce alcohol consumption. Those that have done so generally focused their attention on policy and legislative actions, such as taxation, laws on drunk driving, and restricting alcohol sales to selected places, times, and age limits. Controlled advertising and tightened law enforcement, such as through more widespread breath testing of drivers, have also been imposed. Another successful part of their program was to encourage counseling by healthcare providers through "brief interventions with individual high risk drinkers."[31,p893]

Just as is the case for cigarette taxation, increased taxation on alcohol will likely lead to a decrease in the purchase and consumption of alcohol. Whereas in the case of tobacco, increased taxation can lead to the smuggling of untaxed cigarettes, in the case of alcohol increased taxation can lead to a rise in the consumption of illicit alcohol. This is an issue that countries must take into account when considering raising taxes on alcohol.

In selected high-income countries, studies suggest that reducing the number of hours when alcohol can be sold can lead to a 1.5 to 3 percent decrease in high-risk drinking and to a 1.5 to 4 percent decrease in alcohol-related traffic deaths.[31] Government authorities have to assess the extent to which such measures could be implemented effectively, especially in low- and middle-income countries with weak governance as well as the extent to which such measures might also drive people to seek illicit alcohol.

Bans on alcohol advertising can be put into effect, as discussed for tobacco; however, it appears that such bans have had relatively little effect on the consumption of alcohol.[31] In healthcare settings in a number of countries efforts have been made to engage high-risk drinkers in brief but specific education and counseling about the risks of excessive drinking. Even when taking relapses into account, it appears that such counseling is effective in reducing excessive consumption by 14 to 18 percent, compared to no treatment at all.[31] Although this approach might be effective in middle-income countries, it is unlikely to be effective in many low-income countries, given the scarcity of effective health services, the lack of health providers, and the already excessive demands on their weak health systems.

A recent study that was part of a broader major review of alcohol and health suggested that countries should take a stepwise approach to reducing alcohol consumption. Such an approach would allow countries to implement an increasing number and level of policies on alcohol as their capacity to legislate and enforce such approaches grew. The study recommended, at a minimum, that all countries make alcohol more expensive through excise taxes; reduce availability through regulation, licensing, and controlled sales to minors; check sobriety of drivers; and engage in the brief treatment approach noted above. As countries move to the next level of addressing alcohol abuse, they can, for example, ban sales and drinking in public places, regulate discounts on alcohol, and do random breath testing. At the last level, countries could set high minimum prices for alcohol; ban all forms of product marketing and restrict the design of packaging; and provide mandatory treatment for drunk driving, as well as treatment options for alcoholism.[51]

High Blood Pressure, High Cholesterol, and Obesity

The majority of risks associated with cardiovascular disease relates to a combination of high blood pressure, high cholesterol, high body mass index, low intake of fruits and vegetables, physical inactivity, and tobacco and alcohol use. The single most important risk factor for type II diabetes is obesity. This section comments on measures that can be taken to improve diet and to reduce obesity.

To reduce the burden of CVD and diabetes, healthy eating and maintaining a healthy weight is key. Generally, this requires eating more fruits and vegetables and decreasing the intake of salt and foods that are high in saturated fat and trans fats. It also entails limiting the intake of sugar and replacing refined grains with whole grains. People who are overweight generally need to consume fewer calories each day and need to become more active physically.[52] Tax policies can be used to subsidize healthier foods and tax those that are less healthy.

The lack of regular physical activity, in fact, is associated, among other things, with CVD, stroke, type II diabetes, and colon and breast cancer. Urbanization, motorization, and television watching all reduce physical activity. Countries can use public policies to try to limit the role of automobiles, promote walking and biking, and design communities in ways that encourage healthy lifestyles. In Singapore and London, for example, taxes are levied on cars that enter the center of the city to reduce the use of vehicles and their attendant traffic and pollution. Many cities promote the use of bicycles and have bicycle lanes, as one can see in a number of European cities such as Amsterdam. Some communities in the United States, for example, have no sidewalks, little public transport, and services that are very spread out, all of which provide an incentive for people to use automobiles to get from place to place, rather than to walk or bike.[52]

One way to promote healthier diets is through population-based health education. Large-scale education efforts of this type, often through the mass media, have had mixed results because it is difficult to successfully promote the reduction of obesity on a large scale.[36] Generally, mass programs are more effective when they are combined with direct communication with individuals.

Few efforts to undertake population-based education measures have been studied. However, a study on a project to reduce salt intake among men in one part of China found a reduction in both hypertension and obesity after 5 years. In another effort, the government of Mauritius encouraged the population to switch from cooking with palm oil, which is high in saturated fat, to soybean oil, which has less saturated fat. Over a 5-year period, the intake of saturated fat decreased and the total cholesterol levels of the population fell.[36] Regulations and legislation on labeling food products and the reduction of unhealthy ingredients in commercial food products can also contribute to reducing obesity. New York City, for example, banned the use of trans fats in its restaurants.

Studies suggest that if large-scale health education efforts are to succeed in changing what people eat, then it is important that such programs:[36]

- Have a realistic time frame that takes account of the time it takes to change deeply ingrained behaviors
- Be carried out by a respected organization and headed by a competent manager, with clear responsibility
- Encourage different organizations and agencies to work together to maximize the reach of the program and ensure that messages get disseminated in appropriate ways
- Involve the food industry and enhance food labeling[18]

Even as countries undertake the steps noted, they will still need to treat those who already have CVD or who have some of the key risk factors for CVD, including hypertension. Most low- and some middle-income countries do not have the level of health system or the financial resources needed to carry out sophisticated medical procedures. In such settings,

however, an important reduction in risks and in the burden of disease can be realized through preventive interventions, such as getting people with high cholesterol and hypertension to take inexpensive medicines to lower blood pressure and cholesterol.[36]

Further Addressing Diabetes

There is no evidence that type I diabetes can be prevented; however, avoiding being overweight is the single most important way to prevent type II diabetes. Although large-scale efforts to reduce obesity have generally not been very successful, a pilot project that used intensive personal counseling to promote weight loss through healthier eating and more physical activity was successfully carried out in China, Finland, Sweden, and the United States. The average weight loss after almost 3 years of participation in this study was about 10 pounds more than in the control group. In addition, the study group had a 58 percent lower rate of type II diabetes than the control group.[16]

Treatment for people with diabetes is needed in all countries. Treating people with type I diabetes with insulin is a cost-effective investment, although difficult to afford or manage in the poorest countries, especially for people living outside of the main cities. For all diabetics, it is cost-effective to control hypertension because the combination of the two diseases can produce major vascular complications. Diabetics are also subject to foot problems from circulation difficulties associated with their diabetes, so appropriate foot care is another cost-effective investment. The cost of not doing this can be ulcers and eventual amputation of the foot.[11] Those countries with greater resources and a health system that can deliver additional interventions can also consider other cost-effective measures for treating diabetes, including vaccination against influenza and pneumococcal infections, diagnosis and treatment of retinal problems associated with diabetes, and treating hypertension with ACE inhibitors to prevent kidney problems from getting worse.[16]

Cancer

Tobacco control is overwhelmingly the first priority for preventing cancer, as noted earlier. Countries can also try to reduce the burden of cancer by addressing infectious agents that are associated with cancers, such as hepatitis B, which is vaccine preventable; *Helicobacter pylori*, which is treatable with antibiotics; and schistosomiasis, which is also treatable with drugs.[24] An increasing number of countries are adding the hepatitis B vaccine to their national immunization programs. This is especially important in countries where a relatively large share of the population carries hepatitis B. Many countries have schistosomiasis control programs; some of the most successful efforts against schistosomiasis have been undertaken in Egypt and China. *H. pylori* is important in settings like Japan, China, and Colombia where there is a significant amount of stomach cancer linked with this bacteria. In these settings, it might be cost-effective to carry out a screening and treatment program for *H. pylori*.

However, the prevention and treatment of cancer face many challenges due to the fact that each type of cancer has its own risk factors and the most appropriate form of treatment depends on the type of cancer and the level of resources available. Prevention is the most cost-effective method to reduce the economic burden of cancer because cancer treatment can require very advanced and expensive interventions over a long period of time. The importance of prevention and early detection is highlighted by the fact that the stage of cancer at the time of detection in low- and middle-income countries is, on average, substantially further advanced than in wealthier countries. In some countries, in fact, as much as 80 percent of cancers may already be incurable when first noted. Patients in low- and middle-income countries also tend to have additional health conditions that make their recovery from cancer less likely than patients in high-income countries.[18]

The three main treatments for cancer include surgery, radiation therapy, or systemic therapy (chemotherapy, hormonal therapy, or monoclonal antibody therapy).[53] Because cancer cases can range in severity and aggressiveness and some treatments are very costly, the recommended treatment for a particular cancer varies in different settings. For example, the use of the drug tamoxifen is both feasible and cost-effective for breast cancer in low-income countries and newer hormone treatments can be cost-effective in middle-income countries. The use of classical chemotherapy regimens for breast and cervical cancer is cost-effective in middle-income countries. Where advanced facilities are present, the options can be expanded to include newer regimens for breast and cervical cancer treatment, as well as chemotherapy regimens for colon and oral cancer.[54]

Another aspect of cancer treatment is palliative care. Because many cancer cases are not detected early enough and there is still much left to discover about the disease, there exists a substantial need to limit suffering and discomfort for the many individuals who will die from cancer each year. Unfortunately, low- and middle-income countries generally have only limited access to palliative care. This is despite the fact that two-thirds of cancer patients will suffer from moderate to severe pain and the majority of them will have no access to pain relief. Both medical interventions and psychosocial support comprise palliative care, but oral morphine is underused on a global level and there is a shortage of qualified counselors and therapists for such care.[54]

In addition to preventive measures, improved early detection methods are also critical to reducing the global burden of cancer. The world must continue to devise low-cost, effective screening tests for detecting cancer in low-resource settings. For-example, cervical cancer screening is traditionally done via a Papanicolaou (Pap) smear in higher income countries. However, Pap smear programs can be unfeasible where there is little infrastructure, so a direct visualization method, using visual inspection of the cervix with acetic acid, was developed that allows testing and treatment of precancerous lesions in a single visit.[18]

Other cost-effective screening choices in low-income countries include clinical breast examination and visual inspection for oral cancer in high-prevalence countries. Urban areas in middle-income countries can consider mammography and fecal immunochemical testing for colon cancer, where prevalence patterns suggest a need. Middle-income countries should have the resources to screen in rural areas for liver flukes, if prevalent.[54]

Treatment programs require greater monetary investments but are necessary to reduce the overall cancer burden. There are countries that currently lack any radiation facilities and there are overwhelming shortages of radiation technicians and trained oncologists. Nonetheless, there is evidence that even low-income sub-Saharan African countries, which have some of the greatest resource deficiencies, can acquire and maintain radiation facilities, although ensuring access for patients from remote rural areas may be difficult. After radiation facilities, countries should focus on developing resources for treatments that require sophisticated pathology and laboratory facilities. These more advanced facilities are important for a wide range of medical conditions in addition to cancer and ultimately require a much larger effort and investment to establish and maintain.[17] The cost-effectiveness of initial surgical treatment for treatable breast, cervical, and colorectal cancers can be less than several thousand dollars per year of life saved.[55]

In order to most effectively prevent and treat cancer, monitoring and evaluation of cancer programs must be advanced and knowledge on cost-effective interventions must be furthered. In particular, resources must be developed for risk factor surveillance, collection of cause-specific mortality data, longitudinal studies of chronic disease risk factors, and cancer registries.[18]

Mental Disorders

Unfortunately, despite the enormous and growing importance of mental disorders, there is often an inadequate understanding of the importance of mental health, a lack of funds for mental health, a shortage of people who understand mental health issues, and stigma around mental disorders. As a result, there has been little progress in most low-income countries and many middle-income countries in addressing mental disorders.[24]

Given the important burden of disease associated with mental disorders and the low level of development of mental health services in most low-income and many middle-income countries, the World Health Organization recommends that countries take a number of fundamental steps to address mental health issues. These include:[56]

- Having a mental health policy
- Ensuring there is a unit of government responsible for mental health
- Budgeting for mental health programs—including program development, training, drug procurement, and program monitoring
- Training primary healthcare workers in mental health
- Integrating mental health into the primary healthcare program

In addition, WHO has recommended as part of its mental health gap action program that a package of mental health interventions should be available in each country, tailored to the burden of disease, the mental health resources available, the financing available, and the local context. Some of the core parts of the intervention package would be:[57]

- Childhood mental disorders—Prevent such disorders as far as possible, partly through better maternal nutrition and care and treat children pharmacologically, as appropriate, and offer them psychosocial support
- Depression—Treat with antidepressant medicines and provide psychosocial support
- Schizophrenia and other psychotic disorders—Treat with antipsychotic medicines and family or community-based psychosocial support

Related to these efforts, a number of public health measures can be taken to address some of the risk factors that are associated with mental disorders. Reducing abuse of women and children can reduce the burden of mental illness among the abused. Curtailing bullying of students in schools can also be important. Improving parenting skills is helpful to the healthy development of children. Appropriate care and counseling for children and adults affected by war, conflict, and other complex emergencies can also reduce the risks of mental illness.[58]

A significant amount of the mental health care in low- and middle-income countries is offered in large psychiatric hospitals that consume an overwhelming share of the mental health budget in those countries. Evidence is growing, however, that for $2–$4 per person per year, countries could provide more community-based approaches to care that would offer drug therapy combined with psychosocial support for bipolar disorder, depression, and schizophrenia, and drug therapy for panic disorder. The goal would be to integrate such support into routine primary healthcare services, as far as possible.[58,59]

Given the weak state of health systems in most low-income and many middle-income countries and their lack of attention to mental health, accomplishing these aims will require much greater political attention to mental health issues. In addition, it will require measures to get additional funds for mental health and wiser use of them, including for services for the poor.[60]

There have been few mental health success stories in low- and middle-income countries. However, one of the case studies that follows deals with the efforts to improve mental health services in Uganda, a low-income country. There have also been some interesting efforts to provide community-based care for schizophrenia in India. This has been coupled with shifting of tasks to community-based health workers, given the absence of trained mental health professionals in much of India. In addition, although Chile is now considered a high-income country, it will be important to follow the progress of mental health services for depression in Chile, which has become a model for a national effort to address depression.[58]

It will be essential to keep in mind as one seeks to address mental health issues in low- and middle-income countries that these countries have scarce financial resources and a limited number of mental health professionals. Thus, they are very unlikely to be able to take an approach to mental health that is medically oriented and depends on psychiatrists and psychiatric nurses, as is the case in most high-income countries. Rather, approaches that are cost-effective, scalable, and sustainable will have to depend on the community and family-based efforts being used more and more in India, among other places.[61] Putting such an approach in place will also require that countries:[62]

- Shift financial resources from the large mental hospitals to community-based approaches to diagnosis and treatment
- Train primary care physicians and other staff working in primary care to treat the mentally ill
- Circulate to health workers protocols for brief behavioral and cognitive therapies
- Increase the availability of modern generic drugs

Vision Loss

The World Health Assembly approved in 2013 a global action plan for universal eye health. The plan has three objectives: generate evidence to enhance understanding and commitment; the development of coherent national policies, plans, and programs on eye health; and enhance multisectoral collaboration and partnerships to improve eye health.[63]

The plan sets a global target of reducing preventable blindness globally by 2019, from the 2010 baseline. The plan encourages countries to establish comprehensive eye care programs that are well integrated into their health systems and that focus on cost-effective interventions to address refractive errors and the burden of unoperated cataracts. The plan also encourages countries to continue to work across sectors to help address the infectious and parasitic causes of blindness, as well as the growing threat of blindness related to diabetes. Eye care is an area in which there has been considerable success with task shifting and the plan also comments on the training of personnel for eye care, including allied healthcare personnel.[63] This could include for eye care, for example, ophthalmic assistants who are trained to do cataract surgeries, especially in places where there are an insufficient number of ophthalmologists.

A case study is included later in the chapter that examines the largest coherent effort in any country to address the problem of cataracts: the India Cataract Blindness Program.

Hearing Loss

Despite the substantial burden of disease and economic costs related to hearing loss, the world has not yet adopted any coherent plan or targets to address this problem. WHO suggests, however, that about half of all cases of hearing loss can be addressed by primary prevention:

- Immunizing children against childhood diseases, including measles, meningitis, rubella, and mumps
- Immunizing adolescent girls and women of reproductive age against rubella before pregnancy
- Screening for and treating syphilis and other infections in pregnant women
- Improving antenatal and perinatal care, including promotion of safe childbirth
- Avoiding the use of ototoxic drugs, unless prescribed and monitored by a qualified physician
- Referring babies with high risk factors (such as those with a family history of deafness, those born with low birthweight, birth asphyxia, jaundice, or meningitis) for early assessment of hearing, prompt diagnosis and appropriate management, as required
- Reducing exposure (both occupational and recreational) to loud noises by creating awareness, using personal protective devices, and developing and implementing suitable legislation

WHO also suggests that attention be paid to early diagnosis and appropriate medical or surgical intervention for middle ear infections that can lead to hearing loss.[27]

For that part of hearing loss that cannot be addressed through primary prevention, or for which it is too late, WHO also recommends that countries focus on early detection of hearing loss, accompanied by appropriate management of the problem. In principle, screening and diagnosis can be done in preschools, schools, and the community. However, WHO acknowledges that both diagnosis and appropriate management of hearing loss requires greater attention and resources in most low- and middle-income settings. WHO estimates, for example, that only about 1 in 40 people in low- and middle-income countries who need a hearing aid have one. In addition, the resources available in these settings for speech therapy, training in sign language, cochlear implants, and related efforts are limited.[27]

POLICY AND PROGRAM BRIEFS

Four policy and program briefs follow. The first concerns the costs of addressing noncommunicable diseases in the Pacific islands. The next two briefs deal with mental health—one on the gap between the costs of mental disorders in low- and middle-income countries and the lack of attention to them and the other on the growing costs of dementia. Few countries and few actors in global health have paid much attention to oral health, so the last brief deals with that topic.

The Economic Costs of Noncommunicable Diseases in the Pacific Islands[37]

The World Bank published the report, *The Economic Costs of Non-Communicable Diseases in the Pacific Islands: A Rapid Stocktake of the Situation in Samoa, Tonga, and Vanuatu*, in 2013. The report has three key messages:

- Noncommunicable diseases can impose large health, financial, and economic costs on countries.
- Risk factors in the Pacific are feeding a pipeline of noncommunicable diseases that are potentially very expensive to treat.
- Many of the NCDs are avoidable.

The first key policy point of the report is that noncommunicable diseases can impose large health, financial, and economic costs on countries in the Pacific. According to the World Health Organization, NCDs are already the leading cause of death in the Pacific, accounting for an estimated 70 percent or more of all deaths in 9 out of 12 countries in the region. Life expectancy in Tonga has actually fallen as a result of NCDs. In addition, at least one quarter of NCD deaths are premature in Tonga, Samoa, and Vanuatu, proportions that are higher than in other lower-middle-income countries.

Cardiovascular disease is the leading cause of death in the Pacific. Several factors can explain the particular impact of NCDs in the Pacific, including rapidly changing diets and lifestyles; relatively weak health promotion and prevention strategies; increasing use of tobacco; weak compliance with medication; and a possible genetic predisposition to gain weight, especially in Tonga and Samoa. In addition to premature deaths, NCDs also cause disabilities, including stroke, diabetic amputations, and diabetic related blindness.

NCDs in the Pacific also impose large, but often preventable, costs to government health budgets, thereby squeezing out opportunities for governments to invest in other productive investments. This is a major public policy challenge because in all three countries and much of the Pacific more generally, governments are the dominant source of health funding. In Samoa, Tonga, and Vanuatu, the government finances 87.7, 81.5, and 90.6 percent, respectively, of total expenditure on health. In addition, governments in the Pacific have only limited space in their budgets to increase spending on public health due to low and unpredictable economic growth, a low tax revenue base, and competing demands from other areas such as education.

The rise of NCDs therefore poses a particular public finance challenge to these countries. This is particularly so because NCDs such as heart disease and diabetes can be costly to treat, given their widespread prevalence in the adult population, the fact they are chronic, and specific treatments can be expensive. The cost of diabetes-related dialysis in Samoa, for example, is 12 times the gross domestic product (GDP) per capita per patient per year. This is especially significant light of the fact that WHO suggests that interventions are usually not cost-effective when they exceed three times the GDP per capita of a country.

Moreover, some interventions appear to be simply unaffordable. The cost of insulin for one patient per year, for example, is equal to the cost of the drug allocation for about 76 other citizens in Vanuatu. In fact, only 1.3 percent of the total population could be treated with insulin or 5.3 percent treated with the full regimen of antihypertensive drugs before the total government drug budget for Vanuatu would be fully spent.

A second key policy finding in the report is that risk factors for acquiring NCDs suggest the problem will get worse unless urgent action is taken now. In each of the 10 countries in the Pacific for which data is available, 60 percent or more of the adult population is overweight, and in six countries, more than 75 percent of adults are overweight. Nearly one in four boys and one in five girls in Tonga are obese. Half of the adult population is obese in four countries and in Kiribati,

over two-thirds of people smoke tobacco daily. Over 70 percent of people in the Cook Islands are physically inactive. Only 5 percent of adult females and 10 percent of adult males were free of any of the preventable risk factors for acquiring NCDs in Vanuatu. Even in the face of these substantial risk factors, however, governments have not been putting enough resources toward prevention. In 2005–2006, Tonga's overall health expenditures represented 6.8 percent of GDP but only 1.6 percent of these health funds were used to prevent NCDs. Fortunately, this is now improving.

The third key policy finding in the report is that many of the NCDs are avoidable through affordable and cost-effective prevention strategies. Financial costs to government and health and social costs to patients rise dramatically if an NCD progresses. For example, pharmaceutical costs to government increased more than fourfold from $5.59 per patient per year to $24.55 in Vanuatu in late 2012 as a person moved from regular testing of blood glucose levels to first stage oral medication for diabetes. Pharmaceutical costs increased again to $367 per patient year when insulin and other associated drugs were required. Effective primary and secondary prevention would therefore save the government over $300 per patient per year. This would be substantial when government expenditure on health has recently averaged only around $14 per person per year.

Thus, strategies to prevent NCDs will benefit public health and public finances simultaneously: a win–win for public policy and public health. Preventing NCDs through primary and secondary prevention can be an affordable, cost-effective, and even cost-saving strategy for governments. Moreover, raising the excise duty on tobacco in the Pacific to 70 percent of the retail price is a particularly strategic intervention, given that tobacco use is a major driver of the major NCDs and that raising the excise duty can generate much-needed financial resources for government.

The report outlines key priorities for the ministries of health and finance to consider when trying to reduce NCDs and NCD risk factors in the Pacific Islands. These priorities include improving data on the economics of NCDs, such as the household costs of NCDs and the impact of direct and indirect costs on the poorest quintiles; focusing on high-risk, premature deaths; and improving primary and secondary prevention. The report also suggests prioritizing preventative interventions among young women, because poor maternal health, including obesity and diabetes, can influence the risk of chronic disease in the developing fetus. In addition, the report recommends increasing taxation on foods and drinks that are high in sugar, salt, or saturated fats, as well as on tobacco.

One encouraging sign is that Pacific ministers of health and ministers of finance drew on this and similar reports to endorse a "roadmap" for the prevention and control of NCDs at a joint meeting in 2014.[64]

Mental Disorders—The Unacceptable Gap Between Their Burden and the Lack of Attention Paid to Them[65]

A recent commentary by an eminent psychiatrist and leader of global work on mental health, Dr. Steven Hyman, highlights the large gap between the exceptionally high burden of mental disorders and the lack of attention and financing that most low- and middle-income countries give to them.

First, the commentary reminds the reader of the enormous burden of mental disorders, as discussed earlier in this chapter. It notes that mental disorders represent the leading cause of years of life lived with disability globally among those 15 to 44 years of age. Even taking all age groups into account, mental disorders cause more DALYs than any category of NCD globally, except cardiovascular disease. These disorders also contribute to 35 percent of the loss of economic output among all classes of noncommunicable diseases. Moreover, the prevalence of mental illnesses has increased due to population growth, urbanization, armed conflicts, displacement of populations, and the shift to an increasing burden of noncommunicable diseases.

Second, Dr. Hyman highlights the high health and productivity costs of mental disorders. They impair cognition, emotion, motivation, and ability to function and have a dramatic impact on success in school and the workplace. They also often occur with other NCDs, which further worsens health outcomes and disability. Furthermore, many mental disorders occur in a cycle where they may get better but then get worse again, also making disability worse.

In addition, although the greatest global impact of mental illnesses occurs in the form of disability, mental illnesses do contribute to mortality. According to Hyman's commentary, there are between 800,000 and 1 million suicides per year worldwide, and it is estimated that 90 percent of the people who commit suicide have a mental disorder. In addition, there are high rates of comorbidity between mental illness and NCDs and mood and anxiety disorders can worsen diabetes and cardiovascular disease, shortening one's life.

Another reason to focus attention on mental health is that there *are* cost-effective treatments for a variety of mental disorders. In addition, further progress against mental disorders in low- and middle-income settings could be achieved in cost-effective ways through wider use of generic medicine, more training on mental health of primary healthcare personnel of all types, the transfer of some mental health efforts to community-based mental health workers, and the deconcentration of mental health funding from large mental hospitals to community-based settings for primary care.

Unfortunately, despite the burden of disease, the exceptionally high health and productivity costs of mental illness, and the fact that cost-effective treatments exist for many conditions, 80 percent of the people in low- and middle-income countries with mental illness are not receiving care for their illness.

Moreover, partly because of limited resources and partly because of a lack of priority attention to mental health, about half of the world's population lives in countries that have fewer than one psychiatrist per 200,000 people. In addition, the budget for mental health in many low-resource settings is between 1 and 2 percent of total health expenditure, which is already low in many low- and middle-income countries.

Dr. Hyman notes that the lack of attention to mental disorders stems from a number of factors, including stigma, the lack of strong advocacy groups that can lobby on behalf of people in need of mental health care, and the mistaken ideas that many people hold that mental disorders may not be real and that they can be controlled by the people who have them.

In the end, Dr. Hyman suggests that policymakers must better understand the enormous health burden exacted by mental disorders, the fact that some of them can be addressed in cost-effective ways, and that the costs of continued inaction in ethical human, financial, and productivity terms are already exceptional and will continue to grow.

Dementia

Dementia is a syndrome—usually of a chronic or progressive nature—in which there is deterioration in cognitive function beyond what might be expected from normal aging.[66] The number of people living with dementia in 2013 was estimated to be about 44 million.[67]

Dementia mainly affects older people, and the likelihood of developing dementia after age 65 roughly doubles every 5 years. However, there is a growing awareness of cases with an onset before the age of 65.[68] The most important risk factors for dementia are age, family history, and heredity. Other risk factors include alcohol use, atherosclerosis, obesity, smoking, diabetes, and high cholesterol. Some evidence suggests an association between decreased blood flow conditions and the onset of vascular dementia.[69]

Dementia is a global problem on the rise. The number of people living with dementia is predicted to reach 115 million by 2050. Population aging is the main driver of projected increases in the prevalence of dementia. Low- and middle-income countries going through the demographic transition are predicted to see the largest increase in prevalence, and it is projected that by 2050, 71 percent of dementia patients will live in today's low- and middle-income countries, an increase from 68 percent in 2013. The largest increases are projected in East Asia and sub-Saharan Africa.[67]

The social and economic costs of dementia are great. In 2010, the total global societal cost of dementia was estimated to be $604 billion annually. This corresponds to 1 percent of worldwide gross domestic product (GDP). The total cost of dementia as a proportion of GDP varied from 0.24 percent in low-income countries to 1.24 percent in high-income countries.[66] Costs of informal care provided by families and friends account for about 42 percent of worldwide total costs associated with dementia and the direct costs of care provided by professionals account for 42 percent of costs, as well. Direct medical care costs are much lower and are about 16 percent of worldwide total costs.[68] People with dementia and their families face a significant financial impact from the cost of providing health and social care and from the reduction or loss of income.[70]

Little is known on how to treat dementia, and there is no cure. However, there are many prospective treatments in clinical trials. In the absence of a cure or a treatment to reverse any cognitive loss, emphasis is put on supporting and comforting dementia patients and their families. A high proportion of people with dementia need some care, ranging from support with activities of daily living to full personal care and round-the-clock supervision.

In some high-income countries, between one third and one-half of all people with dementia live in resource- and cost-intensive residential or nursing home care facilities.[67] In the Netherlands, care facilities have reached a new level. Self-contained villages for those experiencing late-stage dementia allow patients to enhance their quality of life by living in a surrogate environment. These villages are set up to allow residents to go about their daily lives of going to the grocery store, shopping, or restaurants safely because everyone working in the village from the storekeeper to the neighbors is trained to be a dementia caregiver.[71] It is known that with appropriate care and support, dementia patients can live many years after the onset of symptoms and can maintain a good quality of life.[70]

Special challenges arise in meeting the needs of dementia patients in low- and middle- income countries. In these settings, there are few social protection programs for the elderly and sick and also fewer overall services for their support and care.[67] In low-resource settings, it is recognized that primary care physicians or community-based workers will be the primary case managers, compared to specialists in more developed settings. With this in mind, primary care physicians and community-based personnel must be properly trained to handle dementia cases in these settings with a focus on continuing care and support rather than curative interventions.[72]

There is an urgent need to develop cost-effective packages for medical and social care that meet the needs of people with dementia and their caregivers across the course of the illness and a need to develop evidence-based prevention strategies. Only by investing now in research and cost-effective approaches to care can future societal costs be anticipated and managed.[67] Moreover, universal social support through pensions and insurance schemes could provide protection to this vulnerable group.[70] Governments and health and social care systems need to be adequately prepared for the future and must seek ways now to improve the lives of the growing number of people with dementia and their caregivers.[68]

Oral Health Among Children in Low- and Middle-Income Countries

The Burden of Disease

Dental caries and periodontal disease are two prominent but often neglected burdens of disease in low- and middle-income countries.[73] Dental caries, commonly known as tooth decay or cavities, are present in 90 percent of the global population,[74] including an estimated 60–90 percent of all school-aged children worldwide.[73] Caries result when naturally occurring oral bacteria break down foods, particularly those containing sugars and starches, into acidic by-products. These acids combine with saliva and food remnants to form plaque, a substance that builds up and adheres to teeth.[75] Without removal, the plaque acids will either degrade the enamel of teeth and create cavities or turn into tartar, which can be removed only with a professional dental cleaning.[76]

Together, plaque and tartar cause gingivitis, or inflammation of the gums. When left untreated, gingivitis advances to periodontitis, a disease characterized by inflammation around the teeth and also gums that retract from teeth to form spaces that are prone to oral infection.[76] Once infection occurs, the body's immune system responds with bacterial toxins that break down the bone and connective tissue, resulting in tooth loss.[74,76] Severe forms of periodontal disease affect 5–15 percent of most populations,[74] including about 2 percent of youth worldwide who suffer from juvenile or early-onset aggressive periodontitis.[73]

Both dental caries and periodontal disease contribute to childhood morbidity and have a negative impact on their quality of life.[74] Research suggests that the discomfort associated with biting and chewing for children who suffer from problems of oral health contributes to school absenteeism. It has been estimated, for example, that 50 million school hours are lost annually due to oral health issues.[77] Malnutrition prevalence rates also increase if children are too pained to eat.[74] A child's psychosocial well-being and ability to smile and speak may also be impaired.[78]

Another oral health disease of importance is noma. This condition originates as an untreated gingival inflammation, which then evolves into a gangrenous lesion that causes necrosis of the lips, chin, and facial tissues.[78,79] Noma has been reported in children, ages 1 to 5, who reside in low-income communities with poor sanitation in Asia, Latin America, and Africa.[73,79] Ninety percent of children who are exposed to this illness die as a result of receiving no medical care,[73] whereas survivors must cope with severe facial disfigurement.[80]

Risk Factors

There are a number of risk factors for pediatric oral health conditions that are prominent in low- and middle-income countries. These include low education levels, low socioeconomic status, poor oral hygiene practices, alcohol and tobacco use, and excessive intake of dietary sugars.[73,81] These often occur in settings with limited access to safe water and modern sanitary facilities, insufficient community infrastructure, and the presence of cultural beliefs that do not support preventive oral health efforts.[81]

Current epidemiological data indicate that the oral health burden for children is most prominent in the Americas and has least affected Africa.[73] However, the prevalence of these diseases is expected to rise in low- and middle-income countries due to increased sugar consumption that accompanies economic growth and globalization of the food industry.[73] Illustratively, Dr. Karen Sokal-Gutierrez, a pediatrician working with the Children's Oral Health Nutrition Project in Latin America and Asia, has noted an "explosion in the availability of soda, chips and other junk food."[82] These products are cheap and contain large amounts of sugars and starches. Unfortunately, children are often exposed to these products without nutrition education to inform them of the potential negative health effects of consuming such food.[82] The result is a pandemic of tooth decay, and Dr. Sokal-Gutierrez estimates that between one-third and one-half of the children she works with in El Salvador, Ecuador, Nepal, Peru, and Vietnam have baby teeth that are black, rotten, and decayed.[82]

Barriers to Treatment and Prevention

In addition to risk factors, there are several barriers to treatment that are prominent in resource-poor countries. In these countries, almost all tooth decay goes untreated.[83] The dental healthcare workforce in these countries is insufficient to satisfy service needs or demands.[74] In high-income countries such as the United States and Germany, for example, the dentist-to-patient ratio is 1 per 1,000 population. In low- and middle-income countries, the ratio increases to 1 per 50,000 population. In some extreme cases in sub-Saharan Africa, the figure is as low as 1 dentist per 900,000 population. To further exacerbate this crisis, dentists in low-resource settings tend to practice in urban settings, neglecting rural populations, as families in these areas are more likely to be of low socioeconomic status and unable to afford dental care.[74]

Another barrier to treatment is the high cost of dental services. In high-income countries, oral diseases rank as the fourth most expensive health condition to treat,[73] yet insurance coverage for oral health is insufficient, even in many high-income countries. For instance, in the United States, about 130 million Americans lack dental coverage under their insurance plan. This includes 22 percent of children ages 1–17. Estimates suggest that, in low-income countries, the cost of treating dental caries in children alone would exceed the total current budget for child health activities.[73]

Some prevention efforts are also hindered by the limited infrastructure in many low- and middle-income countries, as well as constrained family incomes. There is strong evidence that long-term, low exposure to fluoride reduces the prevalence of dental caries in children.[81] Dispersing fluoride treatment in salt and public water systems has proven to be an effective prevention method in many countries.[84] However successful implementation is largely contingent on the capacity of infrastructure of the affected population and most low- and middle-income countries lack the resources to accomplish this.[74] With the world population now over 7 billion, estimates from the British Fluoridation Society's most recent global report suggests that only about 435 million people have access to fluoridated water sources. Moreover, even on a household-level in the poorest countries, fluoridated toothpaste can exceed a family's budget. In the United Kingdom, for example, only 0.02 percent of a household's annual expenditure is accounted for by toothpaste; in Zambia this percentage rises to 4 percent of annual household expenses.[85]

Addressing Oral Health Issues

Interventions focused on cost-effective prevention methods that combine social policy and individual action will have the most impact in low- and middle-income countries.[81] It will be important to include oral health within the scope of comprehensive chronic disease prevention programs.[83] Oral diseases share many risk factors with the four most prominent chronic conditions—CVD, diabetes, cancer, and chronic obstructive pulmonary disease. Using a shared risk factor approach has the potential to address several health issues simultaneously, benefiting resource-poor countries by reducing the required amount of physical and financial resources.[73] Government programs supporting subsidy and taxation relief of fluoridated toothpaste can also help to address financial barriers.[74] The U.S. Centers for Disease Control and Prevention suggest that every dollar spent on community-based fluoridation interventions saves $38 on dental treatment.[87]

Emphasis also needs to be placed on strengthening oral health education and promotional methods in community settings.[86] With an estimated 1 billion children attending primary and secondary schools globally, public schools are an optimal venue for health promotion and education among this population.[76] Oral health education reinforced in this environment can foster productive health attitudes and good oral health habits early in life. Pilot studies conducted in the United States and Ireland have shown that school-based interventions improve knowledge related to oral cleanliness and gingival health among school-age children.[87,88] The World Health Organization also strongly supports similar efforts on a global scale.[76]

CASE STUDIES

Three case studies follow. The first examines efforts to reduce tobacco use in Poland. It is followed by a review of the cataract blindness control program in India. The last case study, which was referred to earlier, is about the program to integrate mental health into primary health care in Uganda.

The Challenge of Curbing Tobacco Use in Poland
Background

More than three quarters of the world's smokers live in low- and middle-income countries, where smoking is on the rise.[89] In the late 1970s, Poland had the highest rate of smoking in the world, with the average Pole smoking 3,500 cigarettes a year and nearly three quarters of Polish men smoking daily. The impact on the nation's health was staggering. In 1990, the probability of a 15-year-old boy in Poland reaching his 60th birthday was lower than in most countries, including China and India.[90] Lung cancer rates were among the highest in the world. But because tobacco

production, run by the state, provided a significant source of revenue, the government did not fully disclose to the population the negative consequences of smoking. The fall of communism further exacerbated smoking because tobacco, the first industry to be privatized, was taken over by powerful multinational corporations who flooded the market with international brands, spent vast sums on advertising, and kept prices so low that cigarettes cost less than a loaf of bread.

The Intervention

As the tobacco epidemic escalated, Poland's scientific community laid the foundation of the anti-tobacco movement. Research in the 1980s by the Marie Sklodowska-Curie Memorial Cancer Centre and Institute of Oncology contributed to the first Polish report on smoking, highlighting the link between tobacco and the country's alarming rise in cancer. A series of international workshops and scientific conferences in Poland further strengthened these findings. Civil society was experiencing a renewal at the time, with the formation of anti-tobacco groups such as the Polish Anti-Tobacco Society that began to interact with international bodies, such as WHO and the International Union Against Cancer. In addition, the Health Promotion Foundation was established to lead public efforts on health issues and anti-tobacco education efforts.

With the fall of the Berlin Wall, the media became free to cover health topics and played an important role in disseminating information, raising awareness about the dangers of smoking, and shaping public opinion. When tobacco control legislation was introduced in 1991, a heated public debate ensued between health advocates and the powerful tobacco lobby, increasingly viewed by the public as a contest between David and Goliath. In 1995, groundbreaking legislation was finally passed, requiring sweeping measures such as large health warnings on cigarette packs and bans on smoking in enclosed workspaces and health centers, on electronic media advertising, and on tobacco sales to minors. A 30 percent increase in taxes levied on cigarettes was subsequently passed in 1999 and 2000, and advertising was completely banned. In parallel, the Health Promotion Foundation also launched extensive health education and consumer awareness efforts. These included an annual "Great Polish Smoke-Out" competition to encourage smokers to quit, with incentives like winning a weeklong stay in Rome and a chance to meet the Polish-born Pope John Paul II. Since the first smoke-out in 1991, more than 2.5 million Poles have permanently snuffed out their cigarettes because of the campaign.

The Impact

Cigarette consumption dropped 10 percent between 1990 and 1998, and the number of smokers declined from 14 million in the 1980s to under 10 million by the end of the 1990s. The reduction in smoking led to 10,000 fewer deaths each year, a 30 percent decline in lung cancer among men ages 20 to 44, a nearly 7 percent decline in CVD, and a reduction in infant mortality and low birthweight.[91] Life expectancy in the 1990s increased by 4 years.

Lessons Learned

Poland's experience shows that once smoking is seen for what it is—the leading cause of preventable deaths among adults worldwide—then governments do act. Working in concert with civil society and using state-of-the-art communication strategies, the Polish government succeeded in countering the powerful economic influence of the tobacco industry and inducing major shifts in smoking, an addictive behavior that was also then an ingrained social norm. Poland's sweeping legislative measures came to serve as a model for other countries. The experience of South Africa provides an interesting parallel: once the African National Congress came to power in 1994, the antismoking movement gained a powerful ally in Nelson Mandela and his first health minister, ultimately leading to the passage of strict tobacco control legislation and dramatic price control measures that increased the real value of cigarette taxes by 215 percent. As a result, cigarette consumption fell by more than 30 percent, from 1.9 billion packs in 1991 to 1.3 billion packs in 2002. As a South African researcher noted, "You need the right combination of science, evidence, and politics to succeed. If you have one without the other, you don't see action."[92] For a more detailed discussion of the Polish efforts, see *Case Studies in Global Health: Millions Saved.*[93]

Cataract Blindness Control in India

This chapter focuses on a limited number of the leading causes of deaths and DALYs due to noncommunicable diseases. As you would expect, few people die of diseases related to vision disorders; however, the burden of disability of these diseases, especially in low- and middle-income countries in which they are not generally treated in a timely manner, is great. In fact, about 39 million people worldwide are blind and another 246 million people are visually impaired.[25]

Background

About one quarter of the total number of people in the world who are blind live in India, and the case study that follows deals with controlling cataract blindness there.[93] The blindness control program in India has been one of the most extensive such programs in a low- or middle-income country for many years. In addition, over the last 20 years or so, this program has emerged, in many respects, as a public health success story. Those wishing to examine this case in greater detail can read further about it in *Case Studies in Global Health: Millions Saved.*[94]

History

Cataracts are the leading cause of blindness in India. About 80 percent of all of the people in India who are blind are blind due to cataracts. In addition, another 10 million people in India are visually impaired due to untreated cataracts.

In the simplest terms, a cataract is a clouding of the lens of the eye. It blurs the image on the retina, producing a visual effect that is like looking through a window that is frosted or fogged with steam. Cataracts form when protein clumps in the lens of the eye. This is associated with age, excessive exposure to sunlight, diabetes, undernutrition, and other risk factors. Cataracts can affect one or both eyes.

Cataracts are treatable through surgery. One form of surgery requires a large incision in the eye and the removal of the lens and lens capsule. This form of surgery (ICCE) is relatively easy to perform and relatively inexpensive; however, it requires that the patient wear thick eyeglasses after surgery, and it has a high rate of complications. Nonetheless, it has been the form of surgery traditionally done in low-income settings. The other form of surgery is more technically sophisticated (ECCE); however, it has a lower rate of complications when done by trained surgeons. In addition, research in India showed that those having ECCE surgery were 2.8 times more likely to have a good outcome than those having ICCE surgery.[95]

Intervention

India's response to the problem of blindness has been impressive in breadth and duration. India's first intervention in 1963 aimed specifically at controlling trachoma, a highly contagious eye infection. By the end of the decade, the government expanded its approach to include all visual impairment. In 1975, the Central Council of Health declared that "one of the basic human rights is the right to see."[96,p99] In 1976, India formed the National Program for the Control of Blindness (NPCB) to expand access to surgical treatment of vision disorders and to increase ophthalmologic services.

India's first international collaboration in eye care was with DANIDA, the Danish International Development

Assistance Agency. Until 1989, DANIDA assisted India in funding the improvement and expansion of its cataract blindness control program through the provision of equipment, mobile units, training, and enhancements of monitoring and evaluation. The program focused then on mass ICCE surgeries in camps that were mostly set up in areas with limited health infrastructure. This demonstrated the ability of the government to lead mass screening and treatment camps, even in rural areas. It also generated enormous demand for cataract surgeries, even among the poor and rural. However, the limited amount of time a camp was stationed in a particular location, as well as the nature of fieldwork, meant that postsurgical follow-up was difficult to implement. Consequently, although the efforts succeeded in reaching many people, only about 75 percent of those who got surgery returned to an acceptable level of vision.[97]

In 1994, building on its experience with DANIDA, the Government of India began to collaborate with the World Bank to finance a 7-year cataract blindness control project. The project focused on seven Indian states that had the highest prevalence of blindness and, in simple terms, it aimed to assist India in moving its cataract blindness control program from a focus on quantity to a focus on quality and outcomes. The aims of the program were to improve surgical outcomes by shifting from ICCE to ECCE, strengthen India's capacity to provide high-quality surgery done by competently trained staff, and increase the coverage of the program to areas that had previously been underserved. Much greater attention was paid than before to monitoring the outcomes of surgery.

The program also focused on trying to achieve its aims through enhancing collaboration between the public and the private sectors. Some surgeries were done in public facilities. The government financed other surgeries that were conducted by the private and NGO sectors. In addition, NGOs such as Sight Savers International, Lions Clubs International, and Christoffel Blinden Mission also financially supported eye hospitals, training institutes, and the development of school vision-screening programs and outreach. The Aravind Eye Hospital in Madurai, India, was a world famous leader in eye care and became increasingly involved in training and other assistance to the NPCB.

Impact

Over 15 million cataract operations were performed in connection with the Cataract Blindness Control Project. In addition, ECCE surgeries increased as a share of the total surgeries from between 15 and 65 percent across different states in 1998–1999 to between 44 and 91 percent in 2001–2002.[97]

Moreover, by 2001, 92 percent of surgeries occurred in fixed facilities where better outcomes can be expected. Most important, surgical outcomes have improved, with the introduction of improved and well-equipped surgical procedures and trained personnel. The ability to see at an acceptable level after surgery grew from 75 percent in 1994 to 82 percent from 1999 to 2002. The number and quality of surgeries was associated with a decrease in the prevalence of cataract blindness by 26 percent.

Cost-Effectiveness

The World Bank–assisted intervention cost $136 million, with close to 90 percent coming from a soft loan from the bank and the remainder from the government of India. When done correctly and in areas of high prevalence, cataract surgery is among the most highly cost-effective interventions.[98] ECCE surgery is estimated to cost about $60 per DALY averted in the South and East Asia regions. Through the combination of serving those most in need and their educational and awareness raising campaigns, NGOs operating under the project used their financial resources very effectively.

Lessons Learned

The efforts in India demonstrate the benefits of collaboration among different public and private sectors and international institutions. The government of India and its political commitment to the problem in the 1960s was a requirement for success, because it offered a big push to combating cataract blindness. In addition, even though the government's early efforts were not always at the level of quality desired, they provided a baseline for further studies on how the program could be improved and expanded in a high quality manner. Finally, the involvement of the NGOs helped to bring innovative approaches to the project and continually encouraged the government to improve and maintain quality services.

Integrating Mental Health into Primary Care in Uganda

Mental disorders are neglected in most low- and middle-income countries. They are difficult to diagnose and treat, they carry considerable stigma, and low-income countries often lack the skilled personnel and financial resources needed to address mental health issues. Uganda is one of the few low-income countries that has made an effort to tackle the important burden of mental disorders, and the case study that follows describes this effort and some of the outcomes associated with Uganda's move to integrate mental health concerns into its primary healthcare program.

Background

In 1986, Uganda came out of a 5-year civil conflict that had been preceded by 8 years of government led by General Idi Amin, which were characterized by misrule and violence. Although the civil conflict was, for the most part, over in the southern parts of the country, the conflict continued in the north, with abduction of children and terrorizing of the communities carried out by the Lord's Resistance Army. At about the same time, Uganda was increasingly being affected by the emerging HIV/AIDS epidemic.

According to the 1995 Uganda Burden of Disease study, over 75 percent of life years lost from premature deaths was the result of preventable communicable disorders.[23] However, it was also recognized that there was a simultaneous surge in the occurrence of noncommunicable disorders, such as hypertension, diabetes, cancer, and mental disorders. It was also becoming clearer that HIV/AIDS and the prolonged armed conflict created an increased need for attention to be paid to mental health.

In order to address the increasing burden of mental disorders, the Ministry of Health decided to promote the integration of mental health into primary health care. This involved developing standards and guidelines for the management of eight priority mental disorders for the community, district, and national referral levels of care. This was part of Uganda's efforts to address health care in an effective and efficient manner through the establishment of a minimum healthcare package.

The Intervention

The process of integrating mental health into primary health care was to be implemented through training all healthcare workers to recognize and manage common mental disorders, as well as establishing and strengthening a referral and supportive supervision system. The initiative was outlined in the Uganda Health Sector Strategic Plan 1999 to 2004.[99]

Central-level activities included the creation of a Mental Health Coordinating Committee whose main responsibilities were the development of standards and guidelines for the management of common mental disorders, developing materials for the training of health workers, and developing and participating in the referral and supervision system. Central-level activities also included participation in the creation of the Core Team on Psychosocial Disorders, a group of representatives of two government sectors—the Ministry of Health and the Ministry of Gender, Labor, and Social Development, which was responsible for child protection—and five NGOs working in the field of psychosocial disorders, and UNICEF.

The Core Team carried out an assessment of the psychosocial situation of the conflict-affected population in eight districts of northern Uganda, disseminated the results to the district leaders, and facilitated the affected districts in the development of psychosocial components to be included in district development plans. The Core Team developed indicators, as well as a monitoring and evaluation plan, that they then implemented. The Core Team was instrumental in the coordinated safe return and reintegration of abducted children into their communities.

As a result of having mental health in the Health Sector Policy and the Health Sector Strategic Plan, a budget line for mental health was created. Although the allocation to mental health from the government of Uganda was only 0.7 percent of the total health budget, having mental health as a budget item made it easier for other funding agencies to support mental health efforts in Uganda.

The African Development Bank (AfDB) provided a loan to the government for support in the integration of mental health into primary health care. This AfDB-assisted project provided $17.73 million to mental health efforts in Uganda over a 5-year period. Activities included rehabilitation of Butabika National Referral Psychiatric Hospital, downsizing it from a 900-bed to a 450-bed hospital, as well as the construction of six regional mental health units. The project included provision of essential mental health medications and support to the training of healthcare workers at all levels of the care system, from training primary healthcare nurses in the recognition and management of common mental disorders, to the training of specialized personnel, such as psychiatrists, psychologists, and psychiatric social workers.[99]

Lessons Learned

It is often thought that mental health is not a priority in low-income countries or that feasible mental health interventions are not available. This case study, however, highlights that mental disorders are of importance in low-income countries, especially those affected by disasters, complex emergencies, and HIV/AIDS. It also demonstrates that countries, even with limited resources, can take measures to considerably improve mental health services.

This case study also suggests that it is possible to design and implement a strategy for dealing with mental disorders that builds on an existing healthcare system. As a result of the investments made, resources for mental health are better allocated in Uganda than before, and funds for mental health have moved from the large psychiatric institution to the regional levels, where services are more accessible to the populations that require them.

Nonetheless, there remain great challenges in trying to provide appropriate mental health services in Uganda. These include the need to strengthen information and public education so the population is aware of what constitutes mental disorders, as well as where help can be sought. A further challenge is likely to be sustainability of the established services. The AfDB project provided the infrastructure and the start-up costs; however, the government of Uganda will have to ensure that recurrent costs for staff, maintenance of equipment and infrastructure, referral and supervision, and other inputs such as drugs are provided for in the long term.

FUTURE CHALLENGES

The world must face a number of challenges if it is to reduce the burden of noncommunicable diseases in low- and middle-income countries. First, the number of people with new cases of noncommunicable diseases will grow in low- and middle-income countries as a result of the aging of the population, urbanization, globalization, and lifestyle changes. In addition, because noncommunicable diseases are chronic, the number of people with these diseases will also rise. The increasing number of people who will be at risk of and living with chronic diseases in low- and middle-income countries will pose a huge challenge to the health of these countries, their health systems, and their national finances.

Related to this, a number of low-income countries will have to deal with the challenge of addressing increasing amounts of noncommunicable disease simultaneously with having to address substantial burdens of communicable diseases. This will severely tax the managerial, technical, and financial capacity of many low- and middle-income countries. It will also require greater attention by low-income countries to noncommunicable diseases and to improved surveillance of these diseases. Low- and middle-income countries will need to strengthen primary care and integrate the prevention and control of noncommunicable diseases into it.

In addition, it will be important to spread as rapidly as possible to low- and middle-income countries the lessons that the high-income countries have already learned about how to address noncommunicable diseases in cost-effective ways. It will also be critical to generate much greater evidence about what works in low- and middle-income countries. This body of evidence, especially for low-cost interventions that have a high payback, needs to be disseminated in low- and middle-income countries as rapidly as possible. Ongoing mechanisms need to be established to ensure that cost-effective diagnostics and drugs get used as early as possible after their development in low- and middle-income countries and not just in high-income countries.

Even as they continue to learn from the experience of the high-income countries, the low- and middle-income countries need to take the measures that are known to prevent noncommunicable diseases, as discussed earlier in the chapter. However, many countries have limited administrative capacity, insufficient financial resources, and major gaps in human resources for health. Thus, lessons will also need to be generated and disseminated on the operational efforts needed to put effective NCD programs in places in low-resource settings. In addition, such countries will almost certainly need to take a stepwise approach to strengthening their NCD programs, starting with those efforts that will have the highest return.

A major goal of public health policy is to try to help people live longer lives that are as healthy as possible. The epidemiologic and demographic changes that are occurring globally suggest this goal can be achieved only if countries take measures now to prevent as much noncommunicable disease as possible. To achieve this aim, countries need to increasingly prepare their health systems to deal with the prevention and treatment of noncommunicable diseases in cost-effective and efficient ways. The failure to address these aims effectively will result in older but unhealthy populations, whose needs for care and cost of care will overwhelm the health systems of a number of countries.[100]

MAIN MESSAGES

Noncommunicable diseases constitute the largest burden of disease worldwide. In all regions of the world, except sub-Saharan Africa, the burden of these diseases is greater than the burden of communicable diseases. Cardiovascular disease is the single largest cause of death worldwide. Diabetes, some forms of cancer, and mental disorders are also major causes of disability and death from noncommunicable diseases. In fact, about 12 percent of the DALYs in 2010 were attributable to CVD, almost 8 percent to cancer, almost 2 percent to diabetes, and about 5 percent to the four mental disorders discussed earlier.[1]

Moreover, economic development, globalization, urbanization, and aging will encourage the growth of noncommunicable diseases globally. In this light, it is projected that by 2030, even in low-income countries, there will be a major epidemiologic shift toward noncommunicable disease. As this happens, it is projected that diarrhea, malaria, and TB will no longer be in the top 10 causes of DALYs in low-income countries. Rather, depression and cardiovascular disease will rise on the list from where they are now, and chronic obstructive pulmonary disease, hearing loss, and refractive errors will make it into the top 10 causes of DALYs for such countries. It is also projected that by 2030 no communicable disease will be in the top 10 causes of DALYs for middle- or upper-income countries.

The leading risk factors for cardiovascular disease are hypertension, obesity, high cholesterol, and tobacco use. A lack of physical activity contributes to CVD and obesity and the main risk factor for diabetes is obesity. Some cancers are associated with an infectious agent, such as hepatitis B, *H. pylori*, or the human papilloma virus. Other cancers are linked with tobacco use. Little is known about the nongenetic risk factors that are associated with mental disorders.

The costs of noncommunicable diseases and the use of tobacco and alcohol abuse are substantial. They have a considerable impact on people in their productive years of life. In addition, mental disorders and diabetes are associated with very large amounts of disability. The costs of trying to prevent the burden of noncommunicable diseases include efforts to promote healthier lifestyles, including a healthy diet, maintaining an appropriate weight, and increasing physical activity, while trying to reduce obesity, cigarette consumption, and excessive drinking. The costs of treating noncommunicable diseases can be high, both because of the high cost of some medical treatments for specific episodes of illness and the need to treat some diseases and conditions for many years. Mental disorders, for example, frequently start early in life and often continue throughout a life. Nonetheless, some medicines used for hypertension and high cholesterol, for example, are highly cost-effective at dealing with CVD, even in low- and middle-income settings.

The single most important step that low- and middle-income countries can take now to reduce the burden of noncommunicable diseases is to reduce the consumption of tobacco. There is good evidence from high-income and some lower- and middle-income countries that taxing cigarettes more heavily, banning smoking from public places, and trying to educate the population about the impact of tobacco on health can all contribute to reducing tobacco consumption.

Reducing the burden of noncommunicable diseases will also require that alcohol-related harm be reduced, which can be done in cost-effective ways by taking measures analogous to those taken for dealing with tobacco. In addition, it is critical that obesity be reduced through healthier diets, fewer calories, increased intake of fruits and green leafy vegetables, and more physical activity. Tax policies can also be used to subsidize healthy foods and tax unhealthy foods. Other measures to reduce obesity can be complemented with food labeling legislation and legislation to encourage the use of healthier ingredients in food products. The intake of salt must also be reduced.

Low-resource countries will need to embed approaches to mental health in their communities and families. This can be coupled with better training of primary healthcare staff at all levels to deal with mental health, improved access to low-cost drugs, and enhanced financing by deconcentrating the budgets so that they are not disproportionately allocated to large psychiatric hospitals.

A number of countries are making important progress in addressing vision loss by reducing the loss from infectious and parasitic causes and taking steps to address unoperated cataracts. To meet the global goals of reduced preventable blindness by 2019, countries will need to take additional measures to establish more comprehensive eye care programs at all levels of their healthcare systems.

There are substantial gaps in attention to hearing loss. However, about 50 percent of all hearing loss can be addressed through primary prevention, including better maternal nutrition and care, enhanced vaccination, and reduction in syphilis. Increasing the attention of resource-poor health systems to the remaining burden of hearing loss will require increases in financial, human, and health system resources with greater attention to early screening and appropriate management.

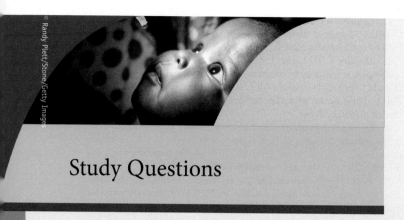

Study Questions

1. How important are noncommunicable diseases to the global burden of disease?

2. Why are noncommunicable diseases less important to the burden of disease in sub-Saharan Africa than in other regions?

3. What are the leading risk factors for cardiovascular disease?

4. What are the most important cancers that affect low-income countries?

5. What are the most important risk factors for cancers?

6. What factors are causing the epidemic of diabetes that is occurring worldwide?

7. Why are mental disorders so important to the burden of disease if so few people die of them?

8. What measures have proven effective in reducing the use of tobacco?

9. What lessons of Uganda's approach to mental health concerns are important for other resource-poor countries?

10. What measures have been effective in reducing the abuse of alcohol?

REFERENCES

1. Institute of Health Metrics and Evaluation. (2015). GBD compare. Retrieved February 15, 2015, from http://vizhub.healthdata.org/gbd-compare/.

2. Institute of Health Metrics and Evaluation. (2013). *The global burden of disease: Generating evidence, guiding policy*. Seattle, WA: Institute of Health Metrics and Evaluation.

3. Lancet. *Global Burden of Disease Study 2010*. Retrieved July 17, 2015, from http://www.thelancet.com/global-burden-of-disease.

4. World Health Organization. (2011). *Global status report on noncommunicable diseases 2010*. Geneva: World Health Organization.

5. Institute of Health Metrics and Evaluation. (2015). GBD 2010 heat map. Retrieved February 15, 2015, from http://vizhub.healthdata.org/irank/heat.php.

6. Nichols, M., Townsend, N., Luengo-Fernandez, R., Leal, J., Gray, A., Scarborough, P., et al. (2012). *European cardiovascular disease statistics 2012*. Brussels, Belgium: European Heart Network; Sophia Antipolis, France: European Society of Cardiology.

7. Institute of Health Metrics and Evaluation. (2015). *GBD 2010 arrow diagram*. Retrieved February 15, 2015, from http://vizhub.healthdata.org/irank/arrow.php.

8. World Health Organization. *Global burden of disease (GBD)*. Retrieved October 20, 2010, from http://www.who.int/healthinfo/global_burden_disease/en/index.html.

9. Gaziano, T. A., Srinath Reddy, K., Paccaud, F., Horton, S., & Chaturvedi, V. (2006). Cardiovascular disease. In D. T. Jamison, J. G. Breman, A. R. Measham, et al. (Eds.), *Disease control priorities in developing countries* (2nd ed., pp. 645–662). New York: Oxford University Press.

10. World Heart Federation. (2015). *Cardiovascular disease risk factors*. Retrieved February 15, 2015, from http://www.world-heart-federation.org/cardiovascular-health/cardiovascular-disease-risk-factors/.

11. National Institutes of Health. Obesity, physical activity, and weight control glossary. Retrieved March 17, 2015, from http://win.niddk.nih.gov/publications/glossary.htm.

12. International Diabetes Federation. (2013). *IDF diabetes atlas* (6th ed.). Brussels: International Diabetes Federation.

13. Ryerson, B., Tierney, E. F., Thompson, T. J., et al. (2003). Excess physical limitations among adults with diabetes in the U.S. population, 1997–1999. *Diabetes Care, 26*(1), 206–210.

14. Global Burden of Disease Study 2013 Collaborators. Global, regional, and national incidence, prevalence, and years lived with disability for 301 acute and chronic diseases and injuries in 188 countries, 1990–2013: a systematic analysis for the Global Burden of Disease Study 2013. *Lancet.* Published Online June 8, 2015 http://dx.doi.org/10.1016/ S0140-6736(15)60692-4

15. Haffner, S. M. (1998). Epidemiology of type 2 diabetes: Risk factors. *Diabetes Care, 21*(Suppl 3), C3–6.

16. Venkat Narayan, K., Zhang, P., Kanaya, A. M., et al. (2006). Diabetes: The pandemic and potential solutions. In D. T. Jamison, J. G. Breman, A. R. Measham, et al. (Eds.), *Disease control priorities in developing countries* (2nd ed., pp. 591–603). New York: Oxford University Press.

17. World Health Organization. (2012). *Assessing national capacity for the prevention and control of noncommunicable diseases: Report of the 2010 global survey*. Geneva: WHO.

18. Sloan, F. A., & Gelband, H. (Eds.). (2007). *Cancer control opportunities in low- and middle-income countries*. Washington, DC: National Academies Press.

19. International Agency for Research on Cancer. (2013). *Latest world global cancer statistics* (Press Release No. 233). Lyon, France: IARC.

20. Veneis, P., & Wild, C. P. (2013, December 16). Global cancer patterns: Causes and prevention. *The Lancet*. Retrieved from http://www.thelancet.com/journals/lancet/article/PIIS0140-6736(13)62224-2/fulltext?_eventId=login.

21. Magrath, I. (2010). Cancer in low and middle-income countries. In M. Carballo (Ed.), *Health G20: A briefing on health issues or G20 leaders* (pp. 58–68). Sutton, UK: Probrook.

22. Centers for Disease Control and Prevention. (2012). *Parasites: Schistosomiasis*. Retrieved March 15, 2015, from http://www.cdc.gov/parasites/schistosomiasis/index.html.

23. Mathers, C. D., Lopez, A. D., & Murray, C. J. L. (2006). The burden of disease and mortality by condition: Data, methods, and results for 2001. In A. D. Lopez, C. D. Mathers, M. Ezzati, D. T. Jamison, & C. J. L. Murray (Eds.), *Global burden of disease and risk factors* (pp. 45–240). New York: Oxford University Press.

24. Hyman, S., Chisholm, D., Kessler, R., Patel, V., & Whiteford, H. (2006). Mental disorders. In D. T. Jamison, J. G. Breman, A. R. Measham, et al. (Eds.), *Disease control priorities in developing countries* (2nd ed., pp. 605–625). New York: Oxford University Press.

25. World Health Organization. (2014). *Visual impairment and blindness* (Fact Sheet No. 282). Retrieved February 16, 2015, from http://www.who.int/mediacentre/factsheets/fs282/en/.

26. Cook, J., Frick, K. D., Baltussen, R., et al. (2006). Loss of vision and hearing. In D. T. Jamison, J. G. Breman, A. R. Measham, et al. (Eds.), *Disease control priorities in developing countries* (2nd ed., pp. 953–962). Washington, DC: The World Bank.

27. World Health Organization. (2015). *Deafness and hearing loss* (Fact Sheet No. 300). Retrieved from February 16, 2015, http://www.who.int/mediacentre/factsheets/fs300/en/.

28. Jha, P., Chaloupka, F. J., Moore, J., et al. (2006). Tobacco addiction. In D. T. Jamison, J. G. Breman, A. R. Measham, et al. (Eds.), *Disease control priorities in developing countries* (2nd ed., pp. 869–885). New York: Oxford University Press.

29. Jha, P., MacLennan, M., Yurkeli, A., et al. (in press). Chapter 10. Global tobacco control. In D. Jamison, H. Gelband, S. Horton, P. Jha, R. Laxminarayan, & R. Nugent (Eds.), *Disease control priorities in the developing world* (3rd ed.). Washington, DC: The World Bank.

30. Jamison, D. T., Breman, J. G., Measham, A. R., et al. (Eds.). *Priorities in health*. Washington, DC: The World Bank.

31. Rehm, J., Chisholm, D., Room, R., & Lopez, A. D. Alcohol. In D. T. Jamison, J. G. Breman, A. R. Measham, et al. (Eds.), *Disease control priorities in developing countries* (2nd ed., pp. 887–906). New York: Oxford University Press.

32. Abegunde, D. O., Mathers, C. D., Adam, T., Ortegon, M., & Strong, K. (2007). The burden and costs of chronic diseases in low-income and middle-income countries. *Lancet, 370*(9603), 1929–1938.

33. Bloom, D. E., Cafiero, E. T., Jané-Llopis, E., Abrahams-Gessel, S., Bloom, L.R., Fathima, S., et al. (2011). *The global economic burden of noncommunicable diseases*. Geneva: World Economic Forum.

34. Bloom, D. E., Cafiero, E. T., McGovern, M. E., Prettner, K., Anderson Stanciole, J. W., Bakkila, S., et al. (2013). *The economic impact of non-communicable disease in China and India: Estimates, projections, and comparisons* (NBER Working Paper No. 19335). Cambridge, MA: National Bureau of Economic Research.

35. World Bank. (2012). The growing burden of non-communicable diseases in the Eastern Caribbean. Human development unit. Washington, DC: World Bank. Retrieved June 19, 2015, from http://documents.worldbank.org/curated/en/2012/01/15978036/growing-burden-non-communicable-diseases-eastern-caribbean.

36. Rodgers, A., Lawes, C. M., Gaziano, T. A., & Vos, T. (2006). The growing burden of risk from high blood pressure, cholesterol, and bodyweight. In D. T. Jamison, J. G. Breman, A. R. Measham, et al. (Eds.), *Disease control priorities in developing countries* (2nd ed., pp. 859–868). New York: Oxford University Press.

37. The brief is based largely on the following sources: Anderson, I. (2013, February 8). The economic costs of non-communicable diseases in the Pacific Islands. *DevPolicyBlog*. Retrieved from http://devpolicy.org/the-economic-costs-of-non-communicable-diseases-in-the-pacific-islands-20130208/; Government of Tonga and the United Nations System in the Pacific Islands. (2013, June). *MDG acceleration framework: Reducing the incidence of non-communicable diseases in Tonga*. Retrieved from http://www.undp.org/content/dam/undp/library/MDG

/MDG%20Acceleration%20Framework/MAF%20Reports/RBAP/Tonga%20-%20october%2004%20WEB.pdf; and World Bank. (2012). *The economic costs of non-communicable diseases in the Pacific Islands: A rapid stocktake of the situation in Samoa, Tonga and Vanuatu.* Retrieved from http://www.worldbank.org/content/dam/Worldbank/document/the-economic-costs-of-noncommunicable-diseases-in-the-pacific-islands.pdf.

38. World Health Organization. (2003). *Investing in mental health.* Geneva: World Health Organization.

39. National Institutes of Health. (2010). *Healthy people 2010. Vision and hearing loss* (Working Paper 28). Retrieved January 16, 2011, from http://www.healthypeople.gov/2010/Document/pdf/Volume2/28Vision.pdf.

40. Rein, D. B., Zhang, P., Wirth, K. E., et al. (2006). The economic burden of major adult visual disorders in the United States. *Archives of Ophthalmology, 124*(12), 1754–1760.

41. Tucci, D. L., Merson, M. H., & Wilson, B. S. (2010). A summary of the literature on global hearing impairment: current status and priorities for action. *Otology & Neurotology, 31*(1), 31–41.

42. Lightwood, J., Collins, D., Lapsley, H., & Novotny, T. E. (2000). Estimating the costs of tobacco use. In P. Jha & F. J. Chaloupka (Eds.), *Tobacco control in developing countries* (pp. 63–104). London: Oxford University Press.

43. Chaloupka, F. J., Tauras, J. A., & Grossman, M. (2007). The economics of addiction. In P. Jha & F. J. Chaloupka (Eds.), *Tobacco control in developing countries* (pp. 107–130). London: Oxford University Press.

44. World Health Organization. (2004). *Global status report on alcohol 2004.* Geneva: World Health Organization.

45. Rehm, J., Mathers, C., Popova, S., Thavorncharoensap, M., Teerawattananon, Y., & Patra, J. (2009). Global burden of disease and injury and economic cost attributable to alcohol use disorders. *Lancet, 373*(9682), 2223–2233.

46. United Nations. (2011). *2011 high-level meeting on the prevention and control of non-communicables diseases.* Retrieved February 20, 2015, from http://www.un.org/en/ga/ncdmeeting2011/.

47. NCD Alliance. (2011). *Political declaration of the high-level meeting on the prevention and control of non-communicable diseases (NCDs): Key points.* Retrieved February 21, 2015, from http://www.ncdalliance.org/sites/default/files/rfiles/Key%20Points%20of%20Political%20Declaration.pdf.

48. Beaglehole, R., Bonita, R., Horton, R., et al., for The Lancet NCD Action Group and the NCD Alliance. (2011). Priority actions for the non-communicable disease crisis. *Lancet, 377*, 1438–1447.

49. Conference of the Parties to the WHO FCTC. (2003). *WHO framework convention on tobacco control.* Geneva: World Health Organization.

50. World Health Organization. (2013). *Tobacco free initiative.* Retrieved February 22, 2015, from http://www.who.int/tobacco/mpower/en/.

51. Casswell, S., & Thamarangsi, T. (2009). Reducing harm from alcohol: A call to action. *Lancet, 373*(9682), 2247–2257.

52. Willett, W. C., Koplan, J. P., Nugent, R., Dusenbury, C., Puska, P., & Gaziano, T. A. (2006). Prevention of chronic disease by means of diet and lifestyle changes. In D. T. Jamison, J. G. Breman, A. R. Measham, et al. (Eds.), *Disease control priorities in developing countries* (2nd ed., pp. 833–850). New York: Oxford University Press.

53. Magrath, I. (2010, March–June). Cancer in low and middle-income countries. *Network: INCTR Magazine, 9*(3).

54. Horton, S. (in press). Cancer in low and middle income countries: An economic overview. In D. Jamison, H. Gelband, S. Horton, P. Jha, R. Laxminarayan, & R. Nugent (Eds.), *Disease control priorities in the developing world* (3rd ed., Chapter 14). Washington, DC: World Bank.

55. Brown, M. L., Goldie, S. J., Draisma, G., et al. (2006). Health service interventions for cancer control in developing countries. In D. T. Jamison, J. G. Breman, A. R. Measham, et al. (Eds.), *Disease control priorities in developing countries* (2nd ed., pp. 569–589). Washington, DC: World Bank. Retrieved from http://www.ncbi.nlm.nih.gov/books/NBK11756/.

56. World Health Organization. (2001). *The world health report 2000. Mental health: New understanding, new hope.* Geneva: WHO.

57. World Health Organization. (2008). *Mental health gap action programme: Scaling up care for mental, neurological, and substance abuse disorders.* Geneva: World Health Organization.

58. Patel, V., Araya, R., Chatterjee, S., et al. (2007). Treatment and prevention of mental disorders in low-income and middle-income countries. *Lancet, 370*(9591), 991–1005.

59. Lancet Mental Health Group. (2007). Scale up services for mental disorders: A call to action. *Lancet, 370*(9594), 1241–1252.

60. Saxena, S., Thornicroft, G., Knapp, M., & Whitford, H. (2007). Resources for mental health: Scarcity, inequity, and inefficiency. *Lancet, 370*(9590), 878–889.

61. Patel, V. (2014). Global mental health: An interview with Vikram Patel. *BMC Medicine, 12*, 44.

62. Hyman, S. (2014). The unconscionable gap between what we know and what we do. *Science Translational Medicine, 6*(253), 1–4.

63. World Health Organization. (2013). *Universal eye health: A global action plan 2014–2019.* Geneva: World Health Organization.

64. Pacific Islands Forum Secretariat. (2014). *NCD roadmap report.* Retrieved March 15, 2015, from http://www.forumsec.org/resources/uploads/attachments/documents/2014JEHM.BackgroundA.NCD_Roadmap_FullReport.pdf.

65. This brief is based on Hyman, S. E. (2014). The unconscionable gap between what we know and what we do. *Science Translational Medicine, 6*(253), 1–4.

66. World Health Organization. (2014). *Dementia* (Fact Sheet No. 362). Retrieved June 26, 2014, from http://www.who.int/mediacentre/factsheets/fs362/en/.

67. Alzheimer's Disease International. (2013). *Policy brief for heads of government: The global impact of dementia 2013–2050.* London: Author.

68. Alzheimer's Disease International. (2010). *World Alzheimer report 2010: The global impact of dementia.* London: Author.

69. Mayo Clinic Staff. (2014). *Dementia: Risk factors.* Retrieved July 6, 2014, from http://www.mayoclinic.org/diseases-conditions/dementia/basics/risk-factors/con-20034399.

70. Alzheimer's Disease International and World Health Organization. (2012). *Dementia: A public health priority.* London: Author.

71. Moisse, K. (2012, April 10). Alzheimer's disease: Dutch village doubles as nursing home. *ABC News.* Retrieved August 13, 2014, from http://abcnews.go.com/Health/AlzheimersCommunity/alzheimers-disease-dutch-village-dubbed-truman-show-dementia/story?id=16103780.

72. Prince, M. J., Acosta, D., Castro-Costa, E., Jackson, J., & Shaji, K. S. (2009). Packages of care for dementia in low- and middle-income countries. *PLoS Med, 6*(11), e1000176. doi:10.1371/journal.pmed.1000176.

73. World Health Organization. (2014). *What is the burden of oral disease?* Retrieved from http://www.who.int/oral_health/disease_burden/global/en/.

74. The Lancet. (2009). Oral health: Prevention is key. *The Lancet, 373*(9657), 1. doi:10.1016/S0140-6736(08)61933-9.

75. Medline Plus. (2014). *Dental cavities.* Retrieved from http://www.nlm.nih.gov/medlineplus/ency/article/001055.htm.

76. National Institute of Dental and Craniofacial Research. (2014). *Periodontal (gum) disease: Causes, symptoms, and treatments.* Retrieved from http://www.nidcr.nih.gov/oralhealth/topics/gumdiseases/periodontalgumdisease.htm.

77. Kwan, S., Petersen, P., Pine, C., & Borutta, A. (2005). Health-promoting schools: An opportunity for oral health promotion. *Bulletin of the World Health Organization, 83*, 677–685.

78. World Health Organization. (2012). *Oral health* (Fact Sheet No. 318). Retrieved from http://www.who.int/mediacentre/factsheets/fs318/en/.

79. Enwonwu, C. O., Falkler, W. A., & Phillips, R. S. (2006). Noma (cancrum oris). *Lancet, 368*(9530), 147–156. doi:10.1016/S0140-6736(06)69004-1.

80. World Health Organization. (2014). *Noma.* Retrieved from http://www.who.int/topics/noma/en/.

81. Peterson, P. (2004). Challenges to improvement of oral health in the 21st century—The approach of the WHO Global Oral Health Programme. *International Dental Journal, 54*(Suppl 6), 329–343.

82. Evert, J., Drain, P. K., Hall, T. (2014). Vignette: Dr. Karen Sokal-Gutierrez and the Children's Oral Health Nutrition Project. In *Developing global health programming: A guidebook for medical and professional schools* (pp. 219–220). Lulu Publishing Services.

83. Benzian, H., Hobdell, M., & Mackay, J. (2011). Putting teeth into chronic diseases. *The Lancet, 377*(9764), 464. doi:10.1016/S0140-6736(11)60154-2.

84. McDonagh, M. S., Whiting, P. F., Wilson, P. M., et al. (2000). Systematic review of water fluoridation. *BMJ, 321*(7265), 855–859.

85. Goldman, A. S., Yee, R., Holmgren, C. J., & Benzian, H. (2008). Global affordability of fluoride toothpaste. *Globalization and Health, 4*(1), 7. doi:10.1186/1744-8603-4-7.

86. Children's Dental Health Project. (2013). *Cost effectiveness of preventive dental services.* Retrieved from https://www.cdhp.org /resources/163-cost-effectiveness-of-preventive-dental-services.

87. Gauba, A., Bal, I., Jain, A., & Mittal, H. (2013). School based oral health promotional intervention: Effect on knowledge, practices and clinical oral health related parameters. *Contemporary Clinical Dentistry, 4*(4), 493. doi:10.4103/0976-237X.

88. Friel, S. (2002). Impact evaluation of an oral health intervention amongst primary school children in Ireland. *Health Promotion International, 17*(2), 119–126. doi:10.1093/heapro/17.2.119.

89. Jha, P., & Chaloupka, F. J. (2000). The economics of global tobacco control. *BMJ, 321*(7257), 358–361.

90. Witold, Z. (1998). *Evolution of health in Poland since 1988.* Warsaw: Marie Sklodowska-Curie Memorial Cancer Center and Institute of Oncology, Department of Epidemiology and Cancer Prevention.

91. Zatonski, W. (2003). Democracy and health: Tobacco control in Poland. In J. de Beyer & L. W. Brigden (Eds.), *Tobacco control policy: Strategies, successes and setbacks* (pp. 97–119). Washington, DC: The World Bank and International Development Research Center.

92. Malan, M., & Leaver, R. (2003). Political change in South Africa: New tobacco control and public health policies. In J. de Beyer, & L. W. Brigden (Eds.), *Tobacco control policy: Strategy, success, and setbacks.* Washington, DC: The World Bank and International Development Research Center.

93. Thomas, R., Paul, P., Rao, G. N., Muliyil, J., & Matahai, A. (2005). Present status of eye care in India. *Survey of Ophthalmology, 50*(1), 85–101.

94. Levine, R., & What Works Working Group. (2007). *Case studies in global health: Millions saved.* Sudbury, MA: Jones and Bartlett.

95. Bachani, D., Gupta, G. K., Murthy, G., & Jose, R. (1999). Visual outcomes after cataract surgery and cataract surgical coverage in India. *International Ophthalmology, 23*(1), 49–56.

96. Sareen, I. B. (2001). National Programme for Control of Blindness. *Health and Population—Perspectives and Issues, 24*(2), 99–108.

97. The World Bank. (2002). *Cataract blindness control project implementation completion report.* Washington, DC: The World Bank.

98. Javitt, J., Venkataswamy, G., & Sommer, A. (1983). The economic and social aspect of restoring sight. In P. Henkind, (Ed.), *ACTA: 24th International Congress of Ophthalmology* (pp. 1308–1312). New York: JP Lippincott.

99. Government of Uganda. (1999). *Uganda health sector strategic plan 1999-2004.* Kampala, Uganda: Government of Uganda.

100. Adeyi, O., Smith, O., & Robles, S. (2007). *Public policy and the challenge of chronic noncommunicable diseases.* Washington, DC: The World Bank.

CHAPTER **14**

Unintentional Injuries

By the end of this chapter the reader will be able to:

- Define the most important types of unintentional injuries
- Describe the burden of disease related to those injuries
- Discuss how that burden varies by age, sex, region, and type of injury
- Outline the costs and consequences of those injuries
- Review measures that can be taken to address key injury issues in cost-effective ways
- Describe some successful cases of preventing unintentional injuries

VIGNETTES

Juan was 25 years old. He was driving his 15-year-old car from Lima, Peru, to a small town in the mountains, where he planned to visit his grandmother. Juan had received only a small amount of driver training. His car was very old, had never been inspected for safety, and had worn tires and poor brakes. The road was very mountainous, did not have good lane markings or signs, and had few safety barriers. As the sun was setting, another car came rapidly around a mountain bend, headed right toward Juan's car. Juan tried to avoid the car but he swerved, slid down the side of the mountain, and was killed in the crash.

Mary was 12 years old and lived in a farming community in northern Tanzania. People in her village used fertilizer and pesticide in their agricultural work. They cooked with kerosene stoves. One day, after coming home from school, Mary was thirsty and saw some of her favorite soft drink near the

area in which her mother cooked. Mary reached for the drink and began to consume it quickly. As she did so, she realized that her mother was storing in the soft drink bottle the kerosene that she used for cooking. Mary lived far from health services, got very sick that evening, and died of kerosene poisoning before she could get proper medical treatment.

Paitoon was a 75-year-old physician in Bangkok, Thailand. He was still practicing medicine but was becoming frail. He fancied himself to be a young man and enjoyed fixing things around his house. While standing on a stool to repair a broken light, Paitoon fell. Like many people his age who suffer falls, Paitoon broke his hip. Paitoon was hospitalized, had surgery, and could not attend to his patients for several months while he recovered.

Shahnaz was a 26-year-old woman in Lahore, Pakistan. She lived in a very small house with a tiny cooking area. While preparing dinner one evening, the sleeve of Shahnaz's clothing dipped into the cooking fire. Before her family could help her, Shahnaz was engulfed in flames. She died the next day from burns.

THE IMPORTANCE OF UNINTENTIONAL INJURIES

Unintentional injuries are exceptionally important and among the leading causes of deaths and disability-adjusted life years (DALYs) worldwide. In 2010, more than 3 million people died of unintentional injuries worldwide.[1] This is fewer than died of ischemic heart disease or stroke that year. However, it is about the same as the number of people who died of chronic obstructive pulmonary disease or lower respiratory infections.[1] In addition, it is almost twice as many as those who died of lung cancer or HIV/AIDS.[1] In fact, unintentional injuries represent about 7 percent of all deaths worldwide.[2] They also represent about 9 percent of total DALYs.[2]

This chapter is about unintentional injuries. It first reviews definitions that are commonly used when discussing unintentional injuries. The chapter then reviews the burden of disease from these injuries and how that burden varies by type of injury, sex, age, and region of the world. After that, the chapter examines the costs and consequences of unintentional injuries. The chapter concludes by examining measures that can be taken to reduce the burden of unintentional injuries in cost-effective ways and by reviewing some cases of successful prevention of unintentional injuries.

KEY DEFINITIONS

As we begin this chapter, it is important to define key terms and the focus of the chapter.

For the purposes of this chapter, we can define an *injury* as:

> the result of an act that damages, harms, or hurts; unintentional or intentional damage to the body resulting from acute exposure to thermal, mechanical, electrical, or chemical energy or from the absence of such essentials as heat or oxygen.[3]

Some injuries, such as being shot by someone trying to do you harm, are intentional injuries.

The *Global Burden of Disease Study 2010* includes a number of causes in the category of "injuries". These are:

- Road injury
- Other transport injury
- Poisonings
- Falls
- Fires
- Drowning
- Exposure to mechanical forces
- Adverse effects of medical treatment
- Animal contact
- Self-harm
- Interpersonal violence
- Collective violence and legal intervention
- Exposure to forces of nature
- Other unintentional injuries not classified elsewhere[3]

Unintentional injuries are "that subset of injuries for which there is no evidence of predetermined intent."[4] When this text refers to unintentional injuries, it refers to everything on the list above, except self-harm, interpersonal violence, and collective violence and legal intervention.

This chapter, however, focuses on the largest causes of unintentional injury globally:

- Road injury
- Poisonings
- Falls
- Fires
- Drownings

The data in this chapter on the burden of disease largely come from the study on the global burden of disease 2010.[1,2]

THE BURDEN OF UNINTENTIONAL INJURIES

Table 14-1 shows the share of deaths globally that can be attributed to unintentional injuries and how that compares with deaths from Group I and Group II causes.

Table 14-2 looks at data on DALYs for unintentional injuries, compared to DALYS from Group I and Group II causes.

There are some countries in which DALYs attributed to unintentional injuries as a share of total DALYs are higher than deaths from unintentional injuries as a share of total deaths. However, globally, in all World Bank regions, except for sub-Saharan Africa, and for all country income groups,[1] DALYs from unintentional injuries represent a larger share of total DALYs than deaths represent as a share of total deaths. Globally, for example, deaths from unintentional injuries constitute 7 percent of total deaths but DALYs from unintentional injuries make up 9 percent of total DALYs.

Although injuries have most commonly been thought of as a problem of high-income countries, about 90 percent of deaths from unintentional injuries in 2010 were in low- and middle-income countries.[1] This is another reminder that low- and middle-income countries simultaneously face the multiple burdens of communicable diseases, noncommunicable diseases, and injuries.

As shown in **Table 14-3**, the leading categorized cause of deaths in low- and middle-income countries from unintentional injuries in 2010 was road traffic accidents. This was followed by falls. Drownings and fires came after falls and led to about the same number of deaths. Only about half as many people died from poisoning as from drownings and fires. The rank order of these causes does not change when considering DALYs related to them.[1] In addition, the share of total DALYs from these causes is very close to the share of total deaths they represent. However, falls make up a larger share of total DALYs globally than they do of deaths.[2]

TABLE 14-1 Deaths from Unintentional Injuries, 2010, Compared to Total Deaths from Group I and Group II Causes for World Bank Regions, Low- and Middle-Income Countries, High-Income Countries, and Globally

Region	Deaths from Group I Causes (Percent of All Deaths)	Deaths from Group II Causes (Percent of All Deaths)	Deaths from Unintentional Injuries (Percent of All Deaths)
East Asia and Pacific	12%	78%	7%
Europe and Central Asia	7%	85%	5%
Latin America and the Caribbean	14%	69%	11%
Middle East and North Africa	18%	73%	7%
South Asia	35%	54%	8%
Sub-Saharan Africa	67%	25%	7%
Low- and Middle-Income Countries	31%	58%	8%
High-Income Countries	7%	87%	4%
Global	25%	65%	7%

Note: Group I = communicable, maternal, neonatal, and nutritional disorders; Group II = noncommunicable diseases.

Data from Institute for Health Metrics and Evaluation (IHME). (2013). *GBD compare*. Seattle, WA: IHME, University of Washington. Retrieved January 14, 2015, from http://vizhub.healthdata.org/gbd-compare.

About 4.2 percent of total deaths in high-income countries in 2010 were a result of unintentional injuries. This compares with about 7.9 percent of total deaths in low- and middle-income countries that year that were a result of unintentional injuries. The lower proportion of unintentional injuries in high-income countries relates to lower rates of such injuries and a greater ability to address them medically than in low- and middle-income countries.[2]

Males more commonly suffer from unintentional injuries than females, and about two-thirds of the deaths from unintentional injuries were among males.[1] In low- and middle-income countries, men were more likely to die than women of all six categories of unintentional injuries, except fires, as shown in **Table 14-4**.

As you can also see from Table 14-4, about three times as many men die in road traffic accidents as women. About two times as many men die as women in all other categories of unintentional injury, except fires, for which women were almost 20 percent more likely to die than men.[1]

When the leading causes of death globally are examined by age, we note that unintentional injuries kill more men ages 15–49 than any other cause. This is also true for low-, middle-, and high-income countries. Globally, only HIV/AIDS kills more women in this age group than unintentional injuries. This is also true for low- and middle-income countries.[2]

Deaths are only part of the injury story. Although the number of deaths is significant, the number of people who suffer disability annually from an injury is much greater than those who actually die from an injury. As an example, a study of fatal and nonfatal injuries in two states in the United States reported 13,052 deaths from injury but also identified over 2 million injuries for which medical care was

TABLE 14-2 DALYs from Unintentional Injuries, 2010, Compared to Total DALYs from Group I and Group II Causes for World Bank Regions, Low- and Middle-Income Countries, High-Income Countries, and Globally

Region	DALYs from Group I Causes (Percentage of All DALYs)	DALYs from Group II Causes (Percentage of All DALYs)	DALYs from Unintentional Injuries (Percentage of All DALYs)
East Asia and Pacific	18%	70%	10%
Europe and Central Asia	13%	75%	9%
Latin America and the Caribbean	18%	63%	13%
Middle East and North Africa	25%	65%	9%
South Asia	43%	46%	9%
Sub-Saharan Africa	69%	24%	6%
Low- and Middle-Income Countries	40%	49%	9%
High-Income Countries	5%	85%	7%
Global	35%	54%	9%

Note: Group I = communicable, maternal, neonatal, and nutritional disorders; Group II = noncommunicable diseases.

Data from Institute for Health Metrics and Evaluation (IHME). (2013). *GBD compare.* Seattle, WA: IHME, University of Washington. Retrieved January 14, 2015, from http://vizhub.healthdata.org/gbd-compare.

sought over the course of the study.[5] In other words, for every person who died from an injury there were approximately 153 people who were injured seriously enough to seek the help of a health professional. Moreover, this figure does not include those injuries for which people did not seek medical help, whether due to the minor nature of the problem, lack of access to care, or other unknown reasons.

A similar study done on children in the United States showed that for each child under 19 years of age who was fatally injured, 45 children required hospitalization, and another 1,300 children sought care in emergency rooms. This study also did not indicate how many injuries were treated at home.[6]

It is apparent that when disability due to injuries is taken into consideration, as well as mortality, the scope of the problem presented by such injuries is magnified. Moreover, these figures likely underestimate the total impact of injuries around the world. The true burden is likely to be much higher than that based on simple reporting of injuries, especially for low- and middle-income countries. Indeed, some authorities have questioned the reliability of disability data from lower income settings where mechanisms to accurately collect and report injury data are lacking and where many injured persons do not seek or do not have access to medical care.[7-9]

When we examine data for unintentional injuries globally, by World Bank region and for the low- and middle-, and high-income countries, we do see some variation. As shown in **Table 14-5**, deaths from unintentional injuries as a share of total deaths in Latin America and the Caribbean are relatively higher than in any other region, largely a reflection of the impact of natural disasters on this region, including the Haiti earthquake in 2010. The share of total deaths represented by unintentional injuries is between 5 percent and 8 percent in all of the other World Bank regions. Deaths from injuries as a share of total deaths are significantly lower, at 4 percent, in high-income countries than in any World Bank region.

TABLE 14-3 Leading Causes of Deaths and DALYs from Unintentional Injuries, Low- and Middle-Income Countries, 2010

	Percentage of Total Deaths from Unintentional Injuries	Percentage of Total DALYs from Unintentional Injuries
Road traffic accidents	37%	36%
Falls	13%	14%
Drownings	10%	10%
Fires	10%	10%
Poisonings	5%	4%

Note: Unintentional injuries are defined here using the *Global Burden of Disease Study 2010* classifications of all unintentional injuries, all transport injuries, and injuries associated with forces of nature.

Data from Institute for Health Metrics and Evaluation (IHME). (2013). *GBD compare.* Seattle, WA: IHME, University of Washington. Retrieved January 20, 2015, from http://vizhub.healthdata.org/gbd-compare.

TABLE 14-4 Distribution of Deaths from Selected Unintentional Injuries, Males and Females in Low- and Middle-Income Countries, 2010 (in Thousands)

	Total Deaths from Unintentional Injuries		
	Males	Females	Total
Drownings	216	94	310
Falls	248	148	395
Fires	142	165	307
Forces of nature	128	68	196
Poisonings	95	50	146
Road traffic accidents	882	284	1,166
Other transport injuries	41	13	54
Other	195	101	296
Total	1,947	923	2,870

Note 1: The classification "Other" includes injuries due to animal contact, mechanical forces, and adverse effects of medicine.

Note 2: The total deaths for both males and females may be different than the sum of the two other columns due to rounding.

Data from Institute for Health Metrics and Evaluation (IHME). (2013). *GBD heat map.* Seattle, WA: IHME, University of Washington. Retrieved January 16, 2015, from http://vizhub.healthdata.org/irank/heat.php.

Road traffic accidents are the largest cause of unintentional injuries in all regions, among low-, middle-income, and high-income countries, and globally. **Table 14-6** reflects the percentage of total deaths by region that is caused by road traffic accidents. As one can see, these also vary by region and between World Bank regions and high-income countries. Only about 1 percent of total deaths in the high-income countries is a result of road traffic accidents. This goes as high, however, as 4 percent for the Middle East and North Africa region.

When considering road traffic accidents, it is especially important to note that in some settings nearly 50 percent of the victims of road traffic accidents are pedestrians. In addition, a larger share of the road traffic victims are pedestrians in low- and middle-income countries than in high-income countries.[10]

CHILDHOOD INJURY

Discussion thus far has centered primarily on older adolescents and adults. However, children throughout the world sustain an alarming number of injuries with high levels of attendant death and disability. About 98 percent of childhood injury deaths occur in the low- and middle-income countries.[1]

Deaths from unintentional injuries for children ages 0–4 in low- and middle-income countries in 2010 were about 5.4 percent of total deaths in this age group. For those 5–14 years of age, these deaths were about 23 percent of total deaths.[3] With regard to specific injuries, children younger than 5 years account for 20 percent of drowning deaths and 19 percent of fire-related deaths globally.[1]

When we look at children 10–14 years of age globally, road traffic accidents are the second leading cause of death.

TABLE 14-5 Percentage of Total Deaths from Unintentional Injuries for World Bank Regions, Low- and Middle-Income Countries, High-Income Countries, and Globally, 2010

Region	Percentage of Total Deaths from Unintentional Injuries and Transport Injuries
East Asia and Pacific	7%
Europe and Central Asia	5%
Latin America and the Caribbean	11%
Middle East and North Africa	7%
South Asia	8%
Sub-Saharan Africa	7%
Low- and Middle-Income Countries	8%
High-Income Countries	4%
Global	7%

Note: Unintentional injuries are defined here using the *Global Burden of Disease Study 2010* classifications of all unintentional injuries, all transport injuries, and injuries associated with forces of nature.
Data from Institute for Health Metrics and Evaluation (IHME). (2013). *GBD compare.* Seattle, WA: IHME, University of Washington. Retrieved January 16, 2015, from http://vizhub.healthdata.org/gbd-compare.

TABLE 14-6 Percentage of Total Deaths from Road Traffic Accident for World Bank Regions, Low- and Middle-Income Countries, High-Income Countries, and Globally, 2010

Region	Percentage of Total Deaths from Road Traffic Accidents
East Asia and Pacific	3%
Europe and Central Asia	2%
Latin America and the Caribbean	3%
Middle East and North Africa	4%
South Asia	3%
Sub-Saharan Africa	3%
Low- and Middle-Income Countries	3%
High-Income Countries	1%
Global	3%

Data from Institute for Health Metrics and Evaluation (IHME). (2013). *GBD compare.* Seattle, WA: IHME, University of Washington. Retrieved January 16, 2015, from http://vizhub.healthdata.org/gbd-compare.

Fires are the 15th leading cause of death and falls are 16th. The rank order of the causes of death in this age group is the same for low- and middle-income countries. In high-income countries, road traffic accidents are the leading cause of death in this age group. Fires were the 10th leading cause, falls, 16th, and poisonings, 23rd.[1]

RISK FACTORS FOR UNINTENTIONAL INJURIES

Numerous reasons are thought to underlie the high prevalence of injuries in young children in low- and middle-income countries. A partial list of factors includes developmental immaturity relative to the dangers these children face within their environments, the influence of poverty on families' ability to provide adult supervision and child care, and exposure to workplaces with unsafe, hazardous, and developmentally inappropriate machinery.[11–13] In support of this last point, a study in the Philippines found that 60 percent of working children were exposed to unsafe conditions, and 40 percent of these had suffered a serious workplace injury.[14]

It might be assumed that as children grow older, they become less susceptible to injury. However, the reality is that as children grow older and better able to maneuver in their environment, the incidence of injuries does not decrease.

More developmentally mature young persons tend to roam more widely within their environments and thus encounter more risks and complex situations, which challenge their reasoning and ability to react.

The risk factors for falls for young people in low- and middle-income countries appear to be associated with physical activity and also may vary with socioeconomic status.[4] The risk factors for injury from falls for older people are mostly related to age and overall physical condition.[4]

Low income, poor housing, and living in a crowded area are all risk factors for burns. Rural dwellers also suffer higher rates of burns than urban people. Children are more likely to suffer burns than any other age group.[4]

The risk factors for drowning in low- and middle-income countries are consistent with what we would expect. Young children are the most likely age group to drown, and males are more likely to drown than females. Most drownings occur during activities in which children regularly engage that take place near water. This is unlike in high-income countries where most drownings are associated with recreational activities. Data suggest that children from poorer and larger families drown more frequently than other children.[4]

Studies done on poisoning in low- and middle-income countries have shed some light on risk factors. Poisoning is more likely in young boys under five than young girls under five.[1] However, it is more likely in girls aged 5 to 14 than boys of that age group.[1] It also tends to be correlated with using nonstandard containers for poisonous goods and storing them within the reach of young children. Lower-income parents who are unable to supervise their children sufficiently around poisons are also more likely to have their children poisoned than better-off parents.[4]

There are several well-known risk factors for road traffic injuries in low- and middle-income countries that are different from those in high-income countries. First is the increasing use of motor vehicles in low- and middle-income countries. Second, in many countries, two-wheeled vehicles, which are especially unsafe, are very common. Third, most low- and middle-income countries pay insufficient attention to road planning, design, engineering, signage, or traffic management. Fourth, enforcement of speed limits is lax in many low- and middle-income countries; studies done on road traffic accidents show that about half of all such accidents are associated with excessive speed. It is also true in low- and middle-income countries that vehicles are less safe than in high-income countries, that many vehicles will not have safety belts or airbags, and that infant seats for cars

are barely known or used. Motorcycle helmets are also used much less than in high-income countries.[4]

THE COSTS AND CONSEQUENCES OF INJURIES

The costs associated with unintentional injuries worldwide are considerable. The economic burden due to such injury includes direct costs such as medical care, hospitalization, rehabilitation, and funeral fees, as well as indirect costs such as lost wages, sick leave from work, disability payments, insurance payouts, and costs associated with family care. These costs may be catastrophic for people within certain socioeconomic strata or those without access to sufficient health insurance. In this case, costs are frequently borne by government or private social services. In all cases, however, injuries represent a significant drain on personal and societal resources. The total costs of injuries in Canada during 1993, for example, were estimated to be $14.3 billion Canadian dollars.[15]

Kenya examined the economic burden due to road traffic injuries and found a rapidly increasing burden over a 12-year period from 1984 to 1996. Costs, including health care, administrative expenses, and vehicle and property damage, increased from 1.5 billion Kenyan shillings in 1984 to 3.8 billion shillings in 1991, which was equal to 5 percent of gross national product (GNP). By 1996, injury-related costs had continued to escalate to between 5 and 10 billion shillings.[16]

The World Health Organization (WHO) estimated in 2006 that the direct costs due to road traffic injuries alone were about $500 billion annually, with the share borne by the low- and middle-income countries estimated at $65–100 billion. WHO also estimated that these costs are 1–2 percent of the GNP of low- and middle-income countries. At the regional level, Asia has the highest direct costs attributable to road traffic injuries at $24.5 billion. Africa, the least affected region by cost, still bears a significant burden, with an estimated $3.7 billion annually in total costs.[17,18]

The consequences of unintentional injury are not limited to financial costs. There are significant social consequences for individuals and families that may be associated with such injury. Numerous studies have documented the long-term physical and psychosocial consequences of unintentional injuries. Persisting problems with pain, fatigue, memory, and psychosocial functioning are common in victims of trauma.[19-21] Moreover, these social consequences may be relatively independent of injury severity and reflect the influence of other noninjury variables.[22] The psychosocial consequences for families of child injury victims may be significant, with difficulties relating to finances, changes in work status required to care for injured children, and altered family dynamics.[23]

ADDRESSING KEY ISSUES OF UNINTENTIONAL INJURIES

One of the key issues in addressing the burden of unintentional injuries is to raise awareness about how to apply rigorous methods of prevention and control to these injury problems. In fact, even among the high-income countries, the prioritization of such injuries as a significant health problem and the application of scientific methods of injury prevention and control are relatively recent phenomena.[8,24] Many public policymakers and public health actors in low- and middle-income countries may not yet appreciate the importance of unintentional injuries to the burden of disease or to understand what can be done to prevent unintentional injuries.

In order to design effective prevention and control activities for unintentional injuries, formal surveillance systems are fundamental to obtain reliable information as to numbers and patterns of injury. Minimal standards for injury morbidity and mortality should be implemented in all countries. In this light, the World Health Organization has published guidelines for collecting, coding, and reporting injury data, which have been specifically developed for use in low-resource settings and do not require the use of technology-intensive data management systems or specialized training.[25,26]

In addition, it will be important to develop local capacity to analyze injury data and design injury prevention and mitigation programs. Injury prevention and control activities from one setting cannot be grafted onto another setting. Rather, planners with an intimate understanding of local knowledge, attitudes, beliefs, and practices are required to design effective interventions for injury prevention in specific settings.

The theoretical foundation of many injury prevention and control efforts is called Haddon's matrix and it is widely used in efforts to understand and address injury issues. Haddon's matrix models the interaction of host, vector, and environment in an injury event. It is dynamic and models the events prior to, during, and after an injury.[24]

The example of road traffic injuries provides a useful learning tool for thinking about injuries using Haddon's matrix and how they can be prevented. The roadway (environment), automobile (vector), and host (human driver and behavior) interact in the moments leading up to a collision, during the collision, and in the moments after the collision.

Measures to prevent unintentional injuries have usually focused on education, enforcement, and engineering in the context of Haddon's matrix. Recent efforts to reduce road traffic injuries have emphasized safer roads, safer vehicles, and safer systems. They have also paid increasing attention to land use and transport planning.[4] A study of the cost-effectiveness of approaches to reducing road traffic injuries in sub-Saharan Africa and South East Asia suggested that combined approaches to enforcement, such as enforcing speed limits, drunk-driving laws, and motorcycle helmet laws, would likely be the most cost-effective approach but that the specifics of the effort would need to be tailored to the local context.[27] In addition, one important new report reminded low- and middle-income countries of the importance of investing in a multidisciplinary approach to road safety as they increase motorization to avoid problems of road traffic accidents later.[28]

Roads can be made safer from the engineering point of view by paying particular attention to building safety into road designs, improving high-risk intersections and routes, providing for slow-moving vehicles and pedestrians, improving barriers and median strips, and enhancing lighting. Ghana was able to reduce road traffic injuries by installing speed bumps at selected places, as discussed later.[4] In countries in which there are many types of vehicles, it would also help to separate those that can travel at high speed from those, like two-wheeled motorized rickshaws, that can only go slowly and that are unsafe in many ways.[4]

Vehicles can be made safer by engineering safety features into them, such as crash protection zones, headrests, seat belts, and daytime running lights. For example, including daytime running lights on motorcycles in China did reduce injuries.[4] People can be encouraged to use vehicles in safer ways through enforcement of speed limits, restricting the driving of those consuming alcohol, limiting the hours allowed for commercial driving, and enforcing the use of bicycle and motorcycle helmets.[4] Although there is considerable corruption in the police forces of many countries, enforcement of driving laws has helped in a number of settings to reduce road traffic injuries by up to 34 percent.[4] The introduction of mandatory seat belt and child restraint laws has been associated in high-income countries with a reduction in deaths and injuries by 25 percent.[4]

Few low- and middle-income countries have taken measures to deal with poisonings. However, South Africa carried out a program in which childproof containers were given to families for free. This program was associated with a cost-effective reduction in child poisonings and deaths.[29] It appears that to reduce poisonings in low- and middle-income countries, it is important to educate families to store poisons away from other household goods and out of the reach of children, to store them in appropriate and marked containers, and to enforce rules that prohibit the sale of poisons in unmarked and inappropriate containers.[4]

It is not easy to prevent falls by older people. It appears, however, that steps that have been taken in high-income countries to address such falls have included working with the elderly to improve their balance and modifying their home environment to reduce risks.[4] In low- and many middle-income countries, it may be that the only cost-effective measure that could be taken to reduce falls among the elderly would be to provide community-based education to families about the risks of falls to their elderly relatives and about measures that are appropriate in that cultural context to reducing those risks.

Few efforts at reducing childhood injuries from falls have taken place in a systematic way in low- or middle-income countries. Here, too, it may be that the most reasonable step initially is community-based education of families about the risks of falling and what can be done to reduce those risks. Of course, if schools do have play equipment, it will be valuable to design that equipment in a way that reduces injury if children fall from it.

There is also little evidence from low- and middle-income countries about what might be done in cost-effective ways to reduce drownings. Perhaps on this front, as well, one has to start with community-based information efforts about increased parental and older sibling supervision and with obvious measures, such as covering wells.[4] A community-based pilot program was carried out in Bangladesh to determine if communities would accept door barriers and playpens as means for protecting children from the risk of being unsupervised around water and drowning. Families provided with a playpen were almost seven times more likely to use it than were the families provided with a door barrier. Further study, however, is needed to determine if such an approach will translate into fewer deaths by drowning of young children.[30]

Not unexpectedly, there is also very little data on effective measures to reduce burns in low- and middle-income countries, despite their importance both generally and especially for women. Separate from the special circumstances of "dowry deaths," it appears that, for this, too, community-based efforts at behavior change must be the starting point for improved action.[4]

EMERGENCY MEDICAL SERVICES

Unintentional injuries will remain an important component of the burden of disease for some time in almost all countries. In addition, that burden may grow in both absolute and relative importance as countries witness economic growth, urbanization, and increasing motorization of transport. Thus, even low-income countries should now examine investments in low-cost but effective ways of improving emergency medical services in their countries.

One important measure would be to arrange for emergency transport. This could be in special vehicles made for low-income or rural communities or it could be advance arrangements with the owner of available transport. A bicycle ambulance was established in Malawi for the transport of obstetric emergencies, and turned out to be used more for medical emergencies and dealing with accident victims.[31] In addition, one could train members of the community who frequently come in contact with road accidents, such as truck drivers, in how to provide first aid and transport to accident victims. This was done with some important successes, for example, in Ghana.[32]

Low-income countries could also begin to invest in better training of healthcare personnel who work in emergency services. They could do the same in emergency transport services based in selected locations known to the public, for example, so that the emergency transport could be hailed quickly, even in environments in which most people would not have a telephone.[33]

CASE STUDIES

Two very brief cases are presented next about efforts that countries have undertaken to reduce the burden of morbidity, disability, and death linked with road traffic accidents. The first concerns the use of a mandatory motorcycle helmet law in Taiwan. The second concerns the use of speed bumps in Ghana, which were meant to slow drivers down and thereby reduce accidents. Both appear to have produced substantial gains in health at relatively low cost, as other countries might wish to do, as well.

Motorcycle Helmet Use in Taiwan

Helmet use for moped and motorcycle riders can help to protect them from death and serious injury. Worldwide, head injuries sustained by a rider are the principal cause of death in riders after a road accident. Yet, the risk of injury if a rider wears a helmet is only one-third the risk of those who do not wear a helmet. Nevertheless, unless a country has a law requiring helmet use, riders will most likely not use one. In addition, helmet use interventions in low- and middle-income countries should be appropriate to the local climate and take account of local manufacturing capability and people's ability to pay.[34]

In Taiwan, more than 60 percent of all motor vehicles registered in the late 1990s were motorcycles. As the number of motorcycles increased, the incidence of motorcycle road traffic injuries rose. Moreover, nearly 80 percent of motor vehicle fatalities in Taiwan, most of which involve motorcycle riders, resulted from serious head injuries.[35]

In 1994, Taipei City began a 6-month pilot program in the use of motorcycle helmets. This resulted in increasing helmet use from 21 percent to 79 percent of motorcycle riders in only 5 months. It also reduced injuries and fatalities by 33 percent and 56 percent, respectively. However, since the intervention was not linked with a mandatory helmet use law, this was a short-lived success that ended soon after it began.[35]

Three years later, Taiwan passed a nationwide law regulating motorcycle helmet use for all riders. In Taipei City, the law was preceded by a 6-month information campaign that was meant to inform residents on the benefits of helmet use. Within 2 months, helmet use was nearly 96 percent nationally, with greater use in Taipei City than in other counties, partly due to greater law enforcement. Furthermore, head injuries decreased by 33 percent and the severity of these injuries also decreased, as indicated by the reduced number of patients with head injuries admitted to intensive care units, as well as those dying or being in a vegetative state following their injury. Linked to the helmet law, head injuries in Taiwan dropped from the fourth to the fifth leading cause of death. Associated with the new law, hospital costs decreased by $3.93 million per month.[35]

As indicated by higher levels of use in Taipei City than in other areas of Taiwan, the passage of a law requiring helmet use is not sufficient to ensure that it will produce the intended benefits. Rather, it is also important that an education campaign be oriented toward getting motorcycle riders to wear their helmets and that the laws requiring helmet use be enforced.

Rumble Strips and Speed Bumps in Ghana

In 2000, speeding contributed to over 50 percent of all motor vehicle accidents in Ghana. In addition, as in other countries, many of those injured as a result of these accidents were pedestrians or passengers in vehicles who had no seat belts or were not using them. Studies in high-income countries demonstrate that reducing speed by 1 km/hr results in a 3 percent reduction in crashes and a higher likelihood of survival if hit by a car. In this light, the government of Ghana decided to put rumble strips and speed bumps at road intersections that had proved to be dangerous.[36]

The Ghanaian authorities first located accident hot spots on the main highway between Accra and Kumasi and installed rumble strips along the highest risk area, the Suhum Junction. In less than a year, this public health measure resulted in a 35 percent decrease in the number of motor vehicle crashes and a 55 percent reduction in related fatalities. The cost of laying rumble strips was $20,900, compared to an estimated $100,000 to redesign lanes or $180,000 to construct a physical division to separate pedestrians from vehicles.[36]

As noted earlier in the chapter, there are other cost-effective measures that countries can take to reduce the burden of road traffic injuries. Nonetheless, it appears that even relatively poor countries, such as Ghana, can avert a considerable toll of injuries, disability, and death from road traffic injuries through the construction of very low-cost speed bumps and rumble strips in selected locations.

FUTURE CHALLENGES

One key challenge for the future will be to ensure that low- and middle-income countries show the political commitment needed to reduce the burden of unintentional injuries. This burden is too large a source of deaths and disabilities to ignore, even in the face of continuing communicable diseases and a growing burden of noncommunicable diseases.

There is increasing information about what works in cost-effective ways to reduce the burden of injury in high-income countries, and this can serve as a starting point for adapting this learning to other settings. It will be important for selected low- and middle-income countries to carry out pilot schemes in preventing injury, especially from road traffic accidents, and then to expand them more broadly as they learn how to make them work effectively in different settings.

As low- and middle-income countries develop economically and become more urbanized and motorized, it will be valuable for them to engineer safety into their newer investments in road transportation. It will also be important to increase efforts to provide information and education to the public about key areas of injury prevention. Governance is weak in many countries. Nonetheless, such countries can take measures in a phased manner to enforce laws concerning road safety that can have a high return with little effort, such as encouraging the use of motorcycle helmets, and enforcing drunk-driving laws and speed limits. As governance improves and people have more knowledge of road safety and trust that enforcement of laws will be honest, the government can enforce additional regulations affecting road safety. The challenge of reducing injuries from falls, burns, and drowning will depend almost completely on informing and educating the public in a community-based manner.

MAIN MESSAGES

Unintentional injuries are an important cause of deaths and DALYs in all regions of the world. In 2010, more than 3 million people died of such injuries. In addition, these injuries are major causes of disability, with many people being disabled by injuries, even if they do not die from them. Moreover, the rate of deaths from unintentional injuries is substantially higher in low- and middle-income countries than in high-income countries.[1]

The leading cause of both deaths and DALYs attributable to unintentional injuries is road traffic accidents. This is followed by deaths from falls, drowning, poisoning, and fires. About three times as many men die in road traffic accidents as women. However, many more women die in fires than men do. Deaths from road traffic accidents as a share of total deaths is particularly high in the Middle East and North Africa region, compared to other regions. Unintentional injuries are an important source of deaths for young children,

who account for about 20 percent of drowning deaths and 19 percent of fire-related deaths globally.[1]

The risk factors for road traffic accidents revolve around education, enforcement, and engineering. The risk factors of other leading causes of unintentional injuries relate largely to lower socioeconomic status, inadequate supervision of children, a failure to store poisons safely, and household cooking arrangements that pay insufficient attention to fire hazards in areas that tend to be crowded and hazardous.

Although there have been few studies of the economic costs of unintentional injuries in low- and middle-income countries, estimates of such costs for road traffic accidents alone have ranged from 1 to 2 percent of GNP.[18] The social costs of dealing with the disabilities caused by accidents can also be very high.

There is increasing evidence from a range of countries of measures that can be taken to improve vehicle operator safety, build safety into vehicles, make plans for land use and traffic, and enforce key traffic rules. These measures can be implemented in a phased manner in low- and middle-income countries and adapted to local settings. Reducing the burden of road traffic injuries and other injuries will require enhancing community-based approaches to providing information about how the community can reduce risk factors for such injuries.

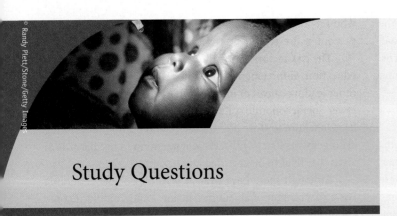

Study Questions

1. How important are unintentional injuries to the global burden of disease?

2. What unintentional injuries cause the most deaths?

3. How does the rate of death from road traffic accidents vary by region and why?

4. What are the most important unintentional injuries that affect children?

5. Do men and women suffer from unintentional injuries at the same rates? Why or why not?

6. What are the risk factors for road traffic accidents?

7. What are the risk factors for drownings?

8. What are the key risk factors for burning, and how do they vary by region?

9. What is Haddon's matrix, and how would you apply it to analyze accidents?

10. What are the most cost-effective steps that low- and middle-income countries can take to reduce the burden of road traffic accidents on health?

REFERENCES

1. Institute for Health Metrics and Evaluation (IHME). (2013). *GBD 2010 heat map*. Seattle, WA: IHME, University of Washington. Retrieved January 26, 2015, from http://vizhub.healthdata.org/irank/heat.php.

2. Institute for Health Metrics and Evaluation (IHME). (2013). *GBD compare*. Seattle, WA: IHME, University of Washington. Retrieved January 26, 2015, from http://vizhub.healthdata.org/gbd-compare.

3. National Highway Traffic Safety Administration. *Trauma system agenda for the future: Glossary*. Retrieved June 23, 2006, from http://www.nhtsa.dot.gov/people/injury/ems/emstraumasystem03/glossary.htm.

4. Norton, R., Hyder, A. A., Bishai, D., & Peden, M. (2006). Unintentional injuries. In D. T. Jamison, J. G. Breman, A. R. Measham, et al. (Eds.), *Disease control priorities in developing countries* (2nd ed., pp. 737–753). New York: Oxford University Press.

5. Wadman, M., Muelleman, R., Coto, J., et al. (2003). The pyramid of injury: Using ecodes to accurately describe the burden of injury. *Annals of Emergency Medicine, 42*, 468–478.

6. UNICEF. (2008). *World report on child injury prevention*. Geneva: World Health Organization.

7. Bangdiwala, S., Anzola-Perez, E., Rommer, C., et al. (1990). The incidence of injuries in young people: I. Methodology and results of a collaborative study in Brazil, Chile, Cuba, and Venezuela. *International Journal of Epidemiology, 19*, 115–124.

8. Bartlett, S. (2002). The problem of children's injuries in low-income countries: A review. *Health Policy and Planning, 17*(1), 1–13.

9. Mohan, D. (1997). Injuries in less industrialized countries: What do we know? *Injury Prevention, 3*, 241–242.

10. World Health Organization & Indian Institute of Technology Delhi. (2006). *Road traffic injury prevention*. Geneva: World Health Organization.

11. Jordan, J., & Valdez-Lazo, F. (1991). Education on safety and risk. In M. Manciaux & C. Romer (Eds.), *Accidents in childhood and adolescence: The role of research* (pp. 106–120). Geneva: World Health Organization.

12. Ljungblom, B.-A., & Köhler, L. (1991). Child development and behavior in traffic. In M. Manciaux & C. Romer (Eds.), *Accidents in childhood and adolescence: The role of research* (pp. 97–105). Geneva: World Health Organization.

13. Leflamme, L., & Diderichsen, F. (2000). Social differences in traffic injury risk in childhood and youth—A literature review and a research agenda. *Injury Prevention, 6*, 293–298.

14. International Labour Office. (1996). *Child labour: Targeting the intolerable*. Geneva: International Labour Office.

15. Ministry of Health—Canada. (1993). *Economic burden of illness in Canada*. Ottawa, Ontario: Canadian Public Health Association.

16. Odero, W., Meleckidzedeck, K., & Heda, P. (2003). Road traffic injuries in Kenya: Magnitude, causes and status of intervention. *Injury Control and Safety Promotion, 10*(1–2), 53–61.

17. Hoffman, K., Primack, A., Keusch, G., & Hrynkow, S. (2005). Addressing the growing burden of trauma and injury in low- and middle-income countries. *American Journal of Public Health, 95*, 13–17.

18. Jacobs, G., Aaron-Thomas, A., & Astrop, A. (2000). *Estimating global road fatalities*. London: Transport Research Laboratory.

19. Depalma, J., Fedorka, P., & Simko, L. (2003). Quality of life experienced by severely injured trauma survivors. *AACN Clinical Issues, 14*(1), 54–63.

20. van der Sluis, C., Eisma, W., Groothoff, J., & ten Duis, H. (1998). Long-term physical, psychological and social consequences of severe injuries. *Injury, 29*(4), 281–285.

21. Landsman, I., Baum, C., Arnkoff, D., et al. (1990). The psychosocial consequences of traumatic injury. *Journal of Behavioral Medicine, 13*(6), 561–581.

22. Mayou, R., & Bryant, B. (2001). Outcome in consecutive emergency department attenders following a road traffic accident. *British Journal of Psychiatry, 179*, 528–534.

23. Osberg, J., Khan, P., Rowe, K., & Brooke, M. (1996). Pediatric trauma: impact on work and family finances. *Pediatrics, 98*(5), 890–897.

24. Haddon, W. (1999). The changing approach to epidemiology, prevention, and amelioration of trauma: The transition to approaches etiologically rather than descriptively based. *Injury Prevention, 5*, 231–235.

25. Holder, Y., Peden, M., Krug, E., et al. (2001). *Injury surveillance guidelines*. Geneva: World Health Organization.

26. McGee, K., Peden, M., Waxweiler, R., et al. (2003). Injury surveillance. *Injury Control and Safety Promotion, 10*, 105–108.

27. Chisholm, D., Naci, H., Hyder, A. A., Tran, N. T., & Peden, M. (2012, March 2). Cost-effectiveness of strategies to combat road traffic injuries in sub-Saharan Africa and South East Asia: Mathematical modelling study. *BMJ, 344*(e612).

28. Global Road Safety Facility The World Bank Group; Institute For Health Metrics and Evaluation, University of Washington. (2014). *Transport for health: The global burden of disease from motorized road transport*. Washington, DC: The World Bank.

29. Krug A., Ellis J. B., Hay I. T., Mokgabudi N. F., & Robertson J. (1994). The impact of child-resistant containers on the incidence of paraffin (kerosene) ingestion in children. *South African Medical Journal, 84*, 730–734.

30. Callaghan, J. A., Hyder, A. A., Blum, L. S, Arifeen, S., & Baqui, A. H. (2010). Child supervision practices for drowning prevention in rural Bangladesh: A pilot study of supervision tools. *Journal of Epidemiology and Community Health, 64*, 645–647.

31. Kobusingye, O. C., Hyder, A. A., Bishai, D., Hicks, E. R., Mock, C., & Joshipura, M. (2005). Emergency medical systems in low- and middle-income countries: Recommendations for action. *Bulletin of the World Health Organization, 83*(8), 626–631.

32. Mock, C., Arreola-Risa, C., & Quansah, R. (2003). Strengthening care for injured persons in less developed countries: A case study of Ghana and Mexico. *Injury Control and Safety Promotion, 10*(1–2), 45–51.

33. Kobusingye, O. C., Hyder, A. A., Bishai, D., Joshipura, E. R. H., & Mock, C. (2006). Emergency medical services. In D. T. Jamison, J. G. Breman, A. R. Measham, et al. (Eds.), *Disease control priorities in developing countries* (2nd ed., pp. 1261–1279). New York: Oxford University Press.

34. Peden, M., Scurfield, R., Sleet, D., Mohan, D., Hyder, A. A., Jarawan, E., et al. (Eds.). (2004). *World report on road traffic injury prevention*. Geneva: World Health Organization. Retrieved February 7, 2015, from http://whqlibdoc.who.int/publications/2004/9241562609.pdf.

35. Chiu, W. T., Kuo, C. Y., Hung, C. C., & Chen, M. (2004). The effect of the Taiwan motorcycle law on head injuries. *American Journal of Public Health, 90*(5), 793–796.

36. Afukaar, F. K. (2003). Speed control in developing countries: Issues, challenges and opportunities in reducing road traffic injuries. *Injury Control and Safety Promotion, 10*(1–2), 77–81.

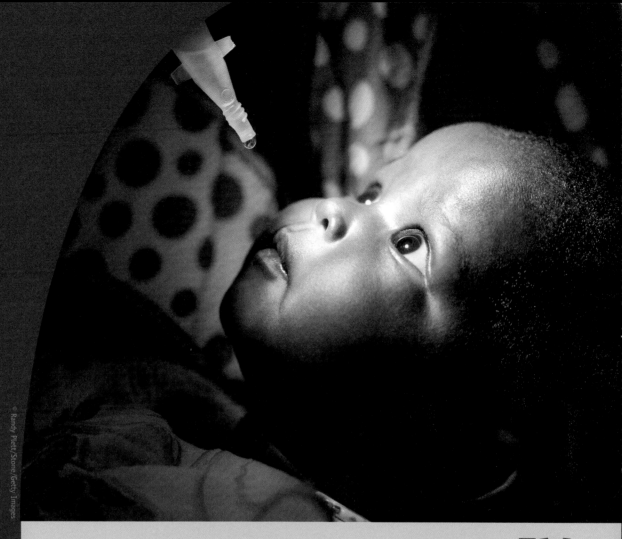
© Randy Plett/Stone/Getty Images

PART IV

Working Together to Improve Global Health

CHAPTER **15**

Natural Disasters and Complex Humanitarian Emergencies

LEARNING OBJECTIVES

By the end of this chapter the reader will be able to:

- Describe several types of disasters that affect human health
- Discuss the health effects of natural disasters and complex humanitarian emergencies
- Review how those health impacts vary by age, sex, location, and type of disaster
- Describe key measures that can be taken to mitigate the health impacts of natural disasters and complex humanitarian emergencies

VIGNETTES

Javad lived in the Pakistani province of Kashmir when the earthquake hit. All the buildings in his village were destroyed. Hundreds of people in the village were killed, mostly a result of being buried in the rubble. Many other people were badly injured from rubble falling on them. Their injuries were overwhelmingly orthopedic in nature. As the earthquake destroyed the village, it also destroyed wells, a health center, and roads leading to and from the village. Javad feared that many of those injured would soon die.

Samuel was living in the eastern part of Sierra Leone when the war started. He did all that he could to protect his family, but it was not enough. In the first year of the conflict, as he and his family were getting ready to flee, a band of armed men stormed the village. As Samuel had heard they would do, they used machetes to kill or take limbs off of many village people. They also raped a large number of women. In addition, they kidnapped some of the children in hopes of making them into sex slaves or soldiers.

As the civil war spread in Rwanda, Sarah and her family fled across the border to what was fast becoming a large refugee camp in Zaire, later called the Democratic Republic of Congo. Although the camp workers did what they could to help the refugees, the circumstances at the camp were not good. There was little shelter, water, or food. In addition, a cholera epidemic spread through the camp not long after Sarah's arrival there. It hit the camp especially hard and led to a large number of deaths.

A number of international organizations rushed staff to refugee camps, just across the border from intense fighting. Some of the agencies involved had many years of experience doing such work and had clear guidelines for their staff concerning relief efforts. Other agencies, however, were not so experienced in this work. They brought to the camps medicine that was not appropriate for the health conditions they found and food to which the local people were completely unaccustomed. Although it would have been most efficient if all of the aid agencies worked together, they did not.

THE IMPORTANCE OF NATURAL DISASTERS AND COMPLEX EMERGENCIES TO GLOBAL HEALTH

Complex emergencies and natural disasters have a significant impact on global health. They can lead to increased death, illness, and disability; and the economic costs of their health impacts can also be very large. Measures can be taken in cost-effective ways, however, to reduce the costs of disasters and conflicts and to address the major health problems that relate to them. These measures would be most effective if those involved in disaster relief would work together according to agreed-upon standards that focus on the most important priorities for action.

This chapter reviews the relationships between natural disasters and health and complex humanitarian emergencies (CHEs) and health. The chapter begins by introducing some key concepts and definitions that relate to these topics. The chapter then reviews the incidence of natural disasters and CHEs. Following that, the chapter describes their main health impacts. Lastly, the chapter examines measures that can be taken in cost-effective ways to prevent and address in some of their effects on health.

KEY TERMS

Understanding the health impacts of natural disasters and complex humanitarian emergencies requires an introduction to several terms and concepts that are examined briefly here.

A disaster is "any occurrence that causes damage, ecological destruction, loss of human lives, or deterioration of health and health services on a scale sufficient to warrant an extraordinary response from outside the affected community area."[1] Another way to think of this would be as "an occurrence, either natural or man made, that causes human suffering and creates human needs that victims cannot alleviate without assistance."[1] Some disasters are natural. These include, for example, the results of floods, volcanoes, and earthquakes. Some, however, are caused by humans, such as the cloud of poisonous gas that rained over the town of Bhopal, India, in 1984 as a result of an industrial accident. Some disasters are rapid onset, such as an earthquake, whereas others are slow onset, such as a drought or famine. Although the long-term effects of these natural and human-made disasters can be substantial, they are often characterized by an initial event and then its aftereffects. Some examples of recent natural disasters that caused a significant loss of life are listed in **Table 15-1**.

In response to the large number of civil conflicts that have taken place, the term *complex emergency* or *complex humanitarian emergency* (CHE) has been established. A complex emergency can be defined as a "complex, multiparty, intra-state conflict resulting in a humanitarian disaster which might constitute multi-dimensional risks or threats to regional and international security. Frequently within such conflicts, state institutions collapse, law and order break down, banditry and chaos prevail, and portions of the civilian population migrate."[2] CHEs have also been described as "situations affecting large civilian populations which usually involve a combination of factors, including war or civil strife, food shortages, and population displacement, resulting in significant excess mortality."[3,p1012]

TABLE 15-1 Selected Natural Disasters, 2010–2013

2010

April: The Gulf of Mexico oil spill leaked 185 million gallons of oil, causing a no-fishing zone in 19 percent of the waters in the Gulf of Louisiana and killing 11 people.

July: Massive flooding in Pakistan after 2 full days of rainfall killed over 1,600 people and left millions homeless.

September: A landslide after a period of rain buried hundreds of homes and killed 11 people in Mexico.

2011

March: An earthquake and tsunami caused an explosion in the Fukushima Daiichi Power Station in Japan. The incident released radioactivity directly into the atmosphere.

August: Hurricane Irene killed 56 people on the East Coast of the Unites States and caused an estimated $15.6 billion in damages.

December: Tropical Strom Washi caused floods that killed 1,268 people in the Philippines.

2012

April: An avalanche hit a Pakistani military base in Pakistan, killing 129 soldiers and 11 civilians.

July: Massive rainfall overnight caused widespread flooding and killed 172 people in Krymsk, Russia.

October: Hurricane Sandy started in the Caribbean and climbed up the East Coast of the United States, causing at least 100 deaths and $30 billion in damages.

2013

September: Flash floods in Colorado, in the United States, caused massive damage to infrastructure and homes and killed at least six people.

October: A powerful earthquake hit the Philippines, killing 144 people and injuring 300 more.

November: Typhoon Haiyan hit many islands in the central, Philippines affecting 4.28 million people in at least 270 towns. The death toll was estimated to be 4,011 and 1,602 people were reported missing.

Data from Infoplease. *World Disasters–2010, 2011, 2012,* and *2013 Disasters.* Retrieved September 10, 2014, from http://infoplease.com/ipa/A0001437.html.

Such emergencies include war and civil conflict. They usually affect large numbers of people and often have severe impacts on the availability of food, water, and shelter. Linked to these phenomena and the displacement of people that often go with them, complex humanitarian emergencies usually result in considerable excess mortality, compared to what would be the case without such an emergency.[4] Some examples of complex humanitarian emergencies are listed in **Table 15-2**.

TABLE 15-2 Selected Complex Humanitarian Emergencies of Importance

Afghanistan: There are currently more than 665,000 internally displaced people (IDP) due to drought and political instability.

Angola: A civil war lasted 27 years and ended in 2002.

Armenia/Azerbaijan: Conflict between the two countries has created almost 250,000 refugees and 600,000 IDPs.

Bosnia and Herzegovina: Between 1992 and 1994, war with various parts of the former Yugoslavia led to more than 100,000 deaths and 1.8 million people displaced.

Burma: Government offensives against a number of ethnic groups have gone on for more than 20 years and produced between 500,000 and 1 million IDP.

The Democratic Republic of Congo: Fighting since the mid-1990s between government forces and rebels has led to more than 2 million displaced people.

Libya: Conflict between pro-Qadhafi and anti-Qadhafi forces led to at least 80,000 IDP with 21,000 displaced in 2014 due to clashes in Sebha alone.

Liberia: Civil war from 1990 to 2004 led to almost 500,000 IDP and more than 125,000 refugees in Guinea alone.

Nepal: Conflict between the government forces and Maoist rebels from 1996 to 2006 led to 100,000–200,000 IDP.

Rwanda: More than 800,000 people were killed in the 1994 genocide, which also produced more than 2 million refugees who fled to Burundi, what is now the Democratic Republic of Congo, Tanzania, and Uganda.

Somalia: Conflict between al-Shabaab and the Transitional Federal Government allied forces has led to 1.1 million civilians displaced.

Sudan: Internal conflicts since the 1980s, including a war with groups in the south and genocide against people in the Darfur region, have displaced 5–6 million people.

Syria: Ongoing civil war since 2011 has created more than 2.8 million Syrian refugees as of 2014, with 6.5 million IDP.

Uganda: Rebellion by the Lord's Resistance Army in the north for almost 20 years has led to between 1 and 2 million displaced people.

Yemen: Clashes between al-Qaeda and government forces have resulted in almost 310,000 IDP.

Zimbabwe: President Mugabe initiated a series of land and political reforms using violent measures, which caused human rights violations, an increase in human trafficking, and 570,000 to 1 million people to be internally displaced.

Data from Central Intelligence Agency (CIA). *The world fact book. Field listing: Refugees and internally displaced persons.* Retrieved September 10, 2014, from https://www.cia.gov/library/publications/the-world-factbook/fields/2194.html.

Complex emergencies create refugees. Under international law, a refugee is a person who is outside his or her country of nationality or habitual residence; has a well-founded fear of persecution because of his or her race, religion, nationality, membership in a particular social group, or political opinion; and is unable or unwilling to avail him- or herself of the protection of that country, or to return there, for fear of persecution. They are a subgroup of the broader category of displaced persons.[5] It is important to note that there are a number of international conventions that define refugees and that accord them rights according to international law, as well. **Table 15-3** notes a number of countries with significant refugee populations and the countries they fled. A United Nations Agency, the United Nations High Commissioner for Refugees (UNHCR), is responsible for protecting the rights of refugees.

TABLE 15-3 Selected Refugee Populations and Source of Refugees, 2015

Country	Number of Refugees	Source Countries
Afghanistan	241,641	Pakistan
Algeria	90,000	Western Saharan Sahrawi
Angola	21,104	Democratic Republic of Congo
Armenia	12,037	Syria (ethnic Armenians)
Austria	31,483	Russia, Afghanistan
Bangladesh	232,565	Burma
Burkina Faso	33,125	Mali
Burundi	53,863	Democratic Republic of the Congo
Cameroon	289,428	Central African Republic, Nigeria
Central African Republic	5,342	Democratic Republic of the Congo
Chad	479,384	Sudan, Central African Republic, Nigeria
China	300,896	North Korea, Vietnam
Ecuador	122,276	Colombia
Egypt	230,653	West Bank and Gaza Strip, Sudan, Somalia, Iraq, Syria
Ethiopia	688,752	Somalia, South Sudan, Eritrea, Sudan
Gaza Strip	1,258,559	Palestine
India	197,451	Tibet/China, Sri Lanka, Burma, Afghanistan
Iran	2,432,000	Afghanistan, Iraq

TABLE 15-3 Selected Refugee Populations and Source of Refugees, 2015 (*continued*)

Country	Number of Refugees	Source Countries
Kenya	583,039	Somalia, South Sudan, Ethiopia, DRC, Sudan, Burundi
Lebanon	1,633,284	Syria, Palestine
Malaysia	92,939	Burma
Nepal	38,059	Tibet/China, Bhutan
Niger	155,071	Mali, Nigeria
Pakistan	3,000,000	Afghanistan
Rwanda	101,575	Democratic Republic of Congo, Burundi
South Sudan	254,978	Sudan, Democratic Republic of Congo
Sudan	295,019	Eritrea, Chad, South Sudan
Syria	526,744	Palestine, Iraq
Turkey	1,864,486	Syria, Iraq
Uganda	416,459	Democratic Republic of Congo, Rwanda, Burundi, South Sudan, Somalia
Venezuela	204,604	Colombia
West Bank	762,288	Palestine
Yemen	250,191	Somalia, Ethiopia

Data from Central Intelligence Agency (CIA). *The world factbook. Field listing: Refugees and internally displaced persons.* Retrieved June 8, 2015, from https://www.cia.gov/library/publications/the-world-factbook/fields/2194.html.

Some of the people who flee or are forced to migrate during a disaster or complex humanitarian emergency leave their homes but stay in the country in which they were living. These are called internally displaced people (IDP). These are more formally defined as "someone who has been forced to leave their home for reasons such as religious or political persecution or war, but has not crossed an international border."[6] The term is a subset of the more general *displaced person*. There is no legal definition of an *internally displaced person*, as there is for refugee, but the thumbnail rule is that if the person was forced to leave and remain away from their home but has not crossed an international border, the IDP label is applicable."[6] **Table 15-4** shows selected examples of countries with large numbers of internally displaced persons. It is important to note that the legal status of IDP is not as well defined as that for refugees.[7] It is also important to understand that, unlike the case for refugees, no agency or organization is responsible for IDPs. Rather, their own government is responsible for them, but that government is often part of the problem as to why these people are fleeing.

TABLE 15-4 Internally Displaced People: Selected Countries of Importance, 2015

Country	Number of IDP
Azerbaijan	568,900
Colombia	6,044,200
Côte d'Ivoire	at least 70,000
Democratic Republic of Congo	2,857,400
India	at least 616,140
Somalia	1,106,000
Sudan	3,100,000
Turkey	954,000–1,200,000
Uganda	30,136

Data from the Central Intelligence Agency (CIA). *The world factbook. Field listing: Refugees and internally displaced persons.* Retrieved June 8, 2015, from https://www.cia.gov/library/publications/the-world-factbook /fields/2194.html.

One of the significant indicators of the health impact of a complex humanitarian emergency is the *crude mortality rate*. This is the proportion of people who die from a population at risk over a specified period of time.[8] For addressing CHEs, the crude mortality rate is generally expressed per 10,000 population, per day. The extent to which diseases might spread in a refugee camp depends partly on the *attack rate* of a disease, which is "the cumulative incidence of infection in a group observed over a period of time during an epidemic."[8,p8] Finally, it is important to understand *case fatality rate*, which is "the number of deaths from a specific disease in a given period, per 100 episodes of the disease in the same period."[9,para2]

THE CHARACTERISTICS OF NATURAL DISASTERS

There are several types of natural disasters. Some of these are related to the weather, including droughts, hurricanes, typhoons, cyclones, and heavy rains. Tsunamis, like the one that occurred in 2011, can also cause extreme devastation, injuries, and death. In addition, earthquakes and volcanoes can have important impacts on the health of various communities. Despite the exceptional nature of tsunamis and the deaths associated with them, earthquakes are the natural disasters that generally kill the most people.

It appears that the number of natural disasters is increasing, affecting larger numbers of people, causing more economic losses than earlier but causing proportionately fewer deaths than before. In addition, the biggest relative impact of natural disasters is in low- and middle-income countries. In fact, more than 90 percent of the deaths from these disasters occur in low- and middle-income countries.[10] The relative impact of natural disasters on the poor, of course, is greater than on the better off because the share of the poorer people's total assets that are lost in these disasters is greater than that lost by higher-income people. Moreover, the poor are often the most vulnerable to losses from natural disasters because they often live in places at risk from such disasters or have housing that cannot withstand such shocks.[10] Climate change could also have an important impact on the number, type, and severity of natural disasters in the future.

Natural disasters can cause significant harm to infrastructure, such as water supply and sewage systems, that are needed for safe water and sanitation, and roads that may be needed to transport people requiring health care. Natural disasters can also damage the health infrastructure itself, such as hospitals, health centers, and health clinics. People can die directly as a result of the natural disaster, such as from falling rubble during an earthquake or drowning during a flood. However, they may also die as an indirect result of the disaster because of epidemics linked to the lack of safe water or sanitation, food, or access to health services.[10] In addition, people affected by the disaster could end up living in camps, which pose a range of health hazards.

THE CHARACTERISTICS OF COMPLEX EMERGENCIES

Over the 10-year period from 1975 to 1985, there were on average about five complex emergencies per year, according to the International Committee of the Red Cross. However, it is estimated that at the end of the 1990s there were about 40 such emergencies per year in countries in which more than 300 million people live.[7] In 2013, there was a major rise in the number of complex humanitarian crises. Linked to this, the number of internally displaced people reached an unprecedented 3.3 million and the number of refugees increased to 16.7 million. This is a stark contrast from 2012, which saw no new major disasters. The United Nations ranked the crises in Central African Republic and Syria as having the highest level of emergency in 2013, with millions of people affected.[11]

Although natural disasters have been associated with considerable death and economic loss, the impact of complex emergencies on health over the last decade has been considerably greater than that of natural disasters.

Complex humanitarian emergencies have a number of features that particularly relate to their health impacts. First, these emergencies often go on for long periods of time. The strife in Sudan, for example, has gone on for more than a decade.[12] In addition, these emergencies are increasingly civil wars, as in Bosnia, Liberia, Sierra Leone, Rwanda, and the Democratic Republic of Congo. As a result of the nature of the conflict, it is quite common that one or more of the groups that are fighting will not allow humanitarian assistance to be provided to other groups. In fact, humanitarian workers have increasingly been the targets of those who are fighting, despite what should be their protected status.

During complex emergencies, combatants often intentionally target civilians for displacement, injury, and death. Many fighters also engage in systematic abuse of human rights, including torture, sexual abuse, and rape as a weapon of war. Those same fighters often intentionally destroy health facilities. Given the nature of some of the fighting and its impact on civilians, large numbers of people have been displaced by some of these conflicts, as noted previously. Sometimes they choose to flee, but sometimes they are forced to flee.[7]

Unfortunately, these are not the only characteristics of complex humanitarian emergencies. The disruption of society often leads to food shortages. Besides the loss of some health facilities, it is also common that the publicly supported health system may break down entirely, as it did, for example, during the civil war in Liberia. Damage may also be done to water supply and sanitation systems.[4] In El Salvador, for example, the shortage of safe drinking water for the poor was a significant health threat.[12]

It is important to understand that the migration of large numbers of people, some of whom will live in camps, brings with it a number of problems, as well. Migrants carry diseases with them, sometimes into areas that did not previously have that disease. When Ethiopian refugees who were living in Sudan returned home, for example, they brought malaria from Sudan. Diseases can also spread faster among refugee populations than they would normally, given the large number of people living in crowded conditions, often without appropriate hygiene and sanitation. In addition, large numbers of migrants, sometimes suddenly, need care from health systems that were weak before and that may now be almost nonexistent after suffering the effects of civil conflict. Finally, one should note that many factions in civil conflicts have used landmines, and their health effects on individuals can be devastating.[12]

THE HEALTH BURDEN OF NATURAL DISASTERS

Although there are very few data available on the morbidity and disability associated with natural disasters, it has been estimated that from 1998 to 2007, about 250 million people each year were affected by climate-related disasters alone.[13] In 2011, natural disasters caused a total of 30,773 deaths and 245 million victims globally. However, there was a decrease in the human impacts of disasters in 2012, during which 9,655 people were killed and 124.5 million people were displaced worldwide.[14]

The direct and indirect health effects of natural disasters depend on the type of disaster. Earthquakes can kill many people quickly. In addition, they can cause a substantial number of injuries in a very short period of time. In the longer term, earthquake survivors face increased risks of permanent orthopedic disabilities, mental health problems, and possibly an increase in the rates of heart disease and other chronic disease. The indirect effect of earthquakes on health depends on the severity and location of the earthquake and the extent to which it damages infrastructure and forces people out of their homes.[10]

In the popular imagination, people are thought to die from the lava flows of volcanoes. In fact, this is rarely the case. About 90 percent of the deaths from volcanoes are due to mud and ash or from floods on denuded hillsides affected by the volcano.[10] In addition, volcanoes can harm health by displacing people, rendering water supplies unsafe, and causing mental health problems among the affected population.[10]

Tsunamis take most of their victims immediately by drowning and cause relatively few injuries, compared to the number of deaths.[10] In storms and flooding, most fatalities occur from drowning and few deaths result from trauma or wind-blown objects. These flood-related events generally lead to an increase in diarrheal disease, respiratory infections, and skin diseases. Most of these problems that relate to natural disasters are relatively short lived, except for drought-related famine. Epidemics do not often spring up as a result of them, except in drought-related famine and when health systems are completely destroyed for long periods of time.

There are few data on the distribution by age and sex of morbidity, disability, and death related to natural disasters. It appears, however, that being very old, very young, or very sick makes one more vulnerable to disasters in which one has to flee for survival. These groups were disproportionately affected by the 1970 tidal wave in Bangladesh and the 2004 tsunami in Asia. Whether men or women suffer the effects of a natural disaster may depend on when and where it occurs and be most related to the kind of work that men or women are doing. Women, however, face considerable risks in the aftermath of natural disasters if housing has been harmed and people are living in camps, as will be discussed further later.[10]

THE HEALTH EFFECTS OF COMPLEX HUMANITARIAN EMERGENCIES

The burden of illness, disability, and death related to complex humanitarian emergencies is large and probably underestimated, given the difficulties of collecting such data. Some of the effects of these CHEs are direct. It has been estimated for example, that between 320,000 and 420,000 people are killed each year as a direct result of these CHEs.[7] In addition, it is estimated that between 500,000 and 1 million deaths resulted from trauma during the genocide in Rwanda in 1994.[7] It is thought that about 4–13 percent of the deaths during CHEs in Northern Iraq, Somalia, and the Democratic Republic of Congo were the direct result of trauma.

Other illness, disability, and death, however, come about as an indirect result of the emergencies. These stem from malnutrition, the lack of safe water and sanitation, shortages of food, and breakdowns in health services. They are exacerbated by the crowded and difficult circumstances in which people have to live when they are displaced. One estimate, for example, suggested that almost 1.7 million more people died in a 22-month period of conflict in the Democratic Republic of Congo than would have died in a normal 22-month period in that country.[7]

The burden of deaths related to wars is also hard to estimate. One estimate suggests that about 200,000 people died in war in 2001 in low- and middle-income countries. Just over 10 percent of these deaths occurred in the South Asia region. Almost 70 percent of these deaths, however, took place in sub-Saharan Africa.[15] Other estimates suggest that between 1975 and 1989 more than 5 million people died in civil conflicts.[16] In terms of deaths from CHEs, some of the most severely affected countries in the last 2 decades have been the Democratic Republic of Congo, Afghanistan, Burundi, and Angola.[7] Iraq, Syria, and Sudan have also been significantly affected and a more recent estimate of annual deaths due to conflict was about 55,000 people per year.[17]

The data on the breakdown of deaths by age in CHEs suggest that child mortality rates early in the CHE are two to three times the rates of adults but that they slowly decline to those of the rest of the population. The data on deaths by gender are limited.[18] About 20 percent of the nonfatal injuries in the Bosnian conflict were among children. Almost 50 percent of the deaths in the Democratic Republic of Congo were among women and children younger than 15 years of age.[7] In European conflicts, the overwhelming majority of those who died have been men between 19 and 50 years of age.[7]

Causes of Death in CHEs

In the early stages of dealing with large numbers of displaced people in CHEs, most deaths occur from diarrheal diseases, respiratory infections, measles, or malaria.[7,19] Generally, diarrheal diseases are the most common cause of death in refugee situations. Major epidemics of cholera occurred in refugee camps in Malawi, Nepal, and Bangladesh, among others, and the case fatality rates from cholera have ranged from 3–30 percent in settings such as these. Dysentery, which refers to severe diarrhea caused by an infection in the intestine, has also commonly occurred in such situations over the last 20 years, including in camps in Malawi, Nepal, Bangladesh, and Tanzania. The case fatality rate for dysentery has been highest among the very old and very young, for whom it reaches about 10 percent.[7,19] In one of the most significant humanitarian crises in the last few decades, tens of thousands of Rwandan refugees poured into the Democratic Republic of Congo during the genocide in Rwanda. Between July and August 1994, 90 percent of the deaths among the refugees in Goma, Democratic Republic of Congo, were from cholera spread by the contamination of a lake from which the refugees got their water.[7,19]

Measles has also been a major killer in camps for displaced persons. This is especially significant in populations that are malnourished and have not been immunized against measles. The risk of a child dying of measles is increased substantially if the child is vitamin A deficient, as would be the case for many refugees. Up to 30 percent of the children who get measles in these situations may die from it.[19]

Malaria is also a significant contributor to death in refugee camps. This is especially the case when refugees move from countries in which there is relatively little malaria to places in which it is endemic. The risk of malaria in such cases is highest in sub-Saharan Africa and a few parts of Asia.[7,19] Acute respiratory infections are also major causes of death in refugee camps. This is to be expected because the camps are crowded, housing is inadequate, and refugees could remain in the camps for many years. Although less common than the problems noted previously, there have also been outbreaks of meningitis in some refugee camps in areas in which that disease is prevalent, such as Malawi, Ethiopia, and Burundi. These outbreaks have generally been contained by mass immunization, as it became clear that there was a risk of epidemic.[4] However, an outbreak in Sudan in 1999 led to almost 2,400 deaths.[7] Outbreaks of hepatitis E have occurred in Somalia, Ethiopia, and Kenya. These led to high case fatality rates among pregnant women, in particular.[4]

The populations that are affected by CHEs are generally poor and not well nourished, and nutritional issues are always of grave concern during CHEs, when there may also be problems of food scarcity. In addition, the relationship of infection and malnutrition also poses risks to displaced populations. In CHEs in sub-Saharan Africa, the rates of acute protein-energy malnutrition during at least the early period of a CHE have been very high, particularly among young children. Reported rates of such malnutrition varied from around 12 percent among internally displaced Liberians[4] to as high as 80 percent among internally displaced Somalis.[7] In CHEs in Bosnia and Tajikistan, the elderly were the group that was the worst affected by acute protein-energy malnutrition.[7]

The underlying nutritional status of the refugees or internally displaced people is often poor, and micronutrient deficiencies can also be very important in CHEs. Vitamin A deficiency can be very important among these populations, given their low stores of vitamin A, the fact that some of the diseases most prevalent in camps, such as measles, further deplete their stores of vitamin A, and the fact that food rations in camps have historically been deficient in vitamin A. There have also been epidemics of pellagra, which is a deficiency of niacin that causes diarrhea, dermatitis, and mental disorders. One such case affected more than 18,000 Mozambican refugees in Malawi, whose rations in the camp were deficient in niacin. Scurvy, from a lack of vitamin C, has also occurred in a number of settings, such as Ethiopia, Somalia, and Sudan. Iron deficiency anemia has also been a problem in some camps and affects primarily women of childbearing age and young children. It appears that women and children who are in the camps without a male adult are at particular risk of not getting enough food in camps and of suffering acute protein-energy malnutrition and micronutrient deficiencies.[19]

Violence Against Women in CHEs

The security conditions during CHEs put women at considerable risk of sexual violence. Rape may be used as a weapon of war. In addition, the chaos and economic distresses of conflict situations place women at risk of sexual violence and sometimes force them to trade sex for food or money, what people call "survival sex." Such women are often very young.

The data on sexual violence against women during CHEs are not good. Some recent data suggest that the rates of violence against women are very high in these circumstances.

A survey carried out in East Timor indicated that 23 percent of the women surveyed after the crisis there reported that they had been sexually assaulted. Fifteen percent of the women in Kosovo who were surveyed reported sexual violence against them during the conflict period. It is estimated that between 50,000 and 64,000 women in Sierra Leone were sexually assaulted during the conflict there, and 25 percent of Azerbaijani women reported sexual violence against them during a 3-month period in 2000.[20]

Mental Health

Those who study CHEs agree that they are associated with a range of social and psychological shocks to affected people due to changes in their way of living, their loss of livelihoods, damaged social networks, and physical and mental harm to them, their families, and their friends. Nonetheless, there is considerable disagreement among those working with CHEs about the validity of defining the impact on people affected by CHEs through the framework of a Western medical model of mental health.[21,22]

Some studies have focused on post-traumatic stress disorder (PTSD) and have shown rates of prevalence for PTSD among adults that ranged from 4.6 percent among Burmese refugees in Thailand to 37.2 percent among Cambodian refugees in Thailand. The rate of PTSD is about 1 percent in the population of the United States. Similar studies showed rates of depression in Bosnian refugees of 39 percent, Burmese refugees of almost 42 percent, and Cambodian refugees of almost 68 percent. By comparison, one estimate of the baseline rate of depression in the U.S. population is 6.4 percent.[23]

Other studies have looked at the mental health impacts of CHEs on children and the extent to which they suffer from both post-traumatic stress and depression. The studies that have been done on such populations have been small ones that cannot be used to draw major conclusions on this question. However, they suggest that children who have been through conflict situations do suffer from high rates of both PTSD and depression. A survey of 170 adolescent Cambodian refugees, for example, indicated that almost 27 percent of them suffered from PTSD. A survey of 147 Bosnian children refugees suggested that almost 26 percent of them suffered from depression.[24]

It should be noted, however, that a number of those involved with the mental health impacts of CHEs believe that the stress placed by some on PTSD is not valid. Rather, they believe that although a small minority of those affected may need psychotropic medication, the most important issue is to help people as rapidly as possible to rebuild their lives and their social networks. This requires a variety of forms of

TABLE 15-5 Guidelines on Mental Health and Psychosocial Support in Emergency Settings

Human Rights and Equity
- Ensure equity and nondiscrimination in the provision of support services to all affected populations, with a special focus on at-risk populations.

Participation
- Promote the participation of the affected population in assistance and reconstruction efforts to improve program quality, equity, and sustainability.

Do No Harm
- Reduce the risk of harm to humanitarian workers through recommended techniques, such as the use of *coordination groups*, the integration of *local knowledge* into interventions, *flexibility* and project *transparency*, *cultural sensitivity*, knowledge of *current research* in emergency response techniques, and an *understanding* of universal human rights, power relations, and participatory approaches.

Building on Available Resources and Capacities
- To improve sustainability, use existing mental health services by building on local capacities, supporting self-help practices, and fortifying available resources.

Integrated Support Systems
- Integrate activities and programs into a broader structure (i.e., general health services or community support mechanisms) to enable programs to have a more extensive reach, improve sustainability, and reduce stigmatization.

Multilayered Supports
- In order to access the majority of the affected population, provide four categories of response: basic services and security, community and family support, focused nonspecialized support, and specialized services.

Data from Inter-Agency Standing Committee. (2007). *IASC guidelines on mental health and psychosocial support in emergency settings*. Geneva: Inter-Agency Standing Committee.

social assistance and help in reuniting families, finding families a place to live, rebuilding social networks, and restoring livelihoods.[21,22] The Inter-Agency Standing Committee of WHO has issued guidelines for planning, establishing, and coordinating integrated responses, across sectors, for mental health and psychosocial well-being in emergencies. The core principles of these guidelines are shown in **Table 15-5**.

ADDRESSING THE HEALTH EFFECTS OF NATURAL DISASTERS

The health effects of rapid-onset natural disasters occur in phases, starting with the immediate impact of the event and then continuing for some time until displaced people can be resettled. It is very important that the health situation be assessed immediately after the disaster has occurred. This assessment will set the basis for the initial relief effort. At the same time, care must begin for those injured in the disaster. Once the immediate trauma cases are taken care of, relief workers and health service providers can turn their attention to other injured people who are in need of early care and treatment. This would include urgent psychological problems. In the earliest stages of the disaster, some important public health functions also need to be carried out, including the establishment of continuous disease surveillance among the affected populations and provision of water, shelter, and food.[10]

Many countries do not have all of the resources needed to cope with the health impacts of the disaster, and they will depend on assistance from other countries to address their health problems. Unfortunately, there have been many instances when such help was poorly coordinated and did not effectively match the conditions on the ground. It has become clear over time, however, that to be most helpful in addressing the impact of natural disasters, external assistance will have to:

- Include all of the external partners
- Be based on a cooperative relationship among the partners

- Have partners working in ways that are complementary to each other
- Be evidence-based and transparent
- Involve the affected communities[10]

In some respects, it is easier to predict places that are at risk of natural disasters than it is to predict where CHEs will occur. There are certain countries that are vulnerable to earthquakes, volcanoes, hurricanes, typhoons, and flooding during major rains. In this light, much can be done to prepare for natural disasters and to reduce their health impact. Disaster preparedness plans can be formulated to:

- Identify vulnerabilities
- Develop scenarios of what might happen and its likelihood
- Outline the role that different actors will play in the event of an emergency
- Train first responders and managers to deal with such emergencies[10]

It is also possible when constructing water systems and hospitals, for example, to take measures that will make them less vulnerable to damage during natural disasters.

Given the way that the health impacts of natural disasters unfurl, what would be the most cost-effective ways for external partners to help in addressing the disaster? There are at least several lessons that have emerged on this front. First, although many countries send search and rescue teams to assist the victims of natural disasters, the efforts of such teams are not cost-effective. Most people who are freed from the rubble of an earthquake, for example, are saved by people in their own community immediately after the event. By the time foreign search and rescue teams arrive, most victims of falling rubble will already have been saved or will be dead. There may be an important humanitarian and foreign policy rationale for external search and rescue teams. However, they will generally save few lives at very high cost per life saved.[10]

It is also common that countries will send field hospitals to disaster areas. The cost of each hospital is about $1 million, and they generally arrive 2 to 5 days after the initial event. Unfortunately, by the time they arrive, they are of little value in addressing the most urgent trauma cases. It appears to be more cost-effective to have fewer field hospitals but to have a few that will remain in place for some time, in addition to building some temporary but durable buildings that can also serve as hospitals.[10]

Countries send different kinds of goods to disaster-affected places. Unfortunately, these goods can be inappropriate to the needs of the problem. This has often been the case, for example, for drugs. Better results occur when the affected country clearly indicates what it needs and other countries send only those goods. Large camps of tents are often established after natural disasters. This is generally also not a cost-effective approach to helping the affected community to rebuild. Providing cash or building materials to affected families allows them to rebuild as quickly as possible, in a manner in line with their cultural preferences. The lack of income, even beyond the cost of rebuilding their home, can be a major impediment to the reconstruction of affected areas. Although it must be managed carefully to avoid abuse, cash assistance to families appears to be a cost-effective way of helping communities rebuild.[10]

ADDRESSING THE HEALTH EFFECTS OF COMPLEX HUMANITARIAN EMERGENCIES

It is difficult to take measures that can prevent complex humanitarian emergencies from occurring and harming human health because these emergencies so often relate to civil conflict. Thus, the key to avoiding such problems lies in the political realm and in the avoidance of conflict, rather than by taking measures that are directly health related. "Primary prevention in such circumstances, therefore, means stopping the violence."[4,p300]

However, if such conflicts continue to occur, are there measures of secondary prevention that can be taken to detect health-related problems as early as possible and take actions to mitigate them? To a large extent, the early warning systems that exist for natural disasters do not exist for political disasters. Although some groups do carry out analyses of political vulnerability in countries, corruption, and the risk of political instability, these analyses are not used to prepare contingency plans for civil conflict.

Given the extent of conflict, however, it would be prudent if organizations, countries, and international bodies would cooperatively establish contingency plans for areas of likely conflict. It would also be prudent to stage near such areas the materials needed to address displacement and health problems that would occur if conflict breaks out. This would be similar to what is done for disaster preparedness in some places, such as those regularly exposed to hurricanes.[4]

As noted earlier in the chapter, complex humanitarian emergencies are characterized by:

- Potentially massive displacement of people
- The likelihood that these displaced people will live in camps for some time
- The need in those camps for adequate shelter, safe water, sanitation, and food
- The importance of security in the camps, especially for women

- The need to address early in the crisis the potentially worst health threats, which are malnutrition, diarrhea, measles, pneumonia, and malaria
- The need to avoid other epidemic diseases, such as cholera and meningitis
- The need as one moves away from the emergency phase of a CHE to deal with longer term mental health issues, primary health care, TB, and some non-communicable diseases

Some of the most important measures that can be taken to address these points are discussed briefly hereafter. It is important to keep in mind that the aim of these efforts is to establish a safe and healthy environment, treat urgent health problems and prevent epidemics, and then to address less urgent needs and establish a basis for longer term health services among the displaced people.[7]

Assessment and Surveillance

As with natural disasters, among the first things that need to be done during the emergency phase of a CHE is to carry out an assessment of the displaced population and establish a system for disease surveillance. Such an assessment would try to immediately gather information on the number of people who are displaced, their age and sex, their ethnic and social backgrounds, and their state of health and nutrition. Although it is difficult to get this information in the chaotic moments of an emergency, it is impossible to rationally plan services for displaced people without this information.

There are a number of health indicators that guide services in CHEs, and a surveillance system needs to be established at the start of the emergency phase of a CHE. Given the difficulties of the emergency, the surveillance system must be simple but still give a robust sense of the health of the affected community. Given the importance of nutrition and the likelihood that a large part of the population will be undernourished, it is essential that the weight for height of all children younger than 5 years of age be checked.[4] It is also important to have surveillance for diseases that cause epidemics among displaced persons, such as measles, cholera, and meningitis.

In general, the daily crude mortality rate is used as an indicator of the health of the affected group; one goal is to keep that rate below 1 death per 10,000 persons in the population per day. Where the daily rate is twice the normal rate, it signifies that a public health emergency is occurring. Say, for example, that the baseline crude mortality rate for sub-Saharan Africa is 0.44/10,000 per day. Thus, if the rate in an affected population were to get to 0.88/10,000 per day, it would signal a public health emergency that would require

urgent attention. For children younger than 5 years, say that the crude mortality rate for sub-Saharan Africa is 1.14/10,000 per day. The goal in a public health emergency, therefore, would be to keep that rate below about 2.0/10,000 per day.[24] Death rates in a large camp are not always easy to get; sometimes people have resorted to innovative ways of getting such data, such as daily reports by gravediggers.

A Safe and Healthy Environment

It is critical in camps and other situations with large numbers of displaced people that efforts be made to ensure that environmental and personal hygiene are maintained. This will be the key to avoiding the potentially serious effect of diarrheal disease. It is recommended that 15 liters of water per person per day should be provided, people should not have to walk more than 500 meters to a water source, and people should not have to wait more than 15 minutes to get their water when they get to a source. Of the 15 liters per day that are recommended, about 2.5 to 3 liters are considered the minimum essential for drinking and food. Another 2 to 6 liters are needed for personal hygiene, and the remainder is needed for cooking.[25]

Providing appropriate sanitation in situations of displaced people is also very challenging. Ideally, every family would have their own toilet. This, however, is certainly impossible in the acute phase of an emergency. The goal instead is one toilet for every 20 people. These should be segregated by sex to provide the most safety to women. They should not be more than 50 meters from dwellings, but must be carefully situated to avoid contamination of water sources.[25]

Many of the displaced people will be poor people with little education and, often, poor hygiene practices. It is very important in these circumstances that efforts be made to make the community aware of the importance of good hygiene and to see that soap is available to all families and used.

Of course, people will also need shelter. The long-term goal is to help them return as quickly as possible to their homes. In the short term, if possible, the goal is to have families be sheltered temporarily with other families. Nonetheless, it is obvious from the tables shown earlier that many displaced people do end up living in camps, often for very long periods of time. When shelter is needed, the goal is to provide 3.5 square meters of covered area per person, with due attention paid in the construction of the shelter to the safety of women. Whenever possible, local and culturally appropriate building materials should be used. In the short run, the aim is to get people into covered areas. When the emergency phase has passed, the need to enhance some of the structures can be prioritized.[26]

Food

It is suggested that each adult in a camp should get at least 2,100 kilocalories of energy from food per day.[27] Food rations should be distributed by family unit, but special care has to be taken, as noted earlier, to ensure that female-headed households and children without their families get their rations. Vitamin A should be given to all children, and the most severely malnourished children may also need urgent nutrition supplementation.[27]

Disease Control

As also suggested earlier, "The primary goals of humanitarian response to disasters are to 1) prevent and reduce excess morbidity and mortality, and 2) promote a return to normalcy."[25] Along these lines, the control of communicable diseases is one of the first priorities in the emergency phase of a disaster, especially a complex humanitarian emergency.

An important priority in the emergency phase of a complex humanitarian emergency is to prevent an epidemic of measles. This starts with vaccinating all children from 6 months to 15 years of age. Another important priority is to ensure that children up to 5 years of age get vitamin A. Systems also need to be put in place so that other epidemics that sometimes occur in these situations, such as meningitis and cholera, can be detected and then urgently addressed. Other priorities will include the proper management of diarrhea in children and the appropriate diagnosis and treatment for malaria, in zones where that is prevalent. Of course, health education and hygiene promotion must take place continuously to try to help families prevent the onset of these diseases in the first place.[24]

Unfortunately, preventing the outbreak of communicable diseases is not the only effort that needs to be taken in the emergency phase of a CHE. Measures need to be in place to handle injuries and trauma, first to stabilize people and then to refer them to where they can receive the additional medical help they need. There will almost certainly be pregnant women among the displaced people, and there will be an immediate need for some reproductive health services. This will generally have to focus on the provision of a minimum package of care that would include safe delivery kits, precautions against the transmission of HIV, and transport and referral in case of complications of pregnancy.[4,24-28]

The care of noncommunicable diseases will be a lower priority in emergency situations than addressing communicable diseases. However, some psychiatric problems will require urgent attention and will need to be treated as effectively as possible with counseling, the continuation of medicines people were taking, and the provision of new medications, if needed. As the emergency recedes, greater attention can be paid to long-term treatment, counseling, and psychosocial support for dealing with mental health problems and the many disruptions that people have faced in their lives.[23] At that time, one can also turn additional attention to ensuring the appropriate medication of people with other noncommunicable diseases.

POLICY AND PROGRAM BRIEFS

This chapter does not contain any case studies that have been based on careful review of the evidence about specific interventions. However, policy and program briefs follow on four CHEs of importance. One concerns the genocide in Rwanda and the plight of Rwandan refugees in Goma, in what is now the Democratic Republic of Congo. A second concerns a major earthquake that hit Pakistan in 2005. A third brief concerns an earthquake in Haiti in 2010. The comments on Haiti largely follow a chronological account of the work done by Doctors Without Borders in the 6 months following the earthquake. The last case is about the impact of Cyclone Nargis on Myanmar in 2008.

The Genocide in Rwanda

In mid-July 1994, nearly 1 million Rwandan Hutus tried to escape persecution from the newly established government of Rwanda that was led by the Tutsis. The border town of Goma, in what is now the Democratic Republic of Congo, situated in the North Kivu region, became the entry point for the majority of the refugees. Many of them settled around Lake Kivu.[29]

Almost 50,000 people died in the first month after the start of the influx, largely as a result of an epidemic of cholera, which was followed by an epidemic of bacillary dysentery. In the first 17 days of the emergency, the average crude mortality rate of Rwandans was 28.1–44.9 per 10,000 per day, compared to the 0.6 per 10,000 per day in prewar conditions inside Rwanda. This crude mortality rate is the highest by a considerable margin over the rate found in any previous CHE. In addition, in Goma, diarrheal disease affected young children and adults alike, whereas normally young children are much more severely affected than adults.[29]

Humanitarian assessments began in the first week of August, 3 weeks after the initial flow of refugees. Rapid surveys conducted in the three refugee camps of Katale, Kibumba, and Mugunga indicated that diarrheal disease contributed to 90 percent of deaths; food shortages were prevalent, especially among female-headed households; and acute malnutrition afflicted up to 23 percent of the refugees. In early August, a meningitis epidemic arose.[29]

The circumstances were complicated by the large numbers of people who fled to Goma in such a short period of time. In addition, the lake represented an easy source of water, but one from which disease could be spread. The soil around Goma was very rocky, which made it very difficult to construct an appropriate number of latrines. In addition, Hutu leaders were given control over the distribution of relief, but this did not provide for the equitable distribution of food that was hoped for.[29]

By early August, the response of the international community was beginning to have the desired effect, under the coordination of the United Nations High Commissioner for Refugees (UNHCR). A disease surveillance network was established. An information system was set up for the camps. Five to 10 liters of safe water per day per person was distributed. Measles immunization was carried out, vitamin A supplements were distributed, and disease problems were attacked using standard protocols.[29]

Despite the exceptional efforts made by many people to deal with the crisis, the events in Goma highlighted a number of shortcomings of the response. First, there was a general lack of preparedness for dealing with this type of emergency, despite the well-known political instability of Rwanda at that time. Second, the medical teams on the ground did not have the physical infrastructure or the experience needed for a task of this magnitude. Many of these staff, for example, were not as knowledgeable about oral rehydration as they needed to be, even though this is fundamental to treating diarrheal disease. Third, the work of the military forces that joined the effort was not integrated into the planning of the other efforts.[29]

Although the Goma crisis was exceptional in many ways, it does suggest a number of lessons for enhancing the response to CHEs in the future. These include the need to:

- Establish early warning systems for CHEs
- Prepare in advance for CHEs
- Strengthen the existing nongovernmental groups with capability to respond to CHEs

The Earthquake in Pakistan

In early October 2005, Pakistan experienced an earthquake measuring 7.6 on the Richter scale. The epicenter was in Kashmir but the earthquake also devastated the North-West Frontier Province (NWFP). Within a matter of minutes, homes and livelihoods were destroyed, leaving over 3 million

people homeless and many individuals buried under the rubble or injured by debris.[30]

It is estimated that 88,000 people, many of whom were children, lost their lives either from instantaneous death, such as severe head injury or internal bleeding; rapid death, such as asphyxia due to dust; or delayed death, such as wound infections. An additional 80,000 people were injured.[31] Moreover, 84 percent of the infrastructure in Kashmir, including 65 percent of all previously existing healthcare facilities, failed to withstand the seismic forces and collapsed. Thus, the immediate needs of the population included medical care, food and water, and sanitation facilities.[30]

To respond to the earthquake, the government of Pakistan created the Federal Relief Commission (FRC) and the Earthquake Rehabilitation and Reconstruction Authority (ERRA) that offered short- and long-term recovery efforts. Furthermore, a week after the initial earthquake, the government presented a plan for relief that included compensation for survivors. The World Bank, along with the Asian Development Bank, conducted assessments to identify vulnerable groups and areas that might hinder early recovery, such as unsanitary environments. Moreover, the South Asia Earthquake Flash Appeal (SAEFA) was created to receive donations for the recovery effort.

Doctors Without Borders (MSF) was an integral part of the interventions, as it provided emergency relief within a day of the earthquake, given that MSF medical teams were already on the ground in Kashmir. These teams focused initially on hygiene promotion; distributing tents, cookware, and mattresses; and treating the injured. They administered 30,000 measles vaccines and later redirected attention to rebuilding medical infrastructure. In NWFP, MSF created hospitals with beds to house patients, and also developed medical villages that were used to treat the overwhelming number of injured people.[30]

Despite national and international efforts to mobilize an effective response, injured individuals flooded hospitals that were still intact but did not have the personnel or the equipment to respond effectively. Thus, many patients suffered more severe secondary complications due to prolonged waiting for medical treatment, a common occurrence when earthquakes significantly affect the medical system.[30,31]

Furthermore, small, remote villages remained inaccessible because of significant road damage. Given the impending winter, the Pakistani military, MSF, and UN agencies used helicopters to distribute basic relief. In addition, the government pledged the provision of tents. People inside and outside of Pakistan responded very generously with donations to help those affected by the disaster. However, many of the donations did not fit what was most needed.[30]

Several valuable lessons emerge from the efforts of the government and military of Pakistan and Pakistan's foreign partners to assist in the rescue and recovery from the earthquake:

- Buildings in rural areas in seismic zones should be built or designed to decrease human injury.
- Governments should analyze existing risks to their ability to rapidly respond to emergencies and prepare emergency plans in advance that take those risks into account.
- Donations of materials and supplies should be managed carefully so that they fit real needs.
- The expertise of nongovernmental organizations (NGOs), like that provided by MSF in Pakistan, can be very helpful in addressing natural disasters, particularly if the involved organizations already have a presence in the affected country.[30,31]

Haiti's 2010 Earthquake[32]

In January 2010, Haiti experienced an earthquake that was centered about 15 miles southwest of Port-au-Prince, the capital city, and measured 7.0 on the Richter scale. Given the magnitude of the earthquake, the poor quality of construction in Haiti, and the exceptionally poor living conditions of many people there, the earthquake caused major devastation. In addition, the country's already weak health system, with only a limited number of trained personnel, was ill equipped to handle the overwhelming health needs stemming from the earthquake. Moreover, with 60 percent of existing health facilities destroyed and 10 percent of medical staff either killed or absent from the country, Haiti was in dire need of external assistance to address the health needs of its people.

Doctors Without Borders (MSF) played a key role in the relief effort. The timeliness and scale of its response was strengthened by the fact that it had already been providing health services in Haiti for 19 years prior to the earthquake. MSF's response to the earthquake provides an informative example of the chronology and focus of health efforts after natural disasters in low-income countries. The actions taken by MSF are also a good reflection of how such external assistance moves through different phases, starting with the acute phase of the emergency and then leading over time toward efforts at reconstruction, rehabilitation, and development.

Providing emergency medical services was the first priority for MSF after the earthquake. In order to perform life-saving surgeries and wound care for people injured by the earthquake, MSF created new emergency facilities. These facilities were needed because so many existing ones had been damaged and because there were so many injured survivors. In addition, MSF sent in more surgical supplies and increased the number of personnel on the ground, which reached 3,500 at its highest point. An inflatable hospital was even constructed, which provided 100 beds and 3 operating theatres. Creating sanitary conditions suitable for performing surgery was one challenge faced in this stage of the emergency response. In total, MSF provided emergency medical care to over 173,000 patients in the 5 months following the earthquake, performing over 11,000 surgeries. The nature of emergency care for earthquake-related injuries soon shifted with time, from lifesaving, often including amputation of limbs, to treating infected wounds.

Provision of emergency obstetric care was also a priority, which is crucial to saving maternal lives. Because MSF's own maternity hospital was demolished, the organization provided support to the Ministry of Health's maternity hospital by providing personnel and critical medicines. MSF helped to deliver 3,752 babies in all its facilities in the first 5 months after the earthquake, spending 4 million euros on maternal health services during this period.

To address the effects of the disaster on mental health, psychological care was integrated with emergency care for trauma patients. Soon after, outreach programs in communities were initiated, reflecting the importance of mental health care both immediately and later in relief efforts. Group counseling sessions and individual consultations were aimed primarily at reducing the anxiety that comes with losing a loved one, coping with injury and poor living conditions, and the fear of an aftershock. MSF delivered psychological care to over 80,000 Haitians in the first 5 months after the earthquake; even so, provision of mental health care remains a great challenge in Haiti due to the lack of psychiatrists to address short- and long-term psychiatric disorders.

Providing primary health care was also a priority for MSF, which was addressed by setting up additional primary health clinics. In the weeks following the earthquake, 400 to 500 people visited each clinic daily (6 months after the earthquake, about 70 people visited daily). In addition to providing basic check-ups, which allowed MSF to monitor common health problems in the area, primary health clinics enabled MSF to screen for disease epidemics. Services provided included ante- and postnatal care, vaccinations, infection treatment, and referrals to mental health services or a hospital.

The delivery of health services consumed the majority of MSF's efforts in Haiti after the earthquake. However, additional efforts to address the health threats of lack of water, sanitation, and shelter as quickly as possible were also needed. Thus, MSF set up sanitation areas in camps surrounding Port-au-Prince, each composed of a latrine, shower, and wash area. In addition to the creation of a waste disposal system, good hygiene was promoted through the distribution of 35,000 hygiene kits that included soap, toothpaste, and a toothbrush. As of May 2010, MSF was distributing about 1,270 cubic meters of water per day by water trucks, in partnership with other organizations.

At the same time, MSF attempted to improve living conditions for the displaced by distributing tents for shelter and nonfood household items, such as cooking materials and sheets. Almost 27,000 tents were distributed, which are supposed to last about 6 months.

MSF also expanded its mobile clinics, which included bringing care to communities and seeking out patients. Mobile clinics are commonly used by MSF. However, the number of such clinics was not expanded immediately because the organization's personnel were already overburdened by the number of patients coming on their own immediately following the disaster to other MSF supported healthcare facilities.

As it tried to carry out this work, particularly its immediate response to the earthquake, MSF confronted the challenge of obtaining landing spots for planes carrying urgently needed medical supplies and personnel. With planes often diverted to the neighboring Dominican Republic, supplies had to be brought to their destination by car, which took an additional 36 hours.

By the second month after the disaster, medical needs shifted from emergency care to longer term care, with an emphasis on recovery and rehabilitation. In addition, hospitals and primary care clinics started to treat conditions not inflicted by the earthquake, which amounted to about half of the cases treated by MSF by early June 2010. During this stage of the response, violence-related injuries and pediatric issues were especially common. During this period, hospitals also had to respond more frequently to conditions such as road traffic accidents, burn injuries, sexually transmitted infections, and illnesses such as TB, HIV, and respiratory infections.

By the third month after the earthquake, MSF was able to replace many of its international workers, who had flown to Haiti for emergency relief, with Haitian workers. By June 2010, the ratio of Haitian to international workers had returned to 10 to 1, the standard before the earthquake.

MSF spent about 53 million euros in Haiti in the first 5 months following the earthquake, with 11 million euros spent on surgical and postoperative care and 8.5 million euros spent on providing shelter.

Despite health improvements in Haiti made possible by MSF, the organization faced some major challenges in the aftermath of the earthquake:

- Proper shelter for earthquake victims will remain an issue, because reconstruction is slow and the makeshift tents distributed are starting to deteriorate.
- MSF is faced with the task of rebuilding medical facilities that were destroyed in the earthquake, in addition to replacing temporary facilities with permanent ones.
- Haiti is subject to natural disasters, including hurricanes, and a serious hurricane could dramatically complicate the already weak infrastructure in Haiti and create additional health problems.

Myanmar: Cyclone Nargis

In early May 2008, a cyclone swept through the southern coastal region of Myanmar. Submerging entire towns, the cyclone killed over 138,000 people and left hundreds of thousands of survivors homeless. Over 50 townships and 2.4 million people were affected.[33] The Irrawaddy Delta, commonly known as the Rice Bowl of Myanmar and populated mostly by farmers, fishermen, laborers, and traders, experienced the worst destruction of infrastructure, water supplies, homes, fuel, and electricity.[34] The livelihoods of the population were swept away with the cyclone, because the coastline and farmlands were in ruins.

Myanmar did not have the resources to adequately respond to the needs of its people after a disaster of such great scale. The health system, for example, was already weak. Myanmar spends only 2.3 percent of gross domestic product on health per year, or about $43 per capita.[35] In addition, the rural population, which made up 70 percent of the total population, had little to no access to basic health and sanitation services or clean water, even before the cyclone. Myanmar also lacked the healthcare professionals needed to deliver critical healthcare services. Moreover, one out of four people live below the poverty line, and Myanmar already suffered from a high burden of communicable disease, including malaria and tuberculosis.[34]

Myanmar was run at the time by a military regime in which elections had been deemed by international standards to be neither free nor fair. In addition, the government was generally perceived as repressive, nontransparent, and limiting of political freedom. These factors had an important impact on the relief effort, as noted later.

In the aftermath of the cyclone, the need for emergency relief efforts was exacerbated by poor health and living conditions. As in any natural disaster, short-term needs included emergency health care for cyclone-related injuries; basic necessities for survival, such as food, shelter, water, and sanitation services; and provision of mental health services for psychological disorders such as depression and anxiety. In the longer term, Myanmar was tasked with reconstruction of infrastructure for health, shelter, food, and transportation.

For about 3 weeks following the disaster, however, the State Peace and Development Council (SPDC) of the Myanmar government did not allow most foreign aid or supplies into the country. Despite the scale of devastation and the country's lack of adequate resources for relief efforts, the government feared foreign influence and possible unrest from civilians if any international assistance groups intervened. Thus, Myanmar relied on local government and community-based organizations to address the acute phase of disaster relief. Even private initiatives by local citizens were subject to government control through mandatory checkpoints.[33] Unfortunately, Myanmar lacked much of the staff capacity it needed to manage logistics and supplies to deal with the crisis, according to the World Food Programme.[34] Thus, initial relief efforts could not possibly provide the food, shelter, sanitation, and emergency health care that was needed.

Many countries and humanitarian relief organizations were outraged by the government's blockage of foreign aid to the people in Myanmar who they thought were in need of additional life-saving assistance.[33] The Association of South East Asian Nations (ASEAN) protested by rapidly deploying medical teams to serve in Myanmar. Following great pressure from the international community, including a visit from the UN Secretary General Ban Ki-moon, the SPDC finally allowed international aid agencies to enter the country in late May.[33]

To facilitate cooperation between foreign assistance groups and the Myanmar government, the Tripartite Core Group (TCG) was created to coordinate and oversee relief efforts. Made up of ASEAN, the United Nations, and the government of Myanmar's Ministry of Health, the TCG created a plan for short-term and long-term rebuilding and pledged to look into measures for increasing preparedness and prevention efforts for future cyclones.

Once let into the country, international aid agencies did not escape tight government controls over their relief efforts. Travel restrictions were placed on many aid workers, and they experienced extensive government monitoring. Each foreign team was assigned a specific township in which to work, where activities were coordinated through a local liaison officer to the government. Differing sharply from previous large-scale disaster relief efforts in other countries, this aid structure lessened the possibility that foreign groups could work together in the same geographical area. In addition, the government restricted communication of information between groups.[33]

Government authorities forced many relief workers to give aid directly to them, according to interviews with cyclone survivors and relief workers in a study conducted by the Johns Hopkins Center for Public Health and Human Rights.[33] According to the same reports, some of the aid was not used as intended. Additionally, foreign aid teams were not allowed to collect data independently.[33]

The same study also confirmed abuses against healthcare workers and cyclone survivors, including land confiscation and forced relocation of survivors. Official assessments conducted by the SPDC have not recognized these occurrences.[33]

With restrictions on communication regarding the disaster throughout the country, the government relied on state-controlled media to disseminate information, which downplayed the extent of the devastation and remaining needs of the people. In effect, the cyclone survivors, and the tragedy of the crisis as a whole, did not receive the attention they deserved within Myanmar.[33]

The types of health conditions treated by foreign relief efforts, once they did arrive in Myanmar, suggest that the delay in international response may have contributed to high rates of early mortality. Instead of deep wound and emergency injuries that would be expected after a cyclone, international relief organizations more commonly treated chronic conditions. For example, one international group that hosted mobile clinics reported that the most common illnesses among adults and children were upper respiratory tract infections and gastritis.[34] The lack of deep wounds and lacerations treated, according to this data, suggests that those people who were severely injured immediately following the cyclone, and who would have required emergency care, most likely did not receive it and lost their lives. The in-country operations lacked the resources to manage the acute phase of emergency response to the scale required.

The mishandling of aid and strict government control of relief efforts prevented aid from reaching many survivors for more than a year after the cyclone. Food, water, and shelter were the most crucial unmet needs 18 months following the cyclone. At that point, an estimated 450,000 people in the Delta still did not have shelter, according to the UN Human Settlements Programme (UN-HABITAT). At the time, food was still in short supply due to the destruction of farmland and farming equipment.[33]

The cyclone in Myanmar raises questions for the international humanitarian assistance community about the appropriate response to emergency situations in which the local government is ill equipped to address the needs of its people with the necessary quality and scale yet blocks outside bodies from helping to address these needs. In addition, the cyclone raises questions about the appropriate degree of autonomy for international relief efforts in the presence of a controlling local government that obstructs aid efforts.

FUTURE CHALLENGES IN MEETING THE HEALTH NEEDS OF COMPLEX HUMANITARIAN EMERGENCIES AND NATURAL DISASTERS

A number of critical challenges confront efforts to address the health effects of natural disasters and complex humanitarian emergencies. One such challenge for the future is how to prevent these from having such negative health impacts. It is difficult in resource-poor settings, many of which are poorly governed, to focus attention on the prevention of disasters and their impacts. Nonetheless, through better mitigation measures, such as water control, better building standards, greater education of the community about how to deal with disasters, and having a disaster preparedness plan for which people are trained, it should be possible, even for very poor countries, to reduce deaths from natural disasters. If these steps are coupled with the development of standard approaches for dealing with health issues when they do arise and the forward staging of medicines, equipment, and materials near to disaster-prone areas, it should be possible to reduce deaths from natural disasters, even in very low-income settings. Bangladesh, which is subject to annual flooding, has reduced the annual deaths from such floods, for example, with a series of the previously mentioned measures.[36]

There has been considerable progress among the international community in the establishment of common standards and protocols for responses to disasters. In fact, a code of conduct has been developed for use by the International Red Cross and Red Crescent Societies and NGOs, to guide their work in emergencies. The core principles of this code are shown in **Table 15-6**. There remains, however, the need to enhance further the coordination of responses. Ideally, the organizations involved in responding to natural disasters and CHEs will:

- Subscribe to a common set of norms, such as the Sphere Project
- Have common protocols for dealing with key issues

TABLE 15-6 The Code of Conduct: Principles of Conduct for the International Red Cross and Red Crescent Movement and NGOs in Disaster Response Programmes

- The humanitarian imperative comes first.

- Aid is given regardless of the race, creed, or nationality of the recipients and without adverse distinction of any kind. Aid priorities are calculated on the basis of need alone.

- Aid will not be used to further a particular political or religious standpoint.

- We shall endeavor not to act as instruments of government foreign policy.

- We shall respect culture and custom.

- We shall attempt to build disaster response on local capacities.

- Ways shall be found to involve programme beneficiaries in the management of relief aid.

- Relief aid must strive to reduce future vulnerabilities to disaster as well as meeting basic needs.

- We hold ourselves accountable to both those we seek to assist and those from whom we accept resources.

- In our information, publicity, and advertising activities, we shall recognize disaster victims as dignified humans, not hopeless objects.

Modified from the International Federation of Red Cross and Red Crescent Societies. *The code of conduct*. Retrieved October 3, 2010 from http://www.ifrc.org/en/publications-and-reports/code-of-conduct/.

- Train their staff to work with those protocols
- Work in close conjunction with the affected communities and local governments[37]

In addition, it is important that responses to disasters focus on cost-effective approaches to the provision of healthcare services in emergencies. We have already seen that search and rescue assistance from abroad is not cost-effective.

The same is true for most field hospitals. Moreover, many agencies have provided health services in emergencies that did not focus on immediate needs and could have waited. Morbidity and mortality can be prevented and reduced more quickly if the agencies involved in disaster relief carefully set priorities for action that would be based on the principle of cost-effectiveness analysis, taking appropriate account of concerns for social justice and equity.[10,37,38]

The continued refinement of indicators that can be used to measure performance of services in disasters will be helpful to gauging the performance of local and international relief efforts.[38]

MAIN MESSAGES

Natural disasters and complex humanitarian emergencies are important causes of illness, death, and disability. They affect large numbers of people, have a huge economic impact, and their aftereffects can go on for some time. Their biggest relative impact is on the poor, who are generally more vulnerable to the effects of these disasters than are better-off people. Some of these disasters are caused by humans. Some are slow onset and some are rapid onset.

Natural disasters, such as droughts, famines, hurricanes, typhoons, cyclones, and heavy rains have important health impacts. Earthquakes and volcanoes are also natural disasters with large potential effects on health. It appears that the number of natural disasters is increasing but the number of deaths from them is decreasing. More than 90 percent of deaths from natural disasters occur in low- and middle-income countries. Climate change could increase the type and severity of natural disasters.

Some deaths are a direct result of natural disasters. However, the impact of those disasters on water supply and sanitation systems, health services, and availability of food can also, indirectly, lead to many more deaths. There are also special health problems associated with living in camps, which sometimes happen to those who survive natural disasters that displace many people from their homes.

In the late 1990s, there were about 40 CHEs each year. There are probably more than 14 million refugees in the world and more than 20 million internally displaced people. Overall, CHEs are associated with considerably larger health impacts than natural disasters. In addition, they may have an acute phase when large numbers of people flee, and they generally go on for long periods of time.

Complex humanitarian emergencies have increasingly been linked to civil conflict. Like natural disasters, they also have direct and indirect impacts on health. They not only take lives directly through war-related trauma but also lead to the destruction of infrastructure. The health effects of some of these conflicts have been dramatic, sometimes because civilians have been targeted by combatants. Women are especially vulnerable in CHEs to sexual violence.

In the emergency phase of a CHE, when large numbers of displaced persons are coming into camps, a number of health risks have to be addressed. Among the most important are diarrhea, measles, malaria, and pneumonia. Malnutrition is also of exceptional importance. Cholera epidemics can also arise and kill large numbers of people quickly.

Countries at risk can take a number of measures to mitigate vulnerability to damage from natural disasters. This could include preparing a disaster plan, building seawalls and levees, and requiring, for example, that buildings in earthquake-prone areas be earthquake proof. It might also be cost-effective to strengthen other infrastructure, such as water supply systems, so that they can withstand significant threats.

Addressing the health impacts of a natural disaster requires that the health situation be assessed quickly and that urgent cases be handled immediately. Less urgent problems can be handled in the following days, weeks, and months. Long-term support for those psychologically affected by the disaster will also need to be provided in the medium and long term.

The health situation of a CHE also needs to be assessed quickly and continuously. Early attention in dealing with large numbers of displaced people must focus on the environment, shelter, water, and food. The next step is the prevention of disease outbreaks, and their treatment if they do occur. Particular attention must be paid to malnutrition, measles, pneumonia, and malaria. Some immediate attention will also have to be paid to a minimum package of reproductive health services and the avoidance of HIV. As the acute phase of the emergency subsides, more attention can be paid to TB, overall primary health care, noncommunicable diseases, and longer-term mental health issues.

There has been some important progress in the coordination and standardization of measures to address CHEs and natural disasters. However, there are still gaps in the preparation and training of staff in some organizations. In addition, there has been inadequate attention to the cost-effectiveness of interventions. There is now enough information about the lessons of CHEs and natural disasters that the priority actions that are needed should be clear and organizations active in relief work need to concentrate their efforts on what will prevent the most deaths, disability, and morbidity, at least cost, with due attention to concerns for social justice.

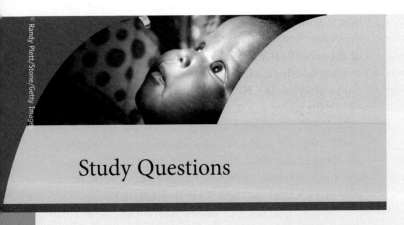

Study Questions

1. How does the annual burden of disease from natural disasters and complex humanitarian emergencies compare with other causes of illness, death, and disability?

2. What is a disaster? A natural disaster? A complex humanitarian emergency?

3. What is an internally displaced person? A refugee? What are the differences between them?

4. What have been some of the most significant natural disasters in the last decade? How many deaths were associated with them? How did people die? How did deaths vary for different types of disasters by age and sex?

5. What countries in sub-Saharan Africa have been the largest sources of displaced people? What countries in sub-Saharan Africa have received the largest numbers of refugees?

6. In the early stages of a complex humanitarian emergency, what are likely to be the most significant health concerns for the refugees? How do those health concerns change over time? Who are the most affected by malnutrition, measles, pneumonia, and cholera?

7. In what ways are women especially vulnerable during complex humanitarian emergencies? What problems do they face as a consequence of these vulnerabilities?

8. What are key steps that can be taken to reduce the vulnerability of certain places to the potential health threats of natural disasters?

9. What are key steps that need to be taken within the first few days of people fleeing to a refugee camp? How do those concerns change over time?

10. How can one try to ensure that relief agencies work together around a common framework and that they focus on the most cost-effective activities?

REFERENCES

1. National Highway Traffic Safety Administration. *Glossary*. Retrieved September 29, 2006, from http://www.nhtsa.dot.gov/people/injury/ems/emstraumasystem03/glossary.htm.

2. Boutros Boutros-Ghali, Concluding Statement of the UN Congress on Public International Law: Towards the Twenty-First Century: International Law as a Language for International Relations, March 13–17, 1995, New York.

3. Burkholder, B. T., & Toole, M. J. (1995). Evolution of complex disasters. *Lancet, 346,* 1012–1015.

4. Toole, M. J., & Waldman, R. J. (1997). The public health aspects of complex emergencies and refugee situations. *Annual Review of Public Health, 18,* 283–312.

5. United Nations High Commissioner for Refugees. (2001). *The 1951 convention relating to the status of refugees and its 1967 protocol.* Retrieved March 29, 2015, from http://www.unhcr.org/4ec262df9.html.

6. Brookings Institute. (2008). Protecting internally displaced persons: A manual for law and policymakers. Retrieved March 29, 2015, from http://www.unhcr.org/50f955599.html/.

7. Brennan, R. J., & Nandy, R. (2001). Complex humanitarian emergencies: A major global health challenge. *Emergency Medicine (Fremantle), 13*(2), 147–156.

8. Last, J. M. (2001). *A dictionary of epidemiology* (4th ed., p. 47). New York: Oxford University Press.

9. UCLA School of Public Health. (n.d.). *Definitions.* Retrieved March 29, 2015, from http://www.ph.ucla.edu/epi/bioter/anthapha_def_a.html.

10. de Ville de Goyet, C., Zapata Marti, R., & Osorio, C. (2006). Natural disaster mitigation and relief. In D. T. Jamison, J. G. Breman, A. R. Measham, et al. (Eds.), *Disease control priorities in developing countries* (2nd ed., pp. 1147–1152). New York: Oxford University Press.

11. Global Humanitarian Assistance. (n.d.). *Global humanitarian assistance report 2014.* Retrieved September 12, 2014, from http://www.globalhumanitarianassistance.org/wp-content/uploads/2014/09/GHA-Report-2014-interactive.pdf.

12. Hansch, S., & Burkholder, B. (1996). When chaos reigns. *Harvard International Review, 18*(4), 10–14.

13. Ganeshan, S., & Diamond, W. (2009). *Forecasting the numbers of people affected annually by natural disasters up to 2015.* Oxford, UK: Oxfam.

14. Guha-Sapir, D., Hoyois, P., & Below, R. (n.d.). *Annual disaster statistical review 2012.* WHO collaborating Centre for Research on the Epidemiology of Disasters (CRED). Retrieved September 12, 2014, from http://reliefweb.int/sites/reliefweb.int/files/resources/ADSR_2012.pdf.

15. Lopez, A. D., Mathers, C. D., & Murray, C. J. L. (2006). The burden of disease and mortality by condition: Data, methods, and results for 2001. In A. D. Lopez, C. D. Mathers, M. Ezzati, D. T. Jamison, C. J. L. Murray (Eds.), *Global burden of disease and risk factors* (pp. 45–93). New York: Oxford University Press.

16. Zwi, A. B., & Ugalde, A. (1991). Political violence in the third world: a public health issue. *Health Policy and Planning, 6,* 203–217.

17. Goldstein, J. S. (2011, August 15). Think again: War. *Foreign Policy.* Retrieved August 24, 2014, from http://www.foreignpolicy.com/articles/2011/08/15/think_again_war.

18. Personal communication, R. J. Waldman to R. Skolnik, March 2007.

19. Waldman, R. J. (2001). Prioritising health care in complex emergencies. *Lancet, 357*(9266), 1427–1429.

20. Marsh, M., Purdin, S., & Navani, S. (2006). Addressing sexual violence in humanitarian emergencies. *Global Public Health, 1*(2), 133–146.

21. Ager, A. (2002). Psychosocial needs in complex emergencies. *Lancet, 360,* s43–s44.

22. Almedom, A., & Summerfield, D. (2004). Mental well-being in settings of "complex emergency": An overview. *Journal of Biosocial Science, 36,* 381–388.

23. Mollica, R. F., Cardozo, B. L., Osofsky, H. J., Raphael, B., Ager, A., & Salama, P. (2004). Mental health in complex emergencies. *Lancet, 364*(9450), 2058–2067.

24. The Sphere Project. (2004). Minimum standards in health services. In *The Sphere handbook 2004: Humanitarian charter and minimum standards in disaster response* (pp. 249–312). Geneva: Oxfam Publishing.

25. The Sphere Project. (2004). Minimum standards in water supply, sanitation, and hygiene promotion. In *The Sphere handbook 2004: Humanitarian charter and minimum standards in disaster response* (pp. 51–102). Geneva: Oxfam Publishing.

26. The Sphere Project. (2004). Minimum standards in shelter, settlements, and non-food items. In *The Sphere handbook 2004: Humanitarian charter and minimum standards in disaster response* (pp. 203–248). Geneva: Oxfam Publishing.

27. UNHCR. (1995). *Refugee health.* Retrieved September 30, 2010, from http://www.unhcr.org/3ae68bf424.html.

28. Krasue, S. K., Meyers, J. L., & Friedlander, E. (2006). Improving the availability of emergency obstetric care in conflict-affected settings. *Global Public Health, 1*(3), 229–248.

29. Goma Epidemiology Group. (1995). Public health impact of Rwandan refugee crisis: What happened in Goma, Zaire, in July 1994? *Lancet, 345*(8946), 339–344.

30. Médicins Sans Frontiéres. *Pakistan—Activity Report 2006.* Retrieved March 29, 2015, from http://www.msf.org/pakistan-activity-report-2006.

31. Noji, E. K. (1997). Earthquakes. In E. K. Noji (Ed.), *The public health consequences of disasters.* New York: Oxford University Press.

32. Doctors Without Borders. (2010). *Emergency response after the Haiti earthquake: Choices, obstacles, activities and finance.* Retrieved October 1, 2010, from http://www.doctorswithoutborders.org/news-stories/special-report/emergency-response-after-haiti-earthquake-choices-obstacles-activities-0.

33. Suwanvanichkij, V., Murakami, N., Lee, C., et al. (2010). Community-based assessment of human rights in a complex humanitarian emergency: The Emergency Assistance Teams—Burma and Cyclone Nargis. *Conflict and Health, 4*(8).

34. Lateef, F. (2009). Cyclone Nargis and Myanmar: A wake up call. *Journal of Emergencies, Trauma, and Shock, 2,* 106–113.

35. BRAC. Pakistan: Health. Available at: http://www.brac.net/content/pakistan-health. Accessed August 17, 2010.

36. ICDDR, B Centre for Health and Population Research. (2004). Documenting effects of the July–August floods of 2004 and ICDDR, B's response. *Health and Science Bulletin, 2*(3), 1–6.

37. The Sphere Project. (2004). *The Sphere handbook 2004: Humanitarian charter and minimum standards in disaster response.* Geneva: Oxfam Publishing.

38. Spiegel, P., Sheik, M., Gotway-Crawford, C., & Salama, P. (2002). Health programmes and policies associated with decreased mortality in displaced people in postemergency phase camps: A retrospective study. *Lancet, 360*(9349), 1927–1934.

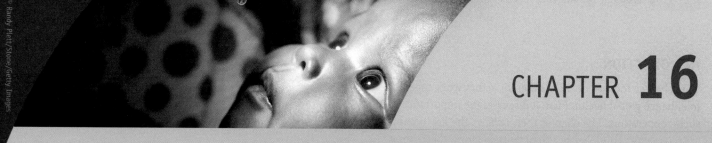

CHAPTER 16

Working Together to Improve Global Health

LEARNING OBJECTIVES

By the end of this chapter the reader will be able to:

- Discuss the value of cooperation in addressing global health problems
- Discuss the most important types of cooperative action in global health
- Describe the major organizational actors in global health and the focuses of their global health efforts
- Discuss the rationale for the creation of public–private partnerships for health
- Outline the key challenges to enhancing cooperative action in global health

VIGNETTES

The world came close to eradicating polio in 2004. However, in 2005, polio spread from northern Nigeria to a number of other African countries, due to the unwillingness of some people in northern Nigeria to immunize their children against polio. By July 2005, polio cases had moved from Africa to Saudi Arabia and Indonesia and then began appearing in Angola, which had not had a case of polio since 2001. By September 2005, cases appeared in Somalia, which had also been free of polio for several years.[1] Stopping new cases of polio and preventing it from spreading from one country to another requires a coordinated global effort.

In 2013, about 9 million people became ill with tuberculosis (TB) and 1.5 million died from it.[2] In fact, TB is one of the leading causes of adult deaths in low-income countries. Despite the importance of TB, however, few new TB

drugs have been developed since the 1960s.[3] TB is a disease that largely affects poor people in low- and middle-income countries. These people have little money to spend on drugs and there is minimal economic incentive for pharmaceutical companies to develop new TB treatments. Can actors in global health work together to encourage the development of new drugs for TB and other neglected diseases? What would they have to do to encourage public and private sector investment in such drugs? What would they have to do to ensure investors that if they are able to develop such drugs that there will be a market for them?

Vaccines are among the most cost-effective investments in health. The basic vaccines for children in low- and middle-income countries have been against six diseases: diphtheria, pertussis, tetanus, TB, measles, and polio. There are also other vaccines that are cost-effective in these countries, including the vaccines for hepatitis B and for *Haemophilus influenza* type B. Yet, throughout the 1990s there were important gaps in coverage of the six basic vaccines in the poorest countries. In addition, the rate of coverage of those vaccines was going down in some countries.[4] Moreover, although the hepatitis B vaccine began to be widely used in high-income countries in the 1980s, almost 20 years later it was still rarely used in low- and middle-income countries. The main reasons behind these gaps included limited money for immunization, a lack of the infrastructure needed to carry out effective immunization programs, and a lack of political interest in immunization. Could key global health actors work together to address gaps in vaccine coverage?

INTRODUCTION

This chapter focuses on how different actors work together to enhance global health. First, it discusses the importance of such cooperation. The chapter then reviews the key organizational actors in global health activities. Third, the chapter examines the roles in cooperation of different types of organizations. The chapter then outlines how the global health agenda is set and how that agenda has evolved historically. The chapter concludes with a number of policy and program briefs, case studies, and an assessment of some of the future challenges to cooperative action in global health.

COOPERATING TO IMPROVE GLOBAL HEALTH[5,6]

There are a number of reasons why different actors cooperate in global health activities and why such cooperation is in everyone's interest. First is the value of cooperating to create consensus around and advocate on behalf of different health causes. Although health is an extremely important issue for both individuals and societies, it does not always receive the political, economic, and financial support that it should. A good example of this is the lack of attention by many countries to nutrition, despite the poor nutritional status of their people. The impact of advocacy efforts is likely to be much greater if numerous actors, across organizations and across countries, work together to promote important health causes. This has been evident in the field of HIV/AIDS, for example, where AIDS activists worldwide have been able to work together to promote the treatment of people who are HIV-positive with antiretroviral drugs.

The need to share knowledge and to set global standards for health activities are other reasons for cooperation in the global health field. It has become clear from trials of different antimalarial drugs, for example, that some drug regimens for malaria are more effective than others. This knowledge is especially important because some malaria is resistant to what has been standard treatment. If lessons like this are to be shared globally, then it is important that technical standards be developed and disseminated by an organization that countries believe is technically sound and internationally representative. As you will read later, helping to define and promulgate such standards is one of the main functions of the World Health Organization.

Another important reason for cooperation to achieve global health aims is the fact that many aspects of global health are global public goods. Thus, it is only through cooperative efforts that the world can ensure that a sufficient amount of these goods is produced and shared. Individual countries, for example, may not have an interest in reducing pollution generated within their borders that causes health problems in adjacent countries, and it is only through collective action that countries will be able to address such problems. A similar issue arises with respect to efforts to reduce the burden of communicable diseases. Individual countries may have little incentive to take the measures needed to effectively address some communicable diseases, despite the fact that the spread of these diseases does not respect national boundaries. Efforts to deal with them, therefore, require cooperative efforts across countries.

The surveillance of disease also has many aspects of a global public good and requires cooperation among many actors to be successful. It is important for all countries to work together to monitor the presence of diseases and to fashion approaches to dealing with them. Surveillance by individual countries, for example, is not sufficient to stem the spread of disease *across* countries. The global effort to address the severe acute respiratory syndrome (SARS) problem in 2003 is an excellent example of the need for close collaboration among countries on surveillance.[7] The fact that Ebola spread more extensively in West Africa in 2014 and 2015 may indicate what happens when early cooperative action does not take place.

Cooperation to achieve better global health outcomes can also take place to assist in financing health efforts in poorer countries. There are multiple motivations for this aid. In one case, wealthier countries may contribute out of humanitarian concern for the well-being of less fortunate people. Richer countries may also wish to assist in addressing these problems because of enlightened self-interest. In an age of travel and extensive contacts among people of different countries, governments may be concerned that the health problems of low- and middle-income countries will endanger their own people if not properly tackled. Many low-income countries, for example, have high burdens of TB but may not have the financial, technical, or institutional resources needed to combat TB effectively. Yet, TB can endanger both their population and that of other countries. Thus, it is in everyone's interest for high-income countries to provide financial and technical assistance to low- and middle-income countries to deal effectively with diseases such as TB.

KEY ACTORS IN GLOBAL HEALTH

The number of actors in the global health arena has grown exponentially. Some of these are international organizations with a global reach. Others are organizations that work globally but are based in individual countries. Some are public organizations. A number are private and for-profit, whereas others are private but operate on a not-for-profit basis.

Foundations are also actively involved in global health activities. Increasingly, there are also organizations that bring the public and private sectors together to work cooperatively on a global health problem. The next section discusses some of the most important organizations that are involved in global health and examples of how they operate in that field.

There are so many actors in global health that it is necessary to think in terms of the type of organizations they represent and the kind of roles they play. **Table 16-1** lists a sample of the types of organizations involved in global health and selected organizations representing those types.

It is also important to consider the activities in which these organizations engage. They could, for example, participate in generating and sharing knowledge. They could engage in advocacy. They might be involved in the setting of technical standards or the provision of technical assistance. In addition, they might provide financing for health efforts. Generally, these organizations work along a continuum, engaging in one or more of the listed activities, but often specializing in only a few of them. When reviewing Table 16-1, readers should also be aware that some of the organizations could be placed into more than one category. The Center for Global Development, for example, does important advocacy work as well as research on global health policy.

Because of the enormity of the topic, this chapter can be only introductory. It is meant to provide an overview of the main types of actors in global health. It is largely descriptive and outlines the stated aims of the organizations that it covers. This chapter does not look critically at these organizations. Students interested in a more critical view may consult the extensive literature that is available on each of these organizations.[8–10]

Agencies of the United Nations

A number of United Nations (UN) agencies work on health and focus on a specific set of public health concerns. Among the most important are the World Health Organization (WHO), the United Nations Children's Fund (UNICEF), the United Nations Population Fund (UNFPA), and the United Nations Development Programme (UNDP). This section examines the three UN agencies most involved in health: the World Health Organization, the United Nations Children's Fund, and UNAIDS.

The World Health Organization

The World Health Organization was established in 1948 and is the United Nations agency that is responsible for health.[11] The headquarters of WHO is located in Geneva, Switzerland, and WHO employs about 7,000 people, including experts on many health topics. The World Health Organization has offices located in each region of the world, with special responsibility for work within that geographic area, as shown in **Table 16-2**. In addition, WHO has 150 field offices in different countries, regions, territories, and areas.[12]

The objective of WHO is to promote "the attainment by all peoples of the highest possible level of health."[11] In pursuit of this goal, WHO largely focuses its attention on the following:

- Advocacy and consensus building for various health causes, such as HIV/AIDS and TB.
- Generating and sharing health knowledge across countries, through studies, reports, conferences, and other forums. The publication of the *World Health Report* on a different topic of global health importance each year is an example of this work.
- Carrying out selected critical public health functions within an international forum, such as the surveillance of epidemics, including influenza, or the outbreak of other potentially dangerous diseases, such as Ebola.
- Setting global standards on key health matters, such as appropriate regimens for drug therapy for leprosy, TB, and HIV. This also includes, for example, WHO certification of quality standards for the manufacturing of vaccines and pharmaceuticals.
- Leading the development of international agreements and conventions, such as the Framework Convention on Tobacco Control and the International Health Regulations.
- The provision of technical assistance to its member states, such as helping China to contain the outbreak of SARS or assistance to countries in managing their child vaccine programs.
- Playing a critical role in of a number of cooperative efforts, such as Stop TB, Roll Back Malaria, and the Tropical Disease Research Program.

WHO is primarily a technical agency that engages in advocacy and the generation and sharing of knowledge. It also plays critical roles in the setting of technical standards and norms. Although WHO does have relatively small country budgets to assist in the financing of selected health projects in low- and middle-income countries, it is not a financing agency.

WHO is governed through its annual World Health Assembly, which sets policy, reviews and approves the budget, and appoints the director-general of the organization. Voting power at the WHO Health Assembly is based on the

TABLE 16-1 Selected Organizational Actors in Global Health, by Type of Organization

United Nations Agencies
UNAIDS
United Nations Development Programme (UNDP)
United Nations Population Fund (UNFPA)
United Nations Children's Fund (UNICEF)
World Health Organization (WHO)

International Health Programs
Gavi, The Vaccine Alliance
The Global Fund to Fight AIDS, TB, and Malaria

Multilateral Development Banks
African Development Bank
Asian Development Bank
Inter-American Development Bank
The World Bank

Bilateral Development Agencies
Australian Agency for International Development
   (AUSAID)
Danish International Development Agency (DANIDA)
Department for International Development of the
   United Kingdom (DFID)
Norwegian Agency for Development Cooperation
   (NORAD)
U.S. Agency for International Development (USAID)

Foundations
The Aga Khan Foundation
The Bill & Melinda Gates Foundation
The Clinton Foundation
The Rockefeller Foundation
The Wellcome Trust

WHO-Related Partnerships
Roll Back Malaria
Stop TB
Tropical Disease Research Program

Public–Private Partnerships for Health/Product Development Partnerships
Aeras
Global Alliance for TB Drug Development
International AIDS Vaccine Initiative
Malaria Vaccine Initiative

National Scientific Organizations
Canadian Institutes of Health Research
Institute of Tropical Medicine, Antwerp, Belgium
National Health and Medical Research Council, Australia
U.S. National Institutes of Health

Nongovernmental Organizations
BRAC
CARE
Catholic Relief Services
Doctors Without Borders
Oxfam
Partners in Health
Save the Children

Advocacy Organizations
Global Health Council
The ONE Campaign
RESULTS

Technical Organizations
International Union Against TB and Lung Disease
KNCV—The Dutch Tuberculosis Foundation
U.S. Centers for Disease Control and Prevention

Consulting Firms
Abt Associates
FHI 360
JSI
PSI

University-Affiliated Programs
Department of Global Health and Development, London
   School of Hygiene and Tropical Medicine
Global Health Leadership Institute, Yale University
Harvard Global Health Institute, Harvard University
Institute for Health Metrics and Evaluation, University
   of Washington
Institute for Global Health and Infectious Diseases,
   University of North Carolina

Think Tanks
Center for Global Development
Results for Development Institute

Human Rights Organizations
Amnesty International
Human Rights Watch
Physicians for Human Rights

TABLE 16-2 WHO Regional Offices

Regional Office	Location
The Americas	Washington, DC, USA
Europe	Copenhagen, Denmark
Eastern Mediterranean	Cairo, Egypt
Africa	Brazzaville, Congo
South-East Asia	Delhi, India
Western Pacific	Manila, Philippines

Data from World Health Organization. About WHO. Available at: http://www.who.int/about/en. Accessed September 13, 2014.

principle of one country–one vote. The overall budget of WHO comes from membership assessments and from voluntary contributions. The latter are mostly from better-off countries but the private sector and foundations also contribute to WHO.

Historically, WHO has helped lead some of the world's most important cooperative efforts in health, including the Health for All program[13] that began with the Declaration of Alma Ata on primary health care. WHO also led the world's smallpox eradication campaign, has played a major role in efforts to expand the coverage of immunization for children in low- and middle-income countries, and is one of the leaders of the world's global polio eradication initiative. More recently, WHO has been instrumental in helping to address issues of tobacco control. WHO also leads the global surveillance of disease and has played an active role in work on avian flu, H1N1 influenza, and SARS, among other emerging and reemerging diseases.

WHO has six priorities:[14]

- Universal health coverage
- The International Health Regulations (2005)
- Increasing access to medical products
- Social, economic, and environmental determinants of health
- Noncommunicable diseases
- Health-related Millennium Development Goals

There is extensive literature on WHO for those who are interested in understanding it in greater detail.

UNICEF

The United Nations Children's Fund was established in 1946 by the UN to respond to the effects of World War II on children in Europe and China. UNICEF is headquartered in New York but has offices in 190 countries.[15] The main function of UNICEF is to enhance the health and well-being of children. In these efforts, UNICEF has been deeply involved in the promotion of family planning, antenatal care, and safe motherhood practices.

UNICEF has an executive board of 36 members who guide all UNICEF work and administration under the leadership of the executive director. All of UNICEF's funding is from voluntary contributions. Governments provide two-thirds of funding, and 36 national committees, consisting of private entities and millions of individuals, raise the remaining third.[15] These national committees are nongovernmental organizations (NGOs) that advocate for children, sell UNICEF products, and raise funds through several well-known campaigns, such as Check out for Children in grocery stores, Change for Good on airplanes, and Trick or Treat for UNICEF on Halloween.[16]

UNICEF is involved in a wide range of activities in support of its mission, including advocacy, knowledge generation and knowledge sharing, and the financing of investments in health. In addition, UNICEF works closely with other development partners such as WHO and the World Bank to help raise the health status of poor women and children globally. UNICEF has carried out significant programs in a number of areas. Traditionally, it has been involved in critical ways in nutrition and early childhood development issues, in which it has generally been considered the world's leader. Immunization and child survival have also been areas of deep UNICEF involvement. In addition, UNICEF has been a major supporter of primary education, especially for poor girls in low- and middle-income countries. More recently, UNICEF has paid particular attention to child protection, child rights, and HIV/AIDS. UNICEF is also deeply involved in emergency relief work.[17]

UNICEF now has a number of focus areas:[18]

- Young child survival and development
- Basic education and gender equality
- HIV/AIDS and children
- Child protection from exploitation and abuse
- Advocacy and partnerships for child rights
- Humanitarian action

In 2013, UNICEF spent about $4.2 billion dollars on its programs and administrative costs.[18]

UNAIDS

In 1996, six agencies joined forces to launch UNAIDS—the Joint United Nations Program on HIV/AIDS. Today, as shown in **Table 16-3**, UNAIDS has 11 cosponsors.[19] The UNAIDS budget was $485 million for its 2014–2015 fiscal year.[20]

UNAIDS is based in Geneva, Switzerland, has offices in many countries in which it is involved, and is guided by a program coordinating board that consists of 22 representatives from country governments, its cosponsors, and 5 NGOs. UNAIDS is the global agency with primary responsibility for dealing with HIV/AIDS. UNAIDS monitors and evaluates the epidemic and the world's response to it. It also advocates on key HIV/AIDS issues and engages civil society, the private sector, and development partners in the fight against HIV/AIDS. In addition, UNAIDS generates and shares knowledge, sets standards, and mobilizes resources. UNAIDS focuses its attention on the regions of the world most affected by HIV/AIDS, particularly sub-Saharan Africa.[21]

Another important emphasis of the work of UNAIDS is to assist countries in developing and implementing national AIDS plans. Technical experts from UNAIDS also help countries build their technical and institutional capacity and mobilize resources to fight against HIV/AIDS. UNAIDS, for example, assists countries in preparing applications for funding from the Global Fund to Fight AIDS, TB, and Malaria, which is discussed further later.[21]

UNAIDS is engaged in a range of HIV/AIDS activities. First, UNAIDS works with countries to strengthen their surveillance of the epidemic. Second, UNAIDS continues to put an important emphasis on prevention of HIV. Third, UNAIDS is also increasingly involved in efforts to increase the number of HIV-positive people worldwide who are treated with antiretroviral therapy. UNAIDS has a particular concern for the extent to which the epidemic affects females and with reducing TB/HIV co-infection.[22] In addition, UNAIDS cooperates with others in the search for technologies, such as microbicides and vaccines, that might be able to help halt the epidemic.

Multilateral Development Banks

There are a number of development banks that lend or grant money to low- and middle-income countries and economies in transition to help promote their economic and social development. These banks are owned by all of their member countries and are referred to as "multilateral." These institutions have some characteristics of real banks; however, these banks do not function to earn money through their lending operations. Rather, their main focus is to serve as a financial intermediary. Essentially, they channel financial resources from high-income countries, through bond sales and grants, to help finance development activities in low- and middle-income countries and countries that are making the transition to more open, market-based economies. All of these banks are involved in work on health, to some degree, but the ones most involved are the African Development Bank, the Asian Development Bank, the Inter-American Development Bank, and the World Bank.

Among the multilateral development banks, the World Bank is the largest, has the broadest scope of activities, and is the most involved in health.[23] The World Bank is located in Washington, DC, and is owned by 187 member countries. The World Bank has about 10,000 staff that work in Washington and in a large number of other country offices.[24,25]

The stated aim of the World Bank is to assist countries in improving the lives of their people and reducing poverty. It seeks to do this by helping them to strengthen the management of their economy and to finance investments in selected areas, including agriculture, transport, private sector development, health, and education. The World Bank lends money at reduced rates to countries with per capita incomes below a certain point, lends money interest free to the poorest countries, and also provides grants to some countries for special activities that affect the poor, such as HIV/AIDS. The World Bank also has relatively generous time periods for repayment of these loans.

The World Bank supports a wide range of efforts in the health sector. It advocates on behalf of important causes, generates and disseminates information and knowledge about

---

TABLE 16-3 UNAIDS Cosponsors

- International Labor Organization
- Office of the United Nations High Commissioner for Refugees
- UNICEF
- United Nations Development Program
- United Nations Educational, Scientific, and Cultural Organization
- United Nations Population Fund
- United Nations Office on Drugs and Crime
- UN Women
- World Bank
- World Food Program
- World Health Organization

Data from UNAIDS. Available at: UNAIDS. UNAIDS Cosponsors. 2014; http://www.unaids.org/en/aboutunaids/unaidscosponsors/. Accessed September 13, 2014.

key health issues, provides technical assistance to countries, and finances specific investments in health and related work in nutrition and family planning. The World Bank focuses its health work largely on the links between health and poverty. It pays considerable attention to health financing, the development of health systems, and universal coverage. The World Bank has also emphasized investments in nutrition, maternal and child health, family planning, HIV/AIDS, malaria, and TB.

The World Bank is also a partner in a number of global health initiatives, including Gavi, Stop TB, Roll Back Malaria, and UNAIDS. In addition, the World Bank has provided financing to other initiatives, such as the International AIDS Vaccine Initiative (IAVI). The World Bank's total lending in its fiscal year 2013 was about $32 billion, of which about $2.41 billion was for health, nutrition, and population."[26,27] From its fiscal year 2005 to fiscal year 2014, total World Bank lending for health, nutrition, and population was more than $21 billion.[27] Until the advent of the Bill & Melinda Gates Foundation and the Global Fund to Fight AIDS, TB, and Malaria, the World Bank was, for many years, the largest provider of development financing for health. Those interested in a more analytical assessment of the World Bank's work both generally and in health can consult extensive literature on those subjects.

Bilateral Agencies

Another set of organizations that are very actively involved in global health are bilateral agencies. These are mostly the development assistance agencies of high-income countries that work directly with low- and middle-income countries to help them enhance the health of their people. Some of the bilateral development agencies that are most involved in the health sector are shown in **Table 16-4**.

USAID is the development assistance agency of the U.S. federal government. USAID promotes U.S. foreign policy goals by advancing economic and social development all over the world. USAID works with other governments and with universities, businesses, international agencies, and NGOs to support its development assistance efforts. In the health field, USAID engages in a wide variety of activities, including advocacy for global health, the generation and sharing of knowledge, and the financing of health investments.

USAID is headquartered in Washington, DC, and has regional field offices for sub-Saharan Africa, Asia, Latin America and the Caribbean, Europe and Eurasia, the Middle East, and Afghanistan and Pakistan. In addition to these geographic bureaus, USAID has functional bureaus for, among other things, economic growth and education, food security,

TABLE 16-4 Selected Bilateral Development Assistance Agencies Involved in Global Health

Australian Agency for International Development
Danish International Development Agency
Department for International Development of the United Kingdom
Dutch Agency for Development Cooperation
United States Agency for International Development

global health; and democracy, conflict, and humanitarian assistance. USAID has offices in many countries, especially poorer countries in Africa, Asia, and Latin America.[28]

USAID's Bureau for Global Health aims to improve health services and enhance the health status of poor and disadvantaged people, particularly in poorer countries. USAID focuses its health work on maternal and child health, HIV/AIDS, other communicable diseases, family planning and reproductive health, nutrition, and health systems. For these purposes, USAID provides grants and technical expertise to other governments, NGOs, and the private sector. In supporting the development of health in other countries, USAID collaborates with other development assistance agencies.[29]

In the 1970s and 1980s, USAID helped support research to develop a number of interventions that are key to saving the lives of poor children in low- and middle-income countries, including oral rehydration therapy, vitamin A supplementation, and immunizations. USAID has also been very supportive of efforts to address malaria, TB, HIV/AIDS, and, more recently, neglected tropical diseases. Traditionally, USAID has also been very involved in supporting family planning.

Foundations

Global health is an area in which foundations have been involved for almost a century. Many of the largest foundations support global health efforts, including, for example, the Ford, Hewlitt, MacArthur, Packard, and Soros Foundations. The Rockefeller Foundation has been among the foundations most involved in global health. The Wellcome Trust has also been engaged in global health activities, primarily through support for scientific research, for more than 70 years. More recently, the UN Foundation was established with a focus on health. The Clinton Foundation and the Bill & Melinda Gates Foundation have also become major actors in the global health arena. This section comments briefly on the health work of the Rockefeller and Gates foundations and the Wellcome Trust.

The Rockefeller Foundation

The Rockefeller Foundation is based in New York City and has offices in Bangkok, Thailand, and Nairobi, Kenya. The foundation aims to "promote the wellbeing of humanity throughout the world."[30] To do so, it seeks to advance health, revalue ecosystems, secure livelihoods, and transform cities.[30] In the health field, the foundation seeks to advance universal health coverage and foster more resilient and equitable health systems—all to enable people to lead healthier lives.[30]

The Rockefeller Foundation has focused considerable attention on the development of knowledge and technology that can be applied to addressing the conditions that most affect the health of the poor globally. The Rockefeller Foundation was instrumental in establishing the first schools of public health in the United States and was also deeply involved in the development of a vaccine against yellow fever. The Rockefeller Foundation does finance a small number of activities in health every year. However, its strength as an organization has been the way in which it uses a relatively small amount of money to invest in the generation of knowledge that can make an important difference to the health of the poor globally.

Over parts of the last 2 decades, the Rockefeller Foundation focused its attention in the health field in three areas. First, the foundation established the framework for developing partnerships between the public and private sectors to meet key health needs that had been neglected. In line with this work, the foundation was instrumental in establishing the first and then a number of additional public–private partnerships for health, including the International AIDS Vaccine Initiative, the International Partnership on Microbicides, and the Global Alliance for TB Drug Development. Second, it tried to help better understand the impact of HIV/AIDS on families and how they might deal with those impacts. Third, the foundation has helped to strengthen the production, deployment, and empowerment of key human resources needed for delivering health services in poor countries. The foundation has also supported improvements in disease surveillance.[31]

More recently, the Rockefeller Foundation has highlighted several initiatives with the aim of improving health

and nutrition. The first initiative aims at strengthening health system performance and expanding universal health coverage. The second aims to improve food security in Africa. The third seeks to enable the development of a private sector industry that can invest in improving social and environmental conditions.[32]

The Wellcome Trust

The Wellcome Trust was founded in London in 1936 with the vision of improving human and animal health through research. Its vision is "improve health by supporting bright minds in science, the humanities and social sciences, and public engagement."[33] It is the second largest charitable foundation in the world, behind the Bill & Melinda Gates Foundation. The trust directly employs about 500 staff and spends about $1.0 billion annually on charitable projects.[34,35]

The trust has a number of focus areas, including biomedical science, innovations, international research and capacity building, "bringing biology and medicine to new areas," supporting research at the interface of medicine, health-related science, and the humanities, and the social and ethical aspects of health and biomedical research.[36]

Although a majority of the independent researchers funded by the Wellcome Trust conduct their work in the United Kingdom, the foundation also funds programs in other countries.[37] Research is conducted either at independent institutions or institutes created by the foundation. The foundation is particularly well known for sequencing one third of the human genome, which has significantly enhanced our understanding of the genes associated with disease. In addition, research funded by the Wellcome Trust has uncovered genetic links to cancer and diabetes, paving the way for future treatments.

Out of the £746 million the trust spent between 2011 and 2012 on grants, direct funding for activities, and support,[37] about 11 percent went toward funding research in low- and middle-income countries.[38] The foundation focuses its international initiatives mainly in sub-Saharan Africa, South Asia, and central Europe and supports research in public health, including communicable and noncommunicable diseases, health services, health systems, and policy. The foundation also supports research in infectious diseases, specifically neglected tropical diseases, animal health, and emerging infections. The foundation invests in both clinical and biomedical research. The foundation has invested more in malaria than any other communicable disease, with £150 million going to malaria over the past 10 years.[39]

The Wellcome Trust has a strong track record in research for antimalarial drugs. In the early 1990s, scientists developed and tested the drug artemisinin in Vietnam and Thailand, which significantly decreased malaria mortality and the incidence of malaria. This drug is now the standard treatment for malaria, when used in combination with other antimalarial drugs.

In addition to funding biomedical research, the Wellcome Trust seeks to improve research facilities and broaden the base for scientific endeavors in low-income countries.[40] For example, the foundation invested £28 million from 2008–2009 in the African Institutions Initiative, which funds over 50 scientific institutions in 18 African countries.[41] In addition, the foundation invested £10 million in improving Kenya and Malawi's research and health policymaking institutions, in partnership with the United Kingdom Department for International Development and the International Development Research Centre, Canada.[42] In doing so, the goal of the Wellcome Trust has been to improve the capacity of low-income countries to do research and make informed health policy decisions.[42]

The Bill & Melinda Gates Foundation

One of the most substantial changes in the key actors involved in global health has been the advent of the Bill & Melinda Gates Foundation. The Gates Foundation is based in the United States in Seattle, Washington. The foundation seeks to help end hunger and extreme poverty.

Toward this aim, the foundation supports two areas of investment that relate most directly to health. The first is its global development work, which aims to help improve people's health and help people lift themselves out of poverty. The second is the global health work of the foundation, which "aims to harness advances in science and technology to save lives in developing countries."[43]

The global development work of the foundation supports investments in both the social determinants of health and directly in health. In support of broader development aims that relate most directly to health, the foundation supports research and investments in agriculture development; financial services for the poor; work on the integrated delivery of development investments; and investments in water, sanitation, and hygiene, including a program to reinvent the toilet.[43] The global development work of the foundation also supports a number of investments more directly related to health, including family planning; maternal, newborn, and child health; nutrition; polio; and vaccine delivery.[43]

The global health work of the foundation focuses on 7 areas:[43]

- Discovery and translational sciences
- Enteric and diarrheal diseases
- HIV
- Malaria
- Neglected infectious diseases
- Pneumonia
- Tuberculosis

The foundation has paid particular attention to supporting the spread of known technologies for improving health, such as immunization, to the places where they are most needed. It has also focused on encouraging the development of new technologies that can meet the most important health needs of the poor globally. The foundation seeks to meet these aims by working with partners to deliver proven tools, including vaccines, drugs, and diagnostics. It also seeks to enable the discovery of affordable, reliable, and innovative solutions to key global health problems that can be brought to those who need them most.[44]

In addition to the substantial funding that the foundation has provided for scientific discovery, the foundation has been a supporter of an array of global health organizations, programs, and projects. The foundation has been a major supporter, for example, of public–private partnerships for health since their inception, and has funded, among others, Aeras, IAVI, the Human Hookworm Vaccine Initiative, and the International Partnership on Microbicides. The foundation has provided considerable funding, as well, for reproductive health issues, such as a $60 million grant that it provided to Johns Hopkins University to improve reproductive health globally. The foundation has also supported major efforts in nutrition, with a focus on breastfeeding, micronutrients, and bio-fortification. The foundation was an early supporter of efforts to save newborn lives, partly through funding to Save the Children. In addition, the Gates Foundation has been a major and continuous financier of Gavi and the Global Fund. The foundation has also financed a major program to address HIV/AIDS in India.[45]

At the end of 2014, the Gates Foundation had an endowment of about $43.5 billion and the foundation is now one of the largest providers of financing for global health efforts. In 2013, the foundation supported total investments of about $3.6 billion, of which about $1.8 was in its global development portfolio and $1.1 billion was in its global health portfolio. Within the global development program, 24 percent of funds went to polio, 19 to vaccines, and 7 to each of family planning and maternal, newborn, and child health. Within the global health program, 21 percent went to HIV/AIDS, 17 to malaria, 14 to TB, and 10 to each of enteric diseases and diarrhea, pneumonia, and neglected tropical diseases.[46]

Research Funders

There are a number of organizations whose primary function is to carry out and fund research, some of which focuses on issues in global health. Although it is a foundation, the Wellcome Trust fits into this category. Funding research is also central to the work of the Gates Foundation. The Howard Hughes Medical Research Institute in the United States and the Institut Pasteur in France are also foundations that are deeply involved in medical research. However, many of the organizations focused on conducting and funding research are supported by national governments. The largest of these is the U.S. National Institutes of Health (NIH). Others include the National Health and Medical Research Council of Australia, the Canadian Institutes of Health Research, the Chinese Academy of Medical Sciences, the South African Medical Council, and the Medical Research Council of the United Kingdom. Some comments follow on the work in global health of the U.S. National Institutes of Health.

The U.S. National Institutes of Health[47]

The National Institutes of Health, part of the U.S. Department of Health and Human Services, is the primary federal agency for conducting and supporting medical research to improve human health. NIH fulfills its mission by performing biomedical and behavioral research in its own laboratories, supporting research conducted by scientists at major academic and research institutions in the United States and around the world, supporting the training of research investigators, and fostering communication of medical and health sciences information.

Research in global health is an integral part of the NIH agenda and one of five priorities for the institutes. As part of these efforts, the Fogarty International Center at NIH seeks to:[48]

- Build research capacity to meet present and evolving global health needs
- Stimulate innovation in technologies that can address global health problems
- Support research and research training in implementation science
- Strengthen research on prevention and control of communicable and noncommunicable diseases
- Build and strengthen partnerships to advance global health research

NIH-funded research, conducted both in the United States and in other countries, has yielded numerous discoveries with global health impact. For example, NIH has supported studies that have aided efforts to address HIV/AIDS.

These have included research on the effectiveness of male circumcision in the prevention of HIV transmission, simplified HIV combination antiretroviral therapies, and the use of nevirapine for prevention of mother-to-child transmission. During the 2009 H1N1 pandemic, NIH scientists played a crucial role in understanding the epidemiology of the H1N1 virus, which led to recommendations that influenza vaccination be targeted at young-to-middle-aged adults. NIH-supported studies conducted in Tanzania and South Africa demonstrated that unless drug treatment for tuberculosis is properly administered, tuberculosis can evolve rapidly to become resistant to available drugs. Another NIH-funded study conducted in Nigeria identified three genes that contribute to high fatality rates and insensitivity to treatment of breast cancer in African women compared with Caucasian women. The NIH has also assisted in the development of a new rotavirus vaccine that India is now adopting.[49]

NIH has also provided substantial support to scientific institutions in low- and middle-income countries that have emerged as research hubs in their own region. For example, in 1983, NIH began funding GHESKIO, a Haitian nongovernmental organization dedicated to clinical service, research, and training in HIV/AIDS and related diseases. In leading Haiti's response to the HIV/AIDS epidemic, GHESKIO is making significant contributions to the understanding of clinical presentation, epidemiology, and transmission of AIDS in that country, as well as in implementation of evidence-based models of care.

Similarly, NIH has supported the International Centre for Diarrhoeal Disease Research, Bangladesh (ICDDR,B) for more than 4 decades. ICDDR,B is a pioneer nonprofit organization that conducts research and is credited with, among other things, developing oral rehydration therapy, which has been used to treat millions of young children with diarrheal disease. In addition, the center has trained more than 20,000 researchers over the past 20 years.

Through the NIH Visiting Program, more than 2,000 foreign scientists conduct research and receive research training every year at NIH.[50] The institutes also support training programs that educate scientists from low- and middle-income countries to conduct health research relevant to their country, primarily through collaborative programs between research institutions in the United States and abroad.

Those wanting a more critical look at research funding for global health can consult the extensive literature on the conduct and financing of research to address the burden of disease in low- and middle-income countries. There is also a Global Forum for Health Research that pays particular attention to this matter.

Nongovernmental Organizations

There are thousands of NGOs in the world today that have as one of their primary aims the improvement of the health of poor people in low- and middle-income countries. Most of these organizations raise money from private sources or receive grants from governments or global health partnerships that they help to invest in activities that address important health issues, such as improving the availability of clean water, strengthening nutrition and immunization programs, or enhancing programs for the treatment of TB and HIV/AIDS. Some of the organizations are small and focus their attention on only a limited number of activities. Other organizations are very large, comprehensive in the topics they cover, and global in their reach. Some NGOs are completely secular, whereas others are faith based. Some of the most important NGOs that operate internationally on health are listed in **Table 16-5**.

Some additional comments are provided in the following sections on BRAC and Doctors Without Borders, two of the most important international NGOs that work on health globally. These are just a few examples of the hundreds of large NGOs that are involved in health efforts in low- and middle-income countries.

BRAC

BRAC was founded in Bangladesh in 1972. It is the largest NGO in the world that is involved in international development work, reaching 135 million people through its staff and volunteers. With the mission "to empower people and communities in situations of poverty, illiteracy, disease, and social injustice," BRAC is currently working in 11 countries in Asia and Africa, including Afghanistan, Bangladesh, Haiti, Liberia, Pakistan, the Philippines, Sierra Leone, Sri Lanka, South Sudan, Tanzania, and Uganda.[51]

TABLE 16-5 Selected Nongovernmental Organizations Involved in Global Health

BRAC
CARE
Catholic Relief Services
Doctors Without Borders
Partners in Health
Save the Children

BRAC was originally responsible for relief projects for refugees in rural northeastern Bangladesh but eventually turned its focus toward long-term development work. Its most established programs are in Bangladesh; however, the organization launched international initiatives in Asia in 2002 and in Africa in 2006.[52]

Broadly speaking, BRAC works in the areas of human rights and social empowerment, education and health, economic empowerment and enterprise development, livelihood training, environmental sustainability, and disaster preparedness.[53] In all its initiatives, women and children are the priority. BRAC is especially well known internationally for its work in reducing infant and child mortality through the spread of oral rehydration therapy, as well as the effectiveness of its community-based approach in other health areas, such as family planning and nutrition.

The main goals of BRAC's health initiatives are to improve maternal, neonatal and child health and decrease vulnerability to communicable diseases and common ailments.[54] Water and sanitation, family planning, immunization, obstetric care, basic services, and education for nutrition and health are some of the health issues BRAC targets. Additionally, the organization seeks to provide prevention and treatment for tuberculosis, malaria, pneumonia, and other common illnesses.[55] More recently, BRAC has developed an eye care program.[56]

The core of BRAC's health programs in Bangladesh is a community-based approach to primary health care, called "Essential Health Care (EHC)." Trained healthcare workers, *shasthya shebika,* are the force behind BRAC's Essential Health Care program that combines promotive, preventive, and basic curative services. These workers are locally recruited women and deliver door-to-door health services in rural areas. They provide health education for families and disseminate health and nutrition messages through health forums, household visits, and community meetings. In collaboration with the Bangladeshi government, BRAC's *shasthya shebika* also work in the areas of immunization, family planning, and basic pregnancy-related care. These workers also provide basic curative care for childhood pneumonia.

The *shasthya shebika* are volunteers who get trained by BRAC and who earn money from health work through the selling of drugs and basic health commodities to their patient population. As of 2013, BRAC was implementing this program in 64 districts, serving 120 million people.[57] Although most of BRAC's health work is done through community outreach, BRAC does operate 19 small clinics offering outpatient services, 11 larger clinics offering both inpatient and outpatient services, and 3 large hospitals.[58]

BRAC is also deeply involved in work on TB, malaria, and nutrition. BRAC heads a consortium of local NGOs that work with the government in promoting TB messages in the community, identifying suspected TB cases, referring patients for testing, and helping to ensure they complete their treatment. BRAC's TB work covers a population of almost 93 million people.[59] For malaria, BRAC's frontline workers provide health education, identification of cases, treatment of simple cases, and referral of complicated cases. They also promote the use of insecticide-treated bednets. BRAC's malaria efforts were associated between 2008 and 2013 with a 90 percent reduction in malaria deaths in Bangladesh.[60]

BRAC has long been involved and known for its work on nutrition, which aims at promoting early and exclusive breastfeeding, community-based treatment of acute malnutrition, the promotion of nutrition in adolescent girls, and nutrition counseling services for pregnant and lactating women. Much of this work is based on home visits by BRAC workers.[61] BRAC also makes and promotes the use of micronutrient powders to reduce anemia and other micronutrient deficiencies. These are sold to most families who can afford them and provided free to indigent families.[62]

Given the evolving burden of disease, BRAC community health workers are increasingly involved in promoting healthy lifestyles, monitoring their patient population for hypertension and diabetes, and referring those people with suspected problems. They also provide follow-up with patients who are under treatment.[63] BRAC's community-based health workers also now carry out vision screening, provision of eyeglasses where appropriate, and referral for those who need it.[64]

BRAC's business model is largely based on raising money from earnings in a variety of social enterprises to help cover the costs of its programs that do not earn revenue. The revenue earning activities include its microfinance program, as well as its social enterprises, which create jobs for poor people in local communities and provide production or marketing support for the enterprises of its microfinance clients. BRAC's social enterprises include selling handicrafts, dairy products, agricultural products, and printing supplies, among other goods. Some enterprises produce a commodity that will aid in improving the health of the community, such as iodized salt in Bangladesh.[65] BRAC's total expenditures in 2013 were about $545 million, of which about 10.5 percent was invested in health activities and 3.6 percent in water, sanitation, and hygiene.[66]

Doctors Without Borders

Doctors Without Borders is usually referred to by its French name, Médicins Sans Frontières, or by the abbreviation of that name, MSF. Doctors Without Borders was founded in 1971 and has an international office in Geneva, Switzerland. It is an umbrella organization made up of affiliated groups in 19 countries. The groups located in Belgium, France, Holland, Spain, and Switzerland carry out health work in more than 70 countries.[67]

Doctors Without Borders is best known for its work in humanitarian crises. It has often been involved in the provision of health services following natural disasters, such as earthquakes and hurricanes, or those humanitarian emergencies related to war and famine.[67] MSF, for example, assisted Nicaragua after an earthquake, Ethiopia during a famine, and Somalia after a war. MSF has also been extensively engaged in health services for refugees and displaced people. In addition, when health services have been severely weakened due to war or conflict, MSF often helps to provide health services temporarily, while trying to help rebuild health system capacity. One example of this was in Liberia after its civil war.

MSF is also involved in a range of nutrition and disease control efforts and efforts to increase access to essential medicines. MSF has also become very involved with prevention, care, and treatment for HIV/AIDS. In this work, MSF has helped to mobilize international support for antiretroviral therapy in poor countries and has become a leader in trying to lower the price of those drugs.[67] Most recently, MSF has been very deeply involved in the 2014–2015 Ebola outbreak in West Africa, where for some time it provided a very substantial share of assistance to the affected countries.[68]

MSF is well known for its commitment to political independence, medical ethics, and human rights. Related to this, MSF has increasingly sought to become a voice in international health policy arenas for the disenfranchised.

Advocacy Organizations

A number of organizations focus their efforts on advocating on behalf of global health issues. Generally, these organizations carry out research and policy studies and then use these and evidence generated by others to carry out advocacy activities for key stakeholders, including the public at large, funding agencies, and national legislatures and governments. Many of these organizations are membership organizations, in whole or in part. Some of these organizations may be aligned with a specific issue, such as the many organizations of this type that focus on HIV/AIDS. These include for example, the International AIDS Alliance and the AIDS Vaccine Advocacy Coalition. Others may work on a cluster of issues, such as communicable diseases. The Global Network on Neglected Tropical Diseases, as another example, focuses an important part of its work on advocacy but also helps to raise funds to address neglected tropical diseases (NTDs) and coordinates some NTD efforts. Other advocacy organizations, however, address a broader range of global health topics. Examples of the better-known advocacy organizations that address a range of issues are the ONE Campaign, RESULTS, and the Global Health Council. Additional comments on the Global Network for Neglected Tropical Diseases are given in the policy and program briefs section of this chapter.

Think Tanks and Universities

A number of organizations focus at least part of their efforts on generating knowledge about key issues in global health. Among the best known of these is the Center for Global Development, based in Washington, DC. The center has a number of staff that are experts in various global health topics. The center carries out an extensive research program on global health, publishes widely on global health matters, and hosts and participates in a wide array of seminars to disseminate the information that it has generated and to highlight important findings by others. The Results for Development Institute, also in Washington, DC, is another think tank that is actively involved in research on policy and program issues in global health. It has recently carried out important work, for example, on the long-term financing of HIV/AIDS in a number of countries. It also focuses important attention on universal health coverage and on innovative approaches to addressing key global health issues. The Center for Strategic and International Studies, also in Washington, DC, has also become involved in a number of ways in global health policy matters.

As interest in global health has spread and the financing for global health has increased, many universities throughout the world have become more involved in teaching, research, and practice on global health issues. Many universities with a public health school, and even some without, have created centers or institutes that bring researchers together from different parts of the university to work on global health. Yale University, for example, has the Global Health Leadership Institute under which it organizes many of its activities in global health. Harvard University has the Harvard Institute for Global Health, which is meant to play an important role in enabling Harvard's work on education and research in global health. The University of Toronto has the Centre for Global Health Research. Many universities also carry out considerable technical assistance for the design, monitoring, and evaluation of global health programs and projects; some universities have established what are essentially consulting firms to engage in this work.

Consulting Firms

A wide array of consulting firms engage in global health work, either as the main focus of their work or as an important part of their activities. Some of these firms are for-profit, such as Abt Associates. Others, however, operate on a not-for-profit basis, such as FHI 360, MSH, JSI, and PSI. Some of the firms may have a broad range of expertise and be able to work, for example, on key management, economic, financing, or policy issues, as well as on critical health programs, such as maternal and child health or the control of communicable diseases. Others, however, have a particular area of expertise, such as supply chain management, nutrition, behavior change communication, or social marketing. Low- and middle-income countries sometimes hire these firms directly; however, the majority of such services provided to low-income countries will be financed by development assistance agencies such as the World Bank, USAID, or DFID. In fact, a substantial share of the development assistance from some agencies, such as USAID, is channeled through consulting firms. The staff of consulting firms is often quite involved in policy work and in program design, monitoring, and evaluation, especially in low-income countries with relatively limited technical capacity of their own.

Specialized Technical Organizations

A number of specialized governmental and nongovernmental technical organizations are important actors in global health. Perhaps the best known of these is the U.S. Centers for Disease Control and Prevention (CDC), based in Atlanta, Georgia. The CDC is part of the U.S. Department of Health and Human Services. Several years ago, CDC stated that its mission is to:

> collaborate to create the expertise, information, and tools that people and communities need to protect their health—through health promotion, prevention of disease, injury and disability, and preparedness for new health threats.[69]

The CDC is deeply involved in helping the United States and other countries to plan and carry out disease surveillance, prevention, and control, across a broad range of disease conditions. CDC staff, for example, collaborate with many countries in work on communicable disease control programs, such as those for HIV, TB, and malaria. In addition, CDC staff are often called upon to assist WHO and individual countries to identify disease threats and address them. This could be for outbreaks of dengue, the Ebola virus, the plague, or other diseases of national and international importance. The CDC has a team of field epidemiologists that are at the forefront of such work and CDC also provides extensive laboratory services to its collaborators. The CDC has also been very involved in technical assistance to build capacity in low- and middle-income countries for improved disease surveillance, prevention, and control, including the strengthening of laboratories.

Two other specialized technical organizations of importance are both nongovernmental and work on TB. KNCV is the Dutch TB foundation and is based in The Hague, the seat of government of the Netherlands.[70] KNCV aims to help address TB both in the Netherlands and in low- and middle-income countries by providing technical assistance in the development and implementation of TB control programs. The International Union Against Tuberculosis and Lung Disease (IUATLD), which is based in Paris, France, is a membership organization that is also deeply involved in TB control efforts.[71] The union has a number of regional offices and works not only on TB, but also on lung health more broadly. Both KNCV and the union have staff with high levels of expertise in all aspects of TB control. Both have been deeply involved in helping many countries to address TB more effectively and efficiently and to build national capacity for addressing TB in the future.

Partnerships Related to WHO

Some global health problems affect an exceptional number of people in a large number of countries. The costs of addressing these problems are great and the skills needed to combat them are substantial. Most of the resource-poor countries cannot tackle these problems without assistance and no individual development partner can provide enough assistance to help deal effectively with the scale of these problems. Therefore, a number of organizations have decided to work together to help address some of the most important burdens of disease. Some of the partnerships that have ensued are closely related to WHO, as noted in **Table 16-6**. Two of the most important such partnerships are Stop TB and Roll Back Malaria.

Stop TB

The Global Partnership to Stop TB was established in 2001. It aims to "eliminate TB as a public health problem, and ultimately, to obtain a world free of TB."[72] Following the

---

TABLE 16-6 Selected WHO-Related Partnerships for Global Health

Global Polio Eradication Initiative
Lymphatic Filariasis Control Program
Roll Back Malaria
Stop TB
Tropical Disease Research Program

Millennium Development Goals (MDGs), it has sought by 2015 to help reduce TB deaths and prevalence by 50 percent compared to 1990 levels. It seeks by 2050 to help reduce prevalence below one person for every million.[73]

Stop TB is composed of 1,300 partners, including countries, development agencies, private sector organizations, and NGOs. WHO plays a prominent role in Stop TB, and the secretariat for the partnership is housed at the United Nations Office for Project Services (UNOPS) in Geneva, Switzerland.

The primary goals of Stop TB are to:[73]

- Ensure that everyone who needs it gets proper diagnosis and treatment
- Stop TB transmission
- Reduce the social and economic costs of TB
- Encourage the development of diagnostics, drugs, and vaccines for TB

The partnership also leads a number of initiatives related to TB, in addition to substantial advocacy on TB. One effort is a grant program to encourage civil society involvement in TB. Stop TB also oversees the Global Drug Facility, which assists countries in procuring high-quality TB medicines at the best possible prices. Stop TB also manages the TB Reach program, aimed at helping to increase TB case detection in low-income settings. Stop TB has several ongoing working groups that aim to encourage progress in key TB areas, such as the expansion of directly observed therapy, short course (DOTS); addressing drug-resistant TB; dealing with TB/HIV co-infection; new TB diagnostics; TB drugs; TB vaccines; laboratories; and TB and human rights.[74]

Roll Back Malaria

Roll Back Malaria was founded in 1998 by WHO, UNDP, UNICEF, and the World Bank to advocate for malaria control, to promote the development of better and more coordinated approaches and technologies for malaria containment, and to help finance and spread appropriate malaria control and treatment.[75] The partnership has expanded since then to include hundreds of public and private actors in a number of countries, who are organized in eight constituencies. The partnership is housed at WHO in Geneva, Switzerland. Roll Back Malaria's vision is to ensure that the world stays below pre-2015 levels of malaria and that in the long term, malaria is eradicated.[76]

The partnership oversees a Commodities Service that assists countries in procuring at the best prices possible the high-quality equipment, materials, and drugs needed for their malaria programs. Stop TB also has a number of working groups on key issues, including advocacy, communication, harmonization, vector control, procurement and supplies management, case management, monitoring and evaluation, and malaria in pregnancy. Roll Back Malaria is also linked with four subregional networks of African countries.[77]

Other Partnerships and Special Programs

In the mid- and late-1990s, a number of global health actors expressed concern about gaps in addressing health issues that affected the poor in low- and middle-income countries. One was the need to strengthen immunization programs for children and for pregnant women. The second was the need to make more rapid progress against HIV/AIDS, TB, and malaria. To address immunization more effectively, the Global Alliance for Vaccines and Immunisation (GAVI), now called Gavi, the Vaccine Alliance, was established. The Global Fund to Fight AIDS, TB, and Malaria, referred to as the Global Fund, was established to make more rapid progress against HIV, TB, and malaria.

Gavi

Gavi is a partnership among public and private sector organizations that was established in 2000.[4] The founding partners of Gavi included WHO, UNICEF, and the World Bank. Gavi is based in Geneva, Switzerland. The Bill & Melinda Gates Foundation made a major grant to help establish Gavi and provide for its operations. Today, about 70 percent of Gavi's funding comes as grants from governments and from philanthropists. About 30 percent comes from innovative financing mechanisms, such as the International Financing Facility for Immunization and the Advance Market Commitment.[78]

Gavi seeks to make vaccines more accessible, affordable, and sustainable. With this in mind, Gavi supports the efforts of eligible countries to strengthen health systems, enhance country capacity to manage and operate vaccine programs, engage civil society in improving immunization activities, and increase the use of new and underused vaccines.[79]

Gavi has tried to improve global health work through two innovative approaches. The first is to tie its financing to the achievement of goals that are agreed to by the countries with which Gavi is working. The second is to work closely with countries to develop plans to sustain the investments that are being supported. Gavi is an organization that advocates for the importance of immunization, provides technical assistance to countries to enhance their immunization efforts, and finances those efforts. Gavi also works internationally to try to ensure that vaccine markets are developing in a way that can get high-quality vaccines in the numbers needed at affordable prices to low- and middle-income countries.

By 2015 Gavi had supported the immunization of more than 500 million children, which had averted more than 7 million deaths. Gavi aims by 2020 to support the vaccination of an additional 300 million children, averting an additional 5–6 million deaths.[80]

The Global Fund

The Global Fund to Fight AIDS, TB, and Malaria was also established in 2002 and is based in Geneva, Switzerland.[81] The driving force behind the establishment of the fund was increasing global concern about HIV/AIDS and an increasing recognition among development partners that measures to address the HIV/AIDS epidemic had been insufficient. Interest in establishing the Global Fund was also heightened by the growing attention to global health more generally, and a special concern for the burden of HIV/AIDS, TB, and malaria in Africa.[82]

The Global Fund is a partnership of the public and private sectors; WHO, UNAIDS, and the World Bank are also key partners. The Global Fund is governed by a board of directors that represents governments, international organizations, civil society, and communities affected by HIV/AIDS, TB, and malaria. The fund is financed by grants that come largely from high-income country governments but also from the private, foundation, and philanthropy sectors, including the Bill & Melinda Gates Foundation.

The Global Fund is primarily a financing agency, but it also engages in advocacy and policy work for global health and the three diseases on which it focuses. The main aim of the fund is to finance proposed investments in these diseases, with an emphasis on HIV/AIDS and Africa. It has had a particular interest in helping to scale up programs for antiretroviral therapy against HIV/AIDS. The fund has taken innovative approaches to a number of aspects of development assistance for health, including the following:[81]

- It is strictly a financing mechanism and not a technical or implementing agency.
- It seeks to raise funds for investments that will be additional to other funding already available.
- It tries to work on the basis of a national plan that is developed by a group representing diverse national interests.
- It evaluates proposals through an independent review process.
- It tries to operate in a performance-based manner by supporting investments that are meeting their targets and reducing or eliminating support for programs that are not meeting their aims.

The Global Fund also assists countries in enhancing the effectiveness and efficiency of their procurement of equipment, materials, supplies, and drugs related to their programs for HIV/AIDS, TB, and malaria. This work focuses on helping countries to improve the planning of procurement, sharing information on prices, maintaining quality assurance standards, and helping them engage in lower cost purchasing through a pooled procurement mechanism.[83]

In 2013, the Global Fund committed more than $29 billion to support large-scale prevention, treatment, and care programs against HIV/AIDS, TB, and malaria and to help the countries it supports to strengthen their health systems. Sixteen billion was for HIV/AIDs, $8 billion for malaria, $4.6 billion for TB, and $750 million for strengthening health systems.[84]

Public–Private Partnerships

As interest in global health rose in the mid-1990s, many of the actors in this field increasingly believed that the mechanisms for developing, manufacturing, and distributing new vaccines, drugs, diagnostics, and medical devices needed to alleviate key global health problems were not sufficient. They noted with growing concern, for example, that the vaccine for TB was over 100 years old and that no new TB drugs had been developed for decades. They saw insufficient attention to the development of vaccines against HIV and malaria in both the public and the private sector and fewer firms willing to engage in vaccine development. They also understood that private pharmaceutical firms did not see a profitable market in the development of low-cost diagnostics, vaccines, drugs, or medical devices that could address the major killers of the poor globally. They knew that without changes in the way the market for these products worked that private sector firms would remain on the sidelines.

In the face of these issues, the Rockefeller Foundation encouraged key global health actors to think creatively about how they could spur the more rapid development of products that could attack global health problems in a low-cost but effective way. One idea that emerged from this was the notion of organizations that would combine the strengths of public and private organizations in a common quest for better health. They would also seek broader sources of financing for these health ventures; try to tackle intellectual property issues that constrained the availability of affordable diagnostics, drugs, medical devices, and vaccines in poor countries; and see how they could encourage more private sector involvement in the search for these products. In some respects, they were conceived of as venture capital firms that would have a social goal rather than a goal that was mostly aimed at maximizing profit. Today, there is a wide array of public–private partnerships for health. The aim of many of

these is to develop new products, and these are often called product development partnerships. Some of the most important of such partnerships are noted in **Table 16-7**. Additional information is provided about the Global Alliance for TB Drug Development in the policy and program briefs section of this chapter.

Pharmaceutical Firms

International pharmaceutical firms have been engaged for several decades in partnerships to try to improve global health at low cost. This has generally been done in one of three ways. First, some firms donate drugs to global health programs. Novartis, for example, donates leprosy drugs to the Global Alliance to Eliminate Leprosy, and today no country needs to purchase such drugs.[85] Pfizer and the Edna McConnell Clark Foundation work with the International Trachoma Initiative by donating an antibiotic, azithromycin, to its efforts to reduce trachoma-related blindness.[86] Merck donates ivermectin to the Onchocerciasis Control Program, which has been successful in reducing river blindness in Africa.[87] These are only some of the many donation efforts now under way.

In addition, a number of drug companies, including Abbott, Boehringer Ingelheim, Bristol Myers Squibb, Gilead, GSK, and Merck, have agreed to sell antiretroviral drugs for HIV/AIDS at greatly discounted prices to low- and middle-income countries affected by the HIV/AIDS epidemic. Some of the drug companies also sponsor programs to address diseases such as HIV/AIDS in particular countries, such as Merck's support for the national HIV/AIDS control program in Botswana.[88] The Eli Lilly Corporation supports a program that helps to address drug-resistant TB.

The role of the major drug companies in global health is a subject of considerable controversy. There is a concern

TABLE 16-7 Selected Public–Private Partnerships for Public Health

Aeras
Global Alliance for TB Drug Development
Human Hookworm Vaccine Institute
International AIDS Vaccine Initiative
International Partnership for Microbicides
Malaria Vaccine Initiative
Medicines for Malaria Venture

among some members of the global health community, for example, that the approach of the branded drug manufacturers to patents raises the price of drugs beyond what people in low- and middle-income countries can afford. Some people also believe that the major manufacturers should be far more generous than they have been in offering their drugs at reduced prices in low- and middle-income countries. Others have expressed concern that these manufacturers have not been open enough in licensing their products to other companies in a way that would reduce their prices in low- and middle-income countries. The role of pharmaceutical firms in global health is very important, complicated, and controversial and goes considerably beyond the scope of this text.

TRENDS IN GLOBAL HEALTH EFFORTS

The notion of cooperating to improve health globally is not a new one. Rather, different countries have realized for more than 100 years that many health problems could not be solved by individual countries and had to be addressed through collective action across countries.

In the ensuing period, in fact, many actors have cooperated in a variety of health activities. This section examines how the themes of those efforts varied over time. The threat of cholera, for example, led to the first international conference on health in 1851.[9] Numerous international conferences on health followed, and by 1903, the International Commission on Epidemics was created.[9] In 1909, the International Office of Public Hygiene was set up in Paris, followed by the establishment of the League of Nations Health Office in 1920 in Geneva, Switzerland. The International Sanitary Bureau was set up in 1924. The Rockefeller Foundation assisted in financing and providing technical support to the League of Nations Health Office. The early international organizations for health focused their efforts on the surveillance of disease, the provision of global standards for drugs and vaccines, and selected technical advice to countries on key health matters, including medical education.[9]

International efforts in health took a substantial leap forward with the establishment of the United Nations agencies after World War II, including WHO and UNICEF. In the more than 60 years since there have been a number of areas of focus for international cooperation on health, as noted hereafter.[5,9,89] Following the establishment of WHO, efforts at international cooperation in health shifted to focus on helping to build capacity for global public health efforts, for health systems development in countries that were newly independent, and in working together to fight disease. Perhaps the greatest single effort at global cooperation in health began in 1966 with the start of the global program to eradicate smallpox. During this period of intensive attention to specific diseases, WHO also led work to combat malaria and other communicable diseases of special importance for the poor, such as leprosy,[90] lymphatic filariasis,[91] and onchocerciasis.[89,92]

Historically, another important area of focus for global cooperation has been family planning. Much of the early work on family planning was led by the United States. Over time, the focus on family planning shifted from one that was centered almost exclusively on limiting family size to an approach that centered much more on reproductive health. This shift was encouraged by and reflected in a series of global conferences on family planning, safe motherhood, reproductive health, and women starting in 1974 in Bucharest, Romania.[93] The 1987 conference on women in Nairobi, Kenya, for example, was used to launch the Safe Motherhood Initiative.[89]

In 1978, the world launched a major effort when it produced the Alma Ata declaration on primary health care, as mentioned earlier. This declaration noted that health was a fundamental human right and that countries had the obligation to ensure that all people had access to appropriate primary health care. The Alma Ata declaration heralded a new global focus on primary health care and on the health needs of the poor. It also led to much greater attention to the needs for health systems that could deliver primary care and to the importance of taking a community-based approach to the health needs of poor people. The Alma Ata Declaration was linked to the world's efforts to achieve what was called globally, "Health for all by the Year 2000."[94]

An immense amount of attention has also been paid to child survival. Early effort was focused on what were called the GOBI interventions: growth monitoring, oral rehydration, breastfeeding, and immunization. UNICEF was the leader of this effort. USAID has also been instrumentally involved in child survival activities, which ultimately became an important focus of attention for the World Bank, WHO, and a variety of bilateral organizations.[5]

As the world moved into the late 1980s and early 1990s, considerable concern arose that despite more than 30 years of global efforts to improve the health of the poor, the unfinished agenda remained very large. Many of those working on health believed that some of the weaknesses stemmed from an approach to health that was too disjointed and that needed to be better grounded in a more systemic view of health that would focus on trying to improve health services more broadly. This led to considerable work being done on health sector reform. At the same time, the *1993 World Development Report* of the World Bank articulated the need to take an approach to decision making on health investments that would be grounded in cost-effectiveness analysis.[95] This framework for analysis soon became the foundation for actions of a number of key actors in global health.

At about the same time, much greater attention began to be paid, even in low-income countries, to the role of the private sector in health. Development partners also created new ways of working together cooperatively within individual countries. Increasingly, for example, development partners would cooperate and jointly help countries to develop and finance investments in health. In much of the work done prior to this period, many development partners worked individually with a country, often leading to a lack of coordination across that country's health sector efforts.

Toward the mid-1990s, the global health community began to pay considerably more attention to HIV/AIDS, as well as to other major killers of the poor in resource-poor countries, including malaria and TB. Particular attention has been paid since then to reducing the cost of AIDS drugs and getting more people treated, raising case finding and cure rates for TB by expanding coverage with DOTS, and strengthening malaria control programs through the use of insecticide-treated bednets, intermittent treatment of pregnant women, more rapid and confirmed diagnosis, and greater use of artemisinin-based combination therapy. There has also been an enormous increase in cooperation through the many health partnerships that have been formed, as noted earlier in the chapter.

More recently there has been a renewed emphasis on some of the topics noted previously, greater interest in others, and considerable attention paid to how countries and their partners work together to enhance health. Driven partly by the Millennium Development Goals, whose targets are for 2015, greater attention is now being paid, for example, to nutrition and maternal health. Considerable effort is being expended to complete polio eradication, which has proven to be more difficult than planned, and attention to measles and the possibility of its eradication has also grown. Much greater attention is being paid than previously to the neglected tropical diseases and how they can be addressed in more coherent ways. There is growing concern about drug-resistant TB and the need to ensure that tools exist to diagnose it more rapidly and treat it more effectively. In fact, there is also much greater focus than ever on the development of new diagnostics, drugs, and vaccines that can address the most important burdens of disease of poor people in poor countries. At the same time, substantial efforts are being directed to helping countries to develop more effective and efficient health systems that can provide universal coverage of key health services in more effective and efficient ways and afford more financial protection to their people from the costs of health care.

Much attention is also being paid to how development partners and countries can work together to achieve these aims, particularly in low-income countries. Increasing focus has been placed on ensuring that development assistance for health is harmonized and aligned with development partners working together on a common platform in each country and ensuring that the processes they use follow the processes of the countries with which they are working. There is also an emphasis on how countries can more effectively and efficiently achieve the intended results from their investments in health, through mechanisms such as results-based financing. Important attention is also being paid to how the investments needed to improve health in low- and middle-income countries, particularly among the poor, can be financed, especially in times of global economic distress. One of these initiatives for addressing this issue, UNITAID, is discussed further in the policy and program briefs section of this chapter.

SETTING THE GLOBAL HEALTH AGENDA

As we think about how different actors cooperate in global health activities and the themes on which they focus, it is important to consider how global health policies get established. This section comments briefly on how the overall global health agenda and the agenda for particular global health topics are set. This is another topic that is quite complicated and often the subject of controversy that readers may wish to explore further.

One important activity in setting global health priorities is the World Health Assembly of the World Health Organization.[96] Once each year, ministers of health of WHO member countries meet in Geneva, Switzerland, to consider important global health matters and resolutions proclaiming their interest in and commitment to addressing key health issues. The World Health Assembly has been the foundation for some of the most important global health efforts undertaken, such as the smallpox eradication campaign.

Some important developments in global health have been encouraged by writings, advocacy efforts, and program activities of WHO, multilateral or bilateral development assistance agencies, and some of the important NGOs involved in health. The *1993 World Development Report* of the World Bank focused on health and was widely read and debated around the world. This document set the basis for the next generation of World Bank-assisted health projects in many countries and for important work done by other development organizations and countries in health, as well. Given the importance of World Bank assistance for health to so many countries, the approaches suggested in the *1993 World Development Report* had a major impact on the world's thinking about health in low- and middle-income countries.

Movement in the policy agenda for global health can also follow significant investments by development partners. This has clearly been the case, for example, as a result of the substantial funds that the Bill & Melinda Gates Foundation has provided to selected global health activities. As noted earlier, the Gates Foundation has focused considerable attention on improving and disseminating technology for improving the health of the poor, as well as selected investments in key health problems, such as HIV/AIDS. The investments the Gates Foundation has made, for example, in immunization and in the development of AIDS vaccines has considerably raised the world's attention to these matters and placed them more firmly on the global health agenda.

Popular action, often led by NGOs or other advocates for health, can also influence the setting of the global health agenda. In the late 1990s, for example, Professor Jeff Sachs, then of Harvard University, began to be actively involved in speaking and writing about the importance of health to economic and social development. His work attracted attention to health issues and led to considerable international engagement and action on the health of poor people globally. At about the same time, some important NGOs, such as Doctors Without Borders, became major advocates for AIDS treatment and the reduction of the prices of AIDS drugs. Their advocacy work and efforts to treat people with antiretroviral drugs, and the efforts of people within the affected countries, attracted considerable attention to these topics and had a major impact on the way the world approached them.

Another good example of how an NGO affected the global health agenda is the impact of Partners in Health, an NGO based in Boston, Massachusetts, in the United States, on the global agenda for TB and for HIV/AIDS. Largely led by the work of Dr. Paul Farmer and Dr. Jim Kim of Harvard University, Partners in Health tried to develop in Peru and Haiti a model of how one could treat drug-resistant TB and then HIV/AIDS at an acceptable cost and in a sustainable way. At the time, the prevailing opinion globally was that drugs for these conditions were so expensive that they could not be used in resource-poor settings. The work of Partners in Health helped to shift global efforts toward finding ways to make treatment affordable for all people.[97]

In other respects, one can think of efforts to set the global health agenda as a kind of ongoing meeting around a negotiating table at which important actors in global health are sitting. The organizations most involved in such discussions will generally be WHO, UNICEF, and the World Bank.

Selected bilateral development agencies will also participate, such as USAID, the Department for International Development of the United Kingdom, and the Norwegian Development Agency. AusAID plays a unique role in some of Asia in the Pacific. The Global Fund has been increasingly involved in policy discussions, as its portfolio has grown, as has UNAIDS, as HIV/AIDS has become more important. The Gates Foundation, the Rockefeller Foundation, and selected NGOs might also participate in setting the agenda. Some other NGOs, such as MSF, may not be present, but through advocacy they do bring their interests to the policy-setting group.

The way in which the agenda is set for specific health topics will be similar to those mentioned previously but will usually also include actors who have particular interests in the topic at hand. WHO and the World Bank will almost always be involved. The key bilateral agencies will also participate. In addition, the agencies working with the topic under discussion and groups representing people affected by particular conditions increasingly have inputs into these discussions. If TB is being discussed, for example, then the key NGOs working globally with TB will be involved, as will the TB programs from representative countries. If leprosy is being discussed, then the leprosy programs of some countries, NGOs working in leprosy, and groups of people affected by leprosy are all likely to be involved.

POLICY AND PROGRAM BRIEFS

This section contains four policy and program briefs that explore some of the concepts discussed in this chapter. The first describes an advocacy organization, the Global Network for Neglected Tropical Diseases. The second concerns a public–private partnership for developing new TB drugs, the TB Alliance. The third is about the innovative financing mechanism, UNITAID. The last concerns Gavi and which countries will get its financing.

The Global Network for Neglected Tropical Diseases[98]

The Global Network for Neglected Tropical Diseases is dedicated to building the political support, funding, and public awareness required to prioritize the most common neglected tropical diseases (NTDs) on the global health agenda and to grow a movement dedicated to their control and elimination.

An initiative of the Sabin Vaccine Institute, the Global Network advocates for wider integration and implementation of mass drug administration to control soil-transmitted helminths (hookworm, ascariasis, trichuriasis), onchocerciasis, and schistosomiasis and to eliminate trachoma and lymphatic filariasis around the world.

For approximately 50 cents per year one person can receive treatment and protection against the seven most common NTDs, making NTD control one of the most cost-effective investments in global health and development. Because most of the pills to treat the seven most common NTDs are donated by leading pharmaceutical companies, the costs are limited to distributing medicine to the people who need them most and setting up treatment programs that communities can run themselves.

Founded in 2006 with six partner organizations striving to better the lives of disadvantaged populations, the Global Network focuses on sustainable, nationally owned, integrated control efforts that are aligned with or supported by a country's ministry of health and the World Health Organization. From the efficient use of financial resources to increasing public support for and compliance with mass drug administration, the Global Network works with endemic country governments to expand NTD programs to reach the control and elimination goals outlined in the 2012 London Declaration on NTDs.

The Global Network promotes the use of integrated platforms, such as water, sanitation, and hygiene; maternal, newborn, and child health; and nutrition as a low-cost means of helping to accelerate the elimination of NTDs. The Global Network also continues to highlight the need to include NTD control and elimination efforts in the post-2015 development agenda to help build support for long-term funding commitments.

The Global Network's advocacy takes many forms—envoys include former presidents and health leaders from Latin America and Africa who leverage access to high-ranking policymakers. In addition, the Global Network's END7 campaign raises funds to directly support NTD treatment programs in endemic countries. Thousands of students around the world have joined END7 chapters at their universities to raise funds to fight NTDs and advocate for their control and elimination.

The Global Network's advocacy work is presently focused on two endemic countries with the highest NTD burden, India and Nigeria. Through this effort, the Global Network aims to demonstrate to other countries that NTD programs—especially those integrated with other health initiatives on water, sanitation, education, and nutrition—represent efficient investments that bring both economic and social returns.

The Global Network's advocacy efforts, in tandem with the NTD community, have raised significant awareness and support for NTDs globally. Funding from the United States and the United Kingdom has increased substantially, as have donations of drugs from leading pharmaceutical companies. However, sustaining this funding and increasing support from Germany and other European nations will be critical to achieve the goals of the London Declaration on NTDS: to control and eliminate 10 NTDs by 2020.

Through its product development partnership (PDP) the Sabin Vaccine Institute is also developing a new generation of NTD vaccines to prevent some of the highest burden diseases, including Chagas disease, hookworm, leishmaniasis, and schistosomiasis.

The TB Alliance

The Global Alliance for TB Drug Development, now called the TB Alliance,[99] was created in 2000 with the mission to accelerate the discovery and development of faster acting and affordable drugs to fight tuberculosis. Its main office is located in New York City, and research is conducted in public and private laboratories around the world.

The TB Alliance is a partnership among governments, nongovernmental organizations, professional organizations, academia, foundations, and pharmaceutical and biotechnology companies that have pledged to work together to accomplish this mission. The TB Alliance comprises the largest effort in history for TB drug development,[100] and the partnership has led to the largest portfolio of TB drug candidates to date.[101] The TB Alliance is funded by governments, foundations, and UNITAID.

The TB Alliance aims to develop a therapy for TB that will "shorten treatment, be effective against susceptible and resistant strains, be compatible with antiretroviral therapies for those HIV-TB patients currently on such therapies, and improve the treatment of latent infection."[99] In doing so, the partnership hopes to increase cure rates overall by improving patient compliance with treatment and lowering toxic side effects. Long-term goals include developing a treatment that could be administered in less than 2 weeks, significantly shorter than the current 6-month treatment for drug-susceptible TB. Developing a drug that could be given once a day orally is another priority.[102] Currently, over 20 projects are under way related to further drug development.[100]

A main concern of the TB Alliance is that treatment for TB, once developed, must be widely available and affordable, especially in low-income countries. To accomplish this goal, the partnership works toward patent and marketing arrangements that will allow any new TB drugs to be sold at affordable prices in low-income countries. It is also working with drug regulatory authorities to ensure that future drugs will get early approval in the countries in which they are to be sold.[102] In addition, the TB Alliance is collaborating with others to ensure that any future TB drugs can be manufactured at the lowest possible cost.[103]

Innovative Financing Mechanisms for Global Health: UNITAID

Within the past decade, there has been significant growth in international development assistance for health. Nonetheless, there remains a substantial gap between the available financing and the estimated financial needs for meeting the MDGs. WHO, for example, earlier estimated that between 2008 and 2015, an additional $251 billion would be necessary to achieve the MDGs in the 49 poorest countries.[104]

Besides being insufficient in amount, conventional development financing for health has a number of shortcomings. First, most countries can allocate such assistance only on a year-to-year basis, which makes it difficult for recipient countries to plan how to use the assistance in the soundest way. Second, this type of assistance may not provide the incentives needed to achieve desired outcomes in the most effective and efficient manner. This relates to the fact that development assistance for health has typically financed health inputs, such as drugs, medical equipment, clinics, training, and technical advice, rather than finance outputs and measurable results on the ground, such as vaccine coverage for childhood diseases or reduction in malaria morbidity and mortality from the use of bednets. There has also been a concern that getting financial assistance from multiple sources can lead to wasteful spending and inefficient duplication of systems for procurement, financial management, and reporting.[104]

In this light, discussion began in 2004 to develop innovative financing mechanisms for development assistance in health that could increase the amount of funding available, and be more predictable and stable than traditional development assistance for health. Such discussions have centered on financial mechanisms that include levies on currency transactions, a voluntary rebate by businesses on their value-added taxes for the use of international development, and other kinds of voluntary consumer contributions. One such effort that has been put into place is UNITAID. [104]

In 2006, Brazil, Chile, France, Norway, and the United Kingdom collaborated to develop an international drug purchase facility, called UNITAID. Officially launched in September 2006, UNITAID was established to scale up access to HIV/AIDS, TB, and malaria treatment for people in low-income countries. UNITAID now has the support of a number of other low-, middle-, and high-income countries, and of the Bill & Melinda Gates Foundation. UNITAID is housed at WHO.

UNITAID is largely financed by a new source of funding: a tax on the purchase of airline tickets in nine countries, plus Norwegian funds from taxing carbon dioxide emissions. UNITAID's business model is based on the idea that this predictable source of financing will allow it to purchase high volumes of diagnostics and drugs for use in low- and middle-income countries, thus encouraging investment in the development of these products and reductions in their prices.[105,106] Since its inception, UNITAID has raised $2.41 billion, of which $1.48 came from the levy on airline tickets.

UNITAID has a number of strategic objectives, including:

- Increase access to simple point of care diagnostics for HIV/AIDS, TB, and malaria
- Increase access to affordable pediatric formulations of drugs for these diseases
- Improve access to new drugs that can address these and related diseases
- Enhance access to drug therapy for malaria
- Improve access to second-line TB drugs
- Increase access to products that can help to prevent HIV, TB, and malaria

UNITAID works closely with other organizations and to fill gaps that other partner organizations have not been able to address effectively.[107]

UNITAID now supports 27 projects with 22 grantees, assisting in 94 countries.[108] It has contributed to the financing of HIV/AIDS treatment and helped to bring down its costs. It has also helped to enhance the quality of drugs being procured. It has assisted in the development of pediatric drugs for TB, the distribution of bednets, and assistance to countries in procuring quality-assured products.[109] In 2013, UNITAID supported investments worth about $300 million.[109]

Prioritizing Gavi Assistance and Sustaining Country Vaccine Programs[110]

Background

Despite the size of Gavi's resources, they are still not sufficient to meet all of the demands on it. Thus, Gavi has decided to prioritize aid for the countries with the least ability to pay. Countries will graduate from Gavi assistance once their gross national income per capita surpasses $1,500. Over the course of the 5-year graduation period, these countries will be gradually weaned off Gavi's assistance for immunization and will take increasing responsibility for their own vaccine financing, procurement, and regulation.

Sixteen countries will pass the income threshold and graduate by 2018. Collectively, these 16 countries must increase their own spending on vaccines from $8 million in 2012 to $90 million in 2018.

In this light, it is important to ask a number of key policy questions, including, for example:

- How will these countries continue to sustain their vaccine programs without foreign aid?
- What are the challenges in transitioning to self-sufficiency?

Addressing the Policy Problem

In a 2012 pilot study, Gavi selected six countries for transition planning in preparation for their graduation in 2018. These countries were Angola, Bhutan, the Republic of Congo, Georgia, Moldova, and Mongolia. Transition planning focused on three key elements: developing a sustainable financing plan, deciding how to procure vaccines, and strengthening regulatory capacity.

Developing a Sustainable Financing Plan

Transition planning teams developed detailed financial projections for each country between 2012 and 2018. Each country's vaccine budget depended on several factors, including:

- The number of new vaccines
- The number of doses required
- Presentation of the vaccine (single dose vs. multidose, liquid vs. freeze-dried, etc.)
- Cofinancing requirements

Under the transition plan, domestic contributions to the vaccine budget would gradually increase over the 5-year graduation period. Meanwhile, Gavi's contribution would steadily decrease until it was phased out entirely.

To assess the feasibility of graduation, Gavi conducted a number of financial analyses. At the most basic level, Gavi examined the projected costs for vaccines over the transition period 2012 to 2018 and how they compared with the country's overall projected health expenditures in each year over that period. The lower the additional costs of vaccines compared to projected health expenditure, the more likely the government would be to finance those vaccine costs from domestic expenditures. Of course, the costs of vaccines in the future will depend partly on the number of new vaccines a country will adopt.

Procuring Vaccines

Countries must decide how they will procure vaccines upon graduating from Gavi assistance. Countries may procure their vaccines through the UNICEF Supply Division, or they can directly procure the vaccines themselves.

Direct procurement of vaccines has been challenging for many countries. It is difficult for some graduating countries to obtain competitive prices for high-quality products because they represent relatively small markets. As a result, they often pay significantly higher prices than the UNICEF Supply Division. Sometimes, because of poor information, countries do not even realize that they are paying higher prices.

To help ensure that countries obtain low prices from vaccine manufacturers even after Gavi support ends, Gavi has sought commitments from vaccine manufacturers to offer Gavi prices to the graduating countries. This commitment has already been secured for the pentavalent, pneumococcal, and rotavirus vaccines. Predictable vaccine prices will also help make more reliable the projections of future country costs for vaccines.

Strengthening Regulatory Capacity

Strong national regulatory agencies are critical to immunization efforts. First, low-quality vaccines put lives at risk. Second, low-quality vaccines damage the public's trust, which in turn hinders future immunization efforts.

Gavi, therefore, made recommendations for strengthening each country's national regulatory agency during the graduation period. For instance, Gavi recommended that Georgia's national regulatory agency respond quickly and effectively to reports of adverse immunization events. Gavi also recommended that regulators monitor the local agents that represent vaccine manufacturers.

Results to Date and Lessons for the Future

The 2012 pilot study found that the six countries studied had diverse capacities to administer and finance their vaccine programs. Most of the graduating countries are projected to experience strong economic growth, which will help ease domestic financing of the vaccine programs. However, many countries have weaknesses in budgeting for vaccine purchase, national procurement practices, performance of national regulatory agencies, and technical capacity for vaccine planning and advocacy.

Gavi will continue to use transition planning in the future. The lessons from the 2012 pilot study will be used for Nicaragua, Papua New Guinea, and Uzbekistan, which started the graduation process in January 2014. Transition planning will also be important for Gavi's largest country, India, which is expected to cross the income threshold in the next several years.

Transition planning is important not just for immunization but also for other initiatives that are donor dependent, such as HIV/AIDS, family planning, and malaria. In fact, transition planning is relevant for development assistance agencies such as the Global Fund, the World Bank, and the U.S. President's Emergency Plan for AIDS Relief (PEPFAR), which seek to promote self-sufficiency in their recipient countries. These lessons are also useful for recipient countries seeking to improve domestic financing for health. Gavi's experience highlights both the opportunities and challenges in achieving sustainable financing in assistance for global health.

CASE STUDY–ONCHOCERCIASIS

The case study that follows deals with the successful effort to eliminate onchocerciasis in Africa. More detailed information on this case is available in *Case Studies in Global Health: Millions Saved.*[111]

Background

Onchocerciasis, or river blindness, is a pernicious disease afflicting approximately 26 million people worldwide. More than 99 percent of its victims are in sub-Saharan Africa.[112] Historically, in the most endemic areas, over a third of the adult population was blind and infection often approached 90 percent.[113] In 11 West African countries in 1974, nearly 2.5 million of the area's 30 million inhabitants were infected with onchocerciasis, and approximately 100,000 were blind. The remaining 19 endemic countries in Central and East Africa were home to 60 million people at risk of the disease.

The Intervention

Onchocerciasis is caused by a worm called *Onchocerca volvulus*, which enters its human victim through the bite of an infected blackfly. The flies breed in fast-moving waters in fertile riverside regions. Once inside a human, the tiny worm grows to a length of 1 to 2 feet and produces millions of microscopic offspring called microfilariae. The constant movement of the microfilariae through the infected person's skin causes torturous itching, lesions, muscle pain, and, in severe cases, blindness. Fertile land is often abandoned for fear of the disease.

Early efforts to control the disease proved ineffective because blackflies cover long distances and cross national borders, rendering unilateral efforts ineffective. An international conference in Tunisia in 1968 concluded that onchocerciasis could not be controlled without regional collaboration and long-term funding of at least 20 years to break the life cycle of the worm. World Bank President Robert McNamara's tour of drought-stricken West Africa in 1972 served as a catalyst to progress. Moved by seeing communities where nearly all the adults were blind and were led by children, McNamara decided to spearhead an international effort against onchocerciasis.[114]

The Onchocerciasis Control Program (OCP), the World Bank's first large-scale health program, was launched in 1974 in conjunction with WHO, the UN Food and Agriculture Organization (FAO), and UNDP. The program included a significant research budget and set out to eliminate onchocerciasis in 7, and eventually in 11, West African countries.[113] Breeding grounds of blackflies were sprayed with larvicide, and the spraying program was able to persist even through regional conflicts and coups. In the 1980s, a Merck drug called ivermectin was included as a powerful new weapon against the disease, a single dose of which could effectively paralyze the tiny worms for up to a full year.[115] The drug proved popular because it quickly reduced uncomfortable symptoms and provided protection against other parasites. Merck donated ivermectin and Dr. William Foege of the Carter Center managed its distribution.

The African Programme for Onchocerciasis Control (APOC) was established in 1995 as a broad international partnership to control the disease throughout Africa and to carry onchocerciasis control to 19 countries in East and Central Africa. These were countries in which long distances and thick forests made spraying difficult. APOC pioneered a system of community-directed treatment (ComDT) with ivermectin to ensure local participation, reach remote villages, and maintain distribution of the drug after donor funding expired in 2010.[116] ComDT workers are often the only health personnel to reach distant villages, and their access could be used for other health interventions in the future.

The Impact

By 2002, OCP halted transmission of onchocerciasis in 11 West African countries, preventing 600,000 cases of blindness, and protecting 18 million children born in the OCP area from the risk of the disease. About 25 million hectares of arable land—enough to feed an additional 17 million people—are now safe for resettlement.[117] APOC is expanding this success to Central and East Africa, where 40,000 cases of blindness are expected to be prevented each year.

Costs and Benefits

OCP operated with an annual cost of less than $1 per protected person. Total commitments from 22 donors amounted to $560 million. The annual return on investment, due mainly to increased agricultural output, was 20 percent, and it is estimated that $3.7 billion will be generated from improved labor and agricultural productivity.[118] APOC coverage cost even less, at just 11 cents per person. The economic rate of return for the program has been estimated at 17 percent for the years 1996 to 2017, and it is estimated that 27 healthy life days will be added per dollar invested.[119]

Lessons Learned

Success in controlling onchocerciasis could not have been attained without a genuinely shared vision among all partners in the program. Commitment among the African governments was critical to coordinating a regional effort across national borders. Long-term commitments from donors, along with Merck's decision to donate ivermectin indefinitely, were essential elements for the program's sustainability. The participation of a wide range of organizations, such as multilateral institutions, private companies, and local NGOs, allowed for a cost-effective and efficient intervention. The ComDT framework, by emphasizing local ownership and participation, proved a cost-effective and self-sustaining means of delivering drugs to remote populations. The onchocerciasis program proved that effective aid programs, implemented with transparency and accountability, can deliver lasting results.

FUTURE CHALLENGES

There are a number of challenges to effective collaborative action in global health. First, the types of health conditions that the world faces are evolving, with an increasing burden of noncommunicable diseases, even in low- and middle-income countries. Second, there have been and will continue to be emerging and reemerging infectious diseases that could challenge the ability of both countries and the global community to respond effectively, as Ebola virus has done in 2014 and 2015. The global community needs to align its assistance with changing burdens of disease and has to be ready, through collaborative efforts, to carry out surveillance, prevention, and treatment of any diseases that emerge or reemerge.

In addition, it will be very important for development partners to work together to help countries strengthen their health systems, as well as to try to combat individual diseases. If countries are to be able to meet their most important health needs in a sustainable manner in the future, then they must have health systems that work. In most low-income countries, this will require better management, more appropriate forms of organization, sounder systems for key public health functions, better trained staff at all levels, and a consistent manner of providing financing for health system needs and for financial protection of the population from the costs of health care. Achieving health system strengthening may not be as attractive politically as working together to fight a specific disease or health problem. Yet, in the long run, a systems approach must be taken to developing health services, and different global health actors will have to work together to achieve this.

Another set of future challenges concerns the need to ensure that actors in global health work together to address the knowledge gaps that prevent sufficient progress against health conditions that cause people to be sick too often and to die prematurely, especially poor people in low-income countries. There will continue to be an important need, for example, for increasing our knowledge of the basic science concerning many diseases, including HIV/AIDS, TB, and malaria. It will not be possible to develop preventive or therapeutic vaccines for these diseases or better treatment for them without significant improvements in scientific knowledge.

There will also be a need for operational research—increasingly called "implementation science"—so that we can learn more about what approaches are effective and efficient. What is the most cost-effective way, for example, to ensure that people take all of their drugs for HIV/AIDS or TB? How should a health system in a low- or middle-income country be organized to ensure that it can operate in a cost-efficient way, while paying sufficient attention to the poor? These questions can only be answered through the generation and sharing of knowledge and experience globally, a process dependent upon cooperation and coordination.

The factors that have encouraged the development of public–private partnerships for health will also continue to challenge the global health community. There are many such partnerships now and it will be very important to learn as quickly as possible which aspects of these partnerships encourage product development in effective and efficient ways and which ones do not. It is also necessary to continue to encourage the development of new and innovative approaches to enabling the development of new diagnostics, vaccines, and therapies that can be affordable in low- and middle-income countries. If any of the public–private partnerships are successful in developing new products, then it will be essential that efforts turn to ensuring that they are used quickly where they are most needed.

The financial needs for addressing global health concerns are very considerable and will continue to have a prominent place on the global health agenda. The multilateral development banks, bilateral aid agencies, and special programs such as Gavi and The Global Fund need continuous financing. In addition, some of the important initiatives that have been started, such as the considerable push for treatment against HIV/AIDS, cannot be sustained in at least the lowest resource settings without many years of additional financing by rich countries, foundations, the private sector, and their partners. There are many risks that donors will develop aid fatigue and not have the political will necessary to continue financing global health efforts at the level needed.

It will be important that any development financing for health be as effective as possible. Although the topic of development effectiveness is considerably beyond the scope of this text, **Table 16-8** summarizes some of the factors most closely associated with the success of development assistance in health.

There are also a number of important challenges to the way that actors in global health cooperate to assist countries in investing in the health sector. In recent years, development assistance agencies have increasingly tried to cooperate closely in their aid work on specific countries. However, there are always tendencies in development agencies to act independently rather than in coordination with other agencies and to focus too much on process issues, such as how they work with others. In the last 2 decades the number of organizations that work on global health has greatly increased. Although we should expect these tensions to continue, it is important if development assistance in health is to be effective that agencies work increasingly in a cooperative fashion and focus on the content of their efforts.

Finally, it will be very important that good leadership in the global health field continues. Different agencies will need to work together in ways that address the challenges noted earlier. New groups and organizations need to join the community of global health actors to continue to inspire innovative and efficient methods of addressing and financing global health needs.

MAIN MESSAGES

It is very important that key actors work together to address global health problems because they may have effects that go beyond one country, they may be expensive to deal with, and they may require technical and managerial resources larger than some poorer countries can bring to bear on their own. In addition, it is very important that there be global standards in some health fields, and these standards need to be broadly developed and widely accepted. Good examples of areas in which it is imperative that different actors work together globally include efforts to carry out disease surveillance, the global fight for polio eradication, and the standards for some disease control programs, such as TB.

There are many actors in global health; among the most actively involved are WHO, UNICEF, UNAIDS, and the World Bank. Most high-income countries have development assistance organizations, such as USAID, AusAID, and DFID, and they often play important roles in global health. The Global Fund and Gavi are also prominent global health actors. A number of foundations are also deeply involved in global health work, and the Bill & Melinda Gates Foundation has become a major actor in global health since the late 1990s. Local NGOs such as BRAC are deeply involved in health efforts in many countries. Many international NGOs are also very engaged in global health activities; Doctors Without Borders is among the best known of these. Organizations like these play one of several roles, singly or in combination, including advocacy, knowledge generation, technical assistance, financing, or program development and implementation.

TABLE 16-8 Factors Associated with Positive Outcomes in Development Assistance

- Strong leadership in the host government and in the development partner agencies
- Close collaboration among governments, donors, and nongovernmental organizations in the design and implementation of the program
- Household and community participation in the design, implementation, and monitoring of programs
- Simple and flexible technologies and approaches that can be adapted to local conditions and do not require complex skills to operate and maintain
- Approaches that help to strengthen health systems, especially human resources for health
- Consistent, predictable funding

Modified with permission from Hecht RM, Shah R. Recent trends and innovations in development assistance in health. In: Jamison DT, Breman JG, Measham AR, et al., eds. Disease Control Priorities in Developing Countries. 2nd ed. Washington, DC and New York: The World Bank and Oxford University Press, 2006:246.

A relatively new form of organization called public–private partnerships for health was created specifically to deal with difficult global health problems. These organizations include, among others, the International AIDS Vaccine Initiative, the International Partnership on Microbicides, and the TB Alliance. Essentially, they try to combine the skills and financing of public and private sector organizations, in order to advocate for specific health issues; develop new vaccines, diagnostics, or drugs; and ensure that what they develop will be appropriate to the health needs of poor countries and affordable to them, as well. Some other new organizations, such as Gavi and the Global Fund have been established to try to dramatically increase the pace of immunizing children and pregnant women and combating HIV/AIDS, TB, and malaria.

The global health community is likely to face many challenges that will continue to require collective action by global health actors. Some of the key challenges will include filling key gaps in knowledge and encouraging public and private sector organizations to develop the diagnostics, vaccines, and drugs needed to address the most important global health issues. They will also include the need for organizations to work together to strengthen health systems, to combat individual diseases, to be ready to address emerging diseases, and to try to ensure that critical global health needs have adequate financing.

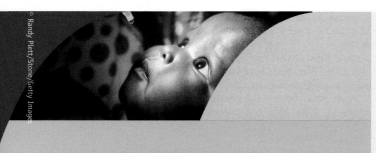

Study Questions

1. What are the most important organizations that work on global health issues?

2. What functions do these organizations play?

3. Why is it important that different actors cooperate to address global health concerns?

4. Name some of the most important successes of cooperative action on global health.

5. What were some of the key factors that led to those successes?

6. What are the lessons of these successes for future global health efforts?

7. What are some of the future challenges that demand continued or strengthened collaboration in global public health?

8. What is a public–private partnership for health, and why might it be valuable?

9. Why is cooperative action needed to address problems like onchocerciasis and Guinea worm?

10. How might the world raise the money needed to further address problems like HIV and the need for drug treatment against AIDS?

REFERENCES

1. UNICEF. (2004, June 22). *Polio experts warn of largest epidemic in recent years, as polio hits Darfur: Epidemiologists "alarmed" by continuing spread of virus.* Retrieved July 12, 2006, from http://www.unicef.org/media/media_21872.html.

2. World Health Organization. (2015). *Tuberculosis* (Fact Sheet No. 104). Retrieved March 17, 2015, from http://www.who.int/mediacentre/factsheets/fs104/en/.

3. Global Alliance for TB Drug Development. *No R&D in 30 years.* Retrieved July 12, 2006, from http://www.tballiance.org/2_3_C_No RandDin30Years.asp.

4. The Gavi Alliance. Gavi Alliance for Vaccines and Immunization. Retrieved July 5, 2006, from http://www.Gavialliance.org.

5. Merson, M. H., Black, R. E., & Mills, A. J. (Eds.). (2001). *International public health: Diseases, programs, systems, and policies.* Gaithersburg, MD: Aspen Publishers.

6. Lele, U., Ridker, R., & Upadhyay, J. (2005). *Health system capacities in developing countries and global health initiatives on communicable diseases.* Retrieved July 12, 2006, from http://www.umalele.org/content/view/85/109.

7. Heymann, D. L., & Rodier, G. (2004). Global surveillance, national surveillance, and SARS. *Emerging Infectious Diseases, 10*(2), 173–175.

8. Walt, G. (2001). Global cooperation in international public health. In M. H. Merson, R. E. Black, & A. J. Mills (Eds.), *International public health* (pp. 667–672). Gaithersburg, MD: Aspen Publishers.

9. Basch, P. (2001). *Textbook of international health* (2nd ed., pp. 486–509). New York: Oxford University Press.

10. Kickbusch, I., & Buse, K. (2001). Global influences and global responses: International health at the turn of the twenty-first century. In M. H. Merson, R. E. Black, & A. J. Mills (Eds.), *International public health* (pp. 701–733). Gaithersburg, MD: Aspen Publishers.

11. World Health Organization. *Constitution of the World Health Organization.* Retrieved June 15, 2015, from http://apps.who.int/gb/DGNP/pdf_files/constitution-en.pdf.

12. World Health Organization. *WHO—Its people and offices.* Retrieved September 13, 2014, from http://www.who.int/about/structure/en/.

13. World Health Organization. *Global Health Declarations.* Retrieved July 16, 2015, from http://www.who.int/trade/glossary/story039/en/.

14. World Health Organization. *About WHO: Leadership priorities.* Retrieved April 8, 2015, from http://who.int/about/agenda/en/.

15. UNICEF. (2012). *The structure of UNICEF.* Retrieved September 13, 2014, from http://www.unicef.org/about/structure/.

16. UNICEF. (2003). *Support UNICEF.* Retrieved October 15, 2010, from http://www.unicef.org/support/14884.html.

17. UNICEF. *What we do.* Retrieved October 15, 2010, from http://www.unicef.org/whatwedo/.

18. UNICEF. (2014). *2013 annual report of the executive director, including on the implementation of the Quadrennial Comprehensive Policy Review.* Retrieved September 13, 2014, from http://www.unicef.org/about/execboard/files/EDAR_presentation-22May2014.pdf.

19. UNAIDS. *Cosponsors.* Retrieved April 8, 2015, from http://www.unaids.org/en/aboutunaids/unaidscosponsors.

20. UNAIDS. (2013). *UNAIDS 2012-2015 unified budget, results and accountability framework (UBRAF).* Geneva: UNAIDS.

21. UNAIDS. *Gap report.* Retrieved May 19, 2015, from http://www.unaids.org/sites/default/files/media_asset/UNAIDS_Gap_report_en.pdf.

22. UNAIDS. *Goals.* Retrieved September 13, 2014, from http://www.unaids.org/en/targetsandcommitments/.

23. World Bank. *Healthy development: The World Bank strategy for health, nutrition, and population results.* Retrieved May 19, 2015, from http://www-wds.worldbank.org/external/default/WDSContentServer/WDSP/IB/2007/09/21/000310607_20070921140425/Rendered/PDF/40928 0PAPER0He101OFFICIAL0USE0ONLY1.pdf.

24. Bretton Woods Project. (2009). *Bank's $100 billion annual lending plan.* Retrieved October 5, 2010, from http://www.brettonwoodsproject.org/art-565290.

25. World Bank. (2006). *Working for a world free of poverty.* Retrieved July 12, 2006, from http://siteresources.worldbank.org/EXTABOUTUS/Resources/wbgroupbrochure-en.pdf.

26. World Bank. *Operational summary fiscal 2008–2013.* Retrieved September 13, 2014, from http://siteresources.worldbank.org/EXTAN-NREP2013/Resources/9304887-1377201212378/9305896-1377544753431/OpSumLendingTables_EN.pdf.

27. World Bank. *World Bank HNP Lending.* Retrieved September 13, 2014, from http://datatopics.worldbank.org/hnp/worldbanklending.

28. USAID. *Who we are: Organization.* Retrieved September 14, 2014, from http://www.usaid.gov/who-we-are/organization.

29. USAID. *Global health.* Retrieved June 29, 2015, from https://www.rockefellerfoundation.org/our-work/topics/advance-health/.

30. The Rockefeller Foundation. Retrieved June 29, 2015, from https://www.rockefellerfoundation.org/our-work/topics/advance-health/.

31. The Rockefeller Foundation. *Disease surveillance networks.* Retrieved April 9, 2015 from http://www.rockefellerfoundation.org/our-work/initiatives/disease-surveillance-network/.

32. The Rockefeller Foundation. *Advance health.* Retrieved March 17, 2015, from http://www.rockefellerfoundation.org/our-work/topics/advance-health/.

33. Wellcome Trust. (2010). *2010–2020 strategic plan: Extraordinary opportunities.* Retrieved July 2, 2010, from http://www.wellcome.ac.uk/Our-vision/index.htm.

34. Wellcome Trust. *Organisation.* Retrieved September 14, 2014, from http://www.wellcome.ac.uk/About-us/Organisation/index.htm.

35. Bill & Melinda Gates Foundation. (2013). *2012 annual report.* Seattle, WA: Author.

36. Wellcome Trust. *Funding.* Retrieved September 14, 2014, from http://www.wellcome.ac.uk/Funding/index.htm.

37. Wellcome Trust. *Current grant portfolio and 2012/2013 grant funding data.* Retrieved September 14, 2014, from http://www.wellcome.ac.uk/stellent/groups/corporatesite/@msh_publishing_group/documents/web_document/wts058353.pdf.

38. Wellcome Trust. *Global health research.* Retrieved November 10, 2013, from http://www.wellcome.ac.uk/stellent/groups/corporatesite/@sf_international_progs/documents/web_document/wtdv026085.pdf.

39. Wellcome Trust. *Funding malaria.* Retrieved July 21, 2010, from http://malaria.wellcome.ac.uk/node40023.html.

40. Wellcome Trust. *Strategic Plan 2010-20.* Retrieved June 14, 2015, from http://www.wellcome.ac.uk/stellent/groups/corporatesite/@policy_communications/documents/web_document/WTDV027438.pdf.

41. Wellcome Trust. *2009 annual report and financial statements.* Retrieved April 9, 2015, from http://www.wellcome.ac.uk/stellent/groups/corporatesite/@msh_publishing_group/documents/web_document/wtx057901.pdf.

42. Wellcome Trust. *Wellcome Trust response to the House of Commons Science and Technology Committee: Science and International Development.* Retrieved June 14, 2015 from http://www.wellcome.ac.uk/stellent/groups/corporatesite/@policy_communications/documents/web_document/wtvm054041.pdf.

43. Bill & Melinda Gates Foundation. *What we do.* Retrieved March 17, 2015, from http://www.gatesfoundation.org/What-We-Do.

44. Bill & Melinda Gates Foundation. *Our Global Health Division.* Retrieved June 15, 2015, from http://www.gatesfoundation.org/what-we-do.

45. Bill & Melinda Gates Foundation. *Grants.* Retrieved April 9, 2015, from http://www.gatesfoundation.org/How-We-Work.

46. Bill & Melinda Gates Foundation. *2013 annual report.* Retrieved March 17, 2015, from http://www.gatesfoundation.org/Who-We-Are/Resources-and-Media/Annual-Reports/Annual-Report-2013.

47. The section on NIH is based on a draft of this section provided by the Fogarty International of Center of NIH and in a series of personal communications with the Fogarty International Center in October 2010 and March 2015.

48. U.S. National Institutes of Health. *Strategic plan of the Fogarty International Center at NIH*. Retrieved March 17, 2015, from http://www.fic.nih.gov/about/pages/strategic-plan.aspx.

49. U.S. National Institutes of Health. (2013). *Results of the ROTAVAC rotavirus vaccine study in India*. Retrieved March 17, 2015, from http://www.nih.gov/news/health/may2013/niaid-14.htm.

50. US National Institutes of Health. *NIH Visiting Program*. Retrieved March 17, 2015, from http://dis.ors.od.nih.gov/visitingprogram/01_vpmain.html.

51. BRAC. *Who we are: Mission & vision*. Retrieved April 9, 2015, from http://www.brac.net/content/who-we-are-mission-vision.

52. BRAC. *Who we are: Evolution*. Retrieved August 17, 2010, from http://www.brac.net/content/who-we-are-evolution.

53. BRAC. *What we do*. Retrieved June 15, 2015, from http://www.brac.net/content/what-we-do#.VX7lLFVViko.

54. BRAC. *Essential Health Care*. June 15, 2015, from http://health.brac.net/essential-health-care-ehc.

55. BRAC. *Essential Health Care (EHC)*. Retrieved May 19, 2015, from http://health.brac.net/essential-health-care-ehc.

56. BRAC. *Overview*. Retrieved March 17, 2015, from http://health.brac.net/overview.

57. BRAC. *Essential health care (EHC)*. Retrieved March 17, 2015, from http://health.brac.net/essential-health-care-ehc.

58. BRAC. *BRAC health facilities*. Retrieved March 17, 2015, from http://health.brac.net/nutrition/82-bhp/brac-projects/169-brac-health-facilities.

59. BRAC. *Tuberculosis Control Programme*. Retrieved March 17, 2015, from http://health.brac.net/tuberculosis-control-programme.

60. BRAC. *Malaria Control Programme*. Retrieved March 17, 2015, from http://health.brac.net/malaria-control-programme.

61. BRAC. *Nutrition activities*. Retrieved March 17, 2015, from http://health.brac.net/nutrition/82-bhp/brac-projects/226-nutrition.

62. BRAC. *Bangladesh Sprinkles Programme*. Retrieved March 17, 2015, from http://health.brac.net/component/content/article/82-bhp/brac-projects/149-bangladesh-sprinkles-programme.

63. BRAC. *Non-Communicable Disease (NCD) Programme*. Retrieved March 17, 2015, from http://health.brac.net/non-communicable-disease-ncd.

64. BRAC. *Eye care interventions*. Retrieved March 17, 2015, from http://health.brac.net/eye-care-intervention.

65. BRAC. *Annual report 2008*. Retrieved August 17, 2010, from http://www.brac.net/oldsite/useruploads/files/BRAC%20Annual%20Report%20-%202008.pdf.

66. BRAC. *Annual report 2013*. Retrieved March 17, 2015, from http://www.brac.net/content/annual-report-and-publications.

67. Doctors Without Borders. *About us*. Retrieved July 12, 2006, from http://www.doctorswithoutborders.org/aboutus/.

68. Doctors Without Borders. *Medical Issues: Ebola*. Retrieved March 17, 2015, from http://www.doctorswithoutborders.org/our-work/medical-issues/ebola.

69. CDC. *About CDC: Mission, role, and pledge*. Retrieved November 6, 2010, from http://www.cdc.gov/about/organization/mission.htm.

70. KNCV. *KNCV Tuberculosis Foundation—An overview*. Retrieved November 6, 2010, from http://www.kncvtbc.nl/Site/Components/SitePageCP/ShowPage.aspx?ItemID=e93456d3-d112-41b4-aac4-973b5b9f7763&SelectedMenuItemID=628a592b-25e8-440b-b04e-6ee3779d13c3.

71. The International Union Against Tuberculosis and Lung Disease. *The Union: Who we are*. Retrieved April 9, 2015, from http://www.theunion.org/who-we-are.

72. World Health Organization. *The Stop TB Department*. Retrieved July 12, 2006, from http://www.who.int/tb/strategy/en/.

73. Stop TB Partnership. *About us*. Retrieved March 17, 2015, from http://www.stoptb.org/about/.

74. Stop TB Partnership. Retrieved March 17, 2015, from http://www.stoptb.org/.

75. Roll Back Malaria. Retrieved April 9, 2015, from http://www.rollbackmalaria.org/.

76. Roll Back Malaria. *RBM mandate*. Retrieved March 17, 2015, from http://www.rollbackmalaria.org/about/about-rbm/rbm-mandate.

77. Roll Back Malaria. *Sub-Regional Networks*. Retrieved June 14, 2015, http://www.rollbackmalaria.org/countries/sub-regional-networks/central-africa-carn.

78. Gavi. *How Gavi is funded*. Retrieved March 17, 2015, from http://www.Gavi.org/funding/how-Gavi-is-funded/.

79. Gavi. *Types of support*. Retrieved March 17, 2015, from http://www.Gavi.org/support/.

80. Gavi. *Gavi's mission*. Retrieved March 17, 2015, from http://www.Gavi.org/about/mission/.

81. The Global Fund to Fight AIDS, Tuberculosis, and Malaria. Retrieved July 6, 2006, from http://www.theglobalfund.org/en.

82. The Global Fund to Fight AIDS, Tuberculosis, and Malaria. *Global Fund: About*. Retrieved May 19, 2015, from http://www.theglobalfund.org/en/about/.

83. The Global Fund. *Procurement and supply management*. Retrieved March 17, 2015, from http://www.theglobalfund.org/en/procurement/.

84. The Global Fund. *Funding and spending*. Retrieved March 17, 2015, from http://www.theglobalfund.org/en/about/fundingspending/.

85. International Federation of Pharmaceutical Manufacturers & Associations. *Ending neglected tropical diseases*. Retrieved May 19, 2015, from http://www.ifpma.org/fileadmin/content/Publication/2012/IFPMA-NTD-NewLogoJUNE2.pdf.

86. National Institutes of Health. (1999). *A leading cause of blindness may be controlled by simple course of oral antibiotic*. Retrieved April 11, 2015, from http://www.niaid.nih.gov/news/newsreleases/Archive/1999/Pages/trachoma.aspx.

87. Benton, B. (2001). *The onchocerciasis (riverblindness) programs: Visionary partnerships* (Findings No. 174). Retrieved April 11, 2015, from http://www-wds.worldbank.org/external/default/WDSContentServer/WDSP/IB/2010/05/31/000334955_20100531073551/Rendered/PDF/547850BRI0Box31740Jan0200101PUBLIC1.pdf.

88. African Comprehensive HIV/AIDS Partnerships. Retrieved July 12, 2006, from http://www.achap.org.

89. Whaley, R. F., & Hashim, T. J. (1994). *A textbook of world health: A practical guide to global health care*. New York: Parthenon.

90. World Health Organization. *Leprosy* (Fact Sheet No. 101). Retrieved July 7, 2006, from http://www.who.int/mediacentre/factsheets/fs101/en.

91. World Health Organization. *Lymphatic filariasis* (Fact Sheet No. 102). Retrieved July 7, 2006, from http://www.who.int/mediacentre/factsheets/fs102/en.

92. World Health Organization. *Onchocerciasis*. Retrieved July 7, 2006, from http://www.who.int/topics/onchocerciasis/en.

93. Bruce, F. C. (2002). Highlights from the national summit on safe motherhood: Investing in the health of women. *Maternal and Child Health Journal, 6*(1), 67–69.

94. World Health Organization. (1978). Declaration of Alma-Ata. *International Conference on Primary Health Care*. Alma-Ata, USSR: WHO.

95. The World Bank. (1993). *World development report 1993*. New York: The World Bank, Oxford University Press.

96. World Health Organization. (2005). Fifty-eighth World Health Assembly. Retrieved April 11, 2015, from http://www.who.int/mediacentre/multimedia/2005/wha58/en/.

97. Kidder, T. (2003). *Mountains beyond mountains*. New York: Random House.

98. This brief is based on a draft provided by the Global Network for Neglected Tropical Diseases. Additional information can be found at their website, http://www.globalnetwork.org.

99. TB Alliance. *Our mission*. Retrieved March 17, 2015, from http://www.tballiance.org/about/mission.php.

100. The Global Alliance for TB Drug Development. (2009). *Accelerating the pace. 2009 annual report*. Retrieved April 11, 2015, from http://www.tballiance.org/downloads/publications/TBA%20Annual%202009.pdf.

101. TB Alliance. *History and impact*. Retrieved March 17, 2015, from http://www.tballiance.org/about/history.php.

102. TB Alliance. *TB Alliance portfolio*. Retrieved April 11, 2015, from http://www.tballiance.org/portfolio/.

103. TB Alliance. *Operating model. 2010*. Retrieved April 11, 2015, from http://www.tballiance.org/about/operating-model.php.

104. Hecht, R., Palriwala, A., & Rao, A. (2010). *Innovative financing for global health: A moment for expanded U.S. engagement?* A Report of the CSIS Global Health Policy Center. Washington, DC: Center for Strategic and International Studies. Retrieved October 7, 2010, from http://csis.org/files/publication/100316_Hecht_InnovativeFinancing_Web.pdf.

105. UNITAID. *Innovative financing for health: Increasing access and affordability of medicines through market impact*. Retrieved October 8, 2010, from http://www.unitaid.eu/images/Factsheets/unitaid_brochure_july_en.pdf.

106. UNITAID. *Innovative financing*. Retrieved March 17, 2015, from http://www.unitaid.eu/en/how/innovative-financing.

107. UNITAID. *Mission and strategy*. Retrieved March 17, 2015, from http://www.unitaid.eu/en/who/mission-and-strategy.

108. UNITAID. *About UNITAID*. Retrieved March 17, 2015, from http://www.unitaid.eu/en/who/about-unitaid.

109. UNITAID. *Results*. Retrieved March 17, 2015, from http://www.unitaid.eu/en/impact/9-uncategorised/425-results.

110. Saxenian, H., Hecht, R., Kaddar, M., et al. (2015). Overcoming challenges to sustainable immunization financing: Early experiences from GAVI graduating countries. *Health Policy and Planning, 30*(2),197–205.

111. Levine, R., & What Works Working Group. (2007). *Case studies in global health: Millions saved*. Sudbury, MA: Jones Bartlett.

112. Global Network Neglected Tropical Diseases. *Onchocerciasis*. Retrieved June 15, 2015, from http://www.globalnetwork.org/onchocerciasis

113. Laolu, A. (2003). Victory over river blindness. *Africa Recovery, 17*(1), 6.

114. Benton, B., Bump, J., Seketeli, A., & Liese, B. (2002). Partnership and promise: Evolution of the African river blindness campaigns. *Annals of Tropical Medicine and Parasitology, 96*(suppl 1), S5–S14.

115. Merck. *25 years: The MECTIZAN® Donation Program*. Retrieved April 11, 2015, from http://www.merck.com/about/featured-stories/mectizan1.html.

116. Amazigo, U., Brieger, W., Katabarwa, M., et al. (2002). The challenges of community-directed treatment with ivermectin (CDTI) within the African Programme for Onchocerciasis Control (APOC). *Annals of Tropical Medicine and Parasitology, 96*(1), S41–S58.

117. The World Bank. *Pushing back neglected tropical diseases in Africa*. Retrieved May 19, 2015 from http://www.worldbank.org/en/news/feature/2012/11/17/pushing-back-neglected-tropical-diseases-in-africa.

118. Hopkins, D., & Richards, F. (1997). Visionary campaign: Eliminating river blindness. In E. Bernstein (Ed.), *Medical and health annual* (pp. 8–23). Chicago: Encyclopaedia Britannica.

119. Benton, B. (1998). Economic impact of onchocerciasis control through the African Programme for Onchocerciasis Control: An overview. *Annals of Tropical Medicine and Parasitology, 92*(Suppl 1), S33–S39.

CHAPTER 17

Science, Technology, and Global Health

LEARNING OBJECTIVES

By the end of this chapter the reader will be able to:

- Articulate the needs for diagnostics, vaccines, and drugs to address high-burden diseases that affect the poor in low- and middle-income countries
- Assess the extent to which existing products meet those needs
- Note the potential of science and technology to develop new products to address high-burden diseases
- State some of the key constraints to investments in such products
- Indicate mechanisms to overcome these constraints and encourage the development and uptake of new diagnostics, vaccines, and drugs
- Outline the lessons for future efforts from selected cases of new product development

VIGNETTES

Juan lived in the highlands of Peru. He had tuberculosis (TB) and was being treated at a local TB clinic. He had to take four drugs for the first 2 months of his treatment and two drugs for 4 months after that. Juan felt better within weeks of starting his drugs and struggled to take the remaining pills because there were so many to take and he had to take them for so long.

Wezi lived in South Africa, where about 19 percent of the adults are HIV-positive.[1,2] Despite intensifying efforts to reduce the spread of new HIV infections in South Africa, the number of these infections is still large. In fact, the latest estimates suggest there were just under 370,000 new infections in 2012[3] and that about 6.3 million people in South Africa are now living with HIV.[2] Many people believe that

stopping transmission of HIV in countries like South Africa will depend on the discovery of a safe, effective, and affordable HIV vaccine.

Mei-Ling was 4 years old and lived in the west of China. Like so many children in her region, Mei-Ling was infected with hookworms. The community had a deworming program, and every 6 months Mei-Ling was given medicine to get rid of the worms. This medicine was generally safe and effective. However, it had to be given twice a year and there was some indication that the hookworms were becoming resistant to it.

David was 7 years old and lived in the eastern part of Kenya. He had a high fever and chills and his mother took him to the local health clinic. The nurse there examined David, decided he had malaria, and prescribed antimalarial medicine. This was the third time in a year that David had malaria. A safe, effective, and affordable malaria vaccine would have prevented him from getting malaria, being sick so often, missing so much school, and spending so much money on medical care.

INTRODUCTION

Scientific and technological progress has contributed substantially to improvements in human health. Such progress has included, for example, vaccines for a number of potential killers; a variety of drugs, such as penicillin; and safer and more effective family planning devices.

In fact, some scientific and technological discoveries have been of exceptional importance to public health. The discovery of the smallpox vaccine led to the first important efforts at vaccination and ultimately to the eradication of smallpox. Jonas Salk's discovery of the polio vaccine began to eliminate the scourge of polio from many societies, and his work was advanced further by Albert Sabin's work on the oral polio vaccine. It is difficult to imagine living in a world without antibiotics, but they emerged only just before World War II.

The enhancement of medical devices has also had an important impact on public health. The invention of the bifurcated needle was instrumental in enhancing the effectiveness of the smallpox eradication campaign. The intraocular lens for cataracts has provided a very low-cost tool for improving visual acuity.

The purpose of this chapter is to examine how science and technology could assist in speeding up the development and dissemination of new products that could address the largest burdens of disease in low- and middle-income countries. First, the chapter examines the characteristics that such products need to possess if they are to have the desired impact. Next, the chapter reviews the extent to which some existing diagnostics, vaccines, and drugs have those traits. The chapter then discusses the potential of science and technology to develop products in selected areas of importance and reviews the constraints to product development. Several policy and program briefs and one case study illustrate the key concepts of the chapter.

As you read this chapter, it is very important that you keep several things in mind. First, you should remember that very substantial gains in health could be obtained from the effective implementation of existing technologies. There are a number of low-cost but highly effective interventions that are well known but not used widely enough, including:

- Reducing maternal disability and deaths by better identification of complications, speedy transport to the hospital, and appropriate emergency obstetric care
- Reducing neonatal deaths by training birth attendants in resuscitation, keeping the baby warm, and the provision of antibiotics for infection
- Reducing young child deaths by expanding vaccination coverage with the six basic antigens and rotavirus and pneumococcal vaccines
- Reducing infant morbidity and mortality by promoting exclusive breastfeeding for 6 months
- Reducing morbidity and mortality from TB by expanding case finding and cure rates and through Directly Observed Therapy, Short Course (DOTS)

In addition, we must remember that better hygiene practices, such as handwashing with soap, do not require the development of any new products but could substantially improve health.

As you read this chapter, it is also important to keep in mind that the development of new products will not be a quick fix. Rather, while supporting the continued search for scientific and technical progress, it is critical to continue to focus on the underlying sources of ill health in low- and middle-income countries. These include poverty, the lack of education, the lack of political interest in the health of the poor, and the place of some minority groups and women in society. Enhancing basic infrastructure, water, and sanitation will also be critical in many settings to sustainable improvements in health.[4]

Finally, you should note that this chapter focuses on a narrow range of the scientific and technological matters that concern global health. It looks largely at new product development, the constraints to it, and what might be done to speed up the process. It does not examine research or operational research. Nor does it focus on the dissemination of existing technologies.

THE NEED FOR NEW PRODUCTS

As we think about the characteristics of diagnostics, drugs, vaccines, and medical devices that could most effectively and efficiently address the critical health problems of low- and middle-income countries, we need to keep several points in mind. First, the most important target groups for these products are poor people. Their financial resources are limited, and the countries in which they live, particularly low-income countries, generally spend little per capita on health. Second, the quality of care in many countries is low and injection safety is often poor. Third, many low- and middle-income countries have health systems that are poorly organized and cannot effectively manage logistics. In addition, transport and storage of goods is weak and the supply of electricity for keeping goods cool is often limited.

In this light, what are some of the ideal characteristics of diagnostics, drugs, vaccines, and medical delivery devices to help address the most critical burdens of disease in low- and middle-income countries? The most important of these characteristics are shown in **Table 17-1**.

As you can see in the table, it is important that diagnostics be specific, sensitive, easy to use, and noninvasive. Ideally, diagnostic tests could be done quickly by relatively untrained workers and would rapidly produce easy-to-read results. They would also be easy to transport, heat stable, inexpensive, and not require refrigeration.

TABLE 17-1 Some Ideal Characteristics of Diagnostics, Vaccines, Drugs, and Delivery Devices

Diagnostics: Affordable; specific and sensitive; provide quick and easy-to-interpret results; easy to store and transport; heat stable

Vaccines: Affordable; safe and effective; require few doses; confer lifelong immunity; easy to transport and store; heat stable

Drugs: Affordable; safe and effective; not easy for pathogens to become resistant to; require small doses over a limited period; easy to store and transport; heat stable

Delivery devices: Affordable; safe and effective; not invasive; easy to transport and store; heat stable

Much the same would be true for the ideal drugs. These drugs would be safe, effective, inexpensive, and have a long shelf life. They could also be used for many years without becoming susceptible to resistance. In addition, the number of pills that patients would have to take would be limited and they would not have to take them for very long.

Vaccines to meet the most important health needs in low- and middle-income countries would also be safe, effective, and inexpensive. They would be easy to transport and store, would be heat stable, and would not require refrigeration. The ideal vaccines would be an inexpensive combination of many antigens, and only one dose would confer lifelong immunity against a number of diseases. It would also be ideal if therapeutic and not just preventive vaccines could be developed for some burdens of disease.

The present state of key products does not meet the ideals noted here. Presently, for example, a child receiving full coverage of the six basic antigens in many countries would require six contacts with the health system to get all of these vaccines.[5] Could vaccines be developed that combine required antigens in such a way that only a few contacts would be needed between the health system and patients?

You read earlier about the cultural preference in many societies for injections, despite problems with injection safety. Could vaccines be delivered in noninvasive ways, such as sprays, air injectors, and skin patches, that would be safe,

effective, heat stable, easy to transport, not very costly and still be culturally acceptable?

There is a vaccine for tuberculosis and drugs that are effective against TB. However, the effectiveness of the TB vaccine against adult pulmonary TB is variable.[6] In addition, the drugs that are used to treat TB require a large pill burden and TB bacteria are increasingly becoming resistant to some of them.[7] What is needed to develop new drugs for TB that could make treatment shorter and easier? Is it possible to develop a safe and effective TB vaccine? Could that vaccine prevent all forms of TB and even prevent latent TB from becoming active TB disease?

Artemisinin-based combination therapy is effective against malaria that is resistant to chloroquine, although resistance to artemisinin is already growing. However, the cost per treatment with this drug, even at globally negotiated prices, is about $1 per child and about $2 per adult.[8] This is about 10 times the cost per treatment with chloroquine for children and 20 times the cost for adults.[9] In addition, although the search for a malaria vaccine has gone on for many years and there has been some progress in developing and testing a vaccine, there is still no approved vaccine for malaria. What would it take to develop additional low-cost and highly effective malaria drugs? What can encourage the development of a safe and effective malaria vaccine?

Drugs for HIV/AIDS can control the virus for most people but cannot cure them of HIV. In addition, people develop resistance to those drugs, and some of the drugs have important side effects. Moreover, there is still no preventive or therapeutic vaccine for HIV/AIDS. How can the world encourage the development of safer and more effective HIV/AIDS drugs, an HIV/AIDS vaccine, and mechanisms, such as microbicides, by which women could protect themselves better from the risk of HIV?

The scientific and technological gaps indicated previously also apply to some of the other neglected diseases. Despite the ubiquity of hookworm, there is no vaccine for hookworm, the drug used to treat it has to be administered regularly, and resistance to it is increasing. Can a vaccine be developed for hookworm and some of the other parasitic diseases?

THE POTENTIAL OF SCIENCE AND TECHNOLOGY

Scientific progress has led to a number of areas in which science could be harnessed to address some of the gaps noted in the previous section and to improve human health. Four such areas, as examples, are noted in this section.

Sequencing the genomes of important pathogens will help scientists better understand why they cause disease, how they develop resistance, and what drugs can best fight them, while reducing the onset of resistance. The genomes have now been sequenced for more than 180 microbial species.[10] The speed with which the SARS virus was sequenced is an indication of the speed with which this can be done, if sufficient priority is given to this work.[11] The sequencing of the mosquito genome may allow scientists to engineer mosquitoes so that they cannot carry malaria and other diseases, such as lymphatic filariasis.[12] Scientists have already sequenced the genome of the *Anopheles stephensi* mosquito, a key vector of malaria throughout the Indian subcontinent. This research has provided new insights into mosquito biology and mosquito–parasite interactions, which have important implications for the prevention of malaria transmission.[13]

Improvements in information technology, chemistry, and robotics, as well as in genetic and molecular epidemiology, will also facilitate the development of new and better drugs. These tools will allow scientists to understand better the nature of disease. They will also enable scientists to more quickly try different chemical compounds to address those pathogens.[14]

In addition, a number of technologies exist that can assist in the design and manufacture of new and improved vaccines.[14] The use of recombinant DNA technology, for example, helped an Indian vaccine company to reduce the cost of hepatitis B vaccine from about $8 to 50 cents.[12] DNA technology should also be very helpful to the development of drugs.[12]

Genetic modification of plants is a controversial subject because, among other things, there are concerns over the environmental and health risks associated with them. Yet, it is possible to engineer plants that can carry higher levels of certain nutrients, such as vitamin A, while being very resistant to disease.[12] In addition, plants can be modified genetically so that they can produce edible vaccines. The most advanced such work is for a vaccine for hepatitis B, but work is under way for other vaccines, as well.[12]

In fact, there is an increasing understanding of the promise of science and technology for improving global health. In one study, the views of 28 experts were sought about the biotechnologies that could help improve health in low- and middle-income countries in the following 5 to 10 years.[15] In particular, these scientists were polled about the extent to which technologies would:[15]

- Improve health
- Be affordable and appropriate in low- and middle-income countries
- Address the most pressing health needs
- Be developed in the next 5 to 10 years

- Advance knowledge
- Have important indirect benefits

They were also asked how they would use science and technology to achieve these aims. As the highest priority, these scientists would use biotechnology to develop new diagnostics, vaccines, and drugs, in that order. They would use technology to improve the environment, including water and sanitation. The scientists also put a premium on the development of products that can help empower women to protect themselves against sexually transmitted diseases, including HIV, such as microbicides.[15]

The Grand Challenges in Global Health aims to engage the world's most innovative researchers in defining and addressing critical research and operational challenges in global health. The initiative was launched in 2003 by the Bill & Melinda Gates Foundation, in conjunction with the Canadian Institute for Health Research, the Foundation for the U.S. National Institutes of Health, and the Wellcome Trust. Several years after it was launched, the Grand Challenges program had already awarded more than $458 million in 45 grants for 33 different countries.[16] The specific goals of this program and the challenges it seeks to address are given in **Table 17-2.**

In 2008, the Bill & Melinda Gates Foundation launched a related initiative, Grand Challenges Explorations, which provides $100 million in financing to encourage the development of bold and unconventional ideas for tackling the need for new tools to address the burden of disease among the poor in low- and middle-income countries. Since 2008, more than 1,140 Grand Challenge Explorations grants were awarded to projects in more than 60 countries.[16]

Grand Challenges Canada was launched in 2010 and is funded by the Government of Canada. Grand Challenges Canada has a similar aim to Grand Challenges in Global Health, which is to support bold ideas that have the potential to make a significant impact in global health. However, Grand Challenges Canada places an emphasis on integrated innovation, meaning the development of ideas that integrate scientific and technical, social, and business innovation. Since its inception, the initiative has supported almost 700 innovations.[17]

In 2011, USAID established the Grand Challenges for Development Initiative. This initiative aims to create and support sustainable solutions to key development issues, including those in health. It focuses specifically on defining problems, identifying constraints, and providing evidence-based analysis for challenges in development. Six Grand Challenges specific to this initiative have been launched: Fighting Ebola, Securing Water for Food, Saving Lives at

TABLE 17-2 Selected Goals of the Grand Challenges in Global Health

Improve Vaccines
- Create effective single-dose vaccines that can be used soon after birth.
- Prepare vaccines that do not require refrigeration.
- Develop needle-free delivery systems.

Create New Vaccines
- Devise reliable tests in model systems to evaluate live attenuated vaccines.
- Solve how to design antigens for effective, protective immunity.
- Learn which immunological responses provide protective immunity.

Control Insect Vectors
- Develop a genetic strategy to deplete or incapacitate a disease-transmitting insect population.
- Develop a chemical strategy to deplete or incapacitate a disease-transmitting insect population.

Improve Nutrition
- Create a full range of optimal, bioavailable nutrients in a single staple plant species.

Limit Drug Resistance
- Discover drugs and delivery systems that minimize the likelihood of drug-resistant microorganisms.

Cure Infection
- Create therapies that can cure latent infection.
- Create immunological methods that can cure chronic infections.

Measure Health Status
- Develop technologies that permit quantitative assessment of population health status.
- Develop technologies that allow assessment of multiple conditions and pathogens at point of care.

Data from Grand Challenges in Global Health. Goals. Retrieved September 28, 2010, from http://www.grandchallenges.org/Pages/BrowseByGoal.aspx.

Birth, All Children Reading, Powering Agriculture, and Making all Voices Count.[18]

Grand Challenges Brazil and Grand Challenges India are the newest Grand Challenges initiatives.[18] Grand Challenges Brazil, launched in 2012, is a partnership framework for the Ministry of Health of Brazil, its National Council on Research, and the Bill & Melinda Gates Foundation. Its goal is to develop joint initiatives to work toward solutions in global health. Grand Challenges India was launched in 2013 and involves a partnership between the Department of Biotechnology in India, the Biotechnology Industry Research Assistance Council, and the Bill & Melinda Gates Foundation. Its aim is to catalyze innovative health and development research within India.[18]

A number of funded projects aim to improve vaccines. For example, one project is attempting to develop a vaccine that can prevent pertussis with a single dose, instead of the current three-dose requirement. Another project is trying to develop a vaccine against pneumococcus that can be given in a single dose, instead of the present four doses. Several projects are seeking to make vaccines more heat stable. Others aim to create vaccine delivery systems that can be eaten, inhaled, or sprayed into the nose. Several projects are working towards the development of a malaria vaccine. Others concern efforts to develop strategies for genetically engineering mosquitoes so they will be unable to spread the dengue virus.[19,20]

Several of the projects that were funded aim to use genetic engineering to biofortify plants. For example, in Uganda, where bananas are a staple food, researchers are attempting to engineer the fruit to contain more usable vitamin A, vitamin E, and iron. Similar work was done on rice with vitamins A and E, iron, zinc, and improved protein quality. Additional projects will focus on the science relating to the development of drugs for addressing latent TB and vaccines for the human papillomavirus.[19] **Table 17-3** lists a small number of examples of the Grand Challenges grants.

The newest initiatives funded by Grand Challenges in Global Health were announced in 2014. The three new initiatives include All Children Thriving, Putting Women and Girls at the Center of Development, and Creating New Interventions for Global Health.[21] These initiatives mark a new focus for Grand Challenges in Global Health on the importance of women and girls in contributing to the health and economic prosperity of their families and communities. The initiatives emphasize developing new tools and holistic approaches to help mothers and children thrive in low- and middle-income countries, supporting new approaches to promote women's and girls' empowerment, and accelerating the safe, effective, and affordable use of vaccines.

TABLE 17-3 Selected Grand Challenges Grants by Goal

Discover New Ways to Achieve Healthy Birth, Growth, and Development
- Azithromycin Administration to Prevent Growth Faltering in Gambian Infants (2012)
- Postpartum Deworming: Improving Breastfeeding and Optimizing Infant Growth (2012)
- Enhancing Infant Immunity: Effect of Early Maternal Treatment for Parasitic Infections (2012)

Discover Biomarkers of Health and Disease
- Development of Human mRNA as a Biomarker for Environmental Enteropathy (2012)
- Disposable Sampling Plate and Breath Test to Identify Patients with Active Tuberculosis (2012)
- Pathogen and Host Metabolites as Diagnostic Signatures of Tuberculosis (2012)

Develop a Chemical Strategy to Deplete or Incapacitate a Disease-transmitting Insect Population
- A New Target for Mosquitocides (2011)
- Molecular Mosquitocides (2011)
- Develop Synthetic Chemical Mimics of Selectively Insecticidal Natural Peptides (2011)

Develop Technologies That Allow Assessment of Multiple Conditions and Pathogens at Point-of-Care
- A Universal One-Step Device to Safely and Painlessly Collect Blood (2011)
- A Multidisciplinary Point-of-Care Laboratory in an Active HIV Treatment Clinic (2011)
- Fabric Chips: A Versatile Platform for Low-Cost, Rapid and Multiplexed Diagnostic Tests (2011)

Learn Which Immunological Responses Provide Protective Immunity
- Biomarkers of Protective Immunity Against TB in the Context of HIV/AIDS in Africa (2005)
- Comprehensive Studies of Mechanisms of HIV Resistance in Highly Exposed Uninfected Women (2005)
- Immunity to Prevent Pneumococcal Transmission: Correlates of Protection and Herd Immunity (2005)

Create a Full Range of Optimal, Bioavailable Nutrients in a Single Staple Plant Species
- Improving Cassava for Nutrition, Health, and Sustainable Development (2005)
- Optimization of Bioavailable Nutrients in Transgenic Bananas (2005)
- Nutritionally Enhanced Sorghum for the Arid and Semiarid Tropical Areas of Africa (2005)

Develop Technologies That Permit Quantitative Assessment of Population Health Status
- Population Health Metrics Research Consortium Project (2005)

Develop Needle-Free Delivery Systems
- Nanoemulsions as Adjuvants for Nasal Spray Vaccines (2005)
- Needle Free Delivery of Stable, Respirable Powder Vaccine (2005)
- Needle Free Vaccination Via Nanoparticle Aerosois (2005)

Data from *Grand Challenges in Global Health Grants*. Retrieved November 12, 2014, from http://gcgh.grandchallenges.org/Pages/GCGHGrantsAwarded .aspx?TDate=TB%20Biomarkers%20-%20February%202012.

CONSTRAINTS TO APPLYING SCIENCE AND TECHNOLOGY TO GLOBAL HEALTH PROBLEMS

Given the strengths of existing scientific knowledge, why is it that some of the products that could make an important difference to the health of the poor globally have not been developed? Beyond the inherent scientific difficulties in some of these efforts, such as the development of HIV and malaria vaccines, there are several common constraints to the development of desired products. First, much of the research and development on new diagnostics, vaccines, drugs, and delivery devices is carried out in the for-profit sector, and that sector has historically believed it could not make a sufficient return from products oriented toward low- and middle-income countries. These firms see the market for their goods in low- and middle-income countries as a small one. They also doubt the ability of governments and individuals in low-income countries to pay prices for their products that would give them a sufficient return on their capital. As evidence of this, for example, they point to the earlier slow uptake in low- and middle-income countries of the vaccines against *Haemophilus influenzae* type b (Hib) and hepatitis B.

Moreover, the costs of research and development on new products can be very high, some suggesting as high as $800 million, to bring a new drug from research to market. Given these costs, profit-making firms will invariably want to use their capital to develop, for example, a potential blockbuster drug against high cholesterol that can be sold in high-income countries, rather than develop a drug for low-income countries on which the firm believes it will not be able to recoup its investment.[22]

In addition, vaccine markets have some particular constraints to entry. Vaccine development requires a considerable amount of upstream investment, the cost of developing vaccine candidates is very high, and governmental regulations may also reduce the potential for sufficient profit from vaccines to attract firms to this market. In addition, the number of firms engaged in vaccine production worldwide is small and production capacity is limited. The development of vaccines for low- and middle-income country markets has also been complicated by the fact that, until recently, vaccine manufacturers often had to produce formulations of vaccines for some low- and middle-income countries that were different from the relatively expensive combination vaccines that were used in other countries. Moreover, pharmaceutical companies can generally earn a higher return on money invested in the development of drugs than money invested in developing vaccines.[23]

Another constraint to greater focus on the health conditions of low- and middle-income countries until recently has been insufficient attention to them by some of the major national research institutions. The basic research that is conducted at places like the U.S. National Institutes of Health often sets a foundation for product development later by the for-profit manufacturers. The greater the attention that national research institutes in high-income countries pay to high-burden problems of low- and middle-income countries, the greater the likelihood that new products for them will eventually be developed.

Some of these constraints are reflected in the extent to which drugs have been developed to address diseases that most affect poor people in low- and middle-income countries.

A study of drugs that were approved for marketing showed that between 1975 and 1999, for example, 1,393 new chemicals were approved but only about 3 percent were relevant to infectious and parasitic diseases that are the most significant burdens of disease in low-income countries. The same study looked at the number of new drugs approved for every million DALYs and found that two to three times more drugs were produced for every million DALYs attributable to diseases of high-income countries, rather than diseases of low- and middle-income countries.[22] Over the same period, only about 1 percent of the drugs approved concerned the neglected tropical diseases and only about 0.2 percent concerned TB.[24]

In 2013, the FDA approved the first new anti-TB drug in 40 years. The new drug, called bedaquiline, will create an alternative to the current regimens for multidrug resistant TB that have high toxicity and inadequate efficiency. Bedaquiline also has the potential to shorten treatment for drug-resistant TB, which could improve patient adherence. Experts estimate that $2 billion must be spent yearly in the future to end the global TB epidemic, yet investment in TB research to develop new drugs, vaccines, and diagnostics was less than one third of this amount in 2013.[25] Moreover, about 90 percent of expenditure on research and development on health has been oriented toward the diseases of the high-income countries and only about 10 percent toward the diseases of the developing world.[26,27] The Global Forum for Health Research called this the "10/90 gap."[27]

ENHANCING NEW PRODUCT DEVELOPMENT

We have seen that gaps in the development of diagnostics, drugs, vaccines, and medical devices that can serve the needs of low- and middle-income countries reflect market failures. In general, the public sector tries to reduce its risks by waiting for such products to be developed by the private sector. However, the private sector generally believes that it is too risky to produce products that are expensive to develop and for which an adequate return on investment cannot be assured. Is it possible to change the market for these products? Can one reduce the cost of product research and development to the point where the private for-profit sector might be interested in such products? What other steps can be taken to speed product development?

Push Mechanisms

A number of steps could encourage a larger share of research and development to focus on the needs of low- and middle-income countries. Some of these are shown in **Figure 17-1**, which depicts push and pull mechanisms and where in the product development cycle they have the most impact.

FIGURE 17-1 Push/Pull Mechanism for Product Development

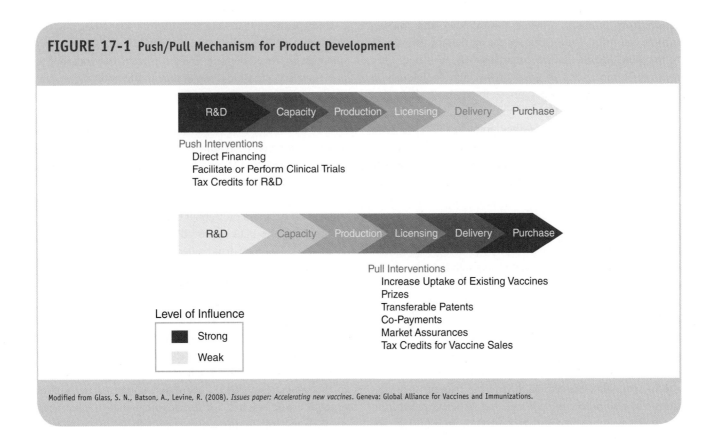

Modified from Glass, S. N., Batson, A., Levine, R. (2008). *Issues paper: Accelerating new vaccines*. Geneva: Global Alliance for Vaccines and Immunizations.

One type of effort is called "push mechanisms." These refer to mechanisms meant to encourage product development by reducing the risks and costs of investments.[23] Push mechanisms could include:[23]

- Direct financing: Government financing or carrying out of research activities needed to develop a product.
- Performing or facilitating clinical trials: This could include government measures to make it easier to carry out clinical trials for the product and to help with the ethical issues involved in such trials.
- Tax credits for research and development: Governments can lower the cost to firms of research and development by giving them credits against their taxes for certain investments.

These push mechanisms operate on the early stages of product development. Such mechanisms have been used successfully before. In addition, they can reduce risk and thereby encourage investment in product development. The disadvantage of push mechanisms, however, is that there is no guarantee that they will produce a product. Even if a product is developed, it may not be the best one, and product developers will then not produce what might have been better candidates. Furthermore, when the money is spent on push mechanisms it is gone whether or not a product has been developed.[23]

Some of the direct financing and facilitation of clinical trials could be done through programs like the U.S. National Institutes of Health or similar institutes in other countries. Additional money could also be channeled, for example, to the Special Program for Research and Training in Tropical Diseases (TDR), which is sponsored by WHO, UNICEF, the United Nations Development Program, and the World Bank.[28] Some of the financing of the Bill & Melinda Gates Foundation, like that for the Grand Challenges, is meant to push new product development.

In conjunction with these efforts, it is important to strengthen the links between researchers in low- and middle-income countries and high-income counties. The links can also be enhanced among researchers in low- and middle-income countries. The aim of these efforts would be to attract more research money to institutions within the low- and middle-income countries that are engaged in research and development on the most important burdens of disease in such countries. A number of low- and middle-income countries, especially India, China, Brazil, South Africa, Mexico, Indonesia, and Cuba, already have the ability to carry out basic research and to develop products that emanate from that research. Additional funding might deepen and speed their research.[29]

It is also important to comment on some aspects of governmental regulation of pharmaceutical and vaccine development. Regulation is necessary, but it is also an important part of the costs of research and development. By arranging to speed drug approvals and harmonize approval processes across countries, the costs of research and development can be reduced to provide some incentives to manufacturers. Granting fast-track approval for generic AIDS drugs, for example, *has* encouraged the development of such drugs.[24]

Pull Mechanisms

A number of mechanisms are intended to help ensure that a future return is provided to those who do develop new products. These are called pull mechanisms.[23,26] Some of the most important pull mechanisms include:[23]

- Increasing the uptake of existing vaccines: Using public funds to increase the use of vaccines that have not been taken up sufficiently, such as the vaccines for Hib and hepatitis B.
- Prizes: Offering monetary rewards to those firms that develop desired products.
- Transferable patents: In exchange for the development of the desired product, providing the manufacturer with the right to extend a patent on another one of their products or patents in markets in high-income countries.
- Copayments: Governments can provide the manufacturer with a payment for every product sold.
- Market assurances: The public sector can promise to buy the products if they are produced.
- Tax credits for vaccine sales: Governments can offer tax credits for products that are sold.

From the point of view of the public sector, pull mechanisms have the advantage of providing funds only when desired products have been developed. However, governments and the private sector have to agree early on what such arrangements would be for any product, and neither party might be satisfied with these arrangements when products do emerge.[23] There has been little experience until recently with financing mechanisms that are meant to exert a pull on new product development and use, but the Advance Market Commitments and the International Finance Facility for Immunisation are now in place and are discussed later in the chapter.

A mechanism that has been used for vaccines for some time and more recently for AIDS drugs is called *tiered pricing*. This is an arrangement by which a firm charges different prices in different markets. The idea behind tiered pricing is that a firm can charge enough to make a profit in high-income markets to offset the fact that the products will not make a profit in low- and middle-income markets. The profits from one market could cross-subsidize the sales at reduced prices in other markets. This is being practiced now for some drugs for which there is a global market. However, tiered pricing is not likely to work effectively for products that are needed exclusively in low- and middle-income countries because the basis for cross-subsidizing will not exist.[24]

In addition, considerable hope is being put into the role that public–private partnerships can play in encouraging the development of the diagnostics, drugs, vaccines, and medical devices that could have a significant impact on the health of the poor in low- and middle-income countries. As indicated earlier, many of these efforts are organized around the search for new products for particular diseases, such as HIV, TB, and malaria. These public–private partnerships are also referred to as product development partnerships (PDPs) and are organized on a not-for-profit basis. They aim to attract private, public, and philanthropic funds to invest in needed research and development, tapping the strengths of the private sector in product development as they do so. There are now PDPs for a large number of vaccines and drugs, including, for example, TB and malaria. A brief is given later in this chapter on the development of TB vaccines.

Meeting product development goals will probably require a combination of these efforts. First, they can start with a greater focus by research institutions in high-income countries on the problems of low- and middle-income countries. They can also promote greater networking of research institutions in low- and middle-income countries. This can help encourage product development, with other push mechanisms. At the same time, it will be important to change the market and perceptions of the market for needed products through pull mechanisms that can ensure that money will be available for products if they are developed. Third, the public and private sectors can collaborate with each other, bringing complementary skills and financing to the partnership.

POLICY AND PROGRAM BRIEFS

This section contains a number of policy and program briefs that highlight some of the different approaches to harnessing science and technology to enhance new product development and use. Mobile technology and telemedicine are increasingly used in health work in many countries, and this section begins with a brief on each of those topics. This is followed by briefs that touch on the development of new diagnostics for TB and a device intended to reduce the risk of maternal hemorrhage.

The next brief discusses a PDP, Aeras, that aims to spur the development of more effective TB vaccines. The last two briefs concern innovative financing mechanisms that are intended to provide a pull on new product development and diffusion, the Advance Market Commitments (AMC) and the International Finance Facility for Immunisation (IFFIm).

mHealth: Using Mobile Technology to Improve the Health of the Poor in Poor Countries

What Is mHealth?

mHealth, or mobile health, is commonly defined as medical and public health practice supported by mobile devices, such as mobile phones, patient monitoring devices, personal digital assistants (PDAs), and other wireless devices that can transmit text messages, photos, and data at the touch of a button. **Table 17-4** lists the different categories of mobile health technologies, potential applications, and selected examples of mHealth programs. mHealth is a rapidly growing area in the development of health technology and is a component of eHealth, or the delivery of health care by electronic means.[30] Over 90 percent of the world is now covered by a mobile network and, as a result, 83 percent of WHO member countries now have mHealth programs. The largest expansion of mHealth has occurred in the Asia-Pacific region due to more extensive mobile data networks. mHealth has seen the largest barriers in Africa, due largely to limited infrastructure, but great progress has been made there, as programs such as SIMpill and Child Count+ demonstrate. Within low- and middle-income countries, mHealth has been more commonly adopted in healthcare areas related to maternal and child health, HIV/AIDS, and primary care.[31] There is hope that mHealth can offer cost-effective programs and interventions to support the performance of health workers and disseminate health education information, especially in places where health systems face significant challenges of human and physical resources.[32]

What Is the Scope of mHealth?

In 2009, the World Health Organization conducted the second global survey of mHealth technologies and used a classification system based on six categories to describe the scope of mHealth initiatives globally.[30]

Although there are many programs that fall within these categories, there is substantial innovation in mHealth, and

TABLE 17-4 WHO Classification of mHealth Technologies

Technology Category	Applications	Example Programs
Communication: individuals to health services	Health call centers; emergency toll-free telephone services	Healthline (Bangladesh); Ligne Verte toll-free hotline (Democratic Republic of the Congo)
Communication: health services to individuals	Appointment reminders; medication reminders; health promotion	On Cue Compliance (South Africa); SIMpill (South Africa)
General consultations	Telemedicine	Mobile Doctors Network (Ghana); Aceh Behar Midwives with Mobile Phone project (Indonesia)
Emergency communication	Referrals; transports	Dial 1298 for Ambulance (India)
Monitoring & surveillance	Mobile surveys; patient reminders	Episurveyor (Senegal); Cam e-WARN (Cambodia)
Health information access	Patient records; population data	Child Count+ (Malawi, Uganda); OpenMRS (many countries)

Data from World Health Organization (WHO) (2014). *mHealth: New horizons for health through mobile technologies: Second global survey on eHealth.* Global Observatory for eHealth series. Vol. 3; Unite for Sight. (2013). *mHealth technology in global health.* Retrieved August 30, 2014, from http://www.uniteforsight.org/global-health-university/mhealth#_ftn27.

there is greater diversity of mHealth than these categories capture. For example, applications have been developed that allow mHealth to help support the diagnostic process, while other applications act as attachments to traditional medical tools such as the stethoscope.[33]

Communication: Individuals to Health Services

One of the most common mHealth initiatives has been the creation of health call centers that allow individuals to call in or text health questions and receive immediate answers. These help lines have been developed with the goal of increasing access to health advice and information, while overcoming potential barriers, such as shortage of healthcare professionals and the costs of service provision and transportation. For example, a medical hotline called Healthline in Bangladesh received more than 3.5 million calls in its first 3 years of operation from individuals seeking answers from a licensed health professional. Similarly, an initiative called the Ligne Verte (Green Line) toll-free hotline was introduced in the Democratic Republic of the Congo to provide confidential family planning information and to refer patients to nearby clinics that offer contraception services. Each call cost $0.36 equivalent. The most successful of these healthcare centers have been operated by for-profit organizations that partner with mobile network operators. As a result, health call centers may not be as accessible to the poor as desired.[30]

Communication: Health Services to Individuals

One of the greatest challenges in many health systems is patient compliance. A 2007 pilot study in South Africa demonstrated that patient compliance could jump to over 90 percent in areas previously recording 22–60 percent compliance when a mobile application technology, SIMpill, was introduced. This application is a medication container that communicates with a patient's mobile phone to remind the patient about the timing of the next medication dose. Repeated or missed dosages are brought to the attention of healthcare workers, who then follow-up with the patient and arrange for an in-person visit.[34]

General Consultations

Telemedicine initiatives have also been widespread and can help improve the quality of care for rural populations by creating more opportunities for interaction with qualified medical professionals in urban settings. Many pilot telemedicine programs have been successful, including a program in Taiwan that had an 85 percent accuracy rate in the remote diagnosis of soft tissue injuries. Other telemedicine programs have attempted to enhance the referral process by facilitating communication between physicians. The Mobile Doctors Network (MDNet) in Ghana was launched in 2008 and was the first program in Africa to provide free mobile-to-mobile voice and text services to all physicians in Ghana. It has been successful in enhancing physician connectivity, the frequency of consultations, the success rate of diagnosis and treatment for populations with limited access to specialized care, the time needed for referral, and the patient's recovery experience.[30] The start-up costs for telemedicine projects can be minimal if telecommunications providers are incentivized to donate the infrastructure and resources such as SIM cards, but the cost-effectiveness of these types of efforts is still being investigated.

Emergency Communication

In emergency situations, a rapid response can be the difference between life and death. Although emergency response systems in high-income countries are established, those in low- and middle-income countries are often limited or nonexistent.[34] Nonetheless, mHealth offers applications that at low cost can capitalize on the mobile network coverage that does exist in these low-resource settings. On a national scale for example, nationwide alert systems can be implemented through these networks. After the 2010 Haitian earthquake, three mHealth organizations—Ushahidi, FrontlineSMS, and SamaSource—created a logistics map using short message service (SMS) alerts for missing people or immediate humanitarian needs that was widely used by aid organizations throughout Haiti. Unfortunately, these types of programs have only been evaluated in a limited manner.[34]

Monitoring and Surveillance

An array of mHealth technologies has been used for health monitoring and surveillance. Senegal piloted a program called Episurveyor that indicated that only 55 percent of the country's health districts were systematically using partograms, graphical tools that monitor the trajectory of labor. Based on the information from this survey, Senegal's Ministry of Health was able to increase the distribution of partograms and institute initiatives that encouraged midwives to use them. A follow-up survey demonstrated that this intervention led to an average increase of 28 percent in partogram use in the applicable regions.[30] This pilot effort was part of a larger mHealth program funded by the UN Foundation and Vodafone Foundation Technology Partnership.[30]

Access to Health Information

Electronic medical records have become a gold standard for health systems. In low- and middle-income countries, electronic records have been implemented slowly but the introduction of mHealth can help reduce the burden on health workers and health facilities by allowing easier access to information and its sharing. For example, OpenMRS allows frontline health workers to access information from a patient's health record using a mobile device and then add information to the health record after a consultation. ChildCount+ has been very successful in sub-Saharan Africa in enhancing the efforts of community health workers. The program offers an integrated system that links individual patient records with population data in order to improve follow-up services and better understand a community's needs.[34] It is important to note, however, that the literature on the outcomes and cost–effectiveness of health information applications is still limited.

The Need for Evaluation

It is important to know whether the investments in time and resources in mHealth have been both impactful and cost-effective and if they are good candidates for scaling up. Despite extensive innovation in the development of mobile health technologies, evaluation of the effectiveness of these technologies has been limited. Although some uses of mHealth appear to be successful and others appear to be promising, only 12 percent of all mHealth activities have been subjected to evaluation.[30] Thus, there are still very few examples of proven impact of mHealth programs.[35] Moreover, many evaluations have been conducted comparing health outcomes of mHealth technologies to the baseline before the introduction of technologies, rather than comparing different mHealth programs or mHealth to other innovations. This type of evaluation is useful, but more widespread comparative evaluations must be made in order to establish best practices and model programs.

Looking Forward

As evidence from well-planned evaluations grows, it is likely that there will be a transition from experimentation with different technologies to strategic implementation of the technologies known to be effective. Currently, more than 50 percent of mHealth programs are in a piloting phase. Moreover, as the application of mHealth continues to advance, it is clear that other issues will also need to be addressed more fully, including data privacy and ways to integrate various applications. Overall, there is hope that mHealth will offer cost-effective solutions to improving health outcomes and access to health information in low- and middle-income countries.

Eliminating Borders: Using Telemedicine to Connect the Medical Community in India

Background

Despite the fact that nearly 75 percent of the people in India live in rural areas, more than 75 percent of Indian health professionals operate in urban areas. Thus, many people in rural areas have particular difficulty accessing specialty care.[36] Aspiring to link rural communities to health professionals in other parts of the country, the Apollo Hospitals Group established the Apollo Telemedicine Networking Foundation (ATNF) in 1997.

Telemedicine is the practice of using information and communication technologies (ICTs) to expand access to care and medical information. In some parts of India, telemedicine has helped connect rural health centers with tertiary care centers and specialists.[37] In the process, distant specialists have diagnosed and treated patients in remote rural settings, patients have begun adhering to treatments earlier, and both patients and specialists have had to travel less to receive and deliver treatments.

ATNF has acted as a champion for bringing telemedicine to South Asia and has inspired similar models in Africa, Kazakhstan, Yemen, and Sudan.[38] Subsequent telemedicine projects by other organizations, for example, have used satellite-enabled mobile vans that travel through villages to connect rural health professionals to diabetes specialists in urban areas. Other uses of telemedicine in India have included neurological consults and psychiatric therapy sessions.

Intervention

In March 1999, ATNF launched the Aragonda Project as a pilot telemedicine initiative in a local hospital in the village of Aragonda, in Andhra Pradesh state. This was the first hospital in India to use ICTs to improve the health of its patients. Working alongside the Department of Space, Government of India, and the Indian Space Research Organization, ATNF's project was unique for two reasons. First, ATNF added videoconferencing technology to the hospital, allowing patients and practitioners to directly interact with specialists located in Chennai. Second, ATNF created databases to store electronic medical records that were made available to patients when they came for appointments.[38]

Since its first center opened 15 years ago, ATNF has also been committed to long-term capacity building of rural health personnel and the sustainability of ATNF's operations. To do this, it has focused heavily on educating rural health practitioners by connecting them with specialists in more urban parts of the country. During teleconsultations, local nurses and health workers in rural regions can seek advice from specialists and be guided through minor procedures. In recent years, ATNF has also developed a disease management module, allowing local practitioners in rural settings to learn about the major burdens of disease in their respective regions and the appropriate symptoms and treatments for different ailments. Because teleconferences serve several different purposes, they have also been used at a community level, allowing tertiary hospitals to connect with rural community health centers and advise them on public health interventions to improve community health.[39] ATNF has also prompted increased knowledge sharing as the first center in India to scan and send images of x-rays and ultrasounds to remote hospitals.

In 2007, ATNF helped organize telemedicine conferences that brought together delegates from all over India and the world. Since then, ATNF has also established certificate programs in Telehealth Technology by collaborating with Anna University in Chennai. These courses have trained over 150 participants and have helped build an expanding network of telemedicine experts across India.[40]

The Impact

Apollo's telemedicine initiatives have had a notable impact on increasing healthcare coverage in parts of rural India. Today, ATNF has 115 peripheral centers across India and 10 overseas. More than 69,000 teleconsultations had been provided through ATNF as of May 2011. These teleconsultations have covered a broad range of medical issues from sexual health to pregnancies and neurosurgeries. In doing so, studies have found that many patients living in rural areas have received diagnoses and treatments earlier than they would have otherwise.[40] Although little data exists on the quality of ATNF's teleconsultations, its use of telemedicine is a promising innovation to connect rural regions with a variety of specialists in urban areas.

Costs and Benefits

Over the last 6 years, the Indian government has spent approximately $100,000 annually per state under the National Rural Health Mission to expand telemedicine networks at the district level. Each teleconsultation costs a patient between $20 and $30. The cost of an Apollo teleconsultation appears to be less than a physical hospital visit for similar services. Including the cost of travel, such physical visits can cost a patient approximately $100–250. The Indian government's recent national health insurance scheme for those below the poverty line, known as Rashtriya Swasthya Bima Yojana (RSBY), has begun to cover some teleconsultation costs for low-income individuals. ATNF is also attempting to make these services more accessible to people who do not have insurance or the means to pay for health services by implementing a cross-subsidization mechanism. Under such a system, patients who are capable of paying for teleconsultations pay higher fees to help subsidize the cost of care for those who cannot afford similar services. Both RSBY and ATNF's cross-subsidization schemes are relatively recent and it will be interesting to see how both the cost and financing of these services evolve.[40]

Lessons Learned

Apollo has placed a strong emphasis on sustainable education and is a leader in Indian telemedicine. From organizing conferences to setting up certificate programs, the foundation is building telemedicine infrastructure in India by encouraging initiatives similar to its own. As part of the government's 11th Five-Year plan, approximately $50 million equivalent was allocated toward building public–private telemedicine partnerships.[41] Today, roughly 500 rural telemedicine centers in India are linked to approximately 50 specialty hospitals.[42] Through an expanding telemedicine network, the Apollo Hospitals group is helping India and the rest of the world reduce geographical barriers and make some healthcare services more affordable and accessible.[43]

New Diagnostics for TB: Xpert MTB/RIF

Although the overwhelming majority of TB deaths could be prevented with early diagnosis and proper treatment, diagnosis of TB has faced substantial challenges.[44] First, the standard for diagnosing pulmonary TB, microscopic examination of sputum samples from a TB suspect, is estimated to correctly diagnose only about 20 to 60 percent of adults who have TB.[45] Second, sputum microscopy cannot be used to diagnose TB in young children, because they cannot produce sputum samples. In addition, substantial training is required for consistently accurate diagnosis of extrapulmonary TB and even skilled clinicians experience significant variability in their results.[46] Finally, the diagnosis of multidrug-resistant TB (MDR-TB) has required that samples be cultured, which can be done only in select laboratories and takes substantial time to produce results.

In light of this situation, the global TB community has long sought improved tools for diagnosing TB, and progress has recently been made in this direction. In 2006, the Foundation for Innovative New Diagnostics (FIND) partnered with Cepheid, Inc. and the University of Medicine and Dentistry of New Jersey to try to develop an enhanced diagnostic tool for TB.[46] They sought to use existing technology to improve the sensitivity and specificity of TB detection—especially in difficult cases involving drug resistance and coinfection with HIV—all while automating the process to reduce interuser variability.

From this collaboration came the Xpert TB test. In just 2 hours, Xpert detects the presence of mycobacterium tuberculosis (MTB) by amplifying and analyzing genetic material in the sputum sample.[44] Furthermore, the technology detects resistance to the first-line drug rifampicin (RIF), which allows doctors to identify and appropriately treat drug-resistant TB. Moreover, the Xpert MTB/RIF system offers high sensitivity and specificity compared to sputum smear microscopy, with rates of 98 to 100 percent and 100 percent, respectively.[47] In addition, clinical trials have shown that the system detects TB in individuals co-infected with HIV with a sensitivity of 70 percent, rather than the 50 percent sensitivity offered by conventional sputum smear microscopy.[48]

FIND and the manufacturer have negotiated prices for use in low- and middle-income countries, with Xpert costing $17,000 for the permanent equipment and $9.98 for each test cartridge, instead of the standard price of $16.86.[49] This concessional pricing is possible because organizations including the President's Emergency Plan for AIDS Relief (PEPFAR), USAID, UNITAID, and the Bill & Melinda Gates Foundation provided financial support and negotiated a discount on each cartridge. Although Xpert's automation means workers will no longer need to spend time examining sputum by microscopy, Xpert does require annual maintenance and is still more expensive than traditional techniques.[50] It is expected that diagnosing a case of TB will now cost $61, about 55 percent more than when using traditional methods.[51] However, given that it costs nearly $2,400 to treat a single case of MDR-TB (compared to $40 for standard TB), more reliable and timely diagnoses may yield significant economic benefits.[52]

Many anticipate Xpert's impact on the global burden of TB will be dramatic. WHO has recommended the technology as the first-line diagnostic tool for both adults and children presenting with symptoms of MDR-TB, those potentially suffering from co-infection with HIV and TB, and patients presumed to have TB meningitis.[44] When countries can afford it, WHO also recommends Xpert as the initial diagnostic for all potential cases of TB. These recommendations, combined with the negotiated lower price per cartridge, have spurred 105 out of 147 countries eligible for discounted pricing to purchase the technology.[53] Given countries' limited resources, Xpert initially will supplement conventional technology in particularly troublesome cases (such as MDR-TB and HIV/TB coinfection) rather than completely replacing sputum smear microscopy.[46]

The development of the Xpert MTB/RIF test owes its success to collaboration across disciplines and organizations. Researchers developed a working technology to improve the efficiency of a common laboratory technique, and a team at the University of Medicine and Dentistry of New Jersey applied the technology to analyze TB in sputum samples.[54] FIND aided in negotiations between funding organizations and Cepheid, Inc. to reduce the price per cartridge for resource-poor countries. By bringing advanced diagnostics at reduced costs to resource-poor settings, Xpert should improve care for TB patients throughout the world.

Saving Women's Lives: The Nonpneumatic Antishock Garment

Postpartum hemorrhages are the largest cause of maternal death worldwide.[55] Especially in resource-poor settings, healthcare workers may lack the training to manage labor appropriately, which can lead to improper uterine muscle tone and subsequent hemorrhage. However, a multitude of other factors also contribute to postpartum hemorrhages (PPH). Ruptured uteruses, vaginal lacerations, and retained placentas are other common causes of PPH that are difficult to manage in resource-poor settings.[55] These problems are particularly troublesome in cases of delayed care, and reducing the rate of blood loss can have a significant effect on the clinical outcome. Thus, there is an important need for treatment of shock and prevention of blood loss among women giving birth.[56] Antishock garments—which inflate to compress the abdomen to prevent blood loss—were developed decades ago, but their price and complexity have been barriers for adoption in low resource settings where they might be particularly helpful.[57,58]

The nonpneumatic antishock garment (NASG), based on technology from the United States National Aeronautics and Space Administration (NASA), offers a simple, cost-effective solution. The product was developed by PATH, the University of California, San Francisco (UCSF) Safe Motherhood Program,[59] Pathfinder International, and the Blue Fuzion Group.[60] Rubber belts with Velcro are tightened around a mother's abdomen to reduce bleeding while the woman is transported to a care provider as quickly as possible. The garment acts to both treat shock and shift blood toward critical organs, stabilizing the mother's condition during delays in care. When WHO originally recommended the NASG for patients with PPH, at $170 per device, the technology was thought to be too expensive for resource-poor countries.[55,60] PATH, a global health organization based in the United States, worked to make manufacturing more cost-effective, which reduced the price to just $54 for each reusable garment.[58] The NASG has been validated in clinical trials analyzed by the UCSF Safe Motherhood Initiative in Egypt, Nigeria, Zambia, Zimbabwe, and India.[61]

The NASG reduces bleeding by 50 percent and is expected to significantly reduce maternal morbidity and mortality due to hemorrhage.[56] Indeed, in a trial in Egypt, mortality was reduced by 20 percent and morbidity by 160 percent when the NASG was applied upon obstetric hemorrhage until time of care.[62] Delays in care happen often in low-resource settings and the rate of bleeding of a woman who has just delivered can mean the difference between life and death. The device is comprised of just rubber and Velcro attachments, so it can be employed in a variety of low-resource settings with minimal need for technical expertise and training.[55]

This promising garment suggests that some existing technologies can be of great use in resource-poor settings after a limited number of simplifying modifications. Indeed, organizations in Pakistan are already conducting training sessions on this device.[63] Inflatable pressure suits were first developed to prevent blood loss during surgery, but they were designed for use only by trained surgeons in the operating room.[57] By developing a nonpneumatic version, UCSF researchers made it easier for untrained personnel to use and also economical for resource-poor countries to purchase. PATH further enhanced the technology by optimizing manufacturing to minimize costs. This simple garment appears likely to be able to buy precious time for dying mothers seeking treatment.

Aeras[64]

Aeras, formerly known as the Aeras Global TB Vaccine Foundation, was founded as the Sequella Global Tuberculosis Foundation in 1998. Aeras's mission is to develop safer, more effective and affordable new vaccine regimens that will prevent tuberculosis—including drug-resistant TB—in all age groups, including people living with HIV/AIDS.

Aeras is one of the most fully integrated of a number of product development partnerships (PDPs) supported by the Bill & Melinda Gates Foundation. It undertakes the full spectrum of vaccine development—vaccine discovery, construction, preclinical research, manufacturing, and clinical development. Like that for other PDPs, the key to success of Aeras's mission is ensuring the availability of new vaccines for all who need them. Aeras seeks to accomplish this through agreements with its vaccine development partners that emphasize affordability and access for poor people in low-income countries of any eventual TB vaccine that might be developed and deployed.

Based in Rockville, Maryland, in the United States, and with an office in Cape Town, South Africa, Aeras employs 140 staff members from 30 different countries. Aeras's operations resemble those of biotech companies, with in-house vaccine discovery laboratories, immunology, clinical trial coordination, data management, and state-of-the-art manufacturing capabilities. Its partners are spread across four continents and include academia, other research institutions, multilateral organizations, biotech and pharmaceutical industries, foundations, governments, patient groups, and advocates. Aeras also works closely with other PDPs focused on new TB drugs and diagnostics to advocate for research and development of new tools, all of which will be needed for better TB control.

Aeras's key accomplishments to date include the establishment of a network of partner clinical trial sites in endemic countries, advancing several vaccine candidates into clinical trials, and the development of backup investigational vaccines. Aeras has sponsored clinical trials in Africa, Europe, India, and the United States of five candidate vaccines originated by external partners. Two of those candidates advanced to the proof-of-concept stage—a phase of development intended to demonstrate that the proposed approach is feasible and capable of providing some protection. A fifth candidate, invented by Aeras, entered a clinical trial in 2010, but development was discontinued because of a safety signal. In addition, Aeras is undertaking epidemiological studies in multiple countries in preparation for possible future trials there. Despite these efforts, it is believed that a new vaccine is unlikely to be deployed before 2025.

One of Aeras's main approaches is to modernize and improve on the existing TB vaccine, known as BCG (Bacille Calmette Guerin), which was introduced in 1921. WHO recommends that the vaccine be given to infants. BCG is widely used and appears to reduce the severity of pediatric TB disease. However, BCG is unreliable at preventing pulmonary TB infection in adults, which accounts for most of the TB transmission and disease burden worldwide. In addition, BCG is not known to protect against latent TB, which is common and a source of many later reactivation TB cases. In addition, it is not recommended for use in infants infected with HIV because of safety concerns. To address these challenges, Aeras scientists and others are working on an improved BCG vaccine that is safer and has the potential to help the immune system respond better to the vaccine. Such a newly developed BCG, or the current BCG, would be used in combination with a different booster vaccine, such as one of the five vaccine candidates that are in clinical development. It is intended that this combination of vaccines would not only enhance the protection afforded by the BCG vaccine but also extend protection over a longer period of time and work well in adolescents and adults.

One of the challenges facing Aeras and other PDPs is mobilizing the resources to fund their work, particularly when candidates are ready for larger and more expensive later stage clinical trials, which are aimed at testing whether investigational vaccines are protective. Scientific hurdles include the lack of immune responses that predict that a person will be protected against TB infection and disease after immunization and the lack of animal models for testing the vaccines that predict protection in humans. Such immune correlates and animal test systems can save time and money in vaccine development. These are also barriers to the development of HIV and malaria vaccines. Collaboration is key to accomplishing Aeras's mission. Like that of all PDPs, Aeras's work is made possible through the involvement of partners in low- and middle-income countries and high-income countries, in industry and the nonprofit sector, and among researchers, government officials, donors, politicians, and volunteers.

Aeras has received funding from the Bill & Melinda Gates Foundation; the governments of Denmark, the Netherlands, the United Kingdom, and the United States; the Research Council of Norway; and the State of Maryland in the United States.

Advance Market Commitments

An advance market commitment (AMC) is a financing mechanism that aims to encourage investment in the development and manufacturing of vaccines that can be sold at affordable prices in low-income countries. The AMC was devised in 2005 and further refined during 2006–2009. It started in 2009 and is housed at Gavi.[65]

The need for a financing mechanism such as the AMC is based on the problem discussed earlier—the unwillingness of vaccine manufacturers to invest in newer vaccines that meet the needs of low-income countries because the manufacturers believe that the market for such vaccines will not be profitable. The high risks and high cost of such an investment ultimately leave suppliers with little incentive to produce. What's more, even if a manufacturer did find reason to supply vaccines, these vaccines would be unaffordable for people in low-income countries at the prices at which they would have to be sold for the manufacturers to make a profit on them.

The AMC can best be thought of as a fund that will make financing available to vaccine manufacturers under certain circumstances they agree to with the AMC management. To erase uncertainties about the market for vaccines and provide an incentive to vaccine manufacturers to produce the needed quantities of the desired vaccines, a pool of money from donors guarantees that the manufacturer will receive a set price per dose produced, provided that the manufacturers will supply a predetermined quantity of vaccines for a certain amount of time at the agreed price.

In addition, manufacturers participating in the scheme must meet certain technical criteria for vaccine quality and safety predetermined by the World Health Organization. The AMC ensures that no single supplier receives all of the funding for a particular vaccine, thereby avoiding the possibility of a monopoly and problems of supply if a sole manufacturer could not meet its production commitments.

The first AMC pilot program for a vaccine against pneumococcal disease was adopted by a group of core donors including Italy, the United Kingdom, Canada, Norway, and the Gates Foundation in 2007 and became fully operational in 2009. The decision to invest in a pneumococcal vaccine for the pilot program was made by a diverse group of experts in epidemiology and vaccine manufacturing. The AMC was projected to save over 500,000 lives by 2015 and over 1.5 million lives by 2020.[66] Gavi has pledged to contribute $1.3 billion to this effort through 2015, with the hope of making the vaccine available to nearly 60 countries by this time.[67]

In exchange for incentives offered by guaranteed purchase and financing, manufacturers who participate in the AMC must sell the vaccine at or below the predetermined price of $7 a dose, to ensure that the vaccine is affordable in low-income countries. The AMC will cover half of this price—$3.50 a dose—and the balance of $3.50 will be paid by Gavi and the participating country as part of its normal cofinancing share. The AMC will eventually discontinue its subsidy to the manufacturer, at which point the manufacturer must continue to sell the vaccine at or below the predetermined, affordable "tail" price of $3.50. This preset price is a more than 90 percent discount on the current price of the vaccine in high-income countries.[67,68]

Setting an appropriate price for the pneumococcal vaccine and subsidy for manufacturers was a major challenge in devising the pilot program. This is largely due to suppliers keeping information about manufacturing costs confidential. To overcome this obstacle, outside consultants helped to assess the cost of manufacturing. The fact that the two main multinational suppliers of the pneumococcal vaccine and several emerging suppliers from India all expressed interest in participating in the AMC suggests that they find the AMC price and the tail price to be reasonably remunerative. Assessing a fair price for vaccines funded by the AMC will continue to be a challenge for this financing mechanism.

The large number of donor and technical organizations that worked together with Gavi and low- and middle-income country partners to develop the AMC and launch the pilot is a testimony to the widespread interest in this innovative mechanism. In addition to the donors mentioned earlier, who committed $1.5 billion to the AMC, the World Bank is providing its financial services, WHO is responsible for technical matters related to the AMC, and UNICEF is leading vaccine procurement efforts.[68]

International Finance Facility for Immunisation

The International Finance Facility for Immunisation (IFFIm) is a financing mechanism that seeks "to rapidly accelerate the availability and predictability of funds for immunization." IFFIm funds are used by the Gavi Alliance to accomplish its mission of "reducing the number of vaccine-preventable deaths and illnesses among children under 5."[69] IFFIm was originally launched in 2006 as a charity by the government of the United Kingdom but now includes Australia, France, Italy, the Netherlands, Norway, South Africa, Spain, and Sweden.[70]

The IFFIm was created to address the lack of secure funding for immunization in low-income countries. Another issue the IFFIm seeks to address is that donors usually provide financing on a year-to-year basis, making it hard for recipient governments to plan their budgets for programs that receive assistance, such as immunization programs. The IFFIm is meant to help ensure longer term and more predictable financing for vaccine programs.

To ensure a reliable stream of funding for Gavi, donor countries pledge a certain amount of money to be paid to Gavi over about 20 years. IFFIm then sells bonds to raise this money in the capital markets of high-income countries. This makes the money available immediately, without having to wait for year-to-year-financing from donor governments. The donor countries repay the bonds over time, based on their initial pledges. The fact that the IFFIm is backed by the promises of these countries allows it to maintain a good credit rating and to sell bonds at rates that are acceptable to the donor countries that have to honor the bonds.

Gavi is using IFFIm funds to purchase and deliver vaccines in countries that receive its support, in addition to working with health services to strengthen immunization programs. With funding from the IFFIm, Gavi has introduced pentavalent vaccines in 73 countries[71] which immunize against diphtheria, pertussis, tetanus, hepatitis B, and Hib in a single vaccine.[72] In fact, the IFFIm enabled Gavi to double its spending between 2006 and 2009. By 2014, the IFFIm had provided Gavi, for example, with $191 million to purchases stockpiles of polio vaccines for use in outbreaks, more than $1 billion for the pentavalent vaccine, and about $100 million for pneumococcal vaccine.[73]

With secure funding, Gavi hopes to deliver reliable aid to countries for the long term, enabling these countries to plan and implement immunization programs more effectively. In addition, having more secure and longer term funding allows Gavi to purchase vaccines in bulk, at lower prices than would otherwise be possible. Thus, the IFFIm hopes to enable the purchase of more vaccines with the same amount of money.

The IFFIm had generated more than $4.5 billion by 2014, and was projected to raise $6.3 billion by 2015.[70]

CASE STUDY

The case study that follows concerns the effort to develop a vaccine for hookworm. It centers on a public–private product development partnership that is being funded by the Bill & Melinda Gates Foundation. This is especially significant, given the burden of disease from hookworm, the fact that treatment has to be repeated every 6 months, and the fact there is no vaccine at the moment for any of the neglected tropical diseases.

The Human Hookworm Vaccine Initiative[74]

Background

The neglected tropical diseases (NTDs) are a group of chronic disabling and poverty-promoting conditions that affect the world's poorest people in rural and peri-urban communities of low-income countries. They include, among other diseases, helminth infections such as ascariasis, hookworm, trichuriasis, schistosomiasis, dracunculiasis (guinea worm), lymphatic filariasis (elephantiasis), and onchocerciasis (river blindness). The NTDs cause human suffering and impede economic development either because of their disfiguring properties or through their impact on child health and development, maternal health and pregnancy outcomes, and worker productivity. The World Health Organization now recognizes 17 major NTDs, and their combined disease burden ranks them with better-known global health conditions. Moreover, because most of the NTDs are chronic and debilitating conditions, their economic impact results in the loss of tens of billions of dollars annually.[75]

Despite their enormous health and economic importance, there has been little interest in developing new drugs or vaccines for the NTDs. A major reason for this situation is the absence of any commercial market for products related to these diseases, because they affect almost exclusively the world's 3 billion people who live on less than $2 per day.[76] As a result, many of the drugs in use for the NTDs were first developed during the early or middle parts of the 20th century.

Similarly, there are no licensed vaccines available for the NTDs even though there have been significant basic research efforts related to their development over the last 20 years. If preventive or therapeutic vaccines could be developed, then they would represent a generation of antipoverty vaccines, which could serve as powerful new tools in achieving the Millennium Development Goals.

Human hookworm infection is an example of an NTD that would benefit from the development of a vaccine. Hookworm affects an estimated 440 million people, almost all of them impoverished individuals living in sub-Saharan Africa, Southeast Asia, and tropical regions of the Americas. The infection is caused by nematode parasites that attach to the inside of the intestine and ingest host blood. When individuals are infected with large numbers of hookworms, the blood loss is sufficient to cause iron-deficiency anemia and protein malnutrition. This is especially a problem for young children and pregnant women.

There are inexpensive drugs available to treat human hookworm infection. The two major drugs for hookworm are the benzimidazoles—albendazole and mebendazole—which are typically administered as single doses to school-age and preschool children in mass drug administration (MDA) programs, sometimes referred to as "deworming" programs. However, deworming does not prevent hookworm reinfection, which can occur within 4–12 months following treatment in areas of high transmission. Moreover, there is evidence that the efficacy of drugs against hookworm diminishes with increasing use and there is concern that the hookworm parasites may develop resistance to them. Single-dose mebendazole is no longer considered an effective drug for hookworm, for example. These concerns have prompted interest in developing complementary or alternative approaches to controlling the infection through vaccination.

The Intervention

The Sabin Vaccine Institute PDP, based at Texas Children's Hospital and Baylor College of Medicine's Texas Medical Center in Houston, is taking the lead on developing the first human hookworm vaccine, as well as other NTD vaccines. Initially financed and supported by the Bill & Melinda Gates Foundation, today development of the human hookworm vaccine is continuing through collaboration with a consortium of European partners known as HOOKVAC (based at the Amsterdam Institute of Global Health and Development and supported by the European Union), with additional key financial support from the Dutch Ministry of Foreign Affairs. Thus the PDP embraces a larger international network of laboratories and clinical trial sites, with program management, manufacturers, toxicology sites, quality assurance, regulatory affairs, and clinical development and oversight units.

The human hookworm vaccine under development includes two recombinant proteins known as *Na*-GST-1 and *Na*-APR-1, together formulated on Alhydrogel and with other immunostimulants known as adjuvants. Each component of the vaccine is in clinical trials in the United States and in Brazil, the latter where hookworm infection is endemic. The clinical development of the vaccine in Brazil is carried out in collaboration with Fundação Oswaldo Cruz (FIOCRUZ), a Brazilian governmental organization that combines research and public health activities. The two antigens will also be tested in a coadministration study in Gabon in collaboration with the Centre de Recherches Médicales de Lambaréné–Cermel, linked to the Albert Schweitzer Hospital.

Impact

Critical to the success of the Sabin PDP is the concept that it is possible to develop and test vaccines in nonprofit and academic settings. This requires the purchase and operation of special equipment and the recruitment of scientists with industrial manufacturing experience, as well as experts in quality control, quality assurance, and documentation. The Sabin Vaccine Institute PDP developed processes for transitioning two target vaccine antigens from discovery through product development, manufacture, toxicology testing, investigational new drug filing, and clinical testing. Ultimately, for the industrial production of the human hookworm vaccine it will likely be necessary to find a large-scale manufacturing partner such as one located in the so-called IDCs—innovative developing countries. IDCs are those with areas of extreme poverty and high endemicity of NTDs but which can "punch above their weight" in terms of their ability to develop pharmaceuticals. Examples of IDCs include countries such as Brazil, India, and China, as well as Mexico and Cuba in the Americas, and Indonesia and Vietnam in Southeast Asia. Indeed, there is a consortium known as the Developing Countries Vaccine Manufacturers Network (DCVMN). It is likely that the industrial scale production of the human hookworm vaccine would include a DCVMN partner, such as one in Brazil where clinical testing is being conducted. FIOCRUZ, for example, also has a prominent public-sector vaccine manufacturer known as BioManguinhos.

Another component of the Sabin Vaccine Institute PDP is its global access plan to ensure that the human hookworm vaccine and its other products are provided to the people who need them the most, such as the poorest people in low- and middle-income countries. This requires that the vaccine is manufactured at extremely low cost and can be integrated into health systems in disease endemic countries. Examples would include adding the human hookworm vaccine to the Expanded Program on Immunization (EPI) by administering it in the first year of life, or working with school-based health systems where deworming and other interventions are provided through child health days. Thus, a human hookworm vaccine could be administered following deworming in a strategy of vaccine-linked chemotherapy. Analyses have been conducted which indicate that combining hookworm vaccination with deworming would be cost-effective, mostly due to the additional reduction in morbidity and the reduced frequency of deworming that would be afforded by vaccination.

Lessons Learned

Several important and useful lessons have been learned so far from the Sabin Vaccine Institute PDP and its program to develop a human hookworm vaccine, including:

- It is feasible to produce and test vaccines in the non-profit sector through product development partnerships (PDPs).
- Partnering with an innovative developing country, like Brazil, represents a new strategy for developing, testing, and distributing neglected disease products.
- Achieving these goals requires strong program management for structuring the partnership, maintaining timelines, and achieving milestones.
- There are important advantages to cooperating with scientifically capable low- and middle-income countries for both manufacture and clinical testing of new products, and looking to these countries as a means to initiate global access for NTD vaccines.
- There is a need to consider how a product will fit into available health systems, or whether novel healthcare delivery systems, such as schools, would be required to ensure that the products will be delivered and will be accessible to the populations who need them the most.

MAIN MESSAGES

Science and technology have the potential to make major contributions to the development of diagnostics, vaccines, drugs, and medical devices that can help address the highest burdens of disease in low- and middle-income countries. Progress in scientific areas like the sequencing of genes, information technology, chemistry, robotics, and

biotechnology can help, for example, to engineer mosquitoes that will not carry disease, discover new drugs much more rapidly than before, and develop less expensive and more effective vaccines.

In a more ideal world, diagnostics, vaccines, drugs, and medical devices would be appropriate to the needs of the health conditions that cause the largest burden of disease in low- and middle-income countries. They would also be appropriate to the ability of countries to manage their health systems. If these were the case, they would be affordable to low-income patients and countries that are unable to spend much on health. They would also be heat stable, not require refrigeration, and be easy to store and transport. The number of pills needed to cure a disease would be few and require a short course of therapy. Ideal vaccines would be a combination of many of the vaccines that exist today, so that children would need fewer vaccinations to be fully covered. Given the risks of injections being unsafe, the delivery devices for vaccines would increasingly rely on noninvasive means, such as nasal sprays, skin patches, or perhaps, vaccines that are edible.

Unfortunately, the needed advances are unlikely to come about on their own. This is largely a reflection of the fact that the for-profit sector has historically been a major developer of diagnostics, vaccines, and drugs but does not believe that the market for these products in low- and middle-income countries is sufficient to give it an adequate return on its investment. In addition, the public sector is risk averse and would prefer to purchase a product developed by the private sector rather than to try to develop these products itself. The failure of the market is reflected, as an example, in the very small number of drugs that have been developed over the last 20 years to address the main burdens of disease among the poor in low- and middle-income countries. Moreover, vaccine development is constrained by the need for substantial investments, limited capacity in an industry with a very small number of producers, and divergence between the vaccines used in high-income countries and those used in low- and middle-income countries.

Overcoming these market failures and encouraging the development of the desired products will probably require a series of measures. Some of these can be push mechanisms that are meant to lower the cost of research and development for the private sector. These could include, for example, direct financing by government of research, the facilitation by government of clinical trials, or governments offering tax credits for research and development. Push mechanisms do lower the cost of research and development, but they provide no certainty that the desired product will be produced.

Another set of efforts could focus on pull mechanisms, which are intended to help assure a satisfactory return to investors in the event that a product is produced. These mechanisms could include funding mechanisms to increase the uptake of existing vaccines, prizes, transferable patents, copayments, market assurances, and tax credits for vaccine sales. Pull mechanisms have the advantage of providing funding only when the desired product is available. However, they have the disadvantage of having to be negotiated far in advance of product availability, and parties may not be satisfied with the terms of their agreement at the time in the future when the products are available.

A mechanism already in use for vaccines and for AIDS drugs is tiered pricing. This is an arrangement in which products are sold at different prices in different markets, with the principle being that the price of sales in high-income country markets will help defray the cost of the products in low- and middle-income country markets. However, these arrangements have generally been put in place only when products were established; efforts are now under way to try to put them in place at the early stages of a product's life.

Considerable hope for new product development is being placed in public–private product development partnerships, such as Aeras, the Global Alliance for TB Drug Development, and the Medicines for Malaria Venture. The aim of these ventures is to bring the strengths of the public and private sector together in complementary ways that can spur the development of new products. In its policy and program briefs and in the case study on hookworm vaccine, the chapter suggests some steps that can be taken both to develop products that are needed and to see that they are widely used once they are developed.

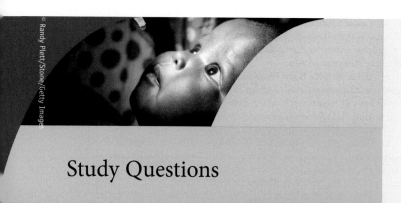

Study Questions

1. What are some of the ideal properties that diagnostics, vaccines, and drugs should have to be most appropriate to the health and health system needs of low- and middle-income countries?

2. To what extent do some of the available vaccines for the six basic antigens and the vaccination schedule for them meet the ideal?

3. What health conditions and risk factors deserve additional attention from science and technology? Why have you chosen those conditions and risk factors?

4. What are some of the specific gaps in diagnostics, drugs, vaccines, and other medical equipment that could most improve global health if filled?

5. What have been some of the major constraints to the development of drugs and vaccines that could better meet health needs in low- and middle-income countries?

6. What steps can be taken to overcome those constraints? What are the roles in this of publicly supported research? What are the roles of public–private partnerships for health?

7. Why does only 10 percent of all research expenditure worldwide focus on the diseases that most affect the poor in low- and middle-income countries? What is the 10/90 research gap?

8. What push and pull mechanisms could most help to encourage the development of new diagnostics, drugs, and vaccines?

9. What lessons does the case study on hookworm suggest for the discovery of other drugs and vaccines?

10. If you were in charge of the Bill & Melinda Gates Foundation, how would you spend money on research and development of new products for global health? Why?

REFERENCES

1. UNAIDS. (2009). *AIDS epidemic update 2009*. Retrieved December 31, 2014, from http://www.unaids.org/en/resources/documents/2009/20091124_jc1700_epi_update_2009_en.pdf.

2. UNAIDS. (n.d.). *South Africa*. Retrieved November 11, 2014, from http://www.unaids.org/en/regionscountries/countries/southafrica.

3. UNAIDS. (2014, January 17). *New HIV report finds big drop in new HIV infections in South Africa*. Retrieved November 11, 2014, from http://www.unaids.org/en/resources/presscentre/featurestories/2014/january/20140117southafrica.

4. Birn, A. E. (2005). Gates's grandest challenge: Transcending technology as public health ideology. *Lancet, 366*(9484), 514–519.

5. UNICEF. (2010). *Facts for life*. Retrieved December 31, 2014, from http://www.factsforlifeglobal.org/resources/factsforlife-en-full.pdf.

6. Centers for Disease Control and Prevention. *BCG vaccine*. Retrieved December 31, 2014, from http://www.cdc.gov/tb/publications/factsheets/prevention/BCG.htm.

7. Global Alliance for TB Drug Development. (2006, May 24). *New TB drugs urgently needed to replace treatment from the 1960s. Second Gates grant to TB Alliance quadruples initial support*. Retrieved December 31, 2014, from http://www.tballiance.org/downloads/pressreleases/PR_GatesGrant_5-23-06.pdf.

8. Roll Back Malaria. (2009). Counting Malaria Out. Retrieved April 2, 2015, from http://archiverbm.rollbackmalaria.org/worldmalariaday2010/docs/fact-sheet-RBM.pdf. (2001).

9. Institute of Medicine Committee on the Economics of Antimalarial Drugs; K. J. Arrow, C. Panosian, & H. Gelband, Eds. (2004). The cost and cost-effectiveness of Antimalarial Drugs. In *Saving lives, buying time: Economics of malaria drugs in an age of resistance* (pp. 61–78). Washington, DC: National Academies Press. Available from: http://www.ncbi.nlm.nih.gov/books/NBK215621/.

10. Ruder, K., & Winstead, E. R. (n.d.). *Quick guide to sequenced genomes*. Genome News Network. Retrieved November 28, 2014, from http://www.genomenewsnetwork.org/resources/sequenced_genomes/genome_guide_p1.shtml.

11. World Health Organization. (2002). *Genomics and world health: A report of the Advisory Committee on Health Research*. Retrieved October 27, 2006, from http://whqlibdoc.who.int/hq/2002/a74580.pdf.

12. Weatherall, D., Greenwood, B., Chee, H. L., & Wasi, P. (2006). Science and technology for disease control: Past, present, and future. In D. T. Jamison, J. G. Breman, A. R. Measham, et al. (Eds.), *Disease control priorities in developing countries* (2nd ed., pp. 119–137). New York: Oxford University Press.

13. Jiang, X., et al. (2014). Genome analysis of a major urban malaria vector mosquito, *Anopheles stephensi. Genome Biology, 15*(9). Retrieved November 11, 2014, from http://genomebiology.com/2014/15/9/459.

14. Fauci, A. S. (2001). Infectious diseases: Considerations for the 21st century. *Clinical Infectious Diseases, 32*(5), 675–685.

15. Daar, A. S., Thorsteinsdottir, H., Martin, D. K., Smith, A. C., Nast, S., & Singer, P. A. (2002). Top ten biotechnologies for improving health in developing countries. *Nature Genetics, 32*(2), 229–232.

16. Grand Challenges in Global Health. *Why the Grand Challenges?* Retrieved November 11, 2014, from http://gcgh.grandchallenges.org/about/Pages/Overview.aspx.

17. Grand Challenges Canada. What is Grand Challenges Canada? Retrieved April 13, 2015, from http://www.grandchallenges.ca/who-we-are/.

18. USAID. *Grand Challenges & Prizes*. Retrieved November 12, 2014, from http://www.usaid.gov/grandchallenges.

19. Bill & Melinda Gates Foundation. (2006). *Grand Challenges in Global Health: Background on the Initiative and Research Projects*. Retrieved April 2, 2015, from http://gcgh.grandchallenges.org/gcghdocs/gcgh_grants_backgrounder_2.pdf.

20. Grand Challenges in Global Health. *Genetic strategies for control of dengue virus transmission*. Retrieved November 14, 2014, from http://gcgh.grandchallenges.org/ControlInsect/Challenges/GeneticStrategy/Pages/DengueTransmission.aspx.

21. Bill & Melinda Gates Foundation. (2014, October 7). *Bill & Melinda Gates Foundation and Grand Challenge Partners commit to innovation with new investments in breakthrough science*. Press Release. Retrieved December 31, 2014, from http://www.gatesfoundation.org/Media-Center/Press-Releases/2014/10/Gates-Foundation-Grand-Challenges-Breakthrough-Science.

22. Mahmoud, A., Danzon, P. M., Barton, J. H., & Mugerwa, R. D. (2006). Product development priorities. In D. T. Jamison, J. G. Breman, A. R. Measham, et al. (Eds.), *Disease control priorities in developing countries* (2nd ed., pp. 139–155). New York: Oxford University Press.

23. Glass, S. N., Batson, A., & Levine, R. (2006). *Issues paper: Accelerating new vaccines*. Geneva: Global Alliance for Vaccines and Immunisation.

24. Trouiller, P., Torreele, E., Olliaro, P., et al. (2001). Drugs for neglected diseases: A failure of the market and a public health failure? *Tropical Medicine and International Health, 6*(11), 945–951.

25. Treatment Action Group. (2014, October 22). *2014 report on tuberculosis research funding trends, 2005–2013*. TB R&D Matters blog. Retrieved November 11, 2014, from http://www.newtbdrugs.org/blog/2014-report-on-tuberculosis-research-funding-trends-2005-2013/.

26. Bloom, B. R., Michaud, C. M., LaMontagne, J. R., & Simonsen, L. (2006). Priorities for global research and development interventions. In D. T. Jamison, J. G. Breman, A. R. Measham, et al. (Eds.), *Disease control priorities in developing countries*. (2nd ed., pp. 103–118). New York: Oxford University Press; 2006.

27. Global Forum for Health Research. Retrieved December 31, 2014, from http://www.globalforumhealth.org/about/1090-gap/.

28. World Health Organization. (2014). *TDR: About us*. Retrieved November 7, 2014, from http://www.who.int/tdr/about/en/.

29. Morel, C. M., Acharya, T., Broun, D., et al. (2005). Health innovation networks to help developing countries address neglected diseases. *Science, 309*(5733), 401–404.

30. World Health Organization. (2011). *mHealth: New horizons for health through mobile technologies: Second global survey on eHealth. Global Observatory for eHealth series: Vol. 3*. Geneva: WHO.

31. Lewis, T., Synowiec, C., Lagomarsino, G., & Schweitzer, J. (2012). E-health in low- and middle-income countries: Findings from the Center for Health Market Innovations. *Bulletin of the World Health Organization, 90*, 332–340. doi: 10.2471/BLT.11.099.

32. Kallander, K. (2013). Mobile health (mHealth) approaches and lessons for increased performance and retention of community health workers in low- and middle-income countries: A review. *Journal of Medical Internet Research, 15*(1), e17. doi: 10.2196/jmir.2130.

33. Mossman, K., McGahan, A., Mitchell, W., & Bhattacharyya, O. (2014). Evaluating high-tech health approaches in low-income countries. *Stanford Social Innovation Review*. Retrieved August 29, 2014, from http://www.ssireview.org/blog/entry/evaluating_high_tech_health_approaches_in_low_income_countries.

34. Unite for Sight. (2013). *mHealth technology in global health*. Retrieved August 30, 2014, from http://www.uniteforsight.org/global-health-university/mhealth.

35. Earth Institute. (2010). Barriers and gaps affecting mHealth in low and middle income countries: A policy white paper. Washington, DC: mHealth Alliance.

36. Bagchi, S. (2006). Telemedicine in rural India. *PLoS Medicine, 3*(3), e82. doi:10.1371/journal.pmed.0030082.

37. Kay, M., Santos, J., & Takane, M. (2009). *Telemedicine: Opportunities and developments in member states. Report on the second global survey on eHealth Global Observatory for eHealth series: Vol. 2*. Geneva: WHO.

38. Bollineni, R. (2011). *Apollo Telemedicine Networking Foundation (ATNF)*. Hyderabad, India: ACCESS Health International.

39. Tarafdar, M., & Scott, N. (2012). Information separation in service supply chains at the bottom of the pyramid: An illustration through telemedicine. *GlobDev 2012*, paper 11. Retrieved December 31, 2014, from http://aisel.aisnet.org/globdev2012/11.

40. Ganapathy, K., & Ravindra, A. (n.d.). Telemedicine in India: The Apollo story. *Telemedicine Journal and E-Health: The Official Journal of the American Telemedicine Association, 15*(6), 576–85. doi:10.1089/tmj.2009.0066.

41. Solberg, K. E. (2008). Telemedicine set to grow in India over the next 5 years. *Lancet, 371*(9606), 17–18. doi:10.1016/S0140-6736(08)60052-5.

42. Pal, A., Mbarika, V. W. A., Cobb-Payton, F., Datta, P., & Mccoy, S. (2005). Telemedicine diffusion in a developing country. *IEEE Transactions on Information Technology in Biomedicine, 9*(1), 59–65.

43. Center for Health Market Innovation. *Apollo Telemedicine Networking Foundation*. Retrieved April 2, 2015 from http://healthmarketinnovations.org/program/apollo-telemedicine-networking-foundation-atnf.

44. World Health Organization. (2014). *Tuberculosis diagnostics: Xpert MTB/RIF Test*. Retrieved December 31, 2014, from http://who.int/tb/features_archive/factsheet_xpert.pdf.

45. Steingart, K. R., Ng, V., Henry, M., Hopewell, P. C., Ramsay, A., Cunningham, J., et al. (2006). Sputum processing methods to improve the sensitivity of smear microscopy for tuberculosis: A systematic review. *The Lancet Infectious Diseases, 6*(10), 664–674. doi: http://dx.doi.org/10.1016/S1473-3099(06)70602-8.

46. World Health Organization. (2010). *Frequently asked questions on Xpert MTB/RIF assay*. Retrieved December 31, 2014, from http://www.who.int/tb/laboratory/xpert_faqs.pdf.

47. Blakemore, R., Story, E., Helb, D., Kop, J., Banada, P., Owens, M. R., et al. (2010). Evaluation of the analytical performance of the Xpert MTB/RIF assay. *Journal of Clinical Microbiology, 48*(7), 2495–2501. doi: 10.1128/jcm.00128-10.

48. Theron, G., Peter, J., van Zyl-Smit, R., Mishra, H., Streicher, E., Murray, S., et al. (2011). Evaluation of the Xpert MTB/RIF assay for the diagnosis of pulmonary tuberculosis in a high HIV prevalence setting. *American Journal of Respiratory and Critical Care Medicine, 184*(1), 132–140. doi: 10.1164/rccm.201101-0056OC.

49. Piatek, A. S., Van Cleeff, M., Alexander, H., Coggin, W. L., Rehr, M., Van Kampen, S., et al. (2013). GeneXpert for TB diagnosis: Planned and purposeful implementation. *Global Health: Science and Practice, 1*(1), 18–23. doi: 10.9745/ghsp-d-12-00004.

50. Schito, M., Peter, T. F., Cavanaugh, S., Piatek, A. S., Young, G. J., Alexander, H., et al. (2012). Opportunities and challenges for cost-efficient implementation of new point-of-care diagnostics for HIV and tuberculosis. *Journal of Infectious Diseases, 205*(suppl 2), S169–S180. doi: 10.1093/infdis/jis044.

51. Meyer-Rath, G., Schnippel, K., Long, L., MacLeod, W., Sanne, I., Stevens, W., et al. (2012). The impact and cost of scaling up GeneXpert MTB/RIF in South Africa. *PLoS One, 7*(5), e36966. doi: 10.1371/journal.pone.0036966.

52. UNITAID. *MDR-TB scale-up initiative*. Retrieved August 30, 2014, from http://www.unitaid.eu/en/mdr-tb-scale-up.

53. World Health Organization. (2013). *WHO monitoring of Xpert MTB/RIF roll-out: Orders of GeneXperts and Xpert MTB/RIF cartridges*. Retrieved August 30, 2014, from http://www.stoptb.org/wg/gli/assets/documents/map/1/atlas.html.

54. Helb, D., Jones, M., Story, E., Boehme, C., Wallace, E., Ho, K., et al. (2010). Rapid detection of mycobacterium tuberculosis and rifampin resistance by use of on-demand, near-patient technology. *Journal of Clinical Microbiology, 48*(1), 229–237. doi: 10.1128/jcm.01463-09.

55. Mourad-Youssif, M., Ojengbede, O., Meyer, C., Fathalla, M., Morhason-Bello, I., Galadanci, H., et al. (2010). Can the non-pneumatic anti-shock garment (NASG) reduce adverse maternal outcomes from postpartum hemorrhage? Evidence from Egypt and Nigeria. *Reproductive Health, 7*(1), 24.

56. Miller, S., Martin, H. B., & Morris, J. L. Anti-shock garment in postpartum haemorrhage. *Best Practice & Research Clinical Obstetrics & Gynaecology, 22*(6), 1057–1074. doi: 10.1016/j.bpobgyn.2008.08.008.

57. Vahedi, M., Ayuyao, A., Parsa, M., & Freeman, H. (1995). Pneumatic antishock garment-associated compartment syndrome in uninjured lower extremities. *Journal of Trauma, 384*(4), 616–618.

58. World Health Organization. (2011). *Non-pneumatic anti-shock garment*. Retrieved December 31, 2014, from http://www.who.int/medical_devices/innovation/new_emerging_tech_30.pdf.

59. ZOEX NIASG. *Zoex non-inflatable anti-shock garment*. Retrieved August 30, 2014, from http://www.zoexniasg.com/.

60. PATH. *Postpartum hemorrhage kills more new mothers than any other cause, but antishock garments can save lives*. Retrieved August 30, 2014, from http://www.path.org/projects/antishock-garment.php.

61. Bixby Center for Global Reproductive Health. *Safe motherhood*. Retrieved August 30, 2014, from http://bixbycenter.ucsf.edu/research/safe_motherhood.html.

62. Sutherland, T., Downing, J., Miller, S., Bishai, D. M., Butrick, E., Fathalla, M. M., et al. (2013). Use of the non-pneumatic anti-shock garment (NASG) for life-threatening obstetric hemorrhage: A cost-effectiveness analysis in Egypt and Nigeria. *PLoS One, 8*(4), e62282. doi: 10.1371/journal.pone.0062282.

63. Syed, S., Manzoor, H., Erum, Siddiqui, S. A., Soomro, H.-u.-R., Safia, & Zafar, F. (2013). *Final report NIASG training*. Pakistan National Forum on Women's Health.

64. Aeras. *About us*. Retrieved November 28, 2014, from http://www.aeras.org/about.

65. Kher U. (2009). A marriage of divergent interests: Partnership in making of the world's first advance market commitment. In *Case studies for global health: Building relationships. Sharing knowledge*. Deerfield, IL: Alliance for Case Studies for Global Health.

66. Gavi Alliance and The World Bank. (2014). *Advance market commitments for vaccines*. Retrieved November 12, 2014, from http://www.gavi.org/library/gavi-documents/amc/fact-sheets/factsheet--advance-market-commitment/.

67. Gavi Alliance. *Advance market commitments (AMCs)*. Retrieved December 31, 2014, from http://www.gavi.org/About/Governance/Secretariat/Innovative-finance.

68. Gavi Alliance. *Pneumococcal AMC vaccine*. Retrieved December 31, 2014, from http://www.gavi.org/funding/pneumococcal-amc/.

69. IFFIm. Retrieved September 21, 2010, from http://www.iff-immunisation.org.

70. IFFim. *Overview*. Retrieved November 12, 2014, from http://www.iffim.org/about/overview/.

71. Gavi Alliance. *Pentavalent vaccine support*. Retrieved November 12, 2014, from http://www.gavi.org/support/nvs/pentavalent/.

72. International Finance Facility for Immunisation (IFFIm). (2013). *Innovative finance. Bringing together capital market investors and children in the world's poorest countries. Both benefit*. Retrieved September 24, 2010, from http://www.iffim.org/Library/Publications/Factsheets/The-International-Finance-Facility-for-Immunisation-(IFFIm)--Brochure/.

73. IFFIm. *Results*. Retrieved November 12, 2014, from http://www.iffim.org/funding-gavi/results/.

74. This update of the case study that appeared in the second edition was prepared by Dr. Peter Hotez and Dr. Maria Bottazi, of the Human Hookworm Vaccine Initiative and the Sabin Vaccine Institute.

75. Hotez, P. J. (2007). Control of neglected tropical diseases. *New England Journal of Medicine, 357*, 1018–1027.

76. Hotez, P. J. (2008). *Forgotten people, forgotten diseases: The neglected diseases and their impact on global health and development*. Washington, DC: ASM Press.

CHAPTER **18**

Working in Global Health

LEARNING OBJECTIVES

By the end of this chapter the reader will be able to:

- Discuss the wide variety of professional opportunities available in the global health field
- Appreciate the skills, knowledge, and experience required to take advantage of those opportunities
- Review some of the many different routes to a career in global health
- Make use of key resources for information about careers in global health
- Articulate career goals in the global health field, as appropriate to their own interests

VIGNETTES

Edith was among the best students in her schools in Kenya, and she had a strong desire to become a scientist. After finishing secondary school and university in her home country, Edith won a fellowship to study HIV/AIDS in graduate school in the United States. Edith's scientific research has focused on people who have contracted HIV but do not develop AIDS. Edith is now working at a research institute in Nairobi, where she focuses her work on nonprogressors, in close collaboration with the International AIDS Vaccine Initiative.[1] The findings from these efforts could be instrumental to the eventual development of an HIV vaccine. Edith remains excited by her research efforts, even in the face of immense scientific challenges.

John is a Canadian civil engineer who works with the development of community-based water supply in poor countries. As a secondary school student, John already

knew that he wanted to use engineering to provide poor people with better water and sanitation. He was inspired to pursue such a career by videos he saw in social studies class about the terrible impact on health of the lack of access to safe water. During his engineering studies, John spent three summers working in Africa with Engineers Without Borders, where he learned much about applying engineering techniques to poor communities.[2] John also learned the importance of working closely with communities in the development and operation of water and sanitation schemes. Through his work as an engineer, John is making important contributions to health.

Vivian is a Filipina. She studied English at the University of the Philippines and then began to work as a journalist for a Manila newspaper. During more than a decade in journalism, Vivian became increasingly familiar with the poor health circumstances of many Filipinos and how they often relate to a lack of knowledge of good health behaviors. As she approached her 35th birthday, Vivian decided to leave journalism and apply her knowledge of communications to working in health. Today, Vivian is the director of communications for a nongovernmental organization (NGO) that focuses on community-based approaches to improving the health of the poor.

Joseph is a graduate of the U.S. Military Academy, a former U.S. Army Ranger, and the former head of logistics for Doctors Without Borders (MSF) in Africa.[3] Joseph grew up in a family with a strong sense of social justice and considered for some time how he might help poor people in low-income countries. When he finished his time in the U.S.

Army, Joseph looked for jobs with NGOs working in Africa, to see if he could bring to them the organizational and management skills he had learned during military service. Logistics management is of great importance to everyone working in health, and this was an area in which Joseph had considerable expertise. This knowledge served him well as he worked with Doctors Without Borders in the Democratic Republic of the Congo, Liberia, Sierra Leone, and Somalia.

John is a 40 year old from Uganda. He works for UNICEF in Kenya on childhood immunization. John studied anthropology in Uganda and then received a graduate degree in public health from the London School of Hygiene and Tropical Medicine. After a number of years working for the Ministry of Health in his own country, John worked for an international NGO that supported Uganda's child health efforts. Noting the exceptional quality of his work, UNICEF in Uganda then asked John to work with them. After several years, the regional UNICEF office asked John if he could work on their Kenya program. John provides technical support to that program, assists Kenya in raising the financing needed to improve child health, and assists in ensuring that UNICEF funds provided to Kenya are used wisely.

Sam is a 45-year-old American. He studied international affairs for his first degree and then spent two years in the U.S. Peace Corps in Niger. Sam then earned an advanced degree in public policy, with a focus on development. Sam is the country director in Madagascar for PSI, a U.S.-based not-for-profit consulting firm that supports health services in 60 countries.[4] Chuck helps PSI to bid for financing proposals, hire the staff to implement those efforts if they win the bid, and supervise the staff. He also has important inputs into the technical work of his international and Malagasy team, as they work with the public and private sectors to improve the maternal health program, the family planning program, and TB control in Madagascar.

INTRODUCTION

Interest in global health has been growing worldwide. As described earlier, there has been an enormous increase over the last decade in financing for global health, the number of public–private partnerships that address global health issues, and the number of students at all levels who are studying global health. With this expansion of global health activities and studies has come a growing interest in careers in global health.

The purpose of this chapter is to introduce you to those careers; the knowledge, skills, and experience you need to work in global health; and how you can acquire the background you need to become a global health professional.

Consistent with the rest of the book, this chapter primarily focuses on careers related to the unfinished agenda—the health issues that confront poor people in poor countries. The chapter is not meant to be a complete guide to job hunting in global health. Rather, it is intended to help you understand whether this is a field in which you would like to work, and if so, how you might pursue such interests. The chapter largely provides the type of information needed by university students who have minimal global health experience.

As you read this chapter, it is important to keep several critical points in mind:

- There is a wide variety of ways to work in global health.
- There are many different areas of global health on which one can work.
- Many organizations, of many different types, work on global health.
- There is a large number of professions that can serve global health needs.

These points may seem trite. However, many people do not understand them and believe that only those people trained in the health professions can work in the field of global health. Of course, you can work in global health as a physician, nurse, or public health graduate; however, you do not need to be trained as a health professional to work in global health. For example, there is also an enormous need for people in global health who understand communications, ecology, economics, engineering, finance, health systems management, law, logistics management, and water and sanitation, as discussed further next.

WHAT KIND OF GLOBAL HEALTH WORK CAN ONE DO?

One can engage in many different types of global health work. Although there is no perfect typology of these efforts, they do fall roughly into several different spheres. These are portrayed in **Table 18-1**.

TABLE 18-1 Selected Areas of Global Health Work

- Research
- Policy
- Program Design and Implementation
- Program Evaluation
- Advocacy

> **TABLE 18-2** Selected Functional Areas of Global Health Work
>
> - Ethics
> - Nutrition
> - Women's Health
> - Reproductive and Sexual Health
> - Children's Health
> - Adolescent Health
> - Immunization
> - Environmental Health
> - Communicable Diseases—TB, HIV/AIDS, Malaria, Neglected Tropical Diseases
> - Noncommunicable Diseases—Heart Disease, Stroke, Diabetes
> - Health Conditions of the Aging
> - Mental Health
> - Unintentional Injuries
> - Complex Humanitarian Emergencies
> - Essential Surgery

THE KEY TECHNICAL AREAS FOR GLOBAL HEALTH WORK

Global health is a rich field, with many different areas of effort. The functional areas in which one might work in global health are suggested by **Table 18-2.**

TYPES OF ORGANIZATIONS WITH WHICH YOU MIGHT ENGAGE IN GLOBAL HEALTH ACTIVITIES

NGOs

Many people want to work with nongovernmental organizations (NGOs) that are engaged in health in low- and middle-income countries. Some of these are local NGOs, such as the Self-Employed Women's Association of India and the Population Foundation of India. Others are international NGOs, such as Oxfam, CARE, and Save the Children. The largest of these organizations support a wide variety of activities, including the delivery of health services and the strengthening of health systems. They may also engage in research, policy, and advocacy activities.

The largest NGOs tend to recruit people with substantial experience and high-level skills for their fieldwork in low- and middle-income countries. However, at their headquarters, these organizations generally have a broader range of positions, and they recruit staff with a variety of skill sets to

carry out this work. These positions range from entry-level program assistants, who coordinate and track program information, to senior technical positions. The latter may include physicians, often with an advanced degree in an area of public health, such as epidemiology. These NGOs also recruit nurses, but usually only those with advanced degrees in public health, as well as experience working in public health in low- or middle-income countries.

In addition, many large NGOs hire public health graduates at the master's and doctoral level. These public health professionals have expertise in some of the key global health issues, such as maternal and child health, family planning, nutrition, communicable diseases, and health systems development. Most large NGOs will also employ a range of social scientists, including economists and anthropologists. Their staff may also include people with knowledge of behavior change and communication. Technical staff are usually involved in research, policy, or advocacy work, or in the design, implementation, monitoring, and evaluation of health programs.

Organizations Involved in the Delivery of Humanitarian Services

A number of organizations, many of which are NGOs, are involved in the delivery of clinical services in low- and middle-income countries, especially related to complex emergencies or other humanitarian efforts. Such organizations would include, for example, Doctors Without Borders or the International Rescue Corps.[3,5] They may also provide services as part of shorter-term medical missions, as in the work of Sightsavers[6] or Operation Smile.[7] In addition, the largest of these organizations are also involved with research, policy, and advocacy work. Many of the people engaged in these organizations are trained in medicine, nursing, and pharmacy; however, these organizations also have staff members who may be trained, for example, in finance or logistics management to support their clinical work, or economics, policy, and communications to support their other efforts. For their humanitarian work overseas, these organizations tend to hire relatively few junior staff that lack clinical training.

Bilateral Organizations and Government Agencies

The leading bilateral aid organizations, such as those from Australia (AUSAID), the United Kingdom (DFID) and the United States (USAID), also support important health programs in low- and middle-income countries. The profiles of staff members recruited by these organizations are similar to those of the largest NGOs. However, the bilateral agencies may include more people with training in economics and finance on their technical staff than most NGOs. In addition, the NGOs tend to focus on a relatively narrow range of technical areas, whereas the bilateral agencies may be involved in a wide range of health activities and require staff with skills in all of those areas. For example, the largest bilateral organizations may simultaneously work on health systems strengthening, maternal and child health, and infectious diseases, among other things. The staff who work with these organizations may be engaged in advocacy, research, or policy activities. They also work on the design, implementation, and evaluation of health programs in developing countries.

Multilateral Organizations and UN Agencies

The multilateral organizations and United Nations (UN) agencies that work on health tend to hire very seasoned professionals for their technical work. Most of these staff are recruited midcareer, after they have already had distinguished careers in their fields. However, many of these organizations also have programs for junior professionals or young professionals. The junior professionals are generally recent graduates of a first degree or an advanced degree program. Other programs, like the World Bank's Young Professionals Program, select people who have advanced degrees, outstanding academic and professional records, and substantial experience compared to most people their age.[8] In addition, these organizations recruit some relatively recent graduates of both first degree and advanced programs to work as program assistants and research assistants.

Multilateral organizations and UN agencies are also involved in a broad range of health sector activities and need professionals with skills in all of these areas. Similar to the work of the bilateral organizations, this generally includes research, policy, and advocacy, as well as program design, implementation, and evaluation. These organizations, however, often place more emphasis on health systems activities and the work of economists and finance specialists than do other organizations working in global health. The World Health Organization, of course, is the most technical of these organizations, and a large share of its staff are trained as physicians.

Public–Private Partnerships for Health

The number of public–private partnerships for health has grown substantially. These organizations, like AERAS, IAVI, and Medicines for Malaria Venture, tend to be highly technical in nature and employ professionals with high-level technical skills. Because the organizations work in science, research, policy, and health services delivery, they recruit staff members with skills in each of these areas. However, their employment needs are frequently determined by new product development efforts, such as for a TB vaccine or a microbicide that could stem the transmission of HIV. In such cases, the organizations hire professionals with the knowledge and skills needed for these specific projects and for the policy, regulatory, and communications efforts needed to support them.

Consulting Firms

There is a wide range of consulting firms, both for-profit and not-for-profit, that work on global health. Many of the largest for-profit firms, such as McKinsey, engage in global health work. However, there is also a wide range of other firms engaged in global health efforts. These include organizations such as FHI, JSI, and PSI. Many of the consulting firms that work on global health also work in a wide variety of health efforts, including research and policy analysis, as well as program development, implementation, and evaluation. To carry out this work, the consulting firms generally require the same skill sets as the bilateral and multilateral organizations. This includes high-level technical expertise from a select number of domains in which the firm wants to specialize. However, they may also recruit younger staff to serve as research assistants, program assistants, and other entry-level positions.

Foundations

In general, the foundations that work in global health have a relatively small number of employees who tend to be very highly trained in their field. However, they often couple these staff with a small number of junior staff. The largest foundations that work in global health, such as the Bill & Melinda Gates Foundation, are generally staffed in a manner similar to the largest bilateral and multilateral organizations.

Academia

A large number of universities throughout the world are involved in education, training, research, and practice in global health. Universities and their associated research programs are generally staffed by faculty that have doctoral-level degrees in a discipline or degrees in law or medicine, frequently in conjunction with a public health degree. These faculty are in a wide variety of academic departments, most often including anthropology, economics, medicine, political science, public health, and sociology.

Many universities now have global health institutes or global health centers that coordinate and bring together faculty research and practice from across different parts of the university. These centers and institutes are often the university organizations that receive grants or contracts for global health projects and recruit people for work in university-affiliated global health activities. These efforts often engage a range of professionals, as well as more junior research assistants and program assistants. Of course, many universities prefer to hire their own students and graduates for such programs.

Policy and Advocacy Organizations

Policy-oriented organizations, such as think tanks, focus on research and analysis of selected policy matters. They often use the conclusions of their analyses to engage with important stakeholders on how key global health issues can be addressed more effectively and efficiently. Organizations with this type of focus include, for example, the Results for Development Institute, the Center for Global Development, and the Council on Foreign Relations.[9–11] For their technical work, they tend to recruit highly skilled and experienced staff.

Advocacy organizations focus on raising awareness and funding for key global health issues. Examples of these types of organizations are RESULTS and ONE.[12,13] These organizations tend to recruit relatively young individuals who have some background in health, communications, and/or advocacy. These organizations are generally looking less for high levels of technical expertise and more for people with a deep sense of commitment to their work, the ability to strategize about how to influence policymakers, and exceptional ability to speak and write well on policy matters.

There is a considerable amount of discussion about social entrepreneurship, and organizations that engage in this type of work might also be of interest. Unfortunately, there is no generally accepted definition of social entrepreneurship, and some people believe that organizations that call themselves social entrepreneurs are just another form of NGO. In any case, most definitions of social entrepreneurship suggest that this includes using business skills and innovation to try to create long-term sustainable social impact. Some would suggest, for example, that Unite for Sight's work on cataract blindness control takes this approach.[14] They might also say that PATH takes this approach as it works in public and private partnerships to promote the development of technologies that can better serve the health needs of poor people in poor countries.[15] A well-documented case of an organization that most people would identify as social entrepreneurs is the Aravind Eye Care Hospital in India.[16] This hospital provides high-quality eye care to people of all social classes and uses fees collected from better-off people to subsidize the cost of its work with less well-off people. In principle, social entrepreneurs who work in health seek to employ creative, innovative staff, who can think out of the box, possess a good knowledge of health, understand a variety of approaches to improving health, and also know something about a range of business practices and how they might be applied to health. Some social entrepreneurs will also employ highly qualified technical staff in a number of areas.

YOUR FUTURE IN GLOBAL HEALTH

Now that you have a better understanding of the broad range of jobs in organizations that work in global health, it is time to establish a framework within which you can consider a possible career in global health. It is also important to provide a basic overview of how you can pursue such a career.

As you begin to think about your professional interests and a possible career in global health, it might be useful to ask yourself the following question: "Ten years from now, what impact do I hope to have on the global health field?" Thinking about this question will help you focus on what you would like to do *and* the impact you would like to make from doing it.

If you are new to the global health field, it may be difficult to know the different types of global health work in which you could engage. You are probably familiar with some of the clinical work that health professionals, such as physicians, engage in to improve global health. However, you may have had little exposure to the work done by other professions. You may never have heard of work like Vivian's on health communications, Joseph's logistics work with Doctors Without Borders, or Edith's use of science to help develop new diagnostics, drugs, or vaccines that could improve the health of the poor in low- and middle-income countries.

Therefore, as you begin to develop your interest in a global health career, it is very important to:

- Become familiar with the opportunities for working in global health
- Understand the background needed for the type of career you may want to pursue and how much of that background you already possess
- Establish a plan to gain the knowledge, skills, and experience you need for such a career, in a manner consistent with your other personal and professional interests and obligations
- Identify people who can serve as role models to help you understand global health professions and how you can pursue them

More is said about each of these topics in the following sections.

What You Need to Know to Work in Global Health

In many respects, careers in global health are just like other careers. Both require a certain type of background to obtain a job and to carry it out effectively. In global health, as in other fields, specific types of knowledge, skills, and experience are usually necessary to gain employment and to grow in the field professionally. If you want to work in global health, it is also important to have a good understanding of how to work in a variety of settings outside of your own country and culture, with humility and an appreciation of one's role in such settings.

If you think broadly about work in low- and middle-income countries, you would generally need to have:

- A good understanding of key political, social, and economic issues in the development of low- and middle-income countries, as well as how these issues might be addressed
- An appreciation for and an understanding of different cultures
- Knowledge of one or more languages commonly used in low- and middle-income countries
- Experience living and working in low- and middle-income countries, ideally close to the grassroots level
- Technical skills that can be used to help address global health issues
- An outstanding ability to write and speak simply and clearly for a wide range of audiences

Developing Your Knowledge, Skills, and Experience

Once you have outlined the knowledge, skills, and experience you are likely to need to pursue your global health career, it is important to assess your progress in each of these areas. You can then determine the gap between where you are and where you need to be. This assessment can serve as the foundation upon which you decide how best to fill that gap. Some of the ways of enhancing your readiness for a career in global health are noted in the following sections.

University Studies

The first step to set the foundation for your future career in global health is to get a good education in the field you want to pursue, if that is already defined. As noted earlier, it could be engineering. It could be anthropology. It could be economics. Whatever field you choose, it is important to master the material and take advantage of every opportunity to link your studies with the field of global health. For an engineering student, this could be a focus on water and sanitation. For an economics student, this could be a focus on the relationship between health and development. For an anthropology student, this could be a focus on medical anthropology.

As you pursue your first or later degrees, it is also important that you engage in the study of development. You do not need to become a development economist; however, you do need to have a good understanding and appreciation of the key issues in development, how they play out in low- and middle-income countries, and how those countries might address them. In addition, it is crucial to understand the many links, in both directions, between health and education and health and development.

It is also essential to master as much as you can of English, Spanish, and French. Several other languages can also be very useful for work on health and development, including Portuguese and some languages commonly used in low-income countries, such as Swahili. It is important to note that the more languages in which you can work efficiently and effectively, the greater the opportunities will be for you in the global health field. The inverse is also important; a lack of knowledge of languages other than your own can be a major obstacle to gaining employment in the global health field.

In the end, the best way to learn about other cultures and languages is to live and work with other culture groups. However, until you can do that, it is essential that you take advantage of opportunities to study other cultures, languages, and development.

Internships and Work Study

One excellent way to build the foundation for a career in global health while you are still a student is to engage in *internships* or *work-study* opportunities in the global health field. By undertaking a variety of internships throughout your studies, you can learn about numerous aspects of global health. This can also help you understand which parts of the global health field are most interesting to you and best suit your strengths. For example, with good planning and some luck, you might be able to work at different times for an NGO that works on health and human rights, another that focuses on the health of women and children, a third that emphasizes TB, and a fourth that is an advocacy organization. Alternatively, if you develop a specific interest at an early stage in your studies, such as HIV/AIDS, you could use your internships to gain a better understanding of the many aspects of HIV/AIDS work.

Most universities provide considerable information on how to find internships. This information may be available in a career office, on a university job or internship website, or through other forms of communication such as mass informational emails and print brochures. Other ways that students obtain internships include searching for advertisements on specialized websites, having faculty connect them to colleagues in global health, word of mouth from student to student, or asking for internships directly from specific organizations of interest to them.

Of course, finding an internship is easiest if you attend a university in a location with a tradition of internships and a wide array of internship opportunities, such as Washington, DC, in the United States or London, in the United Kingdom. If you study somewhere with ongoing global health efforts, you should have opportunities to learn about various aspects of global health throughout the course of your studies.

On the other hand, if you attend a university in a location with few such global health opportunities, you can still prepare yourself for global health work by pursuing internships in areas of domestic health that focus on marginalized populations, such as lower-income or immigrant communities. People in these communities face many of the same challenges that the poor face in low- and middle-income countries, and much can be learned from working with them.

Study Abroad

Another way you can build a foundation for work in global health is by studying for a semester or two in a low- or middle-income country. An increasing number of opportunities exist to study in low-income countries, such as Kenya, Senegal, or Uganda, as well as middle-income countries, such as Brazil, China, South Africa, and Thailand. In addition, some of these programs specifically focus on health and provide students with opportunities to engage in independent research on health topics of their choice. Moreover, many study abroad programs have *homestays*, in which students live with a local family. These opportunities can be transformational and extremely enlightening for university students. The chance to live, even for a short time, with a family in a low- or middle-income country is a unique and invaluable experience.

SIT, for example, has a wide range of study abroad opportunities that focus on health. These include programs in Argentina, Brazil, Chile, China, India, Jordan, Kenya, Madagascar, and South Africa. SIT also operates the International Honors Program that gives students a chance over a semester to visit several countries.[17] The Alliance for Global Education operates a program on global and public health in Manipal, India. There are many other study abroad programs that focus on global health as well.[18]

Work Abroad During Vacation

Another outstanding way to develop a foundation for a career in global health is to work on health in a low- or middle-income country during your university vacations. Some students do this over relatively short breaks, such as the winter break or spring break in the United States. However, others undertake such an experience during their long vacation, which is the summer break in the United States.

You can arrange such a work experience abroad in multiple ways. One possibility is to arrange the work through personal contacts. In many countries, university students are a diverse group, and a student may be able to spend time in the home country of a classmate, working, for example, with a health-oriented NGO. Another way to work in low- or middle-income countries over school vacations is to participate in a variety of programs that are arranged by organizations and firms, such as:

- *Cross-Cultural Solutions:* For more than 15 years, Cross-Cultural Solutions has sent students to volunteer or intern in one of 12 countries in Africa, Asia, Latin America, and Eastern Europe in the fields of education, health, and social service. Trips last anywhere from 1 to 12 weeks.[19]
- *Visions in Action:* Also known as Africa Development Corps, Visions in Action has sent students for over 20 years to work on development projects in Liberia, Tanzania, and Uganda on issues of health, food security, and education. Most health projects in which students participate are related to combating HIV/AIDS, and most programs last anywhere from 6 to 12 months.[20]
- *Global Service Corps:* Located at SUNY Albany (State University of New York at Albany), Global Service Corps sends students to intern in Cambodia and Tanzania. Internships are related to health care, education, and other community development projects and last anywhere from one week to indefinitely.[21]

Unfortunately, one generally has to pay for opportunities such as these. However, many students have found them worthwhile.

Many universities and student groups sponsor short humanitarian visits to low- and middle-income countries during school breaks. The visiting groups may help provide needed health services or may engage in broader aspects of community development, such as home building or the installation of water and sanitation systems.

Some universities also have travel fellowships that support student-led research or practice during the university breaks. Although these fellowships tend to be highly competitive, they represent an excellent opportunity for students to explore research and practice topics in another country.

For example, a student at Yale University recently used such a fellowship to do research on sex trafficking in Mumbai, India. A George Washington University student used a travel fellowship during her winter break to conduct interviews in Mexico on the impact of the *Oportunidades* program on reducing maternal mortality among poor women. This research was part of an honors thesis she did during the final year of her bachelor of science degree program. As part of a practicum for her master of public health degree, a student at George Mason University used such a fellowship to work on infection control in a hospital in Swaziland.

Postgraduate Work Overseas

Although it is very valuable to engage in global health efforts during your university studies, there are also opportunities to gain global health experience after completing your first degree. There are a small number of travel fellowships that can support such activities. These fellowships are sometimes offered by foundations, such as the Luce Foundation Fellowship in the United States.[22] Some universities also have their own fellowship programs for recent graduates. The United States also has a Fulbright scholars program that supports research and teaching in other countries.[23] There are also a large number of teaching fellowships that can help one live and work in a low- or middle-income country. Upon arriving in-country for such teaching fellowships, teachers can find health activities to engage in during their stay. It is possible to conduct valuable global health research or practice through each of these fellowships.

Another popular way of gaining work experience in low- and middle-income countries is through a national overseas volunteer program, such as the U.S. Peace Corps[24] or the British Voluntary Service Overseas.[25] Although one is not guaranteed to work in health, even if one is trained in that area, many volunteers do work in health or a related field. However, even if volunteers do not work specifically on health issues, they can still gain excellent exposure to critical issues in development that will be valuable throughout their global health career.

The Global Health Corps is similar to the Peace Corps in some respects, but places young professionals in global health organizations in Africa and the United States for one year and pairs them with a young professional from the country of their placement.[26] Organizations like the Peace Corps and Global Health Corps have strong alumni networks that can be an excellent resource during job searches. Moreover, many employers place a premium on recruiting ex-volunteers because they believe that such people have personal traits that make them especially productive employees.

Graduate Studies

An important question after completing your first degree is whether you should pursue graduate studies, and if so, in what field. The main point worth reiterating here is that you can work in global health and serve the needs of marginalized people in many ways and with many academic backgrounds. The second point worth repeating is that no matter which field of study you pursue, it is crucial that you bring high-level professional skills to your future work in global health. A third point is that your future field of graduate study could be different from the field of your first degree. A person who studied science can do graduate work in economics or public policy. In North American educational systems, one could study film or English for the first degree and still attend medical school later, provided one also meets the prerequisites for that field.

Indeed, many people who work in global health both clinically and on policy and program issues are trained as physicians. Many of these people also have graduate degrees in public health. Some of them do global health work that is highly technical and requires clinical training. For example, there are physicians who work abroad clinically through organizations like Doctors Without Borders or the International Rescue Committee. However, many of the physicians who work in global health have stopped practicing clinical medicine and now focus on public health work instead. This is the case, for example, for most physicians who work on TB control with the Global Partnership to Stop TB or on HIV/AIDS control with UNAIDS.

Clearly, if you want to work in global health, there is still considerable merit in studying medicine. Indeed, physicians have led many of the most important contributions to global health. For example, Donald "D.A." Henderson, who has MD and MPH degrees, led WHO's Smallpox Eradication Programme. In addition, William Foege, who also has MD and MPH degrees, made substantial contributions to smallpox eradication efforts, directed the U.S. Centers for Disease Control and Prevention (CDC), and has been instrumental in efforts to control neglected tropical diseases. Of course, these comments can also be said of other health professionals, such as nurses, pharmacists, or dentists. It also appears that there will be increasing roles in global health for veterinarians who understand and are trained in public health.

Economists have also made important contributions to global health. They have generally focused their attention on the costs and financing of health systems, the provision of financial protection to the poor, and ways to ensure value for money from health investments. Some economists have made major contributions to research and practice on global health. For example, Dean Jamison, who holds a doctorate in economics, was the main author on a number of global health reports that had a major impact on how low- and middle-income countries invest in health. Ramanan Laxminarayan, who also has a PhD in economics, has conducted important research on cost-effectiveness analysis that is widely used in the global health field. Both Abdo Yazbeck and Rachel Nugent hold PhDs in economics and have had important impacts on global health efforts. Abdo has done seminal work on poverty and health. Among other things, Rachel has done pioneering work on food policy and nutrition and on antimicrobial resistance.

As noted throughout the text, global health issues are inextricably linked with culture. Thus, you might want to study medical anthropology, focusing on selected issues in global health. This might include, for example, the cultural issues that relate to women's health or nutrition. Many people do not know that Paul Farmer and Jim Kim, who have been so involved with the NGO Partners in Health, are both physicians with PhDs in anthropology.

Many people who work in global health have pursued graduate degrees in international affairs or development studies and built strengths in particular areas of global health around those studies. Similarly, many others have gotten advanced degrees in public policy, focusing their work on development, human resources development, or global health issues. There is a risk that degrees in development studies or public policy may leave one without in-depth expertise in any one discipline. They also leave one without a specific professional title. Yet, many employers appreciate the way that graduates of these programs are trained in policy analysis, development, economics, and finance. Keith Hansen, for example, who headed the health program for Latin America at the World Bank, is a graduate of the Woodrow Wilson School at Princeton University, a public policy school. He also has a law degree. His colleague at the World Bank, Tim Johnston, who headed the World Bank's health work in Cambodia, is also a Woodrow Wilson School graduate. Many of the staff of organizations that engage in policy and advocacy work are graduates of public policy programs.

It was noted earlier that many students interested in global health have never thought of pursuing an advanced degree in business and may even see business as something contrary to global health. Yet nothing prevents a business school graduate from devoting his or her life to applying those business skills to work on public health issues. For example, Pape Gaye heads an important nonprofit consulting firm that works on global health. One of the ways that he prepared for this was by obtaining an advanced degree in business. In addition, many people who studied marketing are involved in social marketing for health.

Studying engineering to an advanced level can provide one with an excellent basis for work on global health. For example, designing roads to enhance safety and improve access to social services would have a major impact on health in many countries. Moreover, strengthening water and sanitation systems could make a substantial impact on the burden of disease. Yet, most people do not consider engineering when imagining a career in global health. The late John Briscoe, who was on the faculty of the Harvard Schools of Engineering, Public Health, and Government, was an engineer who made major contributions to work on water supply and sanitation.

As you know, a substantial share of the burden of disease is linked with under- or overnutrition. A number of graduate programs, like those at Tufts University and Cornell University, have excellent education programs in nutrition at both the master's and the PhD level. Proper nutrition is fundamental for the well-being of young children; consistent with this, many UNICEF staff members have obtained a PhD in nutrition.

Those with a strong interest in health and human rights might want to study law or even philosophy. A number of law programs have concentrations in human rights issues, and many staff members who work on health at organizations such as Amnesty International and Human Rights Watch have law degrees. Those who have studied law might also be at the forefront of work on intellectual property issues and trade matters that affect health, such as access to affordable medicines in low- and middle-income countries. Surprising to some people, many of the most distinguished writers on ethical issues in health have a background in philosophy. For example, Norman Daniels, the author of *Just Health*, which focuses on social justice and health, is a philosopher. Toby Ord[27] is a professor of philosophy at Oxford University in the United Kingdom. He established Giving What We Can, a society for charitable giving, and has done research and writing on a number of ethical issues related to global health.[28]

Many people still fail to consider the important role that journalists, filmmakers, and others in media and communications can have in enhancing interest in global health and efforts to improve it. Despite the apparent decline in newspapers in some countries, a number of newspapers continue to have reporters who regularly write on global health issues. For example, Laurie Garrett, now at the Council on Foreign Relations, is a journalist who became interested in global health and wrote several widely read books on public health issues. Documentary films on global health issues, such as

Rx for Survival,[29] as well as popular films, such as *While the Band Played On* or *Philadelphia*, can have a major impact on popular perceptions of key health issues. Many organizations that are involved in global health are now active users of social media, such as Facebook and Twitter.

One last question that will arise as you consider studies in global health is whether you should get a doctoral degree. There is no perfect answer to this question. However, the simplest answer is that a doctoral degree is essential if you wish to engage in research work. However, if you want to work in policy or practice, you may wish to seek additional practical experience instead of taking a substantial number of years to get a doctoral degree.

This list of areas for possible graduate study could include many more fields, such as those related to mental health, which is also an enormous burden of disease. Although the previous comments are only illustrative, they highlight the importance of considering graduate studies as you complete your first degree. It is also crucial to get a sense of the field of study you wish to pursue, knowing that you do not need to compromise your interests in order to work in global health. By contrast, there are many academic paths that can prepare one for a career in global health.

SELECTED ADDITIONAL RESOURCES ON CAREERS IN GLOBAL HEALTH

In this chapter you have been exposed to a framework for thinking about careers in global health. If you are still interested in considering a career in global health, you may want to pursue some additional information on this topic.

Somewhat surprisingly, given the growth of interest in careers in global health, there is still only a limited number of resources available to help guide those interested in pursuing such a career. Some of these include:

- *Building Partnerships in the Americas*[30]
- *Caring for the World: A Guidebook to Global Health Opportunities*[31]
- *Finding Work in Global Health: A Practical Guide for Jobseekers or Anyone Who Wants to Make the World a Healthier Place*[32]

Another book that might be helpful, although it is not specific to global health, is *Idealist Guide to Nonprofit Careers for First-Time Job Seekers*.[33]

In addition, the Consortium of Universities for Global Health has a number of educational modules that touch on careers.[34] Unite for Sight has an online course on careers.[35] Dr. Greg Martin runs an online channel on global health,

which also features a number of videos that relate to careers in the global health field.[36]

There are also a number of websites that list job postings in global health or fields related to global health and development, including the following:

- DEVEX is an organization that focuses on international aid and development. Its web page lists jobs in global health, among other fields.[37]
- The Global Health Council operates a clearinghouse for global health careers that is available to those seeking a position in global health, as well as, for a fee, those recruiting people to work in this field.[38]
- GlobalHealthHub.org has a range of valuable resources on global health broadly and on careers in global health.[39]
- The International Jobs Center is an online weekly publication of international jobs.[40]
- Idealist.org is an "interactive site where people and organizations can exchange resources and ideas, locate opportunities and supporters, and take steps toward building a world where all people can lead free and dignified lives."[41] This website has a number of resources related to jobs in the nonprofit field.
- Zebra Jobs is a resource for jobs in Africa.[42]
- Eldis is a clearinghouse of information on development that has a jobs listing on its website.[43]
- The U.S. government operates a website with information about U.S. government jobs in global health and some related positions.[44]
- The U.S. Centers for Disease Control and Prevention has a website that focuses on its jobs overseas.[45]
- The Public Health Employment Connection is a job clearinghouse operated by the Rollins School of Public Health at Emory University.[46]
- Public Health Career Mart is a website of the American Public Health Association that focuses on jobs for public health professionals.[47]
- The Akili Initiative, an online student initiative for global health, offers a database of organizations that offer global health jobs and links to their career pages.[48]

MAIN MESSAGES

Global health is a growing field, and there are many opportunities to work in it. There are positions, for example, in universities and think tanks, NGOs, social entrepreneurship, bilateral and multilateral aid organizations, and consulting.

Although there is a variety of jobs in the global health field for those trained in the health professions, there are also many opportunities for those trained in other areas, including anthropology, communications, economics, engineering, and logistics management.

If you are considering a career in global health, it is valuable to get a sense of the range of such careers that are available. You will then want to understand better the skills, knowledge, and experience this type of career would entail and how you might fill any gaps you have in terms of the required background for such positions. You will also want to approach potential work in global health with a deep sense of humility.

Most jobs in global health will require a good understanding of economic development; an appreciation of other cultures; an ability to write and speak well, both in English and in other languages; and skills in at least one of the areas important to global health. They often require experience living and working in low- and middle-income countries as well.

If you want to pursue a career in global health, it would be valuable to get your first degree in an area related to the one in which you want to work. It is also important to build on that with internships, fellowships, and other opportunities to live and work abroad. Many different graduate programs can build on your studies and experiences and further prepare you for a career in global health. There are many routes to becoming involved in global health. It is always valuable to learn from the career paths of those already involved in the field and mentors with whom one can work directly.

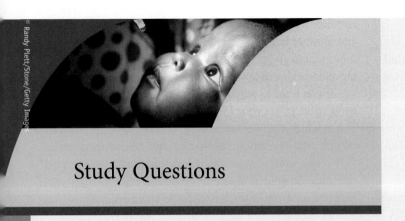

Study Questions

1. What are some of the organizations most involved in global health work?

2. What types of staff carry out their health activities?

3. What types of knowledge and experience are generally essential to working in global health?

4. How can university students get a better understanding of life in low- and middle-income countries?

5. What role might an economist, anthropologist, engineer, or public policy specialist play in global health?

6. What are some of the careers in global health that might be open to physicians?

REFERENCES

1. International AIDS Vaccine Initiative. Retrieved August 16, 2010, from http://www.iavi.org/.

2. Engineers Without Borders—International. Retrieved August 16, 2010 from http://www.ewb-international.org.

3. Doctors Without Borders. Retrieved August 16, 2010, from http://www.doctorswithoutborders.org.

4. PSI. Retrieved August 10, 2014, from http://www.psi.org/.

5. International Rescue Corps. Retrieved August 16, 2010, from http://www.intrescue.org.

6. Sightsavers. Retrieved August 16, 2010, from http://www.sightsavers.org/default.html.

7. Operation Smile. Retrieved August 16, 2010, from http://www.operationsmile.org.

8. The World Bank. *Young Professionals Program*. Retrieved November 20, 2014, from http://web.worldbank.org/WBSITE/EXTERNAL/EXTJOBSNEW/0,,contentMDK:23149336~menuPK:8453554~pagePK:8453902~piPK:8453359~theSitePK:8453353,00.html.

9. Results for Development Institute. Retrieved August 10, 2014, from http://r4d.org/.

10. Center for Global Development. Retrieved August 10, 2014, from http://www.cgdev.org/.

11. Council on Foreign Relations. Retrieved August 10, 2014, from http://www.cfr.org/.

12. RESULTS. Retrieved August 10, 2014, from http://www.results.org/.

13. ONE. Retrieved August 10, 2014, from http://www.one.org/us/.

14. Unite for Sight. (2014). *Module 8: Social entrepreneurship in healthcare*. Retrieved August 8, 2014, from http://www.uniteforsight.org/global-health-careers/module8.

15. PATH. Retrieved August 10, 2014, from http://www.path.org/.

16. Aravind. (2014). Aravind eye care system. Retrieved August 10, 2014, from http://www.aravind.org/.

17. SIT. (2014). *SIT study abroad global health programs*. Retrieved August 8, 2014, from http://studyabroad.sit.edu/sn/programs/critical-global-issues/?cgi=GH.

18. Alliance for Global Education. Study Abroad in Asia. Retrieved June 8, 2015, from http://allianceglobaled.org/programs.

19. Cross-Cultural Solutions. Retrieved August 16, 2010, from http://www.crossculturalsolutions.org.

20. Visions in Action. Retrieved August 16, 2010, from http://africadevcorps.org/.

21. Global Service Corps. Retrieved August 16, 2010, from http://www.globalservicecorps.org/site.

22. Henry Luce Foundation. *Luce Scholars*. Retrieved August 16, 2010, from http://www.hluce.org/lsprogram.aspx.

23. Institute of International Education. *Fulbright Program*. Retrieved August 16, 2010, from http://www.iie.org/en/Fulbright.

24. Peace Corps. Retrieved August 16, 2010, from http://www.peacecorps.gov.

25. Volunteer Service Overseas. Retrieved August 16, 2010, from http://www.vso.org.uk.

26. Global Health Corps. *Why we're here*. Retrieved November 2, 2013, from http://ghcorps.org/why-were-here/mission-vision/.

27. BBC News Magazine. (2010, December 13). *Tony Ord: Why I am giving one million pounds to charity*. Retrieved August 10, 2014, http://www.bbc.co.uk/news/magazine-11950843.

28. Giving What We Can. (2014). *About us*. Retrieved August 10, 2014, http://www.givingwhatwecan.org/about-us.

29. PBS. (2005). *Rx for Survival: A global health challenge*. Retrieved August 16, 2010, from http://www.pbs.org/wgbh/rxforsurvival.

30. Krasnoff, M. (Ed.). (2013). *Building partnerships in the Americas*. Hanover, NH: Dartmouth College Press.

31. Drain, P., Huffman, S., Pirtle, S., & Chan, K. (2009). *Caring for the world: A guidebook to global health opportunities*. Toronto: University of Toronto Press.

32. Ohmans, P., & Osborn, G. (2005). *Finding work in global health: A practical guide for jobseekers or anyone who wants to make the world a healthier place*. Saint Paul: Health Advocates Press.

33. Busse, M. (2008). *Idealist guide to nonprofit careers for first-time job seekers*. Action Without Borders. Retrieved September 3, 2010, from http://idealistcareer.wpengine.netdna-cdn.com/wp-content/uploads/2013/05/IdealistGuideforFirstTimeJobSeekers.pdf.

34. Consortium of Universities for Global Health. (2014). *Educational modules*. Retrieved August 8, 2014, from http://www.cugh.org/resources/educational-modules.

35. Unite for Sight. (2014). *Global health careers online course*. Retrieved August 10, 2014, http://www.uniteforsight.org/global-health-careers/.

36. Martin, G. (2013). *Finding a job in global health*. Retrieved August 10, 2014, from https://www.youtube.com/watch?v=Q5eGIOJhhBA.

37. DEVEX. (2014). International AID and development jobs. Retrieved August 10, 2014, from https://www.devex.com/jobs.

38. Global Health Council. *Global Health Career Network*. Retrieved May 13, 2010, from http://globalhealth.org/resources/job-board/.

39. Global Health Hub. (2014). *Resources*. Retrieved August 10, 2014, from http://www.globalhealthhub.org/resources/.

40. International Jobs Center. Retrieved April 24, 2015, from http://www.internationaljobs.org/.

41. Idealist.Org. Retrieved February 21, 2010, from http://idealist.org.

42. Society for International Development. *Zebra jobs*. Retrieved July 24, 2010, from http://www.zebrajobs.com.

43. Eldis. Retrieved January 12, 2010, from http://www.eldis.org.

44. U.S. Department of Health and Human Services. *U. S. Global Health*. Retrieved September 3, 2010, from http://www.globalhealth.gov.

45. Centers for Disease Control and Prevention. *Global health—Jobs overseas*. Retrieved May 2, 2010, from http://www.cdc.gov/globalhealth/employment/.

46. Emory University Rollins School of Public Health. *Public Health Employment Connection*. Retrieved March 10, 2010, from http://cfusion.sph.emory.edu/PHEC/phec.cfm.

47. American Public Health Association. *Public Health Career Mart*. Retrieved July 30, 2010, from http://www.apha.org/professional-development/public-health-careermart.

48. Akili Initiative. *Global health job opportunities*. Retrieved November 2, 2013, from http://www.mappinghealth.com/akili/.

CHAPTER 19

Profiles of Global Health Actors

LEARNING OBJECTIVES

By the end of this chapter the reader will be able to:

- Articulate a range of global health careers
- Understand the array of people involved in global health
- Appreciate the factors that have inspired people to work in global health and the diverse ways they entered the field
- Identify the types of mentors one might find in global health
- Outline some key lessons of experience from global health work

VIGNETTES

Sarah is an HIV-positive woman from Kenya. She founded and now heads a nongovernmental organization (NGO) in Nairobi that provides support services to other HIV-positive women. Her organization helps them find centers where they can be tested for the virus and get treatment if they are infected. The organization also provides social support for women, to help them overcome the stigma of the disease. In addition, it helps them link with potential employers, so the women can have a source of independent income. Sarah was inspired to establish this NGO by a group of HIV-positive women who helped her when she was diagnosed with HIV. Sarah is now an inspiration to many other people.

John is a Canadian physician who also has a doctorate in public health and tropical medicine. He was trained at outstanding institutions in Canada, the United States, and the United Kingdom. John originally planned to work clinically. However, after taking a 1-month rotation during medical school in Malawi, John decided that he should focus on helping to meet the health needs of poor people in poor countries. He therefore took every opportunity during medical school,

residency, and graduate studies to become especially knowledgeable about newborn health in low- and middle-income countries. Today, John manages a center for global health at a major U.S. hospital. He spends three months each year helping to train health personnel in low-income countries about simple, low-cost ways of saving newborn lives.

Graciella is a Bolivian anthropologist and the director for social development at a multilateral development bank. Graciella completed her first degree in Bolivia and then earned a doctorate in cultural anthropology in the United States. Graciella's doctoral thesis focused on how to build safe motherhood practices in low-income countries on the basis of local birthing practices. Graciella worked for the Ministry of Social Development in Bolivia on the health of indigenous people and then joined a Brazilian consulting firm that worked on international development projects. After 5 years, Graciella joined a nonprofit consulting firm in the United States, focusing largely on health projects serving minority people in different parts of the world. Graciella brought to that work increasing attention to cultural issues. She is now one of the most experienced anthropologists working in development assistance for health.

Joe is an American who has worked in development and health since graduation from university. Between his first and second years in university, Joe spent 3 months working with a small NGO in Mumbai, India, that served the health needs of a large slum. That experience convinced Joe that he should work in development. He majored in international affairs at his university, with a concentration in global health. However, even as he finished at his university, Joe was keen to further enhance his understanding of low- and middle-income countries. Thus, he applied to the U.S. Peace Corps, which gave him a position in Liberia as a community health educator. After two challenging but enlightening years in Liberia, Joe returned to the United States for graduate studies, with a focus on development. Today, Joe is the director of a large project for maternal and child health in Africa.

INTRODUCTION

A common problem when university students think about possible careers is a lack of information about jobs in different fields. Often, they are not familiar enough with specific areas to know if they would be of long-term professional interest. In addition, university students often do not know enough people who work in these fields to learn firsthand from them about the content, challenges, and rewards of the professional's work. As you consider careers in global health, it is essential to explore a variety of global health areas through a combination of coursework, internships, jobs, and research, as suggested earlier. Throughout your experiences in global health, it is also crucial to learn as much as you can from the people with whom you work:

- What inspired them to get involved in global health?
- What knowledge, skills, and experience did they seek to become a global health professional?
- Who were the role models for their global health career?
- Who have been their mentors in this field?
- What have been their greatest work challenges?
- What have been the greatest rewards of their career?
- What are the most important lessons they have learned about having an impact on global health?

The remainder of this chapter provides profiles of 21 people who have made important contributions to the global health field. It also includes their responses to the preceding questions. Those who are profiled come from diverse backgrounds and have become involved in global health in different ways. Some people have contributed locally, by working with community-based organizations in their own country. Some have contributed through work on a national scale. Others have had a global impact through research, practice, and roles at key global institutions.

The profiles that follow are meant to inspire you as well as inform you. Each person featured has a compelling life story that has influenced his or her interest in global health and in serving disadvantaged people. Many of the people highlighted here engaged in one or more transformational experiences at some stage of their life, which helped lead them into the global health arena. Of course, there are tens of thousands of people like those profiled in this chapter who

make exceptional contributions daily to enhancing the health of the poor. The people discussed in the following sections have been selected for profiling because, individually and collectively, their stories provide enlightenment and inspiration to those interested in global health.

The profiles have been compiled largely from interviews and personal communications. Thus, there are no endnotes for this chapter. Readers interested in learning more about the people discussed in this chapter will easily be able to find additional information on all of them.

One of the challenges of presenting these profiles has been the order in which to put them. Should they be in order of length of experience? Region of the world from which they come? The level of position they have attained? In the end, it was decided to arrange the profiles alphabetically. This is meant to encourage the reader to look at each profile individually, without trying to discern the position of the person being profiled.

ELIZABETH (BETSY) BRADLEY

Betsy Bradley is a professor of public health at the Yale School of Public Health, the faculty director for the Yale Global Health Leadership Institute, and director of the Global Health Initiative at Yale University. Professor Bradley's research focuses on improving health delivery systems and the quality of healthcare services. Some of Professor Bradley's work has led to important changes in the organization, delivery, and quality of healthcare in a variety of settings.

Through a Bill & Melinda Gates Foundation grant, Betsy leads the development of an operational framework for the widespread dissemination and implementation of family health innovations. She also works for the Centers for Disease Control and Prevention and the Clinton Health Access Initiative on the Ethiopian Hospital Management Initiative. In addition, Dr. Bradley is involved in several projects that focus on strengthening health systems in Liberia, South Africa, and the United Kingdom.

Betsy grew up in New Britain, Connecticut, in the United States. At the time, New Britain was a manufacturing town, and her father was an engineer. Betsy shared with her father an interest in how things worked. However, rather than being interested in machines, she liked hospitals. At a young age, she began to pursue this interest by volunteering at the New Britain Hospital.

Betsy attended Harvard University, where she received a bachelor of arts degree in economics. At Harvard, Betsy greatly enjoyed studying market failures, and she first became interested in the economics of health care in a six-student seminar that looked at public and private boundaries, with health as one of the topics. Having become excited about work in health, Betsy interned for the chief financial officer of the Dana Farber Cancer Center in Boston, Massachusetts, in the United States after her third year in college. As Betsy gained more experience with health care, she started to ask herself a question she still thinks about regularly—"How do I make a hospital operate more effectively, more efficiently, with the best possible clinical outcomes, and the greatest respect for patients?"

To try to answer that question, Betsy pursued a master of business administration degree at the University of Chicago in the United States, where she specialized in health administration and organizational behavior. Following these studies, Betsy completed a 2-year fellowship at Massachusetts General Hospital (MGH), one of the premier hospitals in the world, and then worked for 5 years as a healthcare administrator. During her time at MGH, Betsy met many outstanding people, including Dr. Donald Berwick, a pioneer on healthcare quality, and she helped Dr. Berwick on his book, *Curing Health Care: New Strategies for Quality Improvement.*

Betsy loved the work she was doing at MGH but faced some large frustrations, such as what to do with uninsured patients. Betsy still vividly remembers a particular patient with cancer and how she advocated getting him treatment. She felt she was good at systems engineering but lacked the skills to help bring about bigger changes in health care in the United States. Therefore, she decided to pursue a PhD in health policy and health economics at Yale University. Through her studies, she also became very interested in the social determinants of health and research on health administration.

Betsy came across global health later in her life, notably when Ed Wood from the Clinton Foundation asked if she would bring to Ethiopia the skills she had used in helping to improve U.S. health care. This experience was very fulfilling and has encouraged Betsy to continue working in global health, as well as on healthcare issues in the United States. In the next 10–15 years, Betsy hopes to use Yale as a platform to help make the world a better and healthier place.

Professor Bradley has received numerous honors and awards during her career. She is a three-time recipient of the Teacher of the Year award from the Department of Epidemiology and Public Health at Yale, as well as a recipient of the John D. Thompson Young Investigator Award and the Investigator Award by the Donaghue Medical Research Foundation. She has served as a fellow with the Gerontological Society of America and is a member of the World Economic Forum. She has authored more than 250 peer-reviewed publications and has just published a book on the U.S. healthcare system and why it seems to get so little in outcomes for such large amounts of expenditure.

When asked what advice she would give to university students studying global health, Betsy stressed the importance of leadership:

- Learn to navigate differences in viewpoints. It is important to recognize differences, let them surface, and manage the inevitable conflict that will emerge. These actions are all core aspects of leadership.
- You need to spend time in the countries you will work on so that you will get the "visual experience" of the country and have an emotional attachment to it. Seeing is believing, and being in the country helps develop greater intuition and subtlety about the country's constraints, realities, and possibilities. Tailoring one's work to adapt to local conditions is fundamental, challenging, and fulfilling.
- Leadership is critical but one must also think about those who work with leaders and "follow" them. To "follow" is to have the capacity of actively supporting the leader. The success of organizations and teams depends not only on how well a leader can lead but also on how well the followers can follow. We often undervalue the role of "followers." Being flexible in playing different roles and wearing different hats, depending on the work to be done, is crucial for global health practitioners. Leaders should also work toward building a team of invested, stable followers. Without an understanding of leadership as depending on "followers," we can end up with big ideas but no action.
- Finding an appropriate balance between reflection and action is a great leadership capacity. We often find unintended consequences from our work. If you develop the habit of reflection, you can sometimes sense potential unintended effects before they become problematic.
- We can learn a lot from low-income settings. In resource-limited areas, people can become exceptionally creative to solve problems. Sometimes these solutions have been missed in high-income settings, where technology or various medicines are readily available. We should not overlook simpler solutions, particularly those that engage the community.

JOANNE CARTER

Joanne Carter is a specialist on global poverty issues, to which she has devoted most of her life. She started her career as a veterinarian, but has worked with RESULTS Education Fund (REF), a grassroots health and poverty alleviation advocacy organization, for the last 22 years. Joanne is an internationally recognized leader of advocacy efforts to support TB, HIV/AIDS, and child survival programs, as well as microfinance. Joanne also plays major roles in a number of international forums. Her career path provides an example of the different routes people take to become involved in global health.

Joanne grew up in Brooklyn, New York, in the United States. Joanne's parents imbued her with a strong sense of social justice and the need to be engaged in making the world a fairer and better place. From an early age, therefore, Joanne had a substantial interest in politics and social causes. She also had a great interest in science.

Joanne received a BS in biology from the State University of New York at Albany, setting what she thought might be the foundation for a career as a veterinarian or researcher. However, still pulled by her social and policy interests, Joanne spent the 2 years immediately following her first degree as a participant in the VISTA program—Volunteers in Service to America. As part of this work, Joanne was engaged in helping to improve access to health services in poor communities outside of Charleston, South Carolina.

Joanne followed her VISTA service by doing coursework and research toward a master's degree program in reproductive physiology, hoping to set an even stronger foundation for veterinary school. Joanne then enrolled in veterinary school and received a doctorate of veterinary medicine (DVM) from the New York State College of Veterinary Medicine at Cornell University. During her studies at Cornell, Joanne was actively involved with a group of faculty and students who were interested in the international and public health aspects of veterinary medicine, and she had the opportunity to spend one summer at an agricultural college in Orissa, India.

Joanne was a practicing veterinarian in the United States from 1987 to 1992. Shortly after starting this work, she took the opportunity to explore her international interests and spent 3 months visiting veterinary training institutions in Africa. Deciding she could have more impact on the root causes of poverty and hunger through changing U.S. policies and priorities rather than practicing as a veterinarian overseas, Joanne returned to New York City and began to explore ways to contribute her personal time to such causes.

In 1988, Joanne began volunteering with RESULTS in New York City. She started as a volunteer coordinator of advocacy efforts for the RESULTS chapter in New York City, and her responsibilities grew to include supporting chapters across the Northeast. Joanne carried out this volunteer work, even as she continued her veterinary practice.

In 1992, pulled by the opportunity to work in these areas full time, despite her continuing appreciation for her work as a veterinarian, Joanne became an employee of RESULTS.

She initially served at RESULTS as legislative director out of its headquarters in Washington, DC. In this capacity, Joanne worked with key congressional allies, U.S. government agencies and members of the executive branch, partner organizations, technical agencies, and international campaigns to combat the diseases of poverty, improve access to education, create economic opportunity for the poor, and reform World Bank and International Monetary Fund policies to best meet the needs of the poor.

Joanne was appointed associate executive director of RESULTS and REF in 2007. Joanne is currently the executive director of REF, a position she assumed in 2008. In addition, Joanne plays a number of other important roles, including vice chair of the global Stop TB Partnership, a partnership of over 1,000 organizations, and member of the boards of the Micronutrient Initiative and the Global Campaign for Education-U.S. In her recent role as a board member and Strategy Committee member for the Global Fund to Fight AIDS, TB and Malaria, Joanne helped shape development of the Global Fund's new funding model.

Joanne is especially proud of the work she and RESULTS have done, with others, to highlight TB as a major public health and poverty issue, build a network of partners together around TB, help focus attention on the links between TB and HIV, and dramatically increase the funding for TB. Joanne feels that these efforts were necessary to overcome the perception in many rich countries that TB was a disease of the past and to reverse the chronic neglect stemming from the fact that TB is a disease that largely affects poor people. Joanne is also extremely gratified by the role she and her organization have played in helping to establish and support the Global Fund to Fight AIDS, TB and Malaria, which was created from the ground up in 2002 and has since mobilized tens of billions of dollars for health in low- and middle-income countries.

Joanne offers the following advice to university students interested in pursuing a career in global health:

- In advocacy and in public health, it is essential to look at where you want to be in the future and then be bold and brave enough to lay out a plan to get there. Work for transformational rather than incremental change.
- Remember that "Hope is not a feeling—it's a decision." We can generate that hope by envisaging what is possible and working with allies to make it happen. As you do this, keep in mind stories of leaders like Jim Grant, the former UNICEF director who helped launch and drive the "child survival revolution." Grant was told during a briefing on progress

in immunization in El Salvador that targets were not being met due to the civil war then raging. Rather than accepting this, Grant replied, "Then stop the war." Indeed, both sides agreed to "Days of Tranquility" so that national immunization campaigns could continue unmolested.

- Work as much as you can with people who give you energy, rather than those who drain it away. Draw as much energy as you can from a network of allies who share your vision and will help you retain that vision in the face of naysayers.
- Follow your passion, even if you start by volunteering in that field. Doors will open.
- Work as much as you can with mentors. Much of what you will learn in life will come from them.

PATRICIA DAOUST

Patricia Daoust is associate director of nursing at Massachusetts General Hospital's Center for Global Health (CGH). She is also the chief nursing officer of Seed Global Health, a partnership program with the U.S. Peace Corps. She lectures on global health at the University of Massachusetts School of Nursing and Health Sciences, cochairs the Global Committee for the Association of Nurses in AIDS Care (ANAC), and serves on the advisory committee for the Global Nursing Caucus.

At CGH, Patricia designs, implements, and provides direction for nursing initiatives related to the organization's mission. She also provides technical assistance and support to nurses working in global health and oversees monitoring and evaluation of the center's nursing programs.

Patricia grew up mostly in Europe, where she lived for 9 years. Her father was in the United States Army and her family moved every 2 to 3 years. Patricia's mother was a nurse and always did volunteer nursing work in the places that they lived. Patricia admired her mother's efforts, thought of nursing as very adventurous, and always knew she wanted to follow in her mothers' footsteps.

Patricia became a registered nurse (RN) in 1968. She started her career by serving as a community health nurse in the Jesuit Volunteer Corps in Copper Valley, Alaska. In this role, she provided health care for the Native American and Eskimo community and students at Copper Valley High School. Upon returning to the U.S. mainland, she became a team leader and staff nurse on a medical-surgical unit at St. Elizabeth Hospital in Brighton, Massachusetts. Patricia found, however, that she struggled with hospital-based nursing. She never had enough time to talk to patients, work with their families, or take the holistic approach to care that she wanted. Her real love was community-based nursing. She

wanted to be creative, have some flexibility, and get to know her patients in the context of their families.

As a result, Patricia decided to take a break from hospital nursing to pursue a bachelor's degree in psychology/rehabilitation counseling at Emmanuel College in Boston, Massachusetts in 1981. She continued to work clinically once a week while she studied. She found that counseling and nursing were a wonderful combination because people often wanted to talk about their health problems with someone who also understood the disease process. After finishing her degree, Patricia worked as a palliative care nurse for a home-based hospice program that primarily served end-stage cancer patients. While she was working there, the hospice received a request from the family of a young gay man dying of AIDS. This was a time in the early 1990s when little was understood about HIV transmission and the potential risk to caregivers. Discrimination and stigma toward those living with HIV/AIDS frequently led to clinicians refusing to care for AIDS patients. When the hospice director refused to accept this referral, feeling that it put the caregivers at risk, Patricia called the AIDS Action Committee (AAC), an AIDS service organization based in Boston, to see if they could help. Although they offered to arrange a training session for her colleagues and supervisors to help alleviate their fears, her supervisor still refused to provide care for AIDS patients. A few weeks later, a similar request came in but this, too was refused.

Disappointed that she could not find help for these families, Patricia left her job with the hospice to work for the AIDS Action Committee. This was the beginning of a long career in nursing related to HIV/AIDS. While working for the AIDS Action Committee, she traveled across the state conducting training in HIV/AIDS for nurses and social workers, providing information about issues of transmission, the importance of universal precautions, and the right to health care for all. She ran a support group for people living with AIDS. Guided by her instincts as a caregiver, she continued with this important work, as she saw close friends pass away from the disease.

This work evolved into a job where Patricia went to parts of the state with no services for people with AIDS and helped to establish them. She became the founder and director of the Metro West AIDS Program in Framingham, Massachusetts, which provided case management and a group program for people affected by HIV/AIDS.

In 2000, Patricia's hero, Larry Kessler, the founding director of the AIDS Action Committee, received a call from a friend at the Harvard AIDS Institute. His friend needed help finding someone to help mobilize people living with

HIV/AIDS in Botswana, Africa. Larry recommended Patricia, and she worked on the Botswana project for the Harvard AIDS Institute for 5 years. Working in Africa, where there are high morbidity rates, many opportunistic infections, and many people living in poverty, made Patricia want to continue working in Africa. Nurses in Africa provide the majority of primary care and Patricia loved the idea of advocating for the profession and improving health outcomes. She has since provided technical assistance to various HIV/AIDS educational, service, treatment, and research organizations. She later worked in Ethiopia where she led a large and innovative project to build nursing capacity and leadership, which is now being replicated in other African countries.

Patricia recently served as director for The Physicians for Human Rights Global AIDS Initiative. In this role, she directed a Gates-funded campaign building a constituency of 10,000 health professionals dedicated to advocating for a comprehensive, evidence-based U.S. response to the global AIDS epidemic. She also developed and implemented national and international educational and advocacy outreach strategies directed toward U.S.- and African-based policymakers. Finally, she coordinated and provided advocacy opportunities for a global health advisory board made up of infectious disease physicians, nurses, public health specialists, and human rights experts.

Patricia has faced many challenges in her work. One of the biggest challenges has been trying to support doctors and nurses within resource-limited settings where mortality is high and essential tools are unavailable. Despite these challenges, Patricia is deeply committed to the field in the same manner she was 30 years ago. She is driven by the impact that she and others have been able to make in the nursing profession and the positive feedback she received from nurses being trained. This provides substantial inspiration to continue what she is doing. Patricia has even produced a film called *The Hawk Takes One Chick* that documents the changing role of grandmothers in family life in Swaziland as a result of the AIDS epidemic.

When asked to point out critical lessons from her own experience for today's students of global health, Patricia offered the following:

- When you do global health—leaving your country and going to another—never think of yourself as an expert. You are there to learn and it is the information sharing and partnerships with people on the ground that make things work. Partnerships, collaboration, and mutual understanding of the local context are extremely important.
- Change takes time. Patience is key.

- Global health is local. You can practice global health in your own backyard by working with vulnerable populations.
- It is essential to bring skills to work in global health. Your interest in global health is critical but without your theoretical and clinical knowledge or skills in other essential areas, you limit your impact.

PAPE GAYE

Pape Gaye, a well-respected leader in global health, is the president and chief executive officer of IntraHealth International, Inc., an organization dedicated to the health workforce. Pape came to this work through a somewhat improbable route. In fact, his story also reflects the many different ways in which people get involved in global health and the many academic backgrounds they bring to it.

Pape is Senegalese. He was born in Dakar, the capital of Senegal. Pape did his primary and secondary schooling and began his university studies in Senegal. Pape's worldview began to open when he befriended a U.S. Peace Corps volunteer who was living in his neighborhood while Pape was in secondary school. Pape met other volunteers and learned of the work they were doing in settings that were often poor, rural, and lacking in basic services. Pape was inspired by the commitment and dedication of these outsiders to helping to improve his own country.

This connection to the U.S. Peace Corps program was transformational for Pape in many other ways, as well. While he was still in secondary school, Pape began to work for the Peace Corps, training their volunteers to speak Wolof and French. In 1971, Pape made his first trip outside of Senegal when he traveled to Benin with the Peace Corps to help train volunteers there. In addition, Pape married one of the volunteers he met in Senegal. Pape's growing experiences with the Peace Corps set the foundation for and sparked a growing interest in development and in bridging gaps across cultures.

Political turmoil in the universities in Senegal made it difficult for Pape to complete his university studies there, so in 1975 Pape and his wife Irene moved to the United States so that he could finish university. Although he wanted to build on his language skills, Pape initially thought after going to the United States that he would work in a large U.S. corporation. With this in mind, Pape received his BA degree in business economics and linguistics from the University of California at Santa Barbara in 1980. Still aiming for a job in the corporate sector, Pape continued his education at the University of California at Los Angeles and received an MBA in Human Resources Management and International Business Management in 1982.

While en route to a job interview for a corporate position, however, Pape decided that his attachment to work in Africa remained strong and that he should return to work there. He immediately withdrew from the interview process and took a position for a year as a management consultant for the Peace Corps Regional Training Resource Office in Togo. In 1984, building on his proficient language skills and passion for cross-cultural understanding, he moved back to the United States and took an assignment with the International Olympic Committee working as a trainer in language services for the Los Angeles Olympic Organizing Committee. In 1985, Pape undertook his first global health assignment as a training consultant for the U.S. Centers for Disease Control and Prevention, working on the Combatting Childhood Communicable Diseases program. Having built a reputation as a leader in the intersecting fields of global health and training, Pape was approached by IntraHealth (then International Training in Health, INTRAH) to establish a regional office in West and Central Africa. From 1986 to 2003, Pape was the regional director for West, Central, and Northern Africa for IntraHealth and served in Abidjan, Lome, and Dakar. In this role, he worked to help countries develop their capacity to train reproductive, maternal, and child health providers. He also developed training programs for clinical and public healthcare workers in project countries.

In 2003, Pape moved to IntraHealth headquarters in Chapel Hill, North Carolina, to serve as senior vice president. Since 2004, Pape has been the chief executive officer of IntraHealth, which now has almost 20 offices and over 600 employees around the world. IntraHealth, originally based out of the University of North Carolina School of Medicine, is now a nonprofit organization that works to build local capacity to deliver health care that is both accessible and sustainable.

Pape is most proud of the work that he carried out building a robust and meaningful program for IntraHealth in Africa, despite the challenges of working in low-resource environments with weak governance structures and unstable leadership. In addition, he found substantial challenges trying to help countries enhance their health work in environments in which their health efforts were often too medically focused and not sufficiently based on the needs or circumstances of local communities.

When asked what advice he has for university students interested in careers in global health, Pape highlighted the following:

- It is essential to bring a global perspective and a deep appreciation of local cultures to work on health and development. Building skills in cultural competencies is therefore crucial.

- There is much to learn. You have to be a life-long learner and remain flexible, as things change constantly.
- The landscape of global health and international development is changing rapidly. There are new actors including social entrepreneurs, students, and members of the private sector, all committed to having their own footprint in the development space. Because of this, it is crucial that new types of partnerships are formed including among donor and "recipient" countries and institutions.

DAVID GOLD

David Gold is a cofounder and principal of Global Health Strategies (GHS), an international global health consulting firm that works with the public, private, and not-for-profit sectors to ensure development and worldwide delivery of health products and technologies. GHS has offices in New York, New Delhi, Rio de Janeiro, and Beijing and works with partners in a wide range of other countries in Africa and Europe. GHS clients include the Bill & Melinda Gates Foundation, the Rockefeller Foundation, the Michael and Susan Dell Foundation, the Paul Allen Foundation, the Gavi Alliance, Johnson & Johnson, GlaxoSmithKline Biologicals, and the Foundation for AIDS Research (Amfar).

In 2011, GHS launched a nonprofit affiliate—GHSi (Global Health Strategies initiatives). GHSi focuses its work on accelerating investment in global health and innovation in emerging economies and developing countries. One of GHSi's most important efforts to date was a report called *Shifting Paradigm: How the BRICS are Reshaping Global Health and Development*, which was released at the 2011 BRICS Heads of State meeting.

David grew up in Long Island, New York, in the United States, and got his bachelor of arts (BA) degree at the State University of New York at Albany. David was always interested in policy and politics. He was president of the student government in college, and as a student, he successfully ran for delegate to the Democratic National Convention. So, it was not surprising that David went to law school, getting a degree from the Boston University School of Law.

After graduating from law school, David started working in real estate to pay back his large student loans. He started a real estate investment company that purchased and owned residential and commercial properties.

Around the same time, David started reading about the first cases of AIDS, which was thought by many at the time to be a "gay disease." David started volunteering at the Gay Men's Health Crisis, where he wrote up wills. This was not what he really wanted to be doing, but his law degree allowed him to provide this much-needed service.

David got started in global health advocacy after hearing Larry Kramer speak. Kramer was a well-known playwright and author and the founder of the Gay Men's Health Crisis and ACT UP (AIDS Coalition to Unleash Power). Kramer suggested that David attend an ACT UP meeting. Because David already knew about working with the private sector, David focused on what could be done to push pharmaceutical companies to accelerate research and development (R&D) efforts on early antiretroviral drugs.

David then became much more active and involved in advocacy work. From 1991 to 1995, he headed the Medical Information Program at the Gay Men's Health Crisis, the world's first and largest AIDS organization, and he edited its newsletter on HIV therapies and treatment issues.

In 1995, David cofounded AVAC (AIDS Vaccine Advocacy Coalition) with a few other treatment activists. AVAC's mission was to speed the development of preventive HIV vaccines by analyzing obstacles to HIV vaccine development and advocating for their removal, without taking resources away from basic research, treatment, or prevention. The idea was to provide an independent, honest, well-informed critique of current efforts toward developing an HIV vaccine.

Prior to cofounding GHS, David was the founding vice-president for global policy and government support at the International AIDS Vaccine Initiative (IAVI). In that position, he oversaw the creation of IAVI's global policy and advocacy programs as well as its regional programs in North America, Europe, Japan, and Latin America. Working closely with IAVI's chief executive officer, David helped IAVI attract political support and financial commitments from governments, multilateral agencies, and the Bill & Melinda Gates Foundation, totaling more than $400 million. David also built partnerships and alliances with the World Health Organization, the European Union, the U.S. National Institutes of Health (NIH), and the Brazilian government. At IAVI, David also developed the *IAVI Report*, a publication devoted to AIDS vaccine research that now reaches more than 8,000 subscribers in 130 countries.

David has written and contributed to a wide range of reports on AIDS research issues. He has also served on research advisory panels for a number of different organizations including UNAIDS and the NIH.

David feels it is a real privilege to work on global health issues, and he has great passion and gratitude for the opportunity to do this work. He also feels driven by the chance to meet with so many committed and talented people working in global health. When asked to point out critical lessons from his own experience for today's students of global health, David offered the following:

- Learn the issues and be open to new approaches; knowledge is power.
- Don't be afraid to make mistakes—there is often more to be learned from failing than from success.
- Be driven by the opportunity to save lives.
- Understand the country/community you are working in and be sensitive to cultural issues.

DAVID HEYMANN

In 2004, U.S. epidemiologist Dr. David Heymann received the American Public Health Association Award for Excellence and was named to the U.S. Institute of Medicine for his contributions to reducing the global burden of infectious diseases. These honors recognized David's important contributions to improving global health.

David always wanted to be a physician, thinking this was the best way he could serve other people. He received his first degree from Pennsylvania State University and then completed medical studies at Wake Forest University.

Just after completing medical studies, David joined the U.S. Public Health Service. As part of this work, David served 1 year on an icebreaker in Antarctica. He served a second year as a family medicine physician in a U.S. Coast Guard Clinic in California. David had taken a rotation during medical school with Project Hope in Tunisia, and, as he considered his professional interests, David decided that the public health work in which he engaged in Tunisia was a better fit for him than clinical medicine.

Thus, after his work with the U.S. Public Health Service, David decided to pursue a public health degree with a specialty in tropical medicine. He had a number of friends who had done such studies at the London School of Hygiene and Tropical Medicine and decided to pursue a 2-year diploma in tropical medicine and hygiene there.

As David was finishing up his program in London, Dr. Donald A. Henderson, who was then the director of the WHO Smallpox Eradication Programme and is widely recognized as a giant in public health, spoke to David's class and requested students to help with smallpox eradication. David traveled that summer to India with Dr. Henderson and then worked as a medical epidemiologist in smallpox eradication for 2 years. As it was for many other prominent actors in public health over the last several decades, David's work with smallpox was an exceptionally formative experience.

David learned many lessons from this program, including the power of public health work and the importance of building country capacity to locally lead and carry out such work.

After completing his work with the Smallpox Eradication Programme, David returned to the United States and joined the Epidemic Intelligence Service of the U.S. Centers for Disease Control and Prevention (CDC). He completed 2 years of practical epidemiology training and during this training traveled to Africa where he worked for the first time on a disease outbreak outside of the United States, which turned out to be the first outbreak of Ebola virus.

David continued to work for the CDC for about 25 years as a medical epidemiologist, mainly on international assignments to Africa and Asia. David's work at the CDC focused on strengthening the surveillance and control of infectious diseases in developing countries, including field research that tested concepts that were just being developed by WHO for the Expanded Programme on Immunization; investigation of outbreaks of hemorrhagic fevers and human monkeypox in West and Central Africa; and applying research to develop methodologies to monitor certain types of antimalarial resistance. During David's work with CDC, he was based in Cameroon, Malawi, and Switzerland. He also spent substantial periods of time in the Democratic Republic of the Congo, Côte d'Ivoire, Burkina Faso, and Thailand.

In 1989, David moved to the World Health Organization (WHO) in Geneva, where he served in a number of key positions. From 1989 to 1995, David was chief of research activities for the WHO Global Programme on AIDS. In October 1995, he became the director of the WHO Programme on Emerging and Other Communicable Diseases. From July 1998 to July 2003, he was the executive director of the WHO Communicable Diseases Cluster. He then became the head of the Polio Eradication Initiative, and WHO's assistant director-general for health security and environment, where he worked on communicable disease issues, food safety, and the health effects of climate change.

While serving at WHO, David was instrumental in strengthening the fight against infectious diseases, establishing the STOP TB partnership and leading the world's efforts to combat the outbreak of SARS in 2002 and 2003. During this period David also authored numerous articles, reports, and chapters within textbooks, making important contributions to global health literature. David especially appreciated the opportunities he had at WHO to help motivate countries effectively address key issues in infectious diseases.

David is currently the chair of the board of Public Health England, head and senior fellow of the Centre for Global Health Security at Chatham House, and a professor at the London School of Hygiene and Tropical Medicine.

When asked what advice he would give to students interested in a career in global health, David offered four key suggestions:

- Get field experience. You need to have an understanding of low-, middle-, and high-income countries to engage in global health work. You must have a deep understanding of these countries if you are to serve their needs effectively.
- Plan your career in 5-year intervals. Look at where you want to be in 5 years and what you need to do to get there. Once you get there, then you can move on to the next steps.
- Keep yourself affiliated, if possible, with an outstanding public health organization, even if you are working on assignment for another organization. This will help provide you with the support you need to carry out your work effectively, such as technical assistance and laboratory services. This will also give you a place to return to after you have finished an overseas experience and an organization in which you can continue to develop your career.
- Always make yourself available to new opportunities. Much of this depends on being in the right place at the right time, but if you remain open and available, you will create opportunities for yourself and develop a network to open doors for further opportunities.

PAUL JENSEN

Paul Jensen is the founder, owner, and sole proprietor of Pivit. This is a consulting firm that assists clients who work in global health in advocacy, strategic communications, and research. Paul serves clients around the world, while operating this firm from Washington, DC, in the United States. He does so in a networked mode. This means that when clients seek Paul's assistance, he assembles a team to work with the client from a variety of other firms and individuals.

Much of Paul's work is with senior executives of organizations involved in global health. Some of Paul's work is to assist clients in advocating for issues of concern to them. An organization, for example, might seek Paul's help in bringing the importance of childhood immunization to the attention of policymakers in selected countries or cities. This might be done through important journals and news media of clear, concise, editorial pieces that are appropriate to the local setting. Other organizations might seek Paul's help in getting out messages about important scientific findings. Many scientific organizations are used to communicating with other science-based organizations but not very experienced at communicating with journalists, the public, or policymakers. One such organization recently asked Paul's firm to help convey to the public and policymakers important findings from scientific research about the optimal timing for treating drug-resistant TB in HIV-positive people. Paul's firm has also been asked to train some global health actors in being more effective communicators.

Paul grew up in the U.S. state of New Jersey. As he approached college age, he had a strong desire to "be of some use to people." At the time, this usually meant a career in medicine, because people Paul's age were not very exposed to the many other ways in which one could try to serve people in need.

Paul entered Franklin and Marshall College, therefore, thinking of a career in medicine and his major field of study was the biological foundations of behavior. After working in a hospital and in a scientific laboratory over summer breaks, however, Paul realized that he was not as interested in medicine as he had thought and not so well suited for it either.

While thinking about what might be next in his academic and professional development, Paul took a course on the public policy aspects of TB control. Paul says that he was transformed by this course. Despite his interests in science and medicine, he found himself shockingly ignorant about TB. In fact, he could not understand how he and others knew so little about one of the most important infectious causes of death in the world.

With this in mind, as well as the desire to make an impact against TB, Paul was fortunate when he finished college to land a job as a trainer on TB with what is now the Global Tuberculosis Institute at Rutgers University. His main task there was to help develop materials for training public health workers about TB control.

As concerns about global health grew, the Bill & Melinda Gates Foundation invested funds in a variety of activities related to TB, including an advocacy effort called ACTION. That effort is based in the NGO RESULTS, which is discussed in the profile of Joanne Carter earlier in this chapter. In 2005, Paul was able to get a position with ACTION.

Paul worked with ACTION from 2005 to 2012. Ultimately he became the deputy director of this program that included 80 staff in 10 countries. During his work with this group, Paul developed advocacy strategies and strategic communications, including talking points, speeches, and op-ed pieces about TB that were intended to influence policymakers and other key stakeholders. He also prepared and managed the preparation of a range of policy reports, fact sheets, and other research

products about TB, that were meant to influence policy and lay the foundation for effective communications about TB. Paul also interacted directly with decision makers about funding and policies for TB. In addition, he helped to develop proposals that would continue to get funding for the ACTION program from the Bill & Melinda Gates Foundation.

Paul enjoyed and appreciated the work he did with ACTION. However, in 2012, Paul decided that at that stage of his career he wanted to be able to work with a broader array of global health topics and with a wider variety of organizations. With these aims in mind, he started his own firm.

Paul offers several lessons from his own experience for those who believe that they want to work in global health:

- Global health work can be inherently fascinating but has unique challenges.
- You do not have to be a scientist or physician to work in global health and to have an impact in the field. There are many opportunities, in many fields to have a substantial impact on global health.
- Learn to write. It is essential that one learns to write with clarity, simplicity, and precision if one wants to have an influence on policymakers.
- You need to appreciate the value of data and the value of learning to analyze it and report clearly on your findings in ways that are packaged to meet the needs of your particular audience.
- Those who are the most successful actors in global health are comfortable with people in many settings, from many walks of life. They can also comfortably work in those settings and put people at ease as they do so.
- If you are interested in global health, you must never forget that the solutions to important global health problems are complex. Even if there is a technological "fix" for a problem, it cannot be put in place unless a range of efforts are aligned. There might be a new and better vaccine for a disease, for example. However, countries have to be able to procure the vaccine at a reasonable price, store it safely, distribute it, ensure that it has the right workers at the right time to make use of it, and then it has to be sure it is properly given to the intended beneficiaries. The new vaccine cannot work unless all of these are in alignment.

GINA LAGOMARSINO

Gina Lagomarsino is cofounder, chief operating officer, and managing director at the Results for Development Institute (R4D) where she focuses on health system design and financing. Gina leads work aimed at expanding health coverage in low- and middle-income countries. She is particularly interested in how to create vibrant health markets that include high-quality, innovative private providers that are accessible to people, regardless of income, through public financing.

At R4D, Gina leads the Center for Health Market Innovations. Gina and her colleagues have collected information on more than 1,000 innovative programs with potential to improve the quality and affordability of care for the poor in 110 countries, and the center is now working to facilitate the scale-up of successful programs. Gina also provides leadership for the Joint Learning Network for Universal Health Coverage, a network of policymakers in low- and middle-income countries who co-develop global knowledge on the practical how-tos of national health insurance reforms.

Gina grew up in Sacramento, California, in the United States. Her parents were teachers and were very public service oriented. Gina was raised thinking that each of us should do what we can to make the world a better place. Gina's mother participated in a program like the U.S. Peace Corps in Mexico, and, as a child, Gina had the opportunity to visit Mexican villages, where she recognized early on that people throughout the world live very different lives.

Gina received a bachelor's degree in public policy from Stanford University. She focused her studies and honor's thesis on international trade policy. Her interest in health began in 1993, when she went to a talk with Alain Enthoven, an eminent economist who helped to craft the Clinton healthcare reform plan in the United States. This talk got Gina thinking about misaligned incentives and overconsumption in health systems. During her junior year at Stanford, Gina had the opportunity to be a summer fellow with U.S. Senator Edward Kennedy while the U.S. Senate was debating the Clinton health reform. Despite her growing involvement in health, however, Gina decided not to pursue work in health policy when she finished her undergraduate degree. The Clinton healthcare reform had been unsuccessful and it did not appear to Gina to be a good time to work on health policy matters.

Instead, Gina sought work on health service delivery and took a job with Kaiser Permanente, a large, private nonprofit integrated healthcare financing and delivery system, in California. Initially, she worked in Kaiser's corporate headquarters on data analysis of consumer surveys, which gave her quantitative skills and taught her about consumer satisfaction in the healthcare industry. Gina later worked in one of Kaiser's large, multispecialty medical centers serving 200,000 members, where she implemented a new model of primary care. The new model was designed to enable doctors, supported by other types of healthcare providers, to manage patients efficiently at a consistently high quality of care. During this time, she learned about many of the challenges associated with healthcare delivery and also learned about what she sees as an encouraging model for healthcare delivery. This work with Kaiser put her on the front lines of healthcare delivery.

Gina went on to get a master's degree in business administration from Harvard, thinking that it would give her good general management skills. She then worked in the healthcare practice of McKinsey & Company, an important consulting firm, where her major clients were U.S. health insurance companies and hospital organizations. This allowed Gina to learn about some of the pitfalls associated with traditional insurance. Her experience at McKinsey furthered her thinking that healthcare delivery and financing should be better integrated.

Gina got married in 1997, and after having her first child in 2003, she was given an unexpected opportunity to work for the mayor of the District of Columbia, Anthony Williams. This gave Gina an opportunity to work on a full range of health policy issues and be deeply involved with the political strategy and operational implementation of the mayor's health priorities. Gina designed and implemented a managed care reform of a public health insurance program serving low-income residents of Washington, DC. She also spearheaded the district's effort to implement the Medical Homes initiative to expand and improve the quality of private community health centers. Gina really appreciated this policy-oriented position, which showed her how policy, financing, and healthcare delivery all came together.

Gina then had her second child, after which she consulted for the Brookings Institution, also in Washington, DC. At the Brookings Institution, she worked on innovative finance for global health, with a focus on malaria. This introduced Gina to the major issues and key players in global health.

Gina had never envisioned herself cofounding a not-for-profit international development organization. However, she eventually found herself in the right place at the right time. While working with David de Ferranti at Brookings, he asked her to help him launch Results for Development (R4D). Gina led R4D's first project, which was funded by the Rockefeller Foundation, on the role of the private sector in health systems in developing countries.

When asked to point out critical lessons from her own experience for today's students of global health, Gina offered the following:

- Gaining experience with different aspects of a healthcare system, such as insurance, service delivery, and pharmaceuticals, as well as the public and private sectors, can give you a unique ability to understand the different components and how they influence each other.

- Developing an understanding of a mature though imperfect health system like that in the United States can offer lessons—about what to do and what not to do—for low- and middle-income countries.

- Within global health, there is a tension between addressing important specific health issues, like HIV/AIDS and child health, and improving overall health systems. It is important to consider how we can integrate these issues. For example, how can national health insurance systems create incentives for doctors to focus on the most cost-effective health interventions?

- With all the recent discussion about "work-life balance" especially for women, it is important to recognize that we can have really interesting and successful careers *and* fulfilling family lives if we choose jobs that we are passionate about and that allow us to have a high degree of ownership of our work and flexibility about how to get it done.

JERKER LILJESTRAND

Jerker Liljestrand is a Swedish obstetrician-gynecologist (OB/GYN) who has been at the forefront of efforts to improve reproductive and maternal and child health in low- and middle-income countries. He is one of a relatively small number of OB/GYNs from high-income countries that have devoted their lives to improving the reproductive health of poor women in poor communities. Jerker's background in both clinical medicine and public health has brought an invaluable perspective to the field of global reproductive health.

Jerker grew up in a family of doctors, which cultivated his interest in health and medicine at a very young age. He attended medical school at Lund University in Sweden and completed residencies in OB/GYN, surgery, and anesthesiology at Västervik Hospital, also in Sweden. During medical school, he became curious about health in low- and middle-income countries and made a concerted effort to meet people working in the global health field.

Jerker worked as a clinical OB/GYN for approximately 20 years. Toward the end of his residency in OB/GYN, he went to Mozambique as a volunteer doctor to train midwives but ended up as head of the Department of OB/GYN at Beira Central Hospital for 2 years. His years in Mozambique were influential—Jerker became curious about why women in labor arrived in the operating room in such bad condition. He started to learn more about the public health issues involved in saving more mothers and newborns.

After Mozambique, Jerker completed his clinical training at Uppsala University. During those years, he also went back and did area-based studies of maternal health in the Mozambican community, exploring the health conditions of pregnant or birthing women at village level. The focus of this work was on the relationship between pregnancy outcomes and risk factors such as anemia, syphilis, nutrition, and socioeconomic conditions. Jerker defended his PhD thesis based on this research in 1985. He thereafter spent 10 years as head of reproductive health for the Blekinge Country Council in Sweden and remained involved with midwifery training. Throughout these experiences, Jerker paid increasing amounts of attention to the social issues that contribute to poor maternal and child health outcomes.

Gradually, Jerker became involved in a variety of other public health activities, including teaching perinatal health in Hanoi, Vietnam; starting an HIV/AIDS campaign in Mozambique; rolling out a sexual education program in a province of Sweden; helping to improve reproductive health in the former Soviet republics; and doing research in Nicaragua.

From 1994 to 1996, Jerker was director of the Blekinge International School of Public Health in Sweden. He then spent 3 years as chief of maternal-newborn health at WHO headquarters in Geneva, Switzerland. From 2000 to 2002, Jerker was the reproductive health advisor at the World Bank, in Washington, DC.

Jerker returned to Sweden, and from 2002 to 2007 helped develop the Department of Community Medicine at Lund University, which focuses on global health. Jerker also began to play a key role in the International Federation of Gynecology and Obstetrics (FIGO). He was treasurer of FIGO from 2003 to 2009 and chair of the FIGO Safe Motherhood Committee from 2003 to 2006. In 2006, he became program manager for an advanced training program in sexual and reproductive health and rights for midwives and OB/GYNs in low-income countries, based at Lund University and sponsored by the Swedish International Development Agency (SIDA).

Jerker's work with the SIDA training program eventually led him to Cambodia, where he now lives and works. From 2009 to 2013, he was team leader for maternal, newborn, and child health with the Better Health Services Project of an organization called URC.

Jerker is most proud of his work training midwives and doctors in low- and middle-income countries. He also considers one of his most meaningful experiences to be the development of WHO's book titled *Managing Complications in Pregnancy and Childbirth*, which he spearheaded.

When asked what advice he would give to university students studying global health, Jerker responded:

- Get a reasonable field experience early in your professional life; don't wait until you are very senior in a high-income country. Go as a volunteer, with an NGO, through the Peace Corps, or something similar. You will learn a lot and will get invaluable experiences and friendships that will carry you through life. Good people are needed in global health, at all ages and from all directions. Getting some solid understanding early on helps you understand key issues from the beginning, and may well influence your life path.
- The world has changed very dramatically in the last 50 years, mostly with very significant improvements in areas such as infant mortality, life expectancy, and poverty reduction. With this in mind, don't despair. If we work well, learning from global mistakes, we can expect more successes ahead. Let us work hard on this; otherwise the world our grandchildren live in will be very different from the world we know today.
- Sexual and reproductive health, in many ways, is a key to development—from gender issues and women's development issues, to helping people achieve their fertility desires, to the excitement of birthing care.
- Get into teaching and you will learn a lot!

ELAINE MURPHY

Elaine Murphy has made major contributions to global health work, especially in areas related to the well-being of women in low- and middle-income countries. Indeed, a paper that Elaine wrote called "Being Born Female Is Dangerous to Your Health," was the inspiration for the women's health chapter of *Global Health 101*. Yet, Elaine's path to working in global health has not been a traditional one, beginning with a liberal arts undergraduate degree, a master's degree in a special program for writers (with a book of poetry as her thesis), and a doctorate in human development. Her career does reflect again, however, that people from many backgrounds can work effectively in global health.

Teaching and learning have inspired Elaine throughout her life. Elaine found that by working with a variety of people and organizations—and through the preparation of research-based briefing papers, articles in peer-reviewed journals, book chapters, academic and training curricula, and presentations at professional meetings—she could help to seize policymakers' and funders' attention and commitment to important areas of public health. Earlier, volunteer work on the environment and population led Elaine to focus attention on global issues, including reproductive health and gender equity. She considered reproductive health and gender equity especially important because global concern about population often seemed to overlook the situation of individual women in low- and middle-income countries and what motivates the attitudes and behavior of such women.

In 1962, Elaine received a bachelor of arts degree from Marquette University with majors in English and French and a minor in education. She then received a master of arts degree in writing from Johns Hopkins University in 1965. Elaine continued her studies at the University of Maryland and received a PhD in human development psychology in 1978.

From 1964 to 1968, Elaine was a high school teacher and counselor in Wisconsin, Minnesota, and Maryland. She then spent a year as a researcher on a project studying learning styles and creativity with the Montgomery County Public Schools in Rockville, Maryland.

Elaine's volunteer work on population and the environment came to the attention of the Population Institute, and she was invited to apply for a fellowship. In 1974, Elaine became a fellow at the Population Institute in Washington, DC, where she developed an interdisciplinary college course on population and reproductive health. Once the University of Maryland agreed to offer the course that Elaine had developed, the Population Institute recommended her to the director of the NGO Zero Population Growth, who was looking for someone to lead a new program that would educate teachers in the United States about population. Beginning in 1975, she led this program for 3 years and then left to become the population education director at the Population Reference Bureau (PRB), a demographic think tank in Washington, DC.

From 1978 to 1983, Elaine was the director of population education at PRB. She organized training workshops and produced training materials on population and the environment for university and high school teachers and students. In addition, she helped initiate PRB's international population education work. Having become an active participant in the population and reproductive health community, Elaine moved to the U.S. Agency for International Development (USAID) where she worked from 1983 to 1985. There, Elaine designed, monitored, and evaluated large-scale family planning communication and training projects for their Office of Population. From 1985 to 1991, Elaine returned to PRB, where she was director of international programs. While at PRB, she directed a project to communicate population and reproductive health research findings to policymakers in low- and middle-income countries.

Elaine then joined the Program for Appropriate Technology in Health (PATH) in Washington, DC and worked on several international programs from 1991 to 2002. She developed and directed the Women's Reproductive Health Initiative (WRHI), a policy project to promote women's reproductive health from a gender and human rights perspective. This program aimed to build a bridge between public health issues and human rights concerns. For example, WRHI highlighted the trafficking of girls and women as a public health issue, not just a human rights violation. At the same time, the project stressed that maternal mortality, although clearly a public health issue, is also a human rights issue.

WRHI disseminated research findings via publications and presentations on the scope of such problems and identified successful programs that address them. WRHI joined other organizations to stress the importance of recognizing and addressing gender inequity, particularly in low- and middle-income countries. This work, along with the efforts of many others, helped to spur action among policymakers and major donors. The landmark 1994 UN Conference on Population and Development was dedicated to these issues for the first time. In addition, continued, concerted advocacy was responsible for the inclusion of women's equality, reproductive health, and maternal mortality issues in the Millennium Development Goals.

From 2002 to 2006, Elaine was a professor of global health and a senior associate in the Center for Global Health at the George Washington University School of Public Health and Health Services.

Elaine is currently a visiting scholar at PRB and a global health consultant. She has done research, writing, and scientific editing for a variety of organizations, including Georgetown University's Institute for Reproductive Health, the Communication for Change Project of the Academy for Educational Development (now FHI 360), the CORE group, and the World Bank Institute's training program in reproductive health. Her work with PRB has included giving seminars, mentoring staff, and writing educational materials about population and reproductive health issues. In addition, she has served as chair of the board of the Willows Foundation, a family planning and reproductive health organization that implements programs in Turkey, Ghana, and Pakistan. She is also a board member of Options for Youth, a holistic teen pregnancy prevention program in Chicago.

When asked what advice she would give university students interested in careers in global health, Elaine offered the following:

- Doing volunteer work in the area of one's concern is not only a good thing to do, but also can be the springboard to an exciting career.

- Of course, just getting the job of your dreams is not enough. One must perform well in the job and bring passion and creativity to it.
- Do not be afraid to "color outside the lines." Having initiative can lead to applying for the funds that will permit your organization to develop expertise in an exciting new area.
- When you rise to a position of leadership within an organization, foster the talent of those whom you supervise. Don't be one of those supervisors who feels threatened by the skills of your staff. Remember the line from the hairdresser Vidal Sassoon: "If you look good, I look good."

POONAM MUTTREJA

Poonam Muttreja is an Indian woman who has been a pioneer in peace promotion, poverty eradication, and women's health efforts in India and elsewhere for many years.

Growing up in New Delhi, India, Poonam was exposed at a young age to poverty, to the disadvantaged position of women in Indian society, and to the discrimination often shown to poor and lower caste people in India. Poonam vividly remembers some of the people with whom she interacted at a young age, whose stories have been an inspiration to her working for social justice ever since. First was the woman who was living on less than $1 a day equivalent, who could not send her children to even a free government school because the cost of transportation, uniforms, and books was more than she could afford. Poonam also remembers the person who cleaned toilets in the homes of middle-class people who was not allowed to touch anything in their homes because the work he did was "unclean" and because he was from the lower castes.

Moved by these experiences, Poonam began to seek ways to help those in need, even as she entered university. She helped, for example, to organize lower caste leather workers into a cooperative, so that they could sell their goods at a better price. She then helped to set up markets in New Delhi so that other poor workers could improve their ability to sell their goods at fair prices. Inspired by Gandhi, Poonam spent much time during this period visiting poor villages in India, always asking if she could stay in the home of the poorest persons, so that she could gain a better understanding of their lives and how she could be helpful to the poor.

Poonam built on her early activities with poor workers and became a social entrepreneur who helped to found, develop, and then pass on a number of nongovernmental organizations of importance. These organizations were oriented toward poverty issues and the development, often through fellowships, of talented people from outside the elite who could become agents of social change and innovation.

From 1979 to 1981, for example, Poonam was the first executive director of the Ashoka Foundation in New Delhi. Poonam cofounded Dastkar—Delhi in 1981, a nonprofit organization that promotes economic opportunities for craftspeople. She then served 2 years as its executive director. In 1983, Poonam founded the Society for Rural, Urban, and Tribal Initiative (SRUTI) in New Delhi. This nonprofit organization provides fellowships to less-known social activists in India. As founding director, she established the office and implemented a fellowship program. In 1984, Poonam was the founding secretary of Nagarik Ekta Manch (Citizen's Unity Forum) in New Delhi. This was established after the 1984 communal riots in Delhi following the assassination of Prime Minister Indira Gandhi. The organization was instrumental in promoting peace and mobilizing volunteers for relief and rehabilitation activities.

In 1986, Poonam moved to the United States with her husband who was to attend graduate school there. From 1986 to 1991, Poonam was the program director for the Coolidge Center for Environmental Leadership in Massachusetts. In that role, Poonam developed training programs on the environment, poverty, and gender for midcareer professionals from low- and middle-income countries. From 1987 to 1988, Poonam was a chairperson for the Harvard–MIT Women in Development Group. In this capacity, Poonam organized programs and seminars on gender issues in low- and middle-income countries. In 1991, Poonam received a master's degree in public administration from Harvard University's Kennedy School of Government.

While still in the United States, Poonam was also invited to teach at two American colleges. She served first as a visiting professor and Packard Fellow in the Peace and Global Studies Program at Earlham College in the state of Indiana. There, she taught a course on international development and offered a faculty seminar series on poverty in low- and middle-income countries. In the spring of 1992, Poonam taught a course on social action, international development, and poverty alleviation at Hampshire College in the state of Massachusetts.

Poonam returned to India in 1993 and for a year she was an advisor to the country representative of the United Nations Development Program in India. Poonam then served 15 years as the country director for the MacArthur Foundation. In 1994, she established the India office for the foundation, which develops and oversees the foundation's grants for programs related to population and reproductive health in India.

Poonam is most proud of the work she did while at the MacArthur Foundation to help build a group of civil society leaders in women's reproductive health who were drawn from outside the establishment. She is also pleased that her work has contributed to moving many Indian stakeholders to a broader and more rights-based approach to reproductive health than would otherwise be the case.

In 2010, Poonam joined the Population Foundation of India (PFI) as its executive director. PFI is a national-level NGO at the forefront of policy, advocacy, and research on population, health, and development issues in the country. As always, Poonam was a catalyst for change. After many passionate conversations with experts and team members, Poonam zeroed in on using popular communication media to change attitudes and behavior by providing positive messages to viewers on women's rights and health. In March 2014, PFI launched a multimedia entertainment education serial (national TV and radio, Internet, mobile phone, outreach) titled Main Kuch Bhi Kar Sakti Hoon—I, a woman, can achieve anything.

Poonam offers a number of lessons for those who would like to work in health and development:

- Get a sense of people's real needs. Get a sense, as well, of what really works and does not work in addressing those needs.
- Guide your decisions on the basis of the life of the poor. Close your eyes and think constantly about how the problem you are trying to address really looks to the poor.
- You have to work at every level, all the time, to address the issues of poverty and ill health. You have to do this in coalition with partners, to whom you must be open. Collective action is better than individual action.
- You must be able to learn from others at all times. You need to doubt the wisdom of your work and test it against people more knowledgeable than you. You also need to learn from failures. Keep an open mind, open eyes, and an open heart at all times.

RACHEL NUGENT

Rachel Nugent is a research associate professor in the Department of Global Health at the University of Washington and the director of the Disease Control Priorities Network Project. Previously, Rachel was the deputy director of global health for the Center for Global Development in Washington, DC. Rachel's research focuses on nutrition-related noncommunicable diseases in low- and middle-income countries and the links between population health and development.

Rachel grew up in the small college town of Bloomington, Indiana. She frequently traveled internationally with her family and learned French and Spanish. These experiences would lead Rachel to pursue international issues in the future. She attended the University of Wisconsin in Madison for her first degree. Rachel was interested in news and current events and loved writing, so she initially decided to major in journalism. However, in college, Rachel took a required economics course, which she unexpectedly loved and she ended up graduating with a BA degree in both economics and journalism.

Economics was a timely issue when Rachel left college, as the United States was in an economic slump. She decided to keep pursuing the discipline, so after 2 years of working in policy development for the state legislature in Indiana, Rachel went on to receive her PhD in economics at The George Washington University in Washington, DC. She combined her interests in current events, practical economics, and international travel into a focus on international policy. Rachel has continued to work in the international realm throughout her career.

Rachel's career path has been characterized by unplanned opportunities. During studies for her PhD, Rachel spontaneously took a job at a think tank called Resources for the Future. She worked as a research analyst in trade and agriculture. Rachel admired the strength of the organization and she thought that she would learn a lot from the experience. Although Rachel did not foresee the significance of this job in her overall career, her experience at Resources for the Future has been a major influence in her life. While in this position, Rachel met a person who would become an important professional mentor and later would hire her for a position at the United Nations. This experience also fed into Rachel's later interest in how agriculture plays a role in health and nutrition. In fact, the topics of international policy issues, economics, and agriculture continued to influence the diverse array of jobs Rachel pursued next and that still contribute to her career today. Her career path, not including her two most recent jobs, includes jobs within the United Nations Food and Agriculture Organization, the Fogarty International Center at the U.S. National Institutes of Health, and the Population Reference Bureau (PRB).

Rachel has worked in all levels of government, from the local to the United Nations, and in both the private and public sectors. She has also been a professor at the Pacific Lutheran University and The George Washington University. She has served on many health, economics, and agriculture advisory and peer review boards and has published numerous reports, articles, and book chapters. Although she has not had an overall plan for her career, Rachel bases her decisions

for the next steps on her main interests. She enjoys change and is always open to new opportunities in which she can make an impact and continue to learn.

What has stayed consistent in her career is Rachel's desire to work on underdog—neglected or unprioritized—issues. In her job at the Center for Global Development, for example, she focused on chronic diseases in low- and middle-income countries and drug resistance. With her present research, Rachel tries to change preconceptions of nutrition and disease in these countries and advocates for an increased understanding of the double burden of undernutrition and obesity. In her current job as director of the Disease Control Priorities Network Project, Rachel finds ways to build capacity in low-income countries to carry out economic evaluation of health activities.

When asked what advice she would give to university students studying global health, Rachel responded:

- Do not be afraid to do things people have not done if they interest you. It is exciting to be on the forefront of rising issues.
- Know where the money is. This sounds contradictory to the first lesson, as people might not have pursued something before because there was no money in it. However, gaining an understanding of funders will make it easier to align your proposals to something in which they would be interested. The sooner you figure this out, the sooner you can influence the funders and put your underdog issues on their agenda.
- There is often a way to do what you want to do even if it is not obvious at first. Try to keep a broad perspective on how things can be connected. For example, there are many different ways to approach work on noncommunicable diseases—nutrition, agriculture, physical activity, to name a few. Think broadly about what areas affect the issue you are interested in and explore opportunities within them.
- Don't worry if the path is not obvious. Sometimes the unplanned path can lead you to exciting opportunities you were unaware of at first. If you have a broad range of interests, try to explore as many as you can in the beginning of your career.

ELLYN OGDEN

In January 2009, Ellyn Ogden was presented with the Heroism Award of the U.S. Agency for International Development (USAID) for her tireless efforts, sometimes in areas of conflict, to help eradicate polio. This important work in global health was the natural outgrowth of experiences Ellyn had at earlier stages of her life and valuable lessons she had learned over almost 30 years of international development efforts.

As a young woman, growing up in the United States, Ellyn developed a strong interest in doing something to make the world a better place for the poor. Initially, Ellyn thought she should become a doctor. Thanks to a secondary school teacher who told her about the Peace Corps, Ellyn aimed initially to become a Peace Corps doctor who would provide medical care to the poor in low-income countries. Ellyn smiles today when talking about this, because at the time she had only limited knowledge of the Peace Corps, of different kinds of public health work, and of international health problems.

During her first 2 years in university, Ellyn's interest in public health grew and she transferred to Tulane University in order to take advantage of its well-known programs in international affairs and public health. Her studies at Tulane further strengthened Ellyn's desire to make a career in public health and to study for an advanced degree in public health, which she completed at Tulane in 1984.

Ellyn also gained valuable experience working in the United States while a student in various hospital roles such as nursing assistant, laboratory phlebotomist, cardiac care aide, and clinical research assistant. Following interests she had entertained since childhood, Ellyn did join the Peace Corps and from 1987–1988 she served as an infectious disease control officer in Papua New Guinea. This was her first international work experience. Ellyn worked in Kavieng, the capitol of the island province of New Ireland, with a population of 80,000 people and very limited medical services. Papua New Guinea was very poor at the time, and Ellyn focused her public health efforts on TB, malaria, leprosy, and sexually transmitted diseases. She paid special attention in her work to women, who were often neglected by public health and medical programs.

Following her stay in Papua New Guinea, Ellyn worked with companies in Washington, DC, that helped to implement health projects financed by USAID. In one of these positions, Ellyn led an evaluation of the child survival activities that had been financed by USAID during a period when this was the focus of important international efforts. Ellyn learned a great deal from this experience about the importance of evaluation, the need for it to be independent, and the value of using the knowledge gained in evaluation to enhance the quality of the programs being reviewed.

Ellyn moved to USAID in 1993, first serving as a child survival fellow for the Latin America and the Caribbean Region and from 1997 to the present, heading up USAID's work on polio eradication. Despite the setbacks in the world's efforts to eradicate polio by 2000, Ellyn remains committed to trying to achieve eradication in the shortest possible time. In her work on polio, Ellyn has helped to negotiate "days of tranquility" in the Eastern Democratic Republic of Congo (DRC), so that warring factions would stop fighting and allow children to be immunized. In Nigeria, Ellyn worked with local leaders to help overcome fears they had of the polio vaccine, which had led to many children not being immunized. With others, she has worked very hard to help India, Afghanistan, and Pakistan immunize all of their children so that polio transmission could be stopped there, as well.

When asked to point out critical lessons from her own experience for today's students of global health, Ellyn offered the following:

- Work on the basis of evidence and be courageous in using evidence to help do things in better ways. Do not accept things as they are if they are not working well. Be gracious to everyone, but don't be afraid to use your evidence to prove people wrong and to highlight more effective and efficient ways of achieving key goals.
- Develop a broad perspective and an ability to work across disciplines. You never know what skills you will need in the future.
- Develop an ability to "flash forward." Imagine how issues will develop in the future and how they might be addressed in that light. Related to this, learn to "envision failure" and what can be done to avoid failure of your efforts over time.
- Understand how business gets done in different places. One cannot succeed in global health without a deep understanding of the cultural context within which you are working.
- Know your audience. It is imperative to know what motivates people in different places, to see how the world looks through their eyes, and to be able to communicate with them in terms they understand.
- Create and seize opportunities to advance your mission. Be alert to the possibilities for positive change.

DAN AND LINDSAY PALAZUELOS

Dan and Lindsay Palazuelos are a married couple who have devoted their lives to improving the health and well-being of marginalized groups in both the United States and Latin America. Dan is a physician who splits his time between clinical medicine, teaching, and education at Harvard Medical

School and global health work with the NGO Partners in Health (PIH) in Mexico. Lindsay is a development specialist, also working with PIH in Mexico.

Dan and Lindsay aspire to listen carefully to the people with whom they work, collaborate closely with others, and show compassion at all times. They recognize the importance, both to their personal and professional aims, of their relationships with the communities with which they are engaged. For this reason, they spend 6 months of each year in Mexico and 6 months in the United States. After years of working with a variety of NGOs in Mexico, they came together with another Mexican doctor (Hugo Flores) to cofound PIH-Mexico, or Compañeros en Salud-México. The organization works to build a model of excellence for primary care in rural Mexico by strengthening the government health system.

Dan and Lindsay work as a husband–wife team in the field of global health equity. Their personal relationship comes first, but they simultaneously support and inspire one another professionally. This may involve helping each other set the strategy for the work in Mexico one day and the next day reflecting together on the range of emotions that are part of working in poor communities.

Dan did not always plan to study medicine. He initially thought he would be a filmmaker, poet, photographer, or other type of "starving artist," as he puts it. In 1999, he received a BA in English and American literature from Brown University as a part of their program in Liberal Medical Education. This program allowed Dan to study the humanities, while guaranteeing him a spot in Brown Medical School, contingent on his maintaining a certain grade point average and meeting certain science requirements. During this time, Dan spent a year at Oxford University in England studying English poetry. In the end, he believes that studying the humanities led him to a career in medicine and taught him invaluable skills such as patience, flexibility, humor, and humility in the face of the profound suffering that so many people experience.

Dan continued his studies at Brown University Medical School and received his MD in 2004. He completed his residency in internal medicine at the Brigham and Women's Hospital (BWH) in Boston, Massachusetts, with a focus on health care for the poor and marginalized. In 2009, he received an MPH with a concentration in clinical effectiveness at the Harvard School of Public Health.

Between his third and fourth years of medical school, Dan spent a year doing independent research in Mexico. Throughout the year, much of which he spent in public hospitals, he interviewed patients on their views of health, dying, and end-of-life care. This experience opened his eyes to pervasive inequity, as well as the complex relationship among race, class, and inequality in health care.

As is often the case with other global health professionals, Dan currently holds a wide variety of positions in addition to his work in Mexico. He is a quarter-time hospitalist physician at BWH and the assistant director of the Howard Hiatt Global Health Equity Residency. At Harvard Medical School, he is the Cannon Society Global Health Fellow and often leads a tutorial section in the mandatory first-year course in global health and social medicine. Increasingly, he is collaborating with a variety of NGOs around the world to study and support best practices in the manner in which community health workers operate. All this work complements his role as chief strategist in Mexico because, as he would say it, "global health is a new field, so we are still constructing what it will be. At this stage, we all need to be the entrepreneurs that will lay down the foundations that others will build upon in the future. There are so many reasons why a career in global health is impossible, but yet indispensable. We may have only this one chance to bridge this gap right."

Lindsay's interest in global health and development began in high school after reading about the parasitic infection schistosomiasis. She was appalled by the enormous number of people it affected, especially considering that she had never heard of the disease. This global inequity mirrored the inequity she saw in her own high school in Austin, Texas, a "magnet" that attracted academic high achievers from around the city to one of the area's poorest neighborhoods. In the high school, specialized coursework coexisted with the state's highest rate of teenage pregnancy. Just as her classmates' reality was marginalized, she was amazed to find that areas beyond Europe and the United States were not covered in her own education. From this point on, Lindsay was drawn to international issues and pursued a variety of internships and volunteer experiences with community-based organizations that aimed at addressing such issues. In 2005, Lindsay received a BA in international development from Brown University. During her studies, Lindsay spent time in rural Ecuador working with a municipal government on community development. Working closely with her supervisor, an agronomist, she worked to create a beekeeping program in collaboration with an association of indigenous communities and found this to be a formative experience.

After graduating, Lindsay worked with a community-based AIDS prevention organization and volunteered with PIH in Boston. There, she learned more about public health concepts such as harm reduction and how to target groups that face stigma. Her volunteer work with PIH expanded, and she took on a position as project coordinator, later progressing to Mexico program officer where her job is to put into practice the strategies set by the program leadership team. Lindsay's role began by working with community health workers to improve access to primary care in marginalized villages. She went on to develop new programs in Guatemala and to cofound CES in Mexico, establishing key programmatic, human resources, and financial frameworks. Today, with an ever-increasing number of talented Mexican physicians and staff at CES, she focuses on helping CES obtain resources and gain greater influence within the Mexican healthcare system.

Dan has several suggestions for those interested in a career in global health:

- Learn from each patient and let them teach you their context. Understanding the social context that they live in and the experiences that helped shape their worldview will allow you to best meet people's needs.
- Remember that you are always only a small part of the larger solution. Progress depends on a wide range of factors and a variety of different actors.
- Always keep reading, listening, learning, and being provoked by a variety of sources. You can do this with diverse media ranging from *This American Life*, a radio show in the United States, to the *New England Journal of Medicine*, one of the elite medical journals. To do more, you must always think more.
- Remember that people must always be at the center of what you are doing. Big ideals, such as justice and equity, always guide us, but the world is much more complex than any single philosophy can fully capture. "Many people, for love of a concept, make terrible decisions that may end up hurting many others."
- When Woody Allen said "80 percent of success is showing up," he might have been talking about global health. You may not get rich or famous from this work, but if you can structure your life to allow for travel and some measured sacrifice, you will quickly find yourself a global health path.

Lindsay also has several suggestions for students interested in global health and development:

- Assume that you do not know the answers. When working in a new context, you will encounter many things that you do not understand. It will be tempting to ascribe your own explanations to them. Instead, talk to people and ask open-ended questions, read widely, and learn the history of the area, so that you may begin to understand what you are seeing.

- You must earn people's trust. The poor may expect powerful people and institutions to make their lives harder. For example, police may harass rather than protect them. You must not only aspire to be different, but follow through in your actions. Always keep your word, despite how challenging it may be.
- Work to make your role dispensable. Low- and middle-income countries are full of optimistic, energetic, and talented people just like you. Use your skills, perspective, and connections to help them gain greater voice, power, and responsibility at all levels.
- Think in terms of decades. Progress takes time and perseverance. If immediate solutions existed, they would have already been put in place. Meaningful change results from incremental and creative collaborative efforts.

KRISTIN PARCO

Kristin Parco is the program manager of the Migration Health Unit of the International Organization of Migration (IOM) in Port Au Prince, Haiti. IOM focuses on migration and response to emergencies, and Kristin manages IOM's health projects. Her most recent projects include cholera elimination; the health of internally displaced persons, including HIV, sexually transmitted infections (STIs), and TB case detection along with mental health; and emergency response to disasters. She works closely with the Haitian government, UN agencies, and NGOs. Kristin is also working with the other health units of IOM, including the WASH (Water, Sanitation, and Hygiene) team, on strategies to fully integrate IOM's emergency response to cholera into the Haitian health system and build the capacity of the national health staff to treat and manage cholera.

Kristin grew up in the Philippines. She developed an interest in health at an early age and had three main experiences that helped her find her career niche. First, when Kristin was young, her parents worked in a camp for Vietnamese, Cambodian, and Laotian refugees. Kristin spent every summer, until she was 18 years old, helping her parents at the camp. She interacted with young refugees in the youth center that her father managed in the refugee camp and shadowed the doctors and nurses in the camp. Second, when Kristin was 12, she was at the hospital when her mother gave birth to Kristin's youngest brother. Her mother suffered from a postpartum hemorrhage, and Kristin was scared she would lose her. Fortunately, her mother survived, and Kristin took care of her during her recovery at home. This experience inspired Kristin to work in hospitals and in women's health. Third, Kristin's grandfather was a medical assistant in World

War II and Kristin's interest in health grew as she listened to the stories of her grandfather and his friends who were also medical professionals.

These experiences inspired Kristin to get a nursing degree from the Aquinas University College of Nursing in the Philippines. After her studies, her first job was as a registered nurse in a maternity ward. She then went to Cambodia to work as a community health trainer for a Save the Children program. She developed training programs and trained Village Health Volunteers. This experience opened more doors for Kristin as she developed skills in managing health programs. She continued to work in Cambodia for MOVI-MONDO, an Italian NGO, and she supervised the implementation of training programs for maternal and child health.

Kristin believes that the drive to never stop learning is important for a career in global health. Although she did not have much experience with TB, she decided to apply for a position as a TB program nurse for IOM in Phnom Penh, the capital of Cambodia. She got the job, and although she was a nurse, Kristin wanted to explore the area of coordinating the different clinical activities. She took on additional responsibilities and tasks for no extra pay. Within a year, she was promoted to health coordinator and medical administrator for IOM, and she organized and implemented all of IOM's activities for refugees and migrants.

After Cambodia, Kristin worked for IOM in Indonesia, acting as the health coordinator for IOM's medical evacuation program in response to the tsunami (2004) and earthquake (2005) in Nias, Indonesia. She continued to work in program management in Indonesia for 5 more years, with a stint in between as an emergency response medical coordinator in typhoon-affected areas of the Philippines. In 2010, she moved to Haiti and began to work on IOM projects, such as implementing health education programs for internally displaced populations, developing health operations, and training health workers in TB, HIV, maternal and child health, STIs, and cholera prevention. She was then promoted to her current position, in which she seeks to build the capacity of the national staff, develop a strong linkage between the local population and health providers, and create long-term impact from her programs with the Ministry of Health.

Kristin enjoys international work because she believes there is much to learn in each country. She takes what she learns in each country to the next country she works in and hopes to one day use the lessons she has gathered to improve health in her home country, the Philippines. She never thinks of her work as dull and is happy she has had the opportunity to develop her career with IOM, as the organization evolved from only aiding in migration to addressing emergencies and a broader array of health and social issues.

The main challenges that Kristin comes across in her work are communities' natural resistance to change; the diminishment of donor interest, funds, and resources that occurs after the first 2 years following an emergency; and the weak capacity of some healthcare providers. Kristin also notes the stress due to deadlines and the demands of many different stakeholders. To address the two latter challenges, she suggests strongly advocating for the needs of the community and leading a healthy life with a strong support system and constant communication with family and friends.

Kristin receives personal satisfaction from working within local communities and seeing the progress of the national health staff. The training programs help the workers become more independent and more confident about their ability to help the Haitian government. Positive feedback from beneficiaries continues to provide her with the joy and inspiration to continue her work.

When asked what advice she would give to university students studying global health, Kristin offered the following lessons:

- Go for global health! There is a huge need for more people to work in global health.
- When implementing projects in specific countries, it is important to focus on health equity, evidence-based decisions, and long-term impact in ways that meet the needs of the local population.
- Community-based programs for health are important. It is critical to focus on the root level of health issues. Understanding the primary needs of the community is integral to sustaining the effectiveness of programs and ensuring long-term impact. Successful community-based programs allow communities' voices to be heard at the national level and their success encourages the national government to implement the program in other regions.
- Reinforce the capacity of existing resources and structures. Work to strengthen and build it, not change it.
- Do not be too idealistic. Change takes time.
- Nurses can, and should, work in global health. All types of medical professionals should be encouraged to pursue global health. If you are such a person, you need a strong commitment and dedication to global health. In addition, experience working in a clinical setting will increase your impact on some types of global health work.

DAVID PETERS

David Peters is a professor at the Johns Hopkins University Bloomberg School of Public Health and also the chair of the Department of International Health. David has devoted all of his professional life to service to the poor and disadvantaged.

David is a Canadian. He was born in Winnipeg, Manitoba, and he did his primary and secondary schooling in Winnipeg as well. David's parents had a strong commitment to social justice, were concerned for the poor globally, and were involved in the work of the Mennonite Central Committee (MCC). Their church supported development projects in poor countries, and David and his family knew people affiliated with the church who worked on these projects. From a young age, David saw the overseas development work that MCC was carrying out as a model for work he should do in public health and development.

With this in mind, David sought to engage in medical studies in Canada and then public health studies overseas because Canada did not have a public health school at the time. David studied chemistry and religious studies in college, receiving a bachelor of science degree from the University of Manitoba in Winnipeg, where he also went to medical school. He spent half a year in medical school in Nepal and remote parts of Canada. David received his MD in 1986. David then did a 1-year medical internship at McGill University in Montreal, Quebec that exposed him to a number of different medical fields.

In 1987 and 1988, David pursued a variety of clinical experiences as a physician in Canada, including work on The Pas, Grand Rapids, and Moose Lake Indian Reserves, and at a nursing home that was also on an Indian reservation. Looking back at those years, David says the experience was inspiring in some regards but humbling in others. On the one hand, David worked with people he considers heroes who devoted themselves to trying to enhance the health of native people. On the other hand, he realized that even good clinical care could not help people overcome the many social problems from which they suffered and that often were at the base of their medical problems, such as poor diets, alcoholism, substance abuse, and domestic violence. In addition, he found it difficult to overcome generations of institutionalized prejudice and poorly performing social programs. Most important, David says he learned that real change will come in the long run only when people are empowered to take charge of their own destinies.

After his work in Canada, and with a constant eye on a career in public health, David carried out a residency in general preventive medicine at the Johns Hopkins University School of Public Health (JHSPH) in Baltimore, Maryland, in the United States between 1988 and 1991. David was especially interested in doing a residency and graduate work in public health at either Johns Hopkins or the London School of Hygiene and Tropical Medicine because these were the premiere places at the time for work on health and development.

While completing his residency, David continued his studies at the JHSPH, receiving a master of public health degree in 1989 and a doctor of public health degree in 1993. David's research for his doctoral dissertation focused on trying to understand how Sri Lankan children could have such high rates of survival when they suffered from relatively high rates of being born underweight. David found answers to this question in the high level of female education in Sri Lanka, the focus of the health system on safe birthing practices, and the emphasis the health system placed on the care of newborns. Related to these and good breastfeeding practices, Sri Lankan children who were born underweight often had catch-up growth that kept them on the path to proper child development.

When David finished his studies, he joined the World Bank and served as a senior public health specialist for the Africa and South Asia Regions from 1993 to 2001. He carried out this work from postings in Washington, DC and New Delhi, India. During this time, he was also an associate in the Department of International Health at the JHSPH and joined as a full-time faculty member in 2002.

From 2006 to 2008, David served as the senior public health specialist for the Human Development Network at the World Bank. In this position, David managed the bank's efforts at assisting low- and middle-income countries in strengthening their capacity for health system reform and management, in an attempt to improve the delivery of health services and health outcomes, especially for the poor. During these years, David split his time between the Johns Hopkins University School of Public Health and the World Bank.

David left the World Bank in 2008 for JHSPH. As the chair of the Department of International Health, David oversees faculty, staff, and students involved in teaching, research, and service in health development in low- and middle-income countries. His own research focuses on ways to make health systems work for the poor, such as providing financial protection, engaging the poor in policy processes, and developing new ways to deliver and regulate health care.

David has found most gratifying the efforts he undertook in a postconflict situation in Sierra Leone to help the country rebuild its health system. He is also pleased with the activities he carried out to help Ghana create a sectorwide approach to health. This included bringing together in a coherent manner the many development partners with which Ghana had been working in fragmented ways that were often at cross-purposes. For the last 10 years in Afghanistan, David led a team that developed the first national balanced scorecard of health services, which annually produced an assessment of performance of health services, focusing on quality and equity of care. David is very excited by the work he is now doing with the Future Health Systems Consortium, which is an unusual multidisciplinary effort across a number of universities to reduce poverty through innovative health and livelihood activities, such as working with informal health providers in Bangladesh, providing health insurance for the poor in China, and testing innovations in health services in Afghanistan, Uganda, and India.

David has also found work in health and development to be challenging. Some of the most important challenges he has faced include the difficulty of ensuring that effective technical interventions can be implemented successfully and in a sustained way in low-income countries. He has also found challenging the "relentless attention that one has to pay to keeping people moving in the same direction," because many institutions do not take a sufficiently long-term view of their work.

David offers the following advice for university students interested in careers in global health:

- Be humble and keep learning. There is always more to learn.
- Take every chance you can find to create positive outcomes for the poor. There is always a chance to innovate, even under the most difficult circumstances, such as in fragile states or states that are emerging from conflict.
- Keep your goals in mind at all times. Think systematically about how vulnerable people experience life and how their lives can be changed for the better. Do not look so much at the way things have always been done, or to rely on formal organizations. Rather, look increasingly to neglected, new, or different ways in which you might be able to encourage the achievement of better health for the poor.

LISA RUSSELL

Lisa Russell is an Emmy Award–winning documentary filmmaker and new media specialist. New media refers to art made with new media technologies usually distributed by use of computers, like computer animation and graphics, digital art, and video games. Her background in humanitarian and international development work has inspired her to produce films about the health and well-being of our global society. She is also a teaching artist for Urban Word NYC, a free after-school program for young writers and poets in New York.

Lisa grew up in a low-resource family in California. She attended the University of California, Santa Barbara, where she majored in cultural anthropology and premedical studies. Lisa thought she wanted to go to medical school to become an emergency room doctor, but halfway through the application process, she decided to take a year off to figure out her plans. Lisa drove across the country to live in Boston, Massachusetts for what she thought would be 1 year.

While she was in Boston, Lisa provided HIV/AIDS education at homeless shelters and took an adult education class on HIV/AIDS at the Harvard School of Public Health. During class one day, her professor showed a short film about the life of the late Jonathan Mann, a leader in the early fight against the HIV/AIDS epidemic. In the film, Jonathan Mann discussed health as a human rights issue and the importance of addressing the social determinants of health, such as gender, ethnicity, and poverty. Something clicked inside Lisa as she watched this film. Jonathan Mann's discussion was a language about health that she had not come across before, but she knew she wanted to pursue the concerns that he spoke about. Lisa immediately looked into master's of public health programs and ended up getting her master's degree (MPH) at Boston University's School of Public Health.

After receiving her MPH, Lisa worked for 2 years in Kosovo and Albania during the Kosovo War. While there, Lisa met women who felt that journalists who came to report on the war were insensitive to their plight and inaccurately represented them. Lisa learned the importance of media representation of social and health issues in low- and middle-income countries, and saw how she could make a difference. She started to help friends with film shoots and fell in love with the art of filmmaking.

Although Lisa is a filmmaker, she never went to film school. Instead, Lisa spent 3 years teaching herself all about cameras, software, and storytelling. She began to make films about maternal health issues in 2005 and focused on obstetric fistula. At the time, not many people knew about women in low- and middle-income countries suffering from obstetric fistula, so she was inspired to put a face on the issue. Lisa still chooses to address issues that are not well known, but should be. She has since collaborated with organizations such as the United Nations Population Fund and produced films in a wide variety of international locations. Her short films, *Love, Labor, Loss*; *Not Yet Rain*; *Youth Zones*; and *In It to Save Lives* have been widely distributed as advocacy tools for students and activists, and she has worked with other leading UN agencies and nongovernmental organizations on various films and creative projects.

Lisa constantly struggles with the ethical issues of a Western filmmaker traveling to low- and middle-income countries and trying to accurately portray other people's stories. As a filmmaker who aims to make socially conscious films that advance positive social change and bring to light issues in the low-income world, she wants to retain the dignity of the people she films and not just focus on their suffering and challenges. Lisa wants to make sure that we see the positive stories as well. In some of her recent work, such as her film *!PODER!*, she emphasizes the power and potential of women and girls, rather than reinforcing the narrative of them as powerless victims. Lisa also acknowledges that she may not always be the most appropriate person to tell a story, so she welcomes other artists from around the world into the creative process. When Lisa travels to another country, she takes time to listen to the intellectuals, artists, and activists who represent the cultures she films. She has realized the strong influence local artists have on their community and that they understand the issues from a cultural context she will never fully understand. Her new media site, mdgfive. tumblr.com/, which she cofounded with Grammy-winning artist Maya Azucena, is a platform that unites artists and activists for maternal health. Visitors to the site are able to remix art from around the world (for example, combining a poem written by a South African, a song from Thailand, and photos taken in Los Angeles) to make their own public service announcement on maternal health.

Lisa believes that there is an important role for artists in global health advocacy. Artists have the power to take intimate situations and tragedies and relate them into universal stories and emotions that everyone can relate to. These stories make the facts and figures of reports and conferences more emotionally moving. Because of the power of artistry and the incredible talent of so many people, Lisa also works on parallel conversations, the growing relationship between artists and the humanitarian communities. She is in the process of launching a new initiative, "I Sell the Shadow," that focuses on artist development and institutional consultations to create more meaningful partnerships between creative professionals and the community of those involved in health and human rights.

Although Lisa comes across many challenges in her work, including financing her projects and the significant amount of time and energy each project requires from her, she loves what she does. She feels rewarded every day knowing that the work she does benefits other people and helps to make the world a better place. She enjoys the many opportunities she has to meet inspiring people around the world and then tell their stories to educate and inspire other people. In addition to filmmaking, Lisa is also a special contributing writer for the Huffington Post "Global Motherhood" platform where she writes on the role of artists in advocacy on issues affecting women and girls. She is also a regular contributor at high-level UN meetings and various global health conferences, and she is a nationally known keynote speaker and presenter at leading universities, youth conferences, and other gatherings.

When asked what advice she would give to university students studying global health, Lisa offered:

- Do what you love. If you do not know what that is yet, don't stress out. Take time off, travel, and get to know yourself. Figure out what you really want to do with your career. You are going to spend a majority of your life working, so you should really love what you do.

- It is wonderful if you want to spend your life working to help other people. However, as outsiders coming into marginalized communities, we must understand our privilege and the responsibility of representing stories accurately. You must understand how your country plays into global problems. You should also be knowledgeable about how aid works, what trade laws are, and why poverty exists. Unfortunately it is not just about raising money and helping the poor; we need to comprehend the political and social forces that keep part of the world in poverty.

JENNIFER STAPLE-CLARK

Jennifer Staple-Clark is the founder and CEO of Unite for Sight, a nonprofit organization that supports eye clinics in Ghana, India, Honduras, the United States, and Canada to improve eye health and eliminate preventable blindness. Due to Jennifer's leadership and focus on entrepreneurial innovation, Unite for Sight is a leader in providing cost-effective eye care to the world's poorest people. Unite for Sight has also become a major actor in education for global health, running online training programs and hosting an annual Global Health and Innovation Conference.

Jennifer grew up in Connecticut. She attended Yale University in New Haven, Connecticut, for her undergraduate education. Jennifer always had an interest in medicine and science, so she planned to major in biology. During her sophomore year, Jennifer took an anthropology class. She loved the class and decided to continue studying anthropology. She felt the small and intimate anthropology classes were a good complement to her biology studies, and she enjoyed learning about the sociocultural aspects of populations and the impact of science on culture. She graduated from Yale University in 2003, with a bachelor of science degree in both biology and anthropology.

During the summer after her first year of college, Jennifer worked as a clinical research assistant in her optometrist's office. She learned that many people do not routinely go to an eye doctor and visit only when their vision has significantly deteriorated. She also realized that many people do not have health insurance and therefore forgo preventative care. Jennifer heard many stories from patients with glaucoma, which, if found too late or left untreated, can cause irreversible blindness. This experience inspired Jennifer to improve eye health in New Haven, and she founded Unite for Sight when she was a second-year college student.

Unite for Sight started as an organization of student volunteers that went to meeting places for disadvantaged people to educate the New Haven community about existing, nationally available healthcare coverage programs, including eye care. Jennifer's two main goals were to educate people about eye disease and assist low-income and homeless patients to obtain affordable eye care. Given the success of the student organization, Jennifer quickly expanded her model of eye care in underserved communities to more than 50 universities across the United States and Canada. Jennifer started to receive inquiries from around the world from people who heard of Unite for Sight from the Internet or word of mouth. One such inquiry came from a refugee camp in Ghana that desperately needed eye care for its inhabitants. This contact became the first overseas partner for Unite for Sight and the organization began to assist in delivering eye care to the camp.

As the CEO for Unite for Sight, Jennifer seeks to improve healthcare delivery programs and offer educational opportunities for people interested in global health. Jennifer has created partnerships with local ophthalmologists in Ghana, India, and Honduras to coordinate outreach to rural communities for patients who are unable to access or afford eye care. Unite for Sight supports local eye care professionals in serving the communities' poorest people by providing necessary human and financial resources. Unite for Sight has helped to provide eye care to more than 1.7 million people living in extreme poverty, including more than 65,000 sight-restoring surgeries. Since the first contact from Ghana, Unite for Sight has partnered with five Ghanaian ophthalmologists who perform half of all cataract surgeries in Ghana.

In addition, Unite for Sight recruits volunteers, has a Global Health University, and hosts an annual conference on global health. Both students and professionals can volunteer as Global Impact Fellows in Unite for Sight's partner clinics to learn how local medical professionals reach the most difficult populations and conduct research projects on healthcare delivery. The Global Health University offers online certificate programs for students and professionals to learn global health strategies to apply to their own work, as well as webinars with leading experts. The Global Health Conference is the world's largest global health conference, and its participants and events reflect various areas of global health, international development, and social entrepreneurship.

Jennifer's greatest challenge is having enough financial resources to continue expanding and sustaining the capacity of the local professionals she works with. She is mindful of the limitations of typical funding sources, like large donors and grants, and is always looking for ways to create sustainable schemes to generate funding. She is constantly rewarded in her work, knowing that thousands of patients receive sight-restoring surgeries every week. She can see the impact of the work she does in New Haven by looking through the data on surgeries and photos of the patients that she receives from Unite for Sight's partners. She is also inspired by the passion and enthusiasm of the students and professionals who participate in the Global Health University and Global Health Conference.

Jennifer and Unite for Sight have received many awards for the organization's programs. Jennifer was the recipient, for example, of the 2007 BRICK Award, the American Institute of Public Service's 2009 National Jefferson Award for Public Service, the 2011 John F. Kennedy New Frontier Award, and the 2013 Praxis Award in Professional Ethics from Villanova University.

When asked about the advice she would offer to students interested in global health, Jennifer said:

- Follow your passion, whatever it may be. You do not necessarily need to study public health or global health to contribute to the field. There are many people that studied or worked in another field and now make significant contributions to global health.
- Understand the importance of quality. The idea that "something is always better than nothing" does not work in global health and can be problematic. Using the example of bed nets, many people may measure the number of bed nets distributed, which is an output. However, this is not the best way to measure your impact. People may not want to sleep under the nets and use them instead for fishing or clothing. Instead, measure education efforts, correct usage of the nets, and outcomes of bed net distribution, such as reduction in malaria. Failure to consider the importance of quality may lead to wasted efforts and even cause harm.

OUK VONG VATHINY

Ouk Vong Vathiny is a Cambodian physician who is head of the Reproductive Health Association of Cambodia (RHAC) and has been at the forefront of efforts to improve reproductive health for the most vulnerable women in Cambodia. Vathiny has carried out this work despite incredible challenges in her personal and professional lives.

Vathiny has always been interested in helping women and children. As a child, her family helped support a number of orphanages, and she dreamed of one day running an orphanage herself. Having many family members who were doctors also inspired Vathiny to become more interested in health.

In 1974, Vathiny began to study medicine at the Faculty of Medicine in Phnom Penh, the capital of Cambodia, with the goal of improving the health of women and children. As with all Cambodian people and students, Vathiny's studies were interrupted when the Khmer Rouge, followers of the Communist Party of Kampuchea, took control of Cambodia in 1975. The Khmer Rouge controlled the country until 1979, evacuated the cities, and forced the population to work in the countryside. They also committed genocide. Like many other Cambodians during this period, Vathiny and her family endured almost 4 years of very difficult labor and starvation in the countryside and a number of Vathiny's family members perished.

Upon returning to Phnom Penh in 1979, Vathiny and her fellow medical students spent about a year reestablishing the medical faculty and the Ministry of Health before continuing their studies. In 1986, Vathiny finally received her MD degree—6 years after she had originally planned.

From 1986 to 1989, Vathiny was chief of the Infectious Disease Ward of the Phnom Penh Municipal Hospital. After 3 years, she switched her focus to obstetrics and gynecology and soon became the head of maternal health within the Maternal and Child Health Department of the Phnom Penh Municipality. She worked in this capacity until 1994 and was responsible for overall staff training and for more specialized training in sexually transmitted diseases and HIV/AIDS counseling. She also organized mobile health teams in surrounding semiurban areas and supervised 47 medical staff.

At the same time, Vathiny was also director of the Toul Kork Dike Community Clinic, where she provided health services for sex workers from the local red light district at the clinic and Toul Kork Dispensary. HIV had begun to spread among certain populations engaging in high-risk behaviors, including sex workers. Because the government was doing little to address this public health challenge, Vathiny and a British colleague started outreach activities for sex workers, and the clinic developed from there.

Although the new clinic was acclaimed by a number of organizations, the Phnom Penh governor tried to ban sex work and closed the brothels around the clinic, leading to the spread of sex workers all over the city. Thus, Vathiny decided to move from the public to the NGO sector. From 1994 to 1997, she worked with Family Planning International Assistance (FPIA/FHSP), initially as a clinic physician and later as deputy director/project director. Her responsibilities with FPIA grew, and as FPIA transitioned into a national NGO, she became the executive director of the RHAC, which she cofounded in 1996.

RHAC currently has about 470 employees and 5,000 volunteers. The organization runs 16 reproductive health clinics and conducts a variety of community-based and outreach programs, especially for high-risk groups such as sex workers, men who have sex with men, and youth in schools and in the community. In addition, RHAC supports approximately a third of the government health centers in Cambodia.

Even as Vathiny has carried out this work, she has continually sought to improve her knowledge and skills. In 1998, she received a graduate certificate in Managing Health Programs in Developing Countries from the Harvard School of Public Health in the United States. In 2002, she received an MBA in Health, Population, and Nutrition in Developing Countries at the University of Keele in the United Kingdom. In 2007, she received a Diploma in Sexual and Reproductive Health and Rights from Lund University in Sweden.

Vathiny is most proud of the work that she and others did during the early 1990s to help control the initial spread of HIV/AIDS in Cambodia. Their approach focused directly on the source of the epidemic. They created programs to help sex workers protect themselves, sometimes even risking their own lives as they did so. For example, they developed the government clinic for sex workers, despite government opposition, and some brothel owners threatened them at gunpoint on more than one occasion.

Vathiny offers the following advice for university students interested in global health:

- Focus on vulnerable populations within your field of interest. If you do not help them, who else will?
- Look for role models—women and men—who have both compassion and knowledge.
- Always remember the relationships among health, nutrition, hunger, poverty reduction, and development. Society needs to address all these links. We are all responsible for the well-being of our society.
- Some things must be changed, such as stigmas, taboos, and violations of people's rights. We must fight for these changes.

- We hope for a world with equity in health care and well-being. In this endeavor, we must especially focus on women and children. Women are the backbone of society. Perhaps it is a dream, but if everyone is involved, it may come true.

ABDO YAZBECK

Abdo Yazbeck is a health economist. He has spent much of his professional life developing innovative strategies for health sector reform to reduce health inequality in low- and middle-income countries.

Abdo always admired those who possess both a social conscience and a diligent work ethic. He remembers being particularly inspired by Mother Teresa's work in Kolkota, India. However, his interest in health and development originated from his experiences growing up during a time of civil conflict.

Abdo was born in Beirut, Lebanon. The Lebanese Civil War began in 1974, when he was 12 years old, and continued long after he left Lebanon to attend graduate school in the United States. Because of the war, Abdo spent part of his early teenage years in Cairo, Egypt, where he first saw extreme poverty and inequality. He recalls seeing very poor children beg for money and depend on scavenging through trash dumps to survive.

When he returned to Lebanon, Abdo volunteered at the American University Hospital in Beirut and helped distribute food to Palestinian refugees in the area. Through these experiences, he learned that there are ways to improve the health of the poor and marginalized without being a physician.

In 1984, Abdo received a BA in economics from the American University of Beirut. He then moved to the United States for graduate studies in economics at Rice University in Houston, Texas. He received an MA in economics in 1988 and a PhD in economics in 1991. His dissertation research focused on health, labor, and applied microeconomics.

While studying in Texas, Abdo conducted research on aging and the relationship between labor choices and health outcomes, funded by the National Institute on Aging. He then began exploring racial and socioeconomic inequality in health, which sparked his lifelong professional focus on health inequality.

In 1987, Abdo participated in a Population, Health, and Nutrition summer internship at the World Bank. He analyzed data related to family size, children's education, and family labor supply. Abdo was inspired to pursue a career in economic development and poverty reduction by what he saw as

the high level of motivation and dedication of the employees at the World Bank.

In the early 1990s, after 2 years lecturing in the Department of Economics at Texas A&M University, Abdo began to solidify his work as a health economist. In 1992, he worked as a health economist for the World Bank, helping to prepare background papers for the 1993 World Development Report, which became an extremely important work globally. From 1993 to 1996, Abdo worked with the consulting firm Abt Associates as a health economist and research manager. In this capacity, he helped develop training programs and provided technical assistance for a variety of health projects in low- and middle-income countries.

Abdo rejoined the World Bank in 1996. From then to 2002, Abdo was a senior health economist for the South Asia Human Development Unit. Abdo's work on South Asia focused on supporting health sector projects and analysis in Bangladesh, India, the Maldives, and Sri Lanka. The work emphasized using economic tools to analyze the health sector and design health policies. He also provided technical and operational assistance to countries with which he was working. From 2002 to 2008, he was program manager and lead health economist for the Health and AIDS Program in the World Bank Institute, a kind of "World Bank University." In this role, he helped develop training programs related to health sector reform, health financing, health inequality, and HIV/AIDS, among other things. Some of the more important publications in which Abdo participated include the World Bank's *World Development Report 1993: Investing in Health*, *Reaching the Poor with Health Nutrition and Population Services* (2005), and *Attacking Inequality in Health* (2009).

Between 2008 and 2011, Abdo was a health sector manager for Europe and Central Asia at the World Bank. In this position, he managed World Bank efforts to strengthen the health sectors of project countries in three main areas: the creation of effective core public health functions; work toward equitable, efficient, and high quality health services; and the integration of the health sector into overall development. Abdo is currently a lead health economist covering the Africa Region.

Abdo is most proud of his efforts that have focused on health inequality in low- and middle-income countries. At the time that he and others started this work, inequality was seen as the poverty of low-income countries compared to higher-income countries. It was generally assumed that all people in poor countries were poor. There was insufficient attention to inequality within countries. Abdo worked with the Reaching the Poor Program to build knowledge of inequality in health outcomes and access to health services, in addition to developing ways to address these issues.

When asked what advice he would offer to current university students interested in global health, Abdo offered the following points:

- Global health and development work is both immensely rewarding and incredibly frustrating. This will require hard work, persistence, and the ability to manage failures and keep your bearing.
- Gain skills in a specific field, such as public health, medicine, economics, finance, business, or law. This will allow you to more effectively improve global health.
- Advocacy is a wonderful thing if it is based on evidence and not just emotions. Advocacy without knowledge is potentially destructive and wasteful.

MAIN MESSAGES

A diverse set of people work in a wide array of global health activities. Many of these people became interested in global health at a young age and oriented their studies and professional experiences around their interest in global health. Others, however, came to global health at a later stage in their career. Many of the people you read about in this chapter had transformative experiences that set the foundation for their global health efforts. Some of these were by design, such as those who sought early in their professional life to work in a low-income country. Some others were encouraged to become active in global health by the people with whom they studied or worked. Some were moved by living in areas of political crisis or among marginalized people.

A number of themes emerge consistently from these profiles:

- Focus on the disadvantaged, the poor, and the marginalized. Social justice and fairness are central to work on global health.
- Be open to learning.
- Seek mentors from whom you can learn.
- Learn from all with whom you work.
- Develop role models, after whom you may want to model parts of your own work.
- Think big. Don't accept things the way they are. Ask instead what it will take to make your vision a reality.
- Work with others in coalitions and alliances. The power of many is greater than the power of one.
- If possible, find a platform from which you can engage in global health efforts, that you can make a home, and to which you can return regularly.
- Global health work requires high levels of humility.

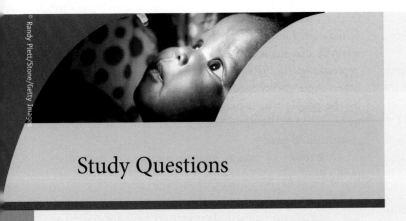

Study Questions

1. What common themes do you see in the lives of the people in the profiles?

2. What different professions are well suited to working in global health?

3. What skills are most valuable in global health work?

4. What personal traits lend themselves well to a career in global health?

5. Where would you like to see yourself in 10 to 15 years?

6. What do you have to do to get to that place?

7. Which of the profiles most aligns with your own interests and needs for further professional growth?

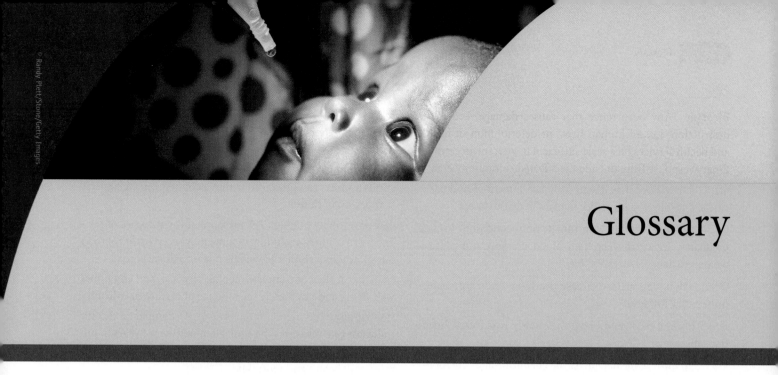

Glossary

Abortion Premature expulsion or loss of embryo, which may be induced or spontaneous

Adolescent A person from 10 to 19 years of age

Anemia Low level of hemoglobin in the blood

Antigen Any substance that can induce an immune response in the body

Asphyxsia A condition of severely deficient supply of oxygen to the body

Bipolar disorder A brain disorder, also known as manic-depressive illness, that brings unusual shifts in mood, energy, activity levels, and the ability to carry out day-to-day tasks

Blood glucose Blood sugar that is transported through the bloodstream to the body cells for energy

Body mass index Body weight in kilograms divided by height in meters squared

Cancer The name given to a range of diseases characterized by body cells that divide without stopping and spread to surrounding tissues

Cardiovascular disease A disease of the heart or blood vessels

Case fatality rate The proportion of cases of a specified condition that is fatal within a specified period of time

Cataract A clouding of the lens of the eye

Cesarean delivery (section) The delivery of a fetus by surgical incision through the abdominal wall and uterus

Child Anyone under 18, unless the laws in their country give them majority status before that

Cholesterol A waxy, fat like substance that is found in all cells of the body

Communicable diseases Illnesses that are caused by a particular infectious agent and that spread directly or indirectly from people to people, from animals to animals, from animals to people, or from people to animals

Control Reduction of disease incidence, prevalence, morbidity, or mortality to a locally acceptable level

Cost-effectiveness analysis In health, a tool for comparing the relative cost of two or more investments with the amount of health that can be purchased with those investments

Culture A set of rules or standards shared by members of a society, which when acted upon by the members, produce behavior that falls within a range of variation that members consider proper and acceptable

Demographic transition The shift from high fertility and high mortality to low fertility and low mortality

Depression A mood disorder in which feelings of sadness, loss, anger, or frustration interfere with activities of everyday life for a significant period

Diabetes Medical illness caused by too little insulin or poor response to insulin

Diarrhea A condition in which the sufferer has frequent and watery or loose bowel movements

Disability The temporary or long-term reduction in a person's capacity to function

Disability adjusted life year A composite measure of premature deaths and losses due to disabilities in a population

Disaster   Any occurrence that causes damage, ecological destruction, loss of human lives, or deterioration of health and health services on a scale sufficient to warrant an extraordinary response from outside the affected community area

Drug resistance   The extent to which infectious and parasitic agents develop an ability to resist drug treatment

Eclampsia   A serious, life-threatening condition in late pregnancy in which very high blood pressure can cause a woman to have seizures

Elimination   Reduction of case transmission to a predetermined very low level

Emerging infectious disease   A newly discovered infectious disease

Environment   External physical, chemical, and microbiological exposures and processes that impinge upon individuals and groups and are beyond the immediate control of individuals

Environmental health   A set of public health efforts that is concerned with preventing disease, death, and disability by reducing exposure to adverse environmental conditions and promoting behavior change. It focuses on the direct and indirect causes of disease and injuries and taps resources inside and outside the healthcare system to help improve health outcomes

Epidemiologic transition   A shift in the pattern of disease from largely communicable diseases to noncommunicable diseases

Equity   Differences in health that are not only unnecessary and avoidable, but also unfair and unjust

Eradication   Termination of all transmission of infection by extermination of the infectious agent

Family planning   The conscious effort of couples to regulate the number and spacing of births through artificial and natural methods of contraception; connotes conception control to avoid pregnancy and abortion, but also includes efforts of couples to induce pregnancy

Female genital mutilation (also called female circumcision and female genital cutting)   A collective term for various traditional practices that are all related to the cutting of the female genital organs; four different forms and grades are usually distinguished

Gestational diabetes   Diabetes that develops during pregnancy because of improper regulation of blood sugar; it usually goes away after delivery, but can increase the woman's risk of developing type II diabetes later

Global health   Health problems, issues, and concerns that transcend national boundaries and may best be addressed by cooperative actions

Gross domestic product   The total market value of all the goods and services produced within a country during a specified period of time

Gross national product   A measure of the incomes of residents of a country, including income they receive from abroad but subtracting similar payments made to those abroad

Health   A state of complete mental, physical, and emotional well-being and not merely the absence of disease or infirmity

Health-adjusted life expectancy   A composite health indicator that measures the equivalent number of years in full health that a newborn can expect to live, based on current rates of ill health and mortality

Health disparities   A type of difference in health that is closely linked with social or economic disadvantage

Health system   The combination of resources, organization, and management that culminate in the delivery of health services to the population

Hemorrhage (related to pregnancy)   Significant and uncontrolled loss of blood, either internally or externally from the body. Antepartum (prenatal) hemorrhage occurs after the 20th week of gestation but before delivery of the baby; postpartum hemorrhage is the loss of 500 ml or more of blood from the genital tract after delivery of the baby; primary postpartum hemorrhage occurs in the first 24 hours after delivery

Hookworm   A parasite that lives in the small intestine of its host, which may be a mammal such as a dog, cat, or human

Hypertension   High blood pressure

Immunization   The process of inducing immunity, usually through vaccination

Incidence rate   The rate at which new cases of a disease occur in a population

Inequality   Differences in health status or in the distribution of health determinants between different population groups

Infant mortality rate   The number of deaths of infants under age 1 per 1,000 live births in a given year

Injury   The result of an act that damages, harms, or hurts; unintentional or intentional damage to the body resulting from acute exposure to thermal, mechanical, electrical, or chemical energy or from the absence of such essentials as heat or oxygen

Internally displaced person   Someone who is forced to flee his home but remains within his own country

Iodine deficiency disorders A number of possible health problems, such as mental retardation, cretinism, goiter, hypoythyroidism, and some developmental abnormalities that stem from an insufficient amount of iodine

Ischemic heart disease Characterized by a reduced blood supply to the heart; also known as coronary heart disease

Life expectancy at birth The average number of years a newborn baby could expect to live if current mortality trends were to continue for the rest of the newborn's life

Low birthweight Birthweight less than 2,500 grams

Malaria A disease of humans caused by blood parasites of the species *Plasmodium falciparum, vivax, ovale, knowlesi,* or *malariae* and transmitted by anopheline mosquitoes

Malnutrition Various forms of poor nutrition, including underweight, stunting, wasting, and overweight or obesity, as well as micronutrient deficiencies

Maternal death The death of a woman while pregnant, during delivery, or within 42 days of delivery, irrespective of the duration and the site of pregnancy; the cause of death is always related to or aggravated by the pregnancy or its management; does not include accidental or incidental causes

Maternal mortality ratio The number of women who die as a result of pregnancy and childbirth complications per 100,000 live births in a given year

Measles A highly communicable disease characterized by fever, general malaise, sneezing, nasal congestion, a brassy cough, conjunctivitis, and an eruption over the entire body, caused by the rubeola virus

Morbidity Illness

Mortality Death

Neonatal mortality rate Number of deaths to children under 28 days of age in a given year per 1,000 live births in that year

Neonatal tetanus A generalized form of a bacterial infection that occurs in newborns as a result of unclean delivery or unhygienic care of the umbilical cord

Noncommunicable disease Illnesses that are not spread by any infectious agent

Nongovernmental organization A nonprofit group or association organized outside of institutionalized political structures to realize particular social objectives, such as environmental protection, or serve particular constituencies, such as indigenous peoples

Obese Body mass index over 30

Obstetric fistula An injury in the birth canal that allows leakage from the bladder or rectum into the vagina, leaving a woman permanently incontinent, often leading to isolation and exclusion from the family and community

Overweight (For an adult) A body mass index between 25 and 30

Panic disorders A mental disorder in which people have attacks of fear that last several minutes or longer

Parasite An animal or vegetable organism that lives on or in another and derives its nourishment therefrom

Pertussis A highly contagious bacterial disease that causes uncontrollable, violent coughing

Pneumonia An inflammation, usually caused by infection, involving the alveoli of the lungs

Poliomyelitis (polio) Infantile paralysis, a viral paralytic disease

Preeclampsia (previously called toxemia) A hypertensive disorder of pregnancy said to exist when a pregnant woman with gestational hypertension develops proteinuria. Originally, edema was considered part of the syndrome of preeclampsia, but presently the former two symptoms are sufficient for a diagnosis of preeclampsia

Prevalence The number of people suffering from a certain condition over a specific time period; *prevalence rate* is the share of the population which is being measured who have the condition

Public health The science and art of preventing disease; prolonging life; and promoting physical health and mental health and efficiency through organized community efforts toward a sanitary environment, control of community infections, education in hygiene, and the development of social machinery to ensure capacity in the community to maintain health

Pull mechanism Interventions that assure a future return in the event that a product is produced

Push mechanism Interventions that reduce the risks and costs of investments

Reemerging infectious disease An existing infectious disease that has increased in incidence or has taken on new forms

Refugee A person who has fled and is outside of his own country because of fear of persecution

Risk factor An aspect of personal behavior or lifestyle, an environmental exposure, or an inborn or inherited characteristic that, on the basis of epidemiologic evidence, is known to be associated with health-related conditions

Schizophrenia A chronic, severe, and disabling brain disorder

Sepsis   Infection in the blood

Severe acute malnutrition   Very low weight for height, below three z scores of the international reference standard

Sex-selective abortion   The practice of aborting a fetus after a determination, usually by ultrasound but also rarely by amniocentesis or another procedure, that the fetus is an undesired sex, typically female

Sexually transmitted infections (STIs)   Diseases, also known as sexually transmitted diseases (STDs), that are commonly transmitted between partners through some form of sexual activity, most commonly vaginal intercourse, oral sex, or anal sex

Social determinants of health   The conditions in which people are born, grow, live, work and age, all of which have an impact on their health

Society   A group of people who occupy a specific locality and share the same cultural traditions

Stroke   Temporary or permanent loss of the blood supply to the brain

Stunting   Failure to reach linear growth potential because of inadequate nutrition or poor health; two z-scores below the international reference

Tetanus   A bacterial and often fatal infection that enters the body through a wound or puncture

Under-5 child mortality rate   The annual number of deaths in children under 5 years, expressed as a rate per 1,000 live births, averaged over the previous 5 years

Undernutrition   The outcome of insufficient food intake and repeated infectious diseases. It includes being underweight for one's age, too short for one's age (stunted), dangerously thin for one's height (wasted) and deficient in vitamins and minerals (micronutrient malnutrition)

Underweight   Low weight-for-age; two z-scores below the international reference for weight-for-age

Unintentional injury   That subset of injuries for which there is no evidence of predetermined intent

Uterine prolapse   A condition in which the uterus protrudes into, and sometimes out of, the vagina

Vitamin A deficiency   An insufficiency of vitamin A in the body that can cause a number of health problems, such as blindness, and which has an important association with excess morbidity and mortality in young children from a number of health conditions such as pneumonia and measles

Wasting   Weight, measured in kilograms, divided by height in meters squared that is two z-scores below the international reference

Youth   A person between the ages of 15 and 24 years

Z-score   A statistical term, meaning the deviation of an individual's value from the median value of a reference population, divided by the standard deviation of the reference population

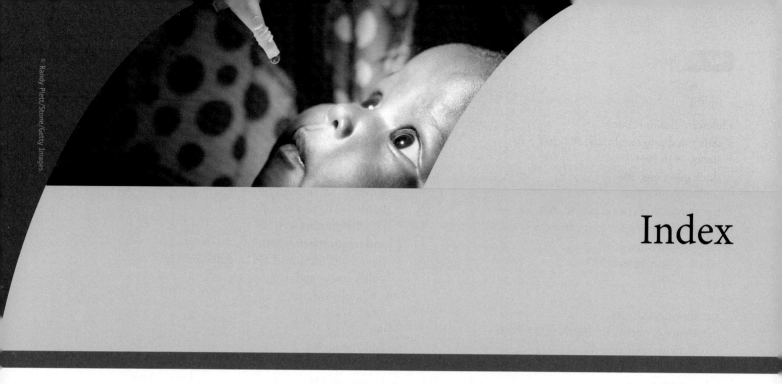

Index

Note: Page numbers followed by *f,* or *t* indicate materials in figures or tables respectively.